Handbook of Pediatric Chronic Pain

Brenda C. McClain • Santhanam Suresh
Editors

Handbook of Pediatric Chronic Pain

Current Science and
Integrative Practice

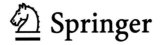 Springer

Editors
Brenda C. McClain, M.D.,
FAAP, DABPM
Director of Pediatric Pain Management
Services
Associate Professor of Anesthesiology
Pediatrics Yale University School of
Medicine
New Haven, CT
USA
brenda.mcclain@yale.edu

Santhanam Suresh, MD
Vice Chairman & Director of Research
& Pain Medicine
Department of Pediatric Anesthesiology
Children's Memorial Hospital
Northwestern University
Feinberg School of Medicine
Chicago, IL
USA
ssuresh@childrensmemorial.org

ISBN 978-1-4939-7922-6   ISBN 978-1-4419-0350-1   (eBook)
DOI 10.1007/978-1-4419-0350-1
Springer New York Dordrecht Heidelberg London

Springer is part of Springer Science+Business Media (www.springer.com)

This book is dedicated to the memory of my parents, Daniel and Celesta McClain, whose support and unconditional love taught me the invaluable life lessons that have made my career a reality.

Brenda C. McClain, M.D.

I would like to dedicate this book to the support from my family, my wife, Nina and my lovely children, Aneesha, Sunitha and Madhav who have been the 'wind beneath my wings' and to my parents, Santhanam and Chandra who encouraged me to always strive for the best, and to my mentor Steven Hall and the members of the Department of Pediatric Anesthesiology at Children's Memorial Hospital who have supported me in all my academic ventures.

Santhanam Suresh, M.D.

Foreword

It was 1:35 AM in the basement of the Hunnewell building. Chuck Berde and I had just finished assembling a long overdue chapter on pediatric pain management for the 2nd Edition of Gregory's textbook on *Pediatric Anesthesia*. It had been an arduous task, marshaling the information on the topic, hand-drawing the figures, battling with the incompatibility of PC and Mac computers, re-numbering all references for the umpteenth time, etc. It was finally done! As we waited for the chapter to print out, we talked about the frustrations of treating children with chronic pain. We talked about why multiple different specialties needed to focus on this problem, otherwise there would be no headway. Midnight musings often lead to great insights. Chuck decided that he would pursue the idea of developing a multidisciplinary pain team focused on the pain problems of children and excitedly started listing the departments that needed to be involved!

Today, 22 years later, the field of chronic pain management in children has mushroomed into a well-developed body of scientific knowledge and a thriving clinical specialty. The editors of this volume, Brenda C. McClain and S. Suresh, have emerged as leaders in this field, not only because of their training pedigree and clinical acumen, but because they have pioneered many of the concepts and techniques used widely today. Their pre-eminence is displayed amply in the pages of this book, which seems destined to become one of the most dog-eared and well-worn references in a Children's Pain Clinic.

What is striking about this book is its practicality, balance and comprehensiveness. The chapters are written by leading scientists and clinicians, derived from multiple disciplines and leading pediatric pain centers, many of whom are at the forefront of research in that specific area. Yet, for all its scientific underpinnings, the contents of each chapter are astonishingly practical. Those who peruse the entire volume will certainly gain a strong education in challenges of treating pediatric chronic pain, but even those who read a small section here and there will find it easy to apply that specific knowledge to the next patient in their clinic! This is because both editors and most chapter authors have distilled the wisdom and practical experience gained from treating many such children; their efforts reflect the sweat equity resulting from spending long hours at a patient's bedside, or from refining the technique of a procedure performed hundreds of times, or from empathic discussions with numerous families at the brink of despair, or from creatively combining different treatment modalities to achieve the same result – the relief of pain and suffering.

The depth of this rich experience will often aid the practitioner, but the broad scope will also satisfy the curiosity of a serious student or scientist.

Frida Kahlo (1907–1954), one of the most influential Mexican painters of the twentieth century, was often called a surrealist because her 55 self-portraits incorporated symbolic portrayals of physical and psychological wounds, but she insisted, "I never painted dreams. I painted my own reality." Chronic pain was a part of her life, but despite the handicaps of childhood polio and serious injuries from a bus accident on September 17, 1925, she achieved a degree of artistic, intellectual, and social success that few of us can imagine. Her story and self-portrayals have provided a poster-child for the scourge of chronic pain, but also remind us of the potential of every child who suffers from chronic pain. We can only speculate how much more Frida could have achieved, had she received the benefits of chronic pain management using the techniques and approaches described in this book. Perhaps the next child who comes into your clinic may achieve something even greater. And that is the motivation that drives people like Drs. McClain and Suresh. We have come a long way from that night in the basement of the Hunnewell building. Or have we? Read the book to find out.

K.J.S. Anand, MBBS, D. Phil., FAAP,
FCCM, FRCPCH
St. Jude Endowed Chair for Critical
Care Medicine
Professor of Pediatrics, Anesthesiology,
& Neurobiology
Division Chief, Pediatric Critical
Care Medicine
Le Bonheur Children's Medical Center
University of Tennessee Health Science
Center at Memphis

June 30, 2010

Preface

The evolution of the concept of this book was to address areas of pediatric chronic pain that have not been traditionally the focus of current literature but still are of great clinical concern. This text is written for pain specialists and pediatric-oriented practitioners who encounter children with persistent and recurrent pain. This book provides an armamentarium for pain management after the acute phase is over and helps in follow-up care. Integration of current philosophy and research are translated to clinical care where possible in this text.

Since evidence-based care in pediatric pain management is not well represented, the scope of this text is intentionally limited to topics that are presently recognized as pain syndromes in children. The spectrum of chronic pediatric pain syndromes is as wide as their adult counterpart and may be greater, as some of the more difficult areas of pediatric chronic pain management do not have adult pain syndromes from which to extrapolate. Children are not little adults and while this dictum is true, we still do not have complete answers with regards as to standardized algorithms for the management of pediatric chronic pain syndromes. While extrapolation from the adult care is not preferred, we would be remiss to deny its use in the management of pediatric chronic pain.

Regional anesthesia is more frequently applied these days in the management of chronic pediatric pain. The chapter on the use of interventional techniques in pediatric chronic pain addresses ultrasound guidance which is relatively new and offers our children additional effective intervention in the armamentarium of pain management.

Pediatric chronic pain is pervasive; yet, specialists in the management of pediatric chronic pain are not plentiful and are limited to university-based facilities. Thus, referrals to pediatric pain specialists are rare and recognition of syndromes or disorders may be beyond one's primary scope of practice. Misdiagnoses, conflicting care plans and lack of standardization of care further complicate management.

The book consists of 23 chapters; however, the reader should realize that this is just the beginning in the frontier of chronic pain in childhood. It is our hope that this book provides insight on chronic pain issues that clinicians face on a consistent basis while dealing with children and adolescents.

We are grateful to all the contributors and their administrative staff who have made this text a reality.

New Haven, CT   Brenda C. McClain, M.D., FAAP
Chicago, IL   Santhanam Suresh, M.D., FAAP

Contents

Contributors

Claude Abdallah Department of Anesthesiology, Children's National Medical Center, Sheikh Zayed Campus for Advanced Children's Medicine, 111 Michigan Avenue, NW Washington, DC 20010, USA

Valerie E. Armstead St. Joseph's Regional Medical Center, 703 Main Street, Paterson, NJ 07503, USA

Lori Brake Department of Physical Therapy, Children's Seashore House, The Children's Hospital of Philadelphia, 34 Civic Center Boulevard, Philadelphia, PA19104, USA

Kathryn Crofton Pediatric Pain Management Services, Yale New Haven Children's Hospital, New Haven, CT 06473, USA; Department of Anesthesiology, Yale University School of Medicine, New Haven, CT, USA

John Curran Director of Neuroradiology, Phoenix Children's Physician Network, 1919 E. Thomas Road, Phoenix, AZ 85016, USA

Jill MacLaren Chorney Pediatric Anesthesia, IWK Health Centre, Halifax, Nova Scotia, Canada; Department of Anesthesiology and Psychology, Dalhousie University, Halifax, Nova Scotia, Canada

Kripa Dholakia Department of Physical Therapy, Children's Seashore House, The Children's Hospital of Philadelphia, 34 Civic Center Boulevard, Philadelphia, PA 19104, USA

Gati Dhroove Divisions of Pediatric Gastroenterology, Children's Memorial Hospital, Northwestern University's Feinberg School of Medicine, Chicago, IL, USA

Genevieve D'Souza Thomas Jefferson University/Jefferson Medical College, 111 S. 11th Street, Suite G5480, 19107 Philadelphia, PA, USA

Jill M. Eckert Department of Anesthesiology, Penn State Milton S. Hershey Medical Center, P.O. Box 850/500, University Drive, Hershey, PA 17033, USA

Maria Fitzgerald Department of Neuroscience, Physiology and Pharmacology, University College London, London, UK

Stephen Robert Hays Monroe Carell, Jr. Children's Hospital at Vanderbilt, Vanderbilt University Medical Center, 2200 Children's Way # 3115, Nashville, TN, USA 37232-9070

Rae Ann Kingsley Pediatric Nurse Practitioner, Pediatric Pain Management Services, Department of Anesthesiology, Yale University, New Haven, CT, USA

Benjamin Howard Lee Johns Hopkins Medical Institutions, 600 North Wolfe Street/Blalock 904A, Baltimore, MD 21287, USA; Pediatric Anesthesiology and Critical Care Medicine, Johns Hopkins Medical Institutions, Baltimore, MD, USA

Victoria Marchese Department of Physical Therapy, Lebanon Valley College, 101 North College Avenue, Annville, PA 17033, USA; Penn State Hershey College of Medicine at The Pennsylvania State University, Hershey, PA, USA

Brenda C. McClain Department of Anesthesiology, Yale University School of Medicine, 333 Cedar Street, TMP-3, 208051, New Haven, CT, USA 06520-8051

Antoun Nader Northwestern Memorial Hospital, Northwestern University, Chicago, IL, USA

Patricia O'Malley Harvard Medical School, Dana–Farber Cancer Institute, Boston, MA, USA

Suzanne Porfyris Anesthesia Pain Service, Department of Anesthesiology, Children's Memorial Hospital, 2300 Children's Plaza, Box 19, Chicago, IL 60614, USA

Sarah E. Rebstock Department of Anesthesiology, Penn State Milton S. Hershey Medical Center, P.O. Box 850/500, University Drive, Hershey, PA 17033, USA

Holly Denise Richter Vanderbilt University Medical Center, 11205 W Sycamore Hills Dr Fort Wayne, IN 46814, Nashville, TN, USA 37232-9070

Lynn M. Rusy Jane B. Pettit Pain and Paliative Care Center, Medical College of Wisconsin, 9000 West Wisconsin Avenue, Milwaukee, WI 53226, USA

Mi-Young Ryee Department of Psychiatry and Behavioral Sciences, Psychology, Northwestern University's Feinberg School of Medicine, Chicago, IL, USA;
Children's Memorial Hospital, Department of Psychiatry and Behavioral Sciences, Chicago, IL, USA

Haleh Saadat Department of Anesthesiology, Yale University School of Medicine, New Haven, CT, USA

Miguel Saps Divisions of Pediatric Gastroenterology, Children's Memorial Hospital, Northwestern University's Feinberg School of Medicine, Chicago, IL, USA

Ali Sephadari Department of Radiology, Northwestern University's Feinberg School of Medicine, Chicago, IL, USA

Hariharan Shankar Department of Anesthesiology, Clement Zablocki VA Medical Center, Milwaukee, WI, USA; Department of Anesthesiology, Medical College of Wisconsin, Milwaukee, WI 53295, USA

Santhanam Suresh Department of Pediatric Anesthesiology, Children's Memorial Hospital, Northwestern University, Feinberg School of Medicine, Chicago, IL, USA

Arlyne Kim Thung Department of Anesthesiology, Yale University School of Medicine, New Haven, CT, USA

Elza Vasconcellos University of Miami, Miller School of Medicine, Miami, FL, USA

Tamara Vesel Dana–Farber Cancer Institute, 450 Brookline Avenue, Boston, MA 02215, USA

Thomas R. Vetter Department of Anesthesiology, University of Alabama School of Medicine, Jefferson Tower 865, 619 19th Street South, Birmingham, AL 35249-6810, USA; Department of Health Policy and Organization, University of Alabama at Birmingham School of Public Health, Birmingham, AL, USA

Shu-Ming Wang Department of Anesthesiology and Perioperative Care, University of California-Irvine School of Medicine, New Haven, CT 06520, USA

Lynda Wells University of Virginia School of Medicine, Charlottesville, VA, USA

Steve D. Wheeler Ryan Wheeler Headache Treatment Center, 5975 Sunset Drive, Suite 501, Miami 33143, FL, USA; University of Miami, Miller School of Medicine, Miami, FL, USA

The Epidemiology of Pediatric Chronic Pain

Thomas R. Vetter

Keywords

Age and Gender • Chronic pain • Musculoskeletal pain • Functional abdominal pain • Complex regional pain syndrome

Introduction

Chronic pain has a substantial adverse impact on the health related quality of life of children and adolescents, resulting in significantly worse physical functioning, psychological functioning, social functioning, lower satisfaction with life, and poorer self-perceived health status (Merlijn et al. 2006; Palermo 2000; Palermo et al. 2008). The current Pediatric Initiative on Methods, Measurement, and Pain Assessment in Clinical Trials (PedIMMPACT) has accordingly recommended that investigators conducting pediatric clinical trials in chronic and recurrent pain consider assessing not only pain intensity but also physical function, emotional function, role function, other condition-related symptoms and adverse events, global judgment of satisfaction with treatment, sleep, and economic factors (www.immpact.org) (McGrath et al. 2008).

T.R. Vetter (✉)
Department of Anesthesiology, University of Alabama School of Medicine, Jefferson Tower 865, 619 19th Street South, Birmingham, AL 35249-6810, USA
and
Department of Health Policy and Organization, University of Alabama at Birmingham School of Public Health, Birmingham, AL, USA
e-mail: tvetter@uab.edu

Chronic pain is very common in the pediatric population and therefore represents both an individual and a public health concern (Vetter 2008). It has been convincingly opined that the health of a nation is largely a reflection of the past and present health of its children, in large part because childhood is an incubation period for many disorders that affect the health of the whole population (Forrest and Riley 2004). This mandates that greater attention be paid to the promotion of pediatric biopsychosocial resilience and adaptability in addition to other approaches to prevent the precursors of future adult health disorders (Forrest and Riley 2004). This vital continuum of health versus disease between childhood, adolescence, and adulthood is intuitively very applicable to the chronic pain experience.

This chapter addresses the epidemiology, including the demographics, natural history, and financial impact of pediatric chronic pain. Attention will initially be focused on the overall prevalence and impact of chronic pain in children and adolescents. Regional differences, the effect of age and gender on the onset, and natural history of pediatric chronic pain will also be examined. Finally, given their predominance in the pediatric age group, the available specific epidemiologic data on headaches, recurrent abdominal pain, chest pain, musculoskeletal pain, and complex regional pain syndrome will be presented.

B.C. McClain and S. Suresh (eds.), *Handbook of Pediatric Chronic Pain: Current Science and Integrative Practice*, DOI 10.1007/978-1-4419-0350-1_1, © Springer Science+Business Media, LLC 2011

The Overall Prevalence and Impact of Chronic Pain in Children and Adolescents

An increasing amount of attention has been focused on the epidemiology of pediatric chronic pain (Huguet and Miro 2008). However, until as recently as 2000, very little was known in North America or Europe about the prevalence of pain in children and adolescents (McGrath et al. 2000; Perquin et al. 2000a). In an attempt to remedy this deficiency, tools such as the Pain Experience Interview have been devised, validated, and applied to provide estimates of the lifetime and point prevalence of various types of pain in children, as well as data on the intensity, effect, duration, and frequency of their pain experiences (McGrath et al. 2000).

A cross-sectional, population-based survey of 5,424 Dutch children and adolescents, 0–18 years of age, drawn randomly from census registries and the enrollment records of 27 primary schools and 14 secondary schools in the greater Rotterdam area revealed that 54% had experienced pain of some type and intensity within the previous 3 months, while 25% of the respondents reported chronic pain, defined as recurrent or continuous pain of more than 3 months duration (Perquin et al. 2000a). A subsequent cross-sectional German study observed a 46% point prevalence of chronic pain of at least 3 months duration in the 10–14-year-old age group (Roth-Isigkeit et al. 2004).

When an expanded-age cohort of 749 German children and adolescents were surveyed in their elementary and secondary school setting, using the Luebeck Pain-Screening Questionnaire, 83% had experienced pain during the preceding 3 months, and pain had been present for greater than 6 months in 31% of the respondents (Roth-Isigkeit et al. 2005). Headache (60%), abdominal pain (43%), limb pain (34%), and back pain (30%) were the rank-ordered most commonly reported types of pain (Roth-Isigkeit et al. 2005). This cross-sectional community sample of children and adolescents also reported a number of perceived chronic pain-related functional issues, including sleep problems (54%), inability to pursue hobbies (53%), eating problems (51%), school absence (49%), and inability to interact with friends (47%). Of note, the prevalence of these restrictions in daily living attributable to pain increased with participant age, and among the children and adolescents with chronic pain, the likelihood of physician visits and medication use also increased with age (Roth-Isigkeit et al. 2005).

A comparable cross-sectional population study of 561 Spanish schoolchildren between the ages of 8 and 16 years revealed a 37% prevalence of chronic pain problems during the previous 3 months; however, only 5.1% of the respondents had experienced moderate or severe chronic pain (Huguet and Miro 2008). The most frequently reported pain locations were the lower limb (47%), the head (43%), and the abdomen (34%), with less common pain locations being the back (11%), the neck (5%), the pelvis (3%), and the chest (2%). Of note, headache and abdominal pain were more frequently reported by girls, whereas lower limb pain was more frequently reported by boys (Huguet and Miro 2008). The children with a chronic pain condition overall reported a worse quality of life, missed more days from school, and were more likely to use pain medicine and to seek medical care for pain relief (Huguet and Miro 2008). This concurs with previous findings that children in the USA who complained often of aches and pains used more health-care services, had more psychosocial problems, missed more days of school, and did worse academically (Campo et al. 2002). However, the above-quoted European studies contrast sharply with a reported 6% lifetime prevalence of chronic pain in a community cohort of 495 Canadian school children, 9–13 years of age (van Dijk et al. 2006).

While a greater understanding thus presently exists regarding the prevalence of pediatric chronic pain, far less is known about to its financial impact. Not surprisingly, children and adolescents suffering from chronic pain utilize various health-care services and require prescription analgesic medications at a significantly greater rate than their healthy peers (Perquin et al. 2000b). The utilization of various health-care services was studied in detail in a subset of 254 Dutch children and adolescents 0–18 years of age, with chronic non-cancer pain (Perquin et al. 2001). During a 3-month period, general practitioners and specialists were consulted for pain symptoms by 31% and 14% of subjects, respectively, and in 53% of the cases a medication was used for pain. Of note, in the preceding year, 6.4% of the sample had been hospitalized due to their pain (Perquin et al. 2001).

Parents and other care providers make significant adjustments to their lives in an attempt to cope with a child or adolescent with chronic pain. These efforts have micro and macro economic consequences. Although more is becoming known about the psychological and social burden of pediatric chronic pain – and despite its considerable prevalence – there are still very few data on the costs of living with, or caring for, a child or adolescent with chronic pain (Sleed et al. 2005). A preliminary retrospective study thus examined the financial burden or cost of illness in 52 families of adolescents with chronic pain (Sleed et al. 2005). Participants were recruited from pediatric rheumatology outpatient clinics and a multidisciplinary outpatient pain management clinic in the UK. The authors used the client service receipt inventory (CSRI), a comprehensive, retrospective, parent self-report inventory of direct and indirect costs, to capture all utilized health services, lost employment, out-of-pocket expenses, and informal care given as a result of the adolescent's pain. Based upon the CSRI, a mean total cost of £8,027/year/adolescent was reported, with a stratified £4,495/year cost for the rheumatology subgroup versus £14,160/year cost for the pain management sub-group. Extrapolating from the prevalence data reported by Perquin et al. (2000a) from the Netherlands, these authors estimated a UK prevalence of 480,000 adolescents/year with severe chronic pain. This equated to a UK societal economic burden of £3,840 million/year due to adolescent pain (Sleed et al. 2005).

The Effect of Age and Gender on the Onset and Natural History of Pediatric Chronic Pain

The British national child development study, a prospective population-based birth cohort study, initially enrolled 17,414 infants, born between March 3 and March 9, 1958 to parents residing in Great Britain (98% of all such births). The study undertook follow-up data collection at the ages of 7, 11, 16, 23, and 33 years. As part of this longitudinal cohort study, parents were interviewed when the subjects were 7 years of age (1965) and 11 years of age (1969), at which time they were asked if their child suffered from frequent headache or migraine (then as now the most common pediatric somatic pain complaint). At 33 years of age (1991), the participants were asked about a variety of specific somatic symptoms, including severe headaches. Children with frequent headache had an increased risk in adulthood of experiencing not only headache (odds ratio of 1.87, 95% CI: 1.58–2.20) but also multiple other physical symptoms (odds ratio of 1.75, 95% CI: 1.46–2.10) and psychiatric morbidity (odds ratio of 1.41, 95% CI: 1.20–1.66) (Fearon and Hotopf 2001). A similar longitudinal British birth cohort study was undertaken from 1946 to 1989 and examined in part the natural history of abdominal pain (Hotopf et al. 1998). While children with persistent and hence chronic abdominal pain on three occasions in childhood (at ages 7, 11, and 15 years) were considerably more likely to suffer from a psychiatric disorder in adulthood (odds ratio of 2.72, 95% CI: 1.65–4.49), they were not more likely to experience recurrent abdominal pain in adulthood (odds ratio of 1.39, 95% CI: 0.83–2.36) (Hotopf et al. 1998).

The aims of a similar but more contemporary longitudinal Swedish study were to determine if headache and back pain were transitory in nature or had became chronic and to identify the predictors of such long-term pain in young adults (Brattberg 2004). A total of 335 children, 8, 11, and 14 years old, were first studied in 1989 and then followed up in 1991 and 2002. The subjects completed questionnaires on pain, the first two times in school, the last via a postal survey. Among those subjects suffering from chronic headache or chronic back pain, 59% of the females and 39% of the males reported similar pain at 21, 24, and 27 years of age. A total of 68 (20%) of the subjects reported pain symptoms at all three study time points. Based upon a multiple logistic regression model, three significant predictors of long-term pain were identified: reported back pain in 8–14-year-olds; reported headaches once a week or more in 8–14-year-olds; and a positive response in the 10–16 year olds to the question: "Do you often feel nervous?" (odds ratio of 2.1, 95% CI: 1.3–3.4). Participants also completed the SF-36 Health Survey, a generic health-related quality-of-life instrument, at the 13-year follow-up point. When compared to normative age-group values, the SF-36 scores of those with pain symptoms were significantly lower scores across all eight physical, social, emotional, and general well-being dimensions, including pain (Brattberg 2004). A similar frequent persistence into adulthood of tension headache (33%), migraine headache (17%), and tension plus migraine headache (23%) was observed in a 20-year follow-up study of an Atlantic Canadian cohort of children (Brna et al. 2005). These collective findings support to the applicability of the above-noted continuum of health versus disease between childhood, adolescence, and adulthood with chronic pain.

Gender and chronological differences in headache have been extensively reported. Pediatric migraine occurs in approximately 11% of children between the ages of 5 and 15 years and in approximately 28% of adolescents between the ages of 15 and 19 years (Hershey 2005). The incidence of migraine with aura in males is 6.6/1,000 and peaks at 5–6 years of age; in females, it is 14/1,000 and peaks at 12–13 years of age. The incidence of migraine without aura in males is 10/1,000 and peaks at 10–11 years of age; in females, it is 18/1,000 and peaks at 14–17 years of age (Stewart et al. 1991). In a population-based study of 10,169 community residents, 12–29-year olds living outside Baltimore, Maryland, 6.1% of males and 14.0%

of females, when interviewed by telephone, reported four or more headaches in the preceding month. The average duration of the subjects' most recent headache was 5.9 h for males and 8.2 h for females; 7.9% of males and 13.9% of the females missed part of a day or more of school or work because of that headache. During the month before the interview, 3.0% of males and 7.4% of females had suffered from a migraine headache (Linet et al. 1989). The majority of patients with so-called chronic daily headache or chronic nonprogressive headache appear to be female adolescents (Gladstein 2004; Koenig et al. 2002; Moore and Shevell 2004; Rothner et al. 2001; Seshia 2004).

As discussed further below, pediatric chest pain is common; however, the preponderance of published data, derived mainly from emergency department visits and cardiology clinic evaluations, have indicated a low incidence of identifiable cardiac pathology in children and adolescents with chest pain (Danduran et al. 2008). However, a recently published report examined not only the role of patient gender, race, and age, but also the association between obesity and physical capacity and chest pain in this age group (Danduran et al. 2008). This is particularly relevant given that the prevalence of children who are overweight or at risk of becoming overweight has reached epidemic proportions in the USA (Danduran et al. 2008). In a cohort of 263 patients (141 males and 122 females, mean age of 13.4 years) with a primary complaint of chest pain, who underwent an extensive cardiopulmonary evaluation at a children's hospital in Milwaukee, Wisconsin, 28% were at risk of overweight (BMI > 85th percentile) and 16% were overweight (BMI > 95th percentile). Preteens and Hispanics in the study cohort were more likely to be overweight. While true cardiac pathology was rare in this study group, reactive airways disease was significantly more prevalent in African American patients, while a significantly decreased exercise tolerance (endurance time) was observed in Hispanics (Danduran et al. 2008).

Musculoskeletal pain in preadolescents does not appear to be a self-limiting phenomenon, and more studies appear warranted to explore its determinants with the goal of improving the long-term outcome of such often widespread symptoms. This conclusion was based on the findings of a rigorous longitudinal study of 1,756 Finnish schoolchildren (El-Metwally et al. 2004). A baseline cross-sectional survey of the study cohort (mean age 10.8 years) identified a 32% prevalence of musculoskeletal pain. Using the same pain questionnaire, the children were reevaluated after 1 year and 4 years (at adolescence). At 1-year follow-up, 54% of the children reported persistent preadolescent musculoskeletal pain and at 4-year follow-up, 64% had musculoskeletal pain. Neck pain was the most persistent/recurrent type of musculoskeletal pain. Those with persistent preadolescent musculoskeletal pain had an approximately three times higher risk of pain recurrence (OR of 2.90 with 95% CI: 1.9–4.4). Female gender, older age (greater than 11 years), hypermobility, coexistence of psychosomatic symptoms (headache, abdominal pain, and depressive feelings), having a high disability index, and reporting multiple types of musculoskeletal pain at baseline were significant predictors of pain recurrence at adolescence (El-Metwally et al. 2004). Subsequent analyses of the Finnish cohort subgroups with neck pain and widespread pain (fibromyalgia) revealed that the co-occurrence of frequent other somatic pain symptoms and markers of psychological stress were predictive risk factors for more persistent pain (Mikkelsson et al. 2008; Stahl et al. 2008). Given that chronic neck pain and fibromyalgia in adulthood may thus originate in childhood, further studies, including preventive interventions, appear indicated (Mikkelsson et al. 2008; Stahl et al. 2008).

There are limited population-based data on the demographics and natural history of pediatric complex regional pain syndrome (CRPS). Nevertheless, valid inferences can be drawn from the published randomized controlled trials of treatment of pediatric CRPS (Berde and Lebel 2005; Dadure et al. 2005; Finniss et al. 2006; Lee et al. 2002; Low et al. 2007; Meier et al. 2006; Sherry et al. 1999), which collectively indicate that the condition tends to afflict disproportionately early adolescent females, with a strong predilection for the lower extremity, particularly the foot. Interestingly, whereas pediatric CRPS predominantly involves the lower extremity, the upper extremity is the more common location in adults (de Mos et al. 2007; Sandroni et al. 2003).

The Types and Characteristics of Patients Referred to a Pediatric Pain Medicine Program

Patients are typically referred to a dedicated, multidisciplinary pediatric pain medicine program when they fail to achieve adequate pain and symptoms relief under the care of their primary care physician or subspecialist(s). Thus any cohort of such patients is innately fraught with selection bias and has limited external generalizability. This notwithstanding, this subset of chronic pain patients is the result of a naturalistic process and worthy of discussion.

The clinical characteristics of a sequential sample of 100 pediatric chronic pain patients, who were previously under the care of another subspecialist and subsequently referred to an anesthesiology-based pediatric chronic pain medicine program have been reported (Vetter 2008). These patients presented with a variety of primary chronic pain-related disorders: abdominal pain (18%), lumbago (14%), fibromyalgia (14%), headache (12%), complex regional pain syndrome (11%), other musculoskeletal pain (11%), and chest and rib pain (6%). These patients were predominantly adolescent females (73%) with frequent coexisting clinically significant anxiety (63%) and depression (84%). The patients in this study reported significantly lower overall health-related quality-of-life scores than those previously reported by pediatric rheumatology, pediatric migraine, and pediatric cancer patients receiving care in a rheumatology, neurology, and oncology subspecialty setting, respectively (Powers et al. 2004; Varni et al. 2002a, b; Vetter 2008).

These observed clinical characteristics are consistent with those previously reported in a diverse group of 207 children and adolescents referred over a 2-year period to a similar multidisciplinary pediatric pain medicine clinic (Chalkiadis 2001). While no formal measurement of health-related quality of life was performed, a substantial majority of these patients exhibited practical evidence of chronic pain-related disability, including school absenteeism (95%), sleep disruption (71%), and an inability to participate in a previous sport (90%) (Chalkiadis 2001). While a different set of measurement instruments were applied, these findings are also consistent with a previous report on the clinical characteristics, effect of maladaptive coping strategies, prevalence of depression, and functional disability in a clinically similar cohort of 73 children and adolescents referred to a dedicated outpatient pediatric pain medicine clinic for further evaluation and treatment (Kashikar-Zuck et al. 2001). These previous authors observed that chronic pain had a substantial adverse impact on functional ability and that coexisting depression was strongly associated with functional disability (Kashikar-Zuck et al. 2001).

Headache

A substantial amount of health care and clinical research has been focused on pediatric headache (Bandell-Hoekstra et al. 2000; Hershey et al. 2007; Kondev and Minster 2003; Lewis et al. 2002; Lipton 1997). This is not surprising in light of the very high and reportedly increasing prevalence of headache in children and adolescents (Brna and Dooley 2006; Winner 2008b). However, pediatric headache disorders, especially migraine, are subject to retrospective patient recall bias (van den Brink et al. 2001). Migraine, the most common headache disorder for which patients see a physician, still remains frequently misdiagnosed, under-diagnosed, and undertreated – this despite standardized, widely published criteria (Winner 2008a; Winner and Hershey 2007). Chronic daily headache or chronic nonprogressive headache (i.e., transformed migraine or tension headache) is increasingly recognized as a problem not only in adults but also in adolescents

and older children (Gladstein 2004; Hershey et al. 2006; Koenig et al. 2002; Moore and Shevell 2004; Rothner et al. 2001; Seshia 2004).

A landmark Scandinavian prevalence study of 9,000 subjects from the early 1960s observed that by 7 years of age, 1.4% of children had migraine headaches, 2.5% had frequent non-migraine headaches, and 35% had infrequent non-migraine headaches (Bille 1962). By 15 years of age, 5.3% of this cohort had migraine headaches, 15.7% had frequent non-migraine headaches, and 54% had infrequent non-migraine headaches (Bille 1962). More recent data from the late 1990s indicate a greater overall prevalence of pediatric headache (Kondev and Minster 2003). A 2002 meta-analysis of five retrospective pediatric headaches studies published between 1977 and 1991, involving a total of 27,606 children, found the prevalence of any type of headache to range from 37% to 51% in 7-year olds, and steadily increasing to 57–82% by age 15 years (Lewis et al. 2002). In a 2001 survey of 2,358 Dutch school children between the ages of 10 and 17 years, 21% of the boys and 26% of the girls in elementary school level, and 14% of boys and 28% of girls in high school reported weekly headaches (Bandell-Hoekstra et al. 2001).

Hunfeld and colleagues (2001) compared a group of adolescents suffering from chronic headaches with a similar group of adolescents suffering from either chronic abdominal pain, back pain, or limb pain. They observed that the adolescent headache patients reported the poorest quality of life, as measured by the Quality of Life Pain-Youth Questionnaire. The headache patients also exhibited the greatest amount of school absenteeism. A subsequent study of children with chronic headaches supported the previously proposed complex relationship between pediatric headache, patient quality of life, coping strategies, and both personal and situational factors (Frare et al. 2002). Affecting between 5% and 7% of adolescents, migraine headaches are especially problematic in the 12–17-year-old age group, due to an even greater reduction in quality of life and attendant patient disability (Hershey 2005; Tkachuk et al. 2003).

Recurrent Abdominal Pain

Pediatric recurrent abdominal pain (RAP) has been clinically recognized for at least 50 years; it was originally defined as a pain syndrome consisting of at least three episodes of abdominal pain over a period of not less than 3 months and severe enough to affect activities (Apley and Naish 1958; Weydert et al. 2003). In the interim, RAP has been extensively studied (Di Lorenzo et al. 2005), with a number of proposed etiologies, including autonomic nervous system instability (Chelimsky et al. 2001), visceral hyperalgesia (Castilloux et al. 2008; Di Lorenzo et al. 2001), intestinal motility disorders (Youssef and Di Lorenzo 2001), and stressful life events and poor coping skills (Robinson et al. 1990).

Chronic abdominal pain is a common pediatric problem encountered by primary care physicians, medical subspecialists, and surgical specialists (American Academy of Pediatrics 2005). RAP has a consistently reported prevalence of 10–20% in school-aged children and adolescents (Duarte et al. 2006). Chronic abdominal pain in children is usually functional, that is, without objective evidence of an underlying organic disorder (American Academy of Pediatrics 2005). Only 5–10% of pediatric patients with RAP in the community setting have an identifiable, underlying organic cause (Weydert et al. 2003), versus approximately 50% who do in a pediatric gastroenterology clinic setting (Croffie et al. 2000). Despite the often functional and ostensibly benign nature of RAP, this often underappreciated disorder has been associated with significant morbidity, including increased school absenteeism, frequent doctor visits, family disruption, and significant anxiety and depression – all leading to a marked reduction in health-related quality of life (Garber et al. 1990; Varni et al. 2006; Weydert et al. 2003; Youssef et al. 2006, 2008).

Beginning in 1994, three evidence-based, international consensus statements on functional gastrointestinal disorders (Rome I, Rome II, and Rome III) have been developed and promulgated (Drossman 2007; Drossman and Dumitrascu 2006). The 2006 Rome III (www.romecriteria. org) standardized criteria for making a diagnosis

of a functional abdominal pain syndrome are: (1) continuous or nearly continuous abdominal pain; (2) no or only occasional relationship of pain with physiological events (e.g., eating, defecation, or menses); (3) some loss of daily functioning; (4) the pain is not feigned (e.g., malingering); (5) insufficient symptoms to meet criteria for another functional gastrointestinal disorder that would explain the pain (Drossman et al. 2006). When applied in a cohort of 368 pediatric patients with no evidence of organic disease, as compared to the Rome II criteria, the Rome III criteria classified a greater percentage of the children as having the diagnosis of irritable bowel syndrome (45%), abdominal migraine (23%), or functional abdominal pain (11%) (Baber et al. 2008). Applying the more inclusive Rome III criteria allowed for the classification of 87% of the patients with medically unexplained chronic abdominal pain (Baber et al. 2008).

Chest Pain

Chest pain is another frequent complaint in the pediatric age group. Although chest pain in children rarely is the result of a serious, organic cardiac condition, it is perceived as "heart pain" by most children and their parents and thus can be physically and emotionally distressing (Evangelista et al. 2000). The typically noncardiac etiology of pediatric chest pain is supported by a prospective study of 50 patients, 5–21 years old, referred to a pediatric cardiology clinic in Boston with a chief complaint of chest pain. All 50 patients underwent a systematic evaluation, and none were found to have a cardiac condition but instead 76% had musculoskeletal or costochondral chest pain, 12% had exercise-induced asthma, 8% had chest pain resulting from gastrointestinal causes, and 4% had chest pain resulting from psychogenic causes (Evangelista et al. 2000). Of 100 consecutive patients, 2–16 years old (54 girls, 46 boys), referred to a pediatric cardiology department in Turkey with the primary complaint of chest pain, 92 cases were concluded to be idiopathic in origin. Interestingly, of the 74 patients who underwent a psychiatric evaluation, 55 of them (74%) had psychiatric symptoms and five required psychiatric care. Anxiety, conversion disorder, and depression were the main psychiatric symptoms (Tunaoglu et al. 1995).

Of 336 consecutive patients presenting to an urban pediatric emergency department in Ottawa, Canada with chest pain, nonspecific chest-wall pain was the most common diagnosis (28%), followed by pain referred from the upper respiratory tract or the abdomen (21%), pulmonary (19%), minor traumatic (15%), idiopathic (12%), and psychogenic (5%) (Rowe et al. 1990). A prospective analysis of 168 pediatric patients, consecutively evaluated in an emergency department in Belgium with a chief complaint of chest pain, also revealed chest-wall pain to be the most common diagnosis (64%), followed by pulmonary (13%), psychological (9%), cardiac (5%), traumatic (5%), and gastrointestinal problems (4%) (Massin et al. 2004). Chest-wall pain was also the most common diagnosis (89%) in a concurrently obtained and reported sample of 69 consecutive pediatric patients referred to the cardiology clinic at the same institution because of chest pain (Massin et al. 2004).

Musculoskeletal Pain

Chronic musculoskeletal pain, either idiopathic or disease-related, is also common in childhood, and the differential diagnosis of such is pain is extensive (Anthony and Schanberg 2005, 2007). The assessment and treatment of pediatric chronic musculoskeletal pain optimally involves a biopsychosocial, interdisciplinary approach, which integrates the biologic, environmental, and cognitive behavioral mechanisms underlying such chronic pain (Anthony and Schanberg 2007; Connelly and Schanberg 2006; Sen and Christie 2006). Of note, as many as 25% of new patients present to pediatric rheumatology clinics with idiopathic musculoskeletal chronic pain, including due to juvenile primary fibromyalgia syndrome – with its often markedly adverse functional and psychosocial impact (Anthony and Schanberg 2001; Connelly and Schanberg 2006;

Sen and Christie 2006). From the 1950s through the early 1990s, the reported point prevalence of musculoskeletal pain in North American and European school-age children ranged from 7% to 15% (de Inocencio 1998; Goodman and McGrath 1991). However, figures as high as 32–40% have more recently been reported, indicating either an overall increasing prevalence or the recognition of juvenile primary fibromyalgia syndrome (or both).

Despite potential selection bias, the prevalence of musculoskeletal pain was determined in a prospective evaluation of 1,000 consecutive clinic visits to an urban general pediatric clinic in Madrid, Spain (de Inocencio 1998). In this convenience sample of 3–14-year olds (mean age of 9.7 years), 6.1% of clinic visits were related to musculoskeletal pain, in keeping with older reports. The presenting complaints included knee arthralgia (33%), other large peripheral joint arthralgias (28%), soft tissue pain (18%), heel pain (8%), hip pain (6%), and back pain (6%). The musculoskeletal pain symptoms were attributed to trauma in 30%, overuse syndromes (e.g., chondromalacia patellae, mechanical plantar fasciitis, overuse muscle pain) in 28%, and skeletal growth variants (e.g., Osgood–Schlatter syndrome, hypermobility, Sever's disease) in 18% of patients (de Inocencio 1998).

The prevalence and persistence of self-reported musculoskeletal pain symptoms was determined using with a structured pain questionnaire in 1756 Finnish third-grade and fifth-grade schoolchildren. In this comprehensive, population-based survey, musculoskeletal pain occurring at least once a week was reported by 32% of the study subjects (Mikkelsson et al. 1997). A cross-sectional study was also performed on an entire private school population of adolescents in the city of São Paulo, Brazil (Zapata et al. 2006a). In this cohort with a male to female sex ratio of 1.1 to 1 and a mean age of 14.2 years, musculoskeletal pain was reported by 40% of the 833 surveyed students. Interestingly, despite frequent computer and video game use in this adolescent cohort, these activities were not associated with the presence of a musculoskeletal pain syndrome (Zapata et al. 2006b). Back pain was instead the most frequently self-reported location (23%) in this Brazilian study (Zapata et al. 2006a). This is consistent with both a previous Icelandic study, in which 21% of a random national sample of 2,173 preteens and teenagers reported recurrent (weekly or more often) back pain (Kristjansdottir and Rhee 2002) and a Danish study, in which recurrent or continuous LBP of a moderate to severe nature was reported by 19% of 1,389 13–16-year-old schoolchildren (Harreby et al. 1999).

Complex Regional Pain Syndrome

CRPS is a neuropathic pain disorder that afflicts all ages (Grabow et al. 2004; Low et al. 2007; Rho et al. 2002; Wilder 2006). Despite over 20 years of focused research and a well-evolved treatment paradigm, the exact mechanism of CRPS remains elusive; however, peripheral sensitization of A-delta and C afferent fibers to noxious stimuli appears to be the basis for CRPS-associated hyperalgesia (Stanton-Hicks 2000, 2003). While it has been posited that enough is now known about its pathophysiology to recommend quantitative sensory and autonomic nervous system testing (Stanton-Hicks 2003), there is no specific diagnostic laboratory test for CRPS, requiring clinicians to rely predominantly upon signs and symptoms. Of note, the presentation, treatment, and prognosis of CRPS can be quite variable in and between pediatric and adult patients, likely related in part to differences in patient populations, referral patterns, and medical practice (Berde and Lebel 2005; Low et al. 2007; Matsui et al. 2000; Sherry et al. 1999).

There is a paucity of large-scale epidemiologic data on pediatric neuropathic pain, including CRPS. However, in recent years there has been an increased reporting of CRPS in children and adolescents (Finniss et al. 2006). Therefore, potentially valid inferences can be drawn from two adult population-based studies of CRPS (de Mos et al. 2007; Sandroni et al. 2003).

As part of the comprehensive Rochester Epidemiology Project, the incidence, prevalence, and outcome of CRPS I between 1989 and 1999 was determined for Olmstead County, Minnesota

(Sandroni et al. 2003). Applying the International Association for the Study of Pain (IASP) criteria for CRPS, 74 cases of CRPS I were identified in a population of 106,470, resulting in an incidence rate of 5.46 per 100,000 person years at risk, and a low period prevalence of 20.57 per 100,000. Interestingly, 74% of these Minnesota patients experienced symptom resolution, often spontaneously, lending the authors to suggest that invasive treatment of CRPS may not be warranted in the majority of adult cases of CRPS I (Sandroni et al. 2003).

As part of the Integrated Primary Care Information project, using a comprehensive search term algorithm, potential CRPS cases were retrospectively identified from the electronic medical records of 600,000 adult patients who received health care throughout the Netherlands from 1996 to 2005 (de Mos et al. 2007). These potential cases were then validated by direct electronic medical record review, supplemented with original specialist letters and information from an inquiry of general practitioners. The estimated overall incidence rate of CRPS in this Dutch cohort was 26.2 per 100,000 person years (95% CI: 23.0–29.7). This observed incidence rate of CRPS in the Netherlands is more than four times higher than the incidence rate observed in the above population-based study, performed earlier in Olmsted County, Minnesota (de Mos et al. 2007).

Conclusions and Health Policy Implications

Chronic pain is a universal and thus multicultural experience that represents a major worldwide threat to health-related quality of life. A disease in its own right, the global burden of pain is substantial (Brennan 2007; Cousins et al. 2004; Lipman 2005). Despite the existence of cost-effective treatment options, pain control has been relatively neglected by national governmental agencies and international nongovernmental organizations (Brennan et al. 2007; Cousins et al. 2004; Lipman 2005). Despite all of the work to date, more information is needed about the prevalence, manifestations, and long-term effects of chronic pain in children (Bhatia et al. 2008). There is likewise a need for increased training and resources for primary care physicians and pain clinicians who manage chronic pain in the pediatric age group (Bhatia et al. 2008).

A major gap presently exists between an increasingly sophisticated understanding of the pathophysiology of pain and the widespread inadequacy of its treatment (Brennan et al. 2007). This gap is most apparent and problematic in the poorest and most socially dysfunctional developing nations, which are contending with widespread poverty, oppression and violence, and war and its aftermath (Brennan et al. 2007). Consequently, in October 2004, the World Health Organization (WHO), the International Association for the Study of Pain (IASP), and the European Federation of the IASP Chapters (EFIC) jointly declared that such widespread, inadequately treated chronic pain must not be tolerated and furthermore that the relief of pain should be a universal human right (Brennan and Cousins 2004; Cousins et al. 2004; Lipman 2005). The two ultimate aims of this global pain initiative were to inform policy makers about the personal burden and the economic costs of chronic pain and to educate physicians and allied health-care professionals about pain assessment and management so as to promote higher standards of care worldwide (Lipman 2005). More recently, similar attention has been focused on effective palliative care being a universal, international human right (Brennan 2007).

Acute, chronic, and cancer pain collectively represent the often unreported and hence silent dimension of many of the worldwide causes of both adult and pediatric morbidity and mortality (Brennan et al. 2007). Specifically, it is generally under-recognized that the pain and other symptom burden experienced by adult and pediatric patients with HIV/AIDS are as complex and widespread as in patients with cancer (Lipman 2005). Greater attention therefore needs to be focused on the pain experience in the developing world, including in the pediatric population.

References

American Academy of Pediatrics. (2005). Chronic abdominal pain in children. *Pediatrics, 115*(3), e370–e381.

Anthony, K. K., & Schanberg, L. E. (2001). Juvenile primary fibromyalgia syndrome. *Current Rheumatology Reports, 3*(2), 165–171.

Anthony, K. K., & Schanberg, L. E. (2005). Pediatric pain syndromes and management of pain in children and adolescents with rheumatic disease. *Pediatric Clinics of North America, 52*(2), 611–639, vii.

Anthony, K. K., & Schanberg, L. E. (2007). Assessment and management of pain syndromes and arthritis pain in children and adolescents. *Rheumatic Diseases Clinics of North America, 33*(3), 625–660.

Apley, J., & Naish, N. (1958). Recurrent abdominal pains: A field survey of 1,000 school children. *Archives of Disease in Childhood, 33*(168), 165–170.

Baber, K. F., Anderson, J., Puzanovova, M., & Walker, L. S. (2008). Rome II versus Rome III classification of functional gastrointestinal disorders in pediatric chronic abdominal pain. *Journal of Pediatric Gastroenterology and Nutrition, 47*(3), 299–302.

Bandell-Hoekstra, I. E., Abu-Saad, H. H., Passchier, J., & Knipschild, P. (2000). Recurrent headache, coping, and quality of life in children: a review. *Headache, 40*(5), 357–370.

Bandell-Hoekstra, I. E., Abu-Saad, H. H., Passchier, J., Frederiks, C. M., Feron, F. J., & Knipschild, P. (2001). Prevalence and characteristics of headache in Dutch schoolchildren. *European Journal of Pain, 5*(2), 145–153.

Berde, C. B., & Lebel, A. (2005). Complex regional pain syndromes in children and adolescents. *Anesthesiology, 102*(2), 252–255.

Bhatia, A., Brennan, L., Abrahams, M., & Gilder, F. (2008). Chronic pain in children in the UK: A survey of pain clinicians and general practitioners. *Paediatric Anaesthesia, 18*(10), 957–966.

Bille, B. S. (1962). Migraine in school children. A study of the incidence and short-term prognosis, and a clinical, psychological and electroencephalographic comparison between children with migraine and matched controls. *Acta Paediatrica, 51*(Supplement 136), 1–151.

Brattberg, G. (2004). Do pain problems in young school children persist into early adulthood? A 13-year follow-up. *European Journal of Pain, 8*(3), 187–199.

Brennan, F. (2007). Palliative care as an international human right. *Journal of Pain and Symptom Management, 33*(5), 494–499.

Brennan, F., & Cousins, M. J. (2004). Pain relief as a human right. *Pain Clinical Updates, 12*(September 2004), 1–4.

Brennan, F., Carr, D. B., & Cousins, M. J. (2007). Pain management: A fundamental human right. *Anesthesia and Analgesia, 105*(1), 205–221.

Brna, P., & Dooley, J. M. (2006). Headaches in the pediatric population. *Seminars in Pediatric Neurology, 13*(4), 222–230.

Brna, P., Dooley, J., Gordon, K., & Dewan, T. (2005). The prognosis of childhood headache: A 20-year follow-up. *Archives of Pediatrics and Adolescent Medicine, 159*(12), 1157–1160.

Campo, J. V., Comer, D. M., Jansen-Mcwilliams, L., Gardner, W., & Kelleher, K. J. (2002). Recurrent pain, emotional distress, and health service use in childhood. *Journal of Pediatrics, 141*(1), 76–83.

Castilloux, J., Noble, A., & Faure, C. (2008). Is visceral hypersensitivity correlated with symptom severity in children with functional gastrointestinal disorders? *Journal of Pediatric Gastroenterology and Nutrition, 46*(3), 272–278.

Chalkiadis, G. A. (2001). Management of chronic pain in children. *Medical Journal of Australia, 175*(9), 476–479.

Chelimsky, G., Boyle, J. T., Tusing, L., & Chelimsky, T. C. (2001). Autonomic abnormalities in children with functional abdominal pain: Coincidence or etiology? *Journal of Pediatric Gastroenterology and Nutrition, 33*(1), 47–53.

Connelly, M., & Schanberg, L. (2006). Latest developments in the assessment and management of chronic musculoskeletal pain syndromes in children. *Current Opinion in Rheumatology, 18*(5), 496–502.

Cousins, M. J., Brennan, F., & Carr, D. B. (2004). Pain relief: A universal human right. *Pain, 112*(1–2), 1–4.

Croffie, J. M., Fitzgerald, J. F., & Chong, S. K. (2000). Recurrent abdominal pain in children–a retrospective study of outcome in a group referred to a pediatric gastroenterology practice. *Clinical Pediatrics, 39*(5), 267–274.

Dadure, C., Motais, F., Ricard, C., Raux, O., Troncin, R., & Capdevila, X. (2005). Continuous peripheral nerve blocks at home for treatment of recurrent complex regional pain syndrome I in children. *Anesthesiology, 102*(2), 387–391.

Danduran, M. J., Earing, M. G., Sheridan, D. C., Ewalt, L. A., & Frommelt, P. C. (2008). Chest pain: Characteristics of children/adolescents. *Pediatric Cardiology, 29*(4), 775–781.

de Inocencio, J. (1998). Musculoskeletal pain in primary pediatric care: Analysis of 1000 consecutive general pediatric clinic visits. *Pediatrics, 102*(6), E63.

de Mos, M., de Bruijn, A. G., Huygen, F. J., Dieleman, J. P., Stricker, B. H., & Sturkenboom, M. C. (2007). The incidence of complex regional pain syndrome: A population-based study. *Pain, 129*(1–2), 12–20.

Di Lorenzo, C., Youssef, N. N., Sigurdsson, L., Scharff, L., Griffiths, J., & Wald, A. (2001). Visceral hyperalgesia in children with functional abdominal pain. *Journal of Pediatrics, 139*(6), 838–843.

Di Lorenzo, C., Colletti, R. B., Lehmann, H. P., Boyle, J. T., Gerson, W. T., Hyams, J. S., et al. (2005). Chronic abdominal pain in children: A technical report of the American Academy of Pediatrics and the North American Society for Pediatric Gastroenterology, Hepatology and Nutrition. *Journal of Pediatric Gastroenterology and Nutrition, 40*(3), 249–261.

Drossman, D. A. (2007). Introduction. The Rome Foundation and Rome III. *Neurogastroenterology and Motility, 19*(10), 783–786.

Drossman, D. A., & Dumitrascu, D. L. (2006). Rome III: New standard for functional gastrointestinal disorders. *Journal of Gastrointestinal and Liver Diseases, 15*(3), 237–241.

Drossman, D. A., Corazziari, E., Delvaux, M., Spiller, R. C., Talley, N. J., Thompson, W. G., et al. (Eds.). (2006). *Rome III: the functional gastrointestinal disorders* (3rd ed.). McLean: Degnon Associates.

Duarte, M. A., Penna, F. J., Andrade, E. M., Cancela, C. S., Neto, J. C., & Barbosa, T. F. (2006). Treatment of non-organic recurrent abdominal pain: Cognitive-behavioral family intervention. *Journal of Pediatric Gastroenterology and Nutrition, 43*(1), 59–64.

El-Metwally, A., Salminen, J. J., Auvinen, A., Kautiainen, H., & Mikkelsson, M. (2004). Prognosis of non-specific musculoskeletal pain in preadolescents: A prospective 4-year follow-up study till adolescence. *Pain, 110*(3), 550–559.

Evangelista, J. A., Parsons, M., & Renneburg, A. K. (2000). Chest pain in children: Diagnosis through history and physical examination. *Journal of Pediatric Health Care, 14*(1), 3–8.

Fearon, P., & Hotopf, M. (2001). Relation between headache in childhood and physical and psychiatric symptoms in adulthood: National birth cohort study. *British Medical Journal, 322*(7295), 1145.

Finniss, D. G., Murphy, P. M., Brooker, C., Nicholas, M. K., & Cousins, M. J. (2006). Complex regional pain syndrome in children and adolescents. *European Journal of Pain, 10*(8), 767–770.

Forrest, C. B., & Riley, A. W. (2004). Childhood origins of adult health: A basis for life-course health policy. *Health Affairs, 23*(5), 155–164.

Frare, M., Axia, G., & Battistella, P. A. (2002). Quality of life, coping strategies, and family routines in children with headache. *Headache, 42*(10), 953–962.

Garber, J., Zeman, J., & Walker, L. S. (1990). Recurrent abdominal pain in children: Psychiatric diagnoses and parental psychopathology. *Journal of the American Academy of Child and Adolescent Psychiatry, 29*(4), 648–656.

Gladstein, J. (2004). Children and adolescents with chronic daily headache. *Current Pain and Headache Reports, 8*(1), 71–75.

Goodman, J. E., & McGrath, P. J. (1991). The epidemiology of pain in children and adolescents: A review. *Pain, 46*(3), 247–264.

Grabow, T. S., Christo, P. J., & Raja, S. N. (2004). Complex regional pain syndrome: Diagnostic controversies, psychological dysfunction, and emerging concepts. *Advances in Psychosomatic Medicine, 25*, 89–101.

Harreby, M., Nygaard, B., Jessen, T., Larsen, E., Storr-Paulsen, A., Lindahl, A., et al. (1999). Risk factors for low back pain in a cohort of 1389 Danish school children: An epidemiologic study. *European Spine Journal, 8*(6), 444–450.

Hershey, A. D. (2005). What is the impact, prevalence, disability, and quality of life of pediatric headache? *Current Pain and Headache Reports, 9*(5), 341–344.

Hershey, A. D., Kabbouche, M. A., & Powers, S. W. (2006). Chronic daily headaches in children. *Current Pain and Headache Reports, 10*(5), 370–376.

Hershey, A. D., Winner, P., Kabbouche, M. A., & Powers, S. W. (2007). Headaches. *Current Opinion in Pediatrics, 19*(6), 663–669.

Hotopf, M., Carr, S., Mayou, R., Wadsworth, M., & Wessely, S. (1998). Why do children have chronic abdominal pain, and what happens to them when they grow up? Population based cohort study. *British Medical Journal, 316*(7139), 1196–1200.

Huguet, A., & Miro, J. (2008). The severity of chronic pediatric pain: An epidemiological study. *Journal of Pain, 9*(3), 226–236.

Hunfeld, J. A., Passchier, J., Perquin, C. W., Hazebroek-Kampschreur, A. A., van Suijlekom-Smit, L. W., & van der Wouden, J. C. (2001). Quality of life in adolescents with chronic pain in the head or at other locations. *Cephalalgia, 21*(3), 201–206.

Kashikar-Zuck, S., Goldschneider, K. R., Powers, S. W., Vaught, M. H., & Hershey, A. D. (2001). Depression and functional disability in chronic pediatric pain. *Clinical Journal of Pain, 17*(4), 341–349.

Koenig, M. A., Gladstein, J., McCarter, R. J., Hershey, A. D., & Wasiewski, W. (2002). Chronic daily headache in children and adolescents presenting to tertiary headache clinics. *Headache, 42*(6), 491–500.

Kondev, L., & Minster, A. (2003). Headache and facial pain in children and adolescents. *Otolaryngologic Clinics of North America, 36*(6), 1153–1170.

Kristjansdottir, G., & Rhee, H. (2002). Risk factors of back pain frequency in schoolchildren: A search for explanations to a public health problem. *Acta Paediatrica, 91*(7), 849–854.

Lee, B. H., Scharff, L., Sethna, N. F., McCarthy, C. F., Scott-Sutherland, J., Shea, A. M., et al. (2002). Physical therapy and cognitive-behavioral treatment for complex regional pain syndromes. *Journal of Pediatrics, 141*(1), 135–140.

Lewis, D. W., Ashwal, S., Dahl, G., Dorbad, D., Hirtz, D., Prensky, A., et al. (2002). Practice parameter: Evaluation of children and adolescents with recurrent headaches: Report of the Quality Standards Subcommittee of the American Academy of Neurology and the Practice Committee of the Child Neurology Society. *Neurology, 59*(4), 490–498.

Linet, M. S., Stewart, W. F., Celentano, D. D., Ziegler, D., & Sprecher, M. (1989). An epidemiologic study of headache among adolescents and young adults. *Journal of the American Medical Association, 261*(15), 2211–2216.

Lipman, A. G. (2005). Pain as a human right: The 2004 Global Day Against Pain. *Journal of Pain & Palliative Care Pharmacotherapy, 19*(3), 85–100.

Lipton, R. B. (1997). Diagnosis and epidemiology of pediatric migraine. *Current Opinion in Neurology, 10*(3), 231–236.

Low, A. K., Ward, K., & Wines, A. P. (2007). Pediatric complex regional pain syndrome. *Journal of Pediatric Orthopedics, 27*(5), 567–572.

Massin, M. M., Bourguignont, A., Coremans, C., Comte, L., Lepage, P., & Gerard, P. (2004). Chest pain in pediatric patients presenting to an emergency department or to a cardiac clinic. *Clinical Pediatrics, 43*(3), 231–238.

Matsui, M., Ito, M., Tomoda, A., & Miike, T. (2000). Complex regional pain syndrome in childhood: Report of three cases. *Brain and Development, 22*(7), 445–448.

McGrath, P. A., Speechley, K. N., Seifert, C. E., Biehn, J. T., Cairney, A. E., Gorodzinsky, F. P., et al. (2000). A survey of children's acute, recurrent, and chronic pain: Validation of the pain experience interview. *Pain, 87*(1), 59–73.

McGrath, P. J., Walco, G. A., Turk, D. C., Dworkin, R. H., Brown, M. T., Davidson, K., et al. (2008). Core outcome domains and measures for pediatric acute and chronic/recurrent pain clinical trials: PedIMMPACT recommendations. *Journal of Pain, 9*(9), 771–783.

Meier, P. M., Alexander, M. E., Sethna, N. F., De Jong-De Vos Van Steenwijk, C. C., Zurakowski, D., & Berde, C. B. (2006). Complex regional pain syndromes in children and adolescents: Regional and systemic signs and symptoms and hemodynamic response to tilt table testing. *Clinical Journal of Pain, 22*(4), 399–406.

Merlijn, V. P. B. M., Hunfeld, J. A. M., van der Wouden, J. C., Hazebroek-Kampschreur, A. A. J. M., Passchier, J., & Koes, B. W. (2006). Factors related to the quality of life in adolescents with chronic pain. *Clinical Journal of Pain, 22*(3), 306–315.

Mikkelsson, M., Salminen, J. J., & Kautiainen, H. (1997). Non-specific musculoskeletal pain in preadolescents. Prevalence and 1-year persistence. *Pain, 73*(1), 29–35.

Mikkelsson, M., El-Metwally, A., Kautiainen, H., Auvinen, A., Macfarlane, G. J., & Salminen, J. J. (2008). Onset, prognosis and risk factors for widespread pain in schoolchildren: A prospective 4-year follow-up study. *Pain, 138*(3), 681–687.

Moore, A. J., & Shevell, M. (2004). Chronic daily headaches in pediatric neurology practice. *Journal of Child Neurology, 19*(12), 925–929.

Palermo, T. M. (2000). Impact of recurrent and chronic pain on child and family daily functioning: A critical review of the literature. *Journal of Developmental and Behavioral Pediatrics, 21*(1), 58–69.

Palermo, T. M., Long, A. C., Lewandowski, A. S., Drotar, D., Quittner, A. L., & Walker, L. S. (2008). Evidence-based Assessment of Health-related Quality of Life and Functional Impairment in Pediatric Psychology. *Journal of Pediatric Psychology, 33*(9), 983–996.

Perquin, C. W., Hazebroek-Kampschreur, A. A., Hunfeld, J. A., Bohnen, A. M., van Suijlekom-Smit, L. W., Passchier, J., et al. (2000a). Pain in children and adolescents: A common experience. *Pain, 87*(1), 51–58.

Perquin, C. W., Hazebroek-Kampschreur, A. A., Hunfeld, J. A., van Suijlekom-Smit, L. W., Passchier, J., & van der Wouden, J. C. (2000b). Chronic pain among children and adolescents: Physician consultation and medication use. *Clinical Journal of Pain, 16*(3), 229–235.

Perquin, C. W., Hunfeld, J. A., Hazebroek-Kampschreur, A. A., van Suijlekom-Smit, L. W., Passchier, J., Koes, B. W., et al. (2001). Insights in the use of health care services in chronic benign pain in childhood and adolescence. *Pain, 94*(2), 205–213.

Powers, S. W., Patton, S. R., Hommel, K. A., & Hershey, A. D. (2004). Quality of life in paediatric migraine: Characterization of age-related effects using PedsQL 4.0. *Cephalalgia, 24*(2), 120–127.

Rho, R. H., Brewer, R. P., Lamer, T. J., & Wilson, P. R. (2002). Complex regional pain syndrome. *Mayo Clinic Proceedings, 77*(2), 174–180.

Robinson, J. O., Alverez, J. H., & Dodge, J. A. (1990). Life events and family history in children with recurrent abdominal pain. *Journal of Psychosomatic Research, 34*(2), 171–181.

Roth-Isigkeit, A., Thyen, U., Raspe, H. H., Stoven, H., & Schmucker, P. (2004). Reports of pain among German children and adolescents: An epidemiological study. *Acta Paediatrica, 93*(2), 258–263.

Roth-Isigkeit, A., Thyen, U., Stoven, H., Schwarzenberger, J., & Schmucker, P. (2005). Pain among children and adolescents: Restrictions in daily living and triggering factors. *Pediatrics, 115*(2), e152–e162.

Rothner, A. D., Linder, S. L., Wasiewski, W. W., & O'Neill, K. M. (2001). Chronic nonprogressive headaches in children and adolescents. *Seminars in Pediatric Neurology, 8*(1), 34–39.

Rowe, B. H., Dulberg, C. S., Peterson, R. G., Vlad, P., & Li, M. M. (1990). Characteristics of children presenting with chest pain to a pediatric emergency department. *Canadian Medical Association Journal, 143*(5), 388–394.

Sandroni, P., Benrud-Larson, L. M., McClelland, R. L., & Low, P. A. (2003). Complex regional pain syndrome type I: Incidence and prevalence in Olmsted county, a population-based study. *Pain, 103*(1–2), 199–207.

Sen, D., & Christie, D. (2006). Chronic idiopathic pain syndromes. *Best Practice & Research Clinical Rheumatology, 20*(2), 369–386.

Seshia, S. S. (2004). Chronic daily headache in children and adolescents. *Canadian Journal of Neurological Sciences, 31*(3), 319–323.

Sherry, D. D., Wallace, C. A., Kelley, C., Kidder, M., & Sapp, L. (1999). Short- and long-term outcomes of children with complex regional pain syndrome type I treated with exercise therapy. *Clinical Journal of Pain, 15*(3), 218–223.

Sleed, M., Eccleston, C., Beecham, J., Knapp, M., & Jordan, A. (2005). The economic impact of chronic pain in adolescence: Methodological considerations and a preliminary costs-of-illness study. *Pain, 119* (1–3), 183–190.

Stahl, M., Kautiainen, H., El-Metwally, A., Hakkinen, A., Ylinen, J., Salminen, J. J., et al. (2008). Non-specific neck pain in schoolchildren: Prognosis and risk factors for occurrence and persistence. A 4-year follow-up study. *Pain, 137*(2), 316–322.

Stanton-Hicks, M. (2000). Complex regional pain syndrome (type I, RSD; type II, causalgia): Controversies. *Clinical Journal of Pain, 16*(2 Suppl), S33–S40.

Stanton-Hicks, M. (2003). Complex regional pain syndrome. *Anesthesiology Clinics of North America, 21*(4), 733–744.

Stewart, W. F., Linet, M. S., Celentano, D. D., Van Natta, M., & Ziegler, D. (1991). Age- and sex-specific incidence rates of migraine with and without visual aura. *American Journal of Epidemiology, 134*(10), 1111–1120.

Tkachuk, G. A., Cottrell, C. K., Gibson, J. S., O'Donnell, F. J., & Holroyd, K. A. (2003). Factors associated with migraine-related quality of life and disability in adolescents: A preliminary investigation. *Headache, 43*(9), 950–955.

Tunaoglu, F. S., Olgunturk, R., Akcabay, S., Oguz, D., Gucuyener, K., & Demirsoy, S. (1995). Chest pain in children referred to a cardiology clinic. *Pediatric Cardiology, 16*(2), 69–72.

van den Brink, M., Bandell-Hoekstra, E. N., & Abu-Saad, H. H. (2001). The occurrence of recall bias in pediatric headache: A comparison of questionnaire and diary data. *Headache, 41*(1), 11–20.

van Dijk, A., McGrath, P. A., Pickett, W., & VanDenKerkhof, E. G. (2006). Pain prevalence in nine- to 13-year-old schoolchildren. *Pain Research & Management, 11*(4), 234–240.

Varni, J. W., Burwinkle, T. M., Katz, E. R., Meeske, K., & Dickinson, P. (2002a). The PedsQL in pediatric cancer: Reliability and validity of the Pediatric Quality of Life Inventory Generic Core Scales, Multidimensional Fatigue Scale, and Cancer Module. *Cancer, 94*(7), 2090–2106.

Varni, J. W., Seid, M., Knight, T. S., Burwinkle, T., Brown, J., & Szer, I. S. (2002b). The PedsQL (TM) in pediatric rheumatology - reliability, validity, and responsiveness of the Pediatric Quality of Life Inventory (TM) generic core scales and rheumatology module. *Arthritis and Rheumatism, 46*(3), 714–725.

Varni, J. W., Lane, M. M., Burwinkle, T. M., Fontaine, E. N., Youssef, N. N., Schwimmer, J. B., et al. (2006). Health-related quality of life in pediatric patients with irritable bowel syndrome: A comparative analysis. *Journal of Developmental and Behavioral Pediatrics, 27*(6), 451–458.

Vetter, T. R. (2008). A clinical profile of a cohort of patients referred to an anesthesiology-based pediatric chronic pain medicine program. *Anesthesia and Analgesia, 106*(3), 786–794.

Weydert, J. A., Ball, T. M., & Davis, M. F. (2003). Systematic review of treatments for recurrent abdominal pain. *Pediatrics, 111*(1), e1–e11.

Wilder, R. T. (2006). Management of pediatric patients with complex regional pain syndrome. *Clinical Journal of Pain, 22*(5), 443–448.

Winner, P. (2008a). Classification of pediatric headache. *Current Pain and Headache Reports, 12*(5), 357–360.

Winner, P. (2008b). Pediatric headache. *Current Opinion in Neurology, 21*(3), 316–322.

Winner, P., & Hershey, A. D. (2007). Epidemiology and diagnosis of migraine in children. *Current Pain and Headache Reports, 11*(5), 375–382.

Youssef, N. N., & Di Lorenzo, C. (2001). The role of motility in functional abdominal disorders in children. *Pediatric Annals, 30*(1), 24–30.

Youssef, N. N., Murphy, T. G., Langseder, A. L., & Rosh, J. R. (2006). Quality of life for children with functional abdominal pain: A comparison study of patients' and parents' perceptions. *Pediatrics, 117*(1), 54–59.

Youssef, N. N., Atienza, K., Langseder, A. L., & Strauss, R. S. (2008). Chronic abdominal pain and depressive symptoms: Analysis of the national longitudinal study of adolescent health. *Clinical Gastroenterology and Hepatology, 6*(3), 329–332.

Zapata, A. L., Moraes, A. J., Leone, C., Doria-Filho, U., & Silva, C. A. (2006a). Pain and musculoskeletal pain syndromes in adolescents. *Journal of Adolescent Health, 38*(6), 769–771.

Zapata, A. L., Moraes, A. J., Leone, C., Doria-Filho, U., & Silva, C. A. (2006b). Pain and musculoskeletal pain syndromes related to computer and video game use in adolescents. *European Journal of Pediatrics, 165*(6), 408–414.

The Neurobiology of Chronic Pain in Children

Maria Fitzgerald

2

Keywords

Nociceptor • Central sensitization • Cortex and chronic pain • Dorsal horn • Early pain exposure and long term effects

Chronic pain arises from plastic changes in the peripheral and central nervous system. These changes are triggered and may be maintained by an insult to tissues, organs or to the nervous system itself. Because neural connections within the sensory and nociceptive systems have been altered, pain can take on a 'life of its own' and no longer require the presence of tissue damage. As a result, chronic pain will often persist beyond the resolution of the original injury. Thus, chronic pain has a clear biological origin, but that origin lies within the nervous system itself and if we are to prevent or treat it effectively, we need to understand these neural changes. The poor pain recovery following the resolution of a physical insult can lead to the conclusion that patients, especially children, are catastrophizing or have aberrant health beliefs, while in fact defined neurobiological changes in neural pain pathways are the source of the problem.

M. Fitzgerald (✉)
Department of Neuroscience, Physiology and Pharmacology, University College London, London, UK
e-mail: m.fitzgerald@ucl.ac.uk

Chronic Pain Mechanisms

Neural Plasticity and Chronic Pain

Several excellent reviews cover the neural basis of chronic pain in adults (Woolf 2004; Latremoliere and Woolf 2009; Costigan et al. 2009; Sandkuhler 2009). These reviews explain the biological basis for long-lasting changes that can occur in pain pathways following a peripheral trauma. Many of these reviews focus on trauma that involves damage to a peripheral nerve which can result in neuropathic pain, a particularly unpleasant chronic pain which is especially difficult to treat. Figures 2.1–2.3 illustrate some of the key changes that occur in the peripheral and central nervous system following tissue injury that contribute to chronic pain. Figure 2.1 shows how prolonged activation or sensitization of nociceptor and mechanosensitive sensory neurons can arise from the local peripheral immune reaction and release of cytokines, increased sympathetic activity within the dorsal root ganglion and upregulation of ion channels and receptor molecules in the cell bodies and terminals of damaged sensory neurons. All these changes cause increased action potentials or altered

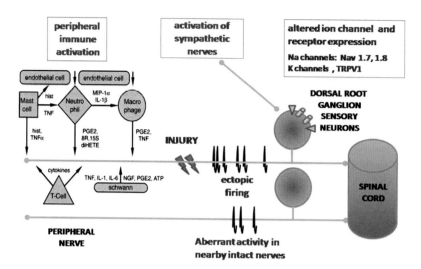

Fig. 2.1 Peripheral events that contribute to the generation and maintenance of chronic pain following nerve injury

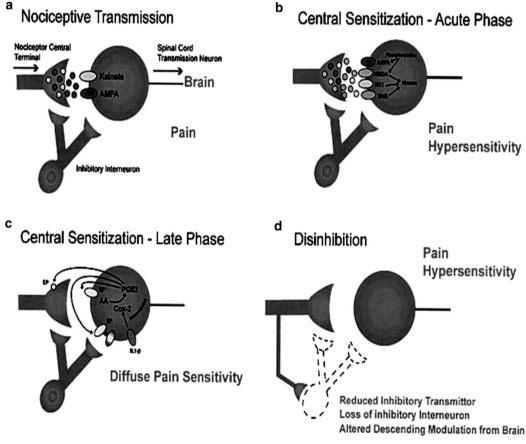

Fig. 2.2 Different synaptic mechansims underlying nociception, acute and chronic pain. (**a**) Normal nociceptive transmission in the spinal cord is carried out by glutamate released from central nociceptive terminals acting on AMPA (α-amino-3-hydroxy-5-methyl-4-isoxazole propionate) and NMDA (*N*-methyl-d-aspartic acid) receptors on central sensory neurons, controlled by inhibitory neurons. (**b**) Strong nociceptor input, such as follows tissue trauma, involves other neurotransmitter receptors, NK1 (neurokinin 1) and trkB (tyrosine kinase B) to activate intracellular kinases that phosphorylate ion channels and receptors, altering their distribution and function and increasing excitability and thereby pain sensitivity. (**c**) Longer lasting pain arises when changes in transcription in dorsal horn neurons occur, such as the induction of cyclooxygenase 2 (Cox-2) via interleukin (IL1β), arachidonic acid (AA) and prostaglandin E2 (PGE2) acting on prostaglandin receptors (EP). (**d**) After peripheral nerve lesions, there is also a reduction in the activity of inhibitory interneurons which increases nociceptive signals across the synapses (From Woolf 2004)

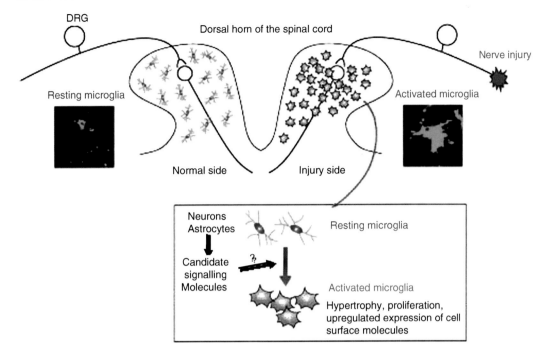

Fig. 2.3 Processes causing activation of microglia in the dorsal horn of the spinal cord following injury to a nerve in the periphery. On the normal side of dorsal horn, microglia have small somas, bearing thin and branched processes, and are homogeneously distributed (i.e. they are 'resting microglia'). After peripheral nerve injury, microglia in the spinal cord ipsilateral to the nerve injury transform from the resting to the 'activated microglia' phenotype, which is characterized by hypertrophy, proliferation and expression of cell-surface molecules (e.g. CR3, CB2, CD14, MHC proteins, TLR4 and the P2X4 receptor). Photographs show resting (*left*) and activated (*right*) microglia staining for CR3. Activation of microglia in the dorsal horn occurs predominantly in the central projection area of the injured peripheral nerve, which implies contribution of signals from injured nerve and/or affected dorsal horn neurons or astrocytes. Candidate signalling molecules include MCSF, IL-6, CD200, ATP, substance P and fractalkine (From Tsuda et al. 2005)

patterns of action potentials in the damaged nerves and in nearby undamaged nerves, which will, in turn, cause aberrant neuronal firing in the central nervous system (CSN) and pain.

Chronic pain also has a major central component. Unlike other sensory stimuli, relatively brief trains of activity in peripheral nociceptors have the ability to trigger long-term changes in CNS circuitry and cause prolonged states of hypersensitivity. This 'central sensitization' contributes to an amplification of the noxious input and a spread of pain into areas outside the original damaged region (hyperalgesia) and the onset of pain from normally innocuous stimuli (allodynia). The central sensitization arises from prolonged increases in membrane excitability, strengthened excitatory synaptic inputs, and reduction of inhibitory interneuronal activity, which in turn are regulated by shifts in gene expression, the production

and trafficking of key receptors, channels and downstream neuronal signalling pathways. It may be relatively short-lasting but in cases of chronic pain, new mechanisms come into play that act to maintain this central sensitization for prolonged periods or even permanently. Figure 2.2 shows some of the mechanisms by which this can occur.

All these changes contribute to an increase in the number and pattern of action potentials generated by spinal nociceptive circuits which, when transmitted to higher centres in the brain, increase pain sensitivity.

Major Shifts in CNS Function in Chronic Pain

Recent evidence suggests that the cellular, synaptic and molecular events underlying central sensitization and chronic pain, illustrated in Fig. 2.2, are driven by several major shifts in CNS function.

One shift is in the functional activity of pain-modulating circuits in the brainstem that normally control nociceptive processing in the spinal cord (Heinricher et al. 2009; Porreca et al. 2002; Gebhart 2004; Suzuki et al. 2004; Vanegas and Schaible 2004). A defined area of the medullary brainstem, called the rostroventral medulla (RVM), plays a key role in this descending brainstem control. The neurons in the region receive afferent input from spinal cord sensory projection neurons and, in turn, send projections back down to spinal sensory circuits, forming a powerful feedback loop. The RVM is itself controlled by higher brainstem and subcortical areas such as the periaqueductal grey (PAG), the amygdala and the hypothalamus, thus making it a strong candidate for mediating the modulatory effects of stress, attention and reward upon pain perception and behaviour. The ability of the RVM to suppress nociceptive transmission is well-documented but at some intensities and sites, stimulation of RVM can also be facilitatory. In normal animals, the balance of RVM descending control is inhibitory, but the situation changes in persistent pain states when the balance of RVM activity becomes facilitatory, probably due to a change in the balance of activity from sub-populations of RVM neurons. Thus, there is an altered balance of inhibition/facilitation or pro-nociceptive/anti-nociceptive mechanisms in chronic pain sates. Evidence for this has been found in both animal models and human imaging studies (Bingel and Tracey 2008). The potential importance of this cannot be overstated; normal CNS pain processing depends upon a system of endogenous control that modulates nociceptive activity through descending fibres and endogenous opioids that represent a homeostatic feedback mechanism of control. These descending and endogenous pain modulatory pathways controls are the mechanisms by which factors such as anticipation, distraction, suggestion, context and past experience can influence pain responses (Fairhurst et al. 2007). If the balance of this mechanism is shifted, then pain processing may effectively become 'out of control'.

The second important shift is in the cellular immune system. While it is well-established that neuronal circuits are sensitized in chronic pain, it has recently become evident that central glia and immune cells also play a key role in chronic pain states (Scholz and Woolf 2007; Milligan and Watkins 2009; DeLeo et al. 2004; Tsuda et al. 2005). The CNS normally contains resident, quiescent, microglial cells, but tissue and nerve injury outside the CNS changes this situation. Resident microglia become swollen and activated and new microglia infiltrate and migrate through the neuropil to join them; all focused upon CNS areas of intense neural activity. Activation of microglia by chemokines, purines, cytokines and complement anaphylotoxins (DeLeo et al. 2004; Tsuda et al. 2005; DeLeo and Yezierski 2001; Watkins et al. 2001; Griffin et al. 2007) leads to release of signal molecules which alter excitability or synaptic transmission in the dorsal horn which leads to ongoing pain and hypersensitivity. As yet it is not known exactly what signals lead to central glial activation after injury and how exactly they cause pain, but there is no doubt that this is an important mechanism (Wei et al. 2008). Indeed it has been argued that neuropathic pain has many features of a neuroimmune disorder and that immunosuppression and blockade of the reciprocal signalling pathways between neuronal and non-neuronal cells may be a successful approach to the management of pain (Scholz and Woolf 2007).

The Cortex and Chronic Pain

Pain is an emotional/affective process requiring higher-level cortical activity. As such, the neural pathways under consideration go beyond circuits in the spinal cord and brain stem and require the involvement of specific regions of the cortex and other higher brain centres. Extensive research on the central mechanisms regarding the sensory-discriminative dimensions of pain have revealed a complex network of cortical and subcortical brain structures involved in the transmission and integration of pain, the so-called pain matrix, and there is evidence from imaging studies that chronic pain is associated with changes in this central matrix for pain processing (Bingel and Tracey 2008; Seifert and Maihofner 2009; Apkarian 2008). Chronic pain appears to involve both structural and functional changes in the matrix. Thus, an important component of the pain involves a change in wiring of cortical networks in addition to and perhaps in consequence of the peripheral, spinal cord and brainstem plasticity described above (Zhuo 2008).

Individual Variation in Chronic Pain

Thus far the reader might be forgiven for concluding that everyone who suffers a peripheral injury, especially if it involves a peripheral nerve, will automatically develop maintained hypersensitivity and chronic pain. In reality this is not so. The individual variability in the incidence of chronic pain is very great. While acute post-operative pain is followed by persistent pain in 10–50% of individuals after common operations, chronic pain is severe in only about 2–10% of these patients (Kehlet et al. 2006). Striking interindividual variability in pain sensitivity, the propensity to develop chronic pain conditions and the response to analgesic manipulations, is currently a major focus of chronic pain research. The explanation is likely to be a classic genetic–environmental interaction; that is, the injury itself, an earlier history of injury (see below) and an innate propensity act together to increase the chance of an acute pain changing into a chronic one. The advances, problems and pitfalls of human pain genetic research have recently been discussed in an excellent review by Mogil (Lacroix-Fralish and Mogil 2009). The next few years will no doubt provide a clearer picture of the genetic components of chronic pain.

Much of our knowledge of chronic pain mechanisms is extrapolated from inbred rat and mouse strains, chosen for study because of behavioural signs of long-lasting mechanical hypersensitivity or allodynia, guarding or withdrawal of the affected area and behavioural anxiety and altered decision- making in the presence of tissue or nerve injury. While providing information on the physiology of pain, they cannot model the full human pain experience. The strengths and limitations of these animal models have been recently reviewed (Mogil 2009) and we should not forget, especially with respect to higher pain processing, that 'a rat is not a monkey is not a human' (Craig 2009).

Chronic Pain in Children

While the neurobiology of chronic pain in adults has been the subject of intensive research over the last two decades, the neural mechanisms underlying chronic pain in children have received little attention. Many of the neural mechanisms may be similar to those in adults, but the fundamental differences in the immature and mature pain systems suggest that a number of key differences are likely to arise in the incidence, pattern, time course and treatment of chronic pain in children. Paediatric pain pathways are not simply less efficient forms of adult pathways – they function differently, undergoing a series of transitional functional states before reaching maturity (Fitzgerald 2005). This affects nociceptive and acute pain (Fitzgerald and Walker 2009) and thus is likely to impact on the natural history of chronic pain in childhood as well.

Figure 2.4 shows a developmental time line for laboratory rats to help interpret data from young laboratory animals and translate the findings to children. It shows that data from the first two post-natal weeks in rats are likely to be relevant to human infancy, while post-natal day (P) 21–35 are especially relevant to childhood. It is taken from an excellent review that discusses how CNS developmental changes can be qualitative or quantitative in nature, involving gradual changes, rapid switches, or inverted U-shaped curves. Thus, single phenomena may be governed by different mechanisms at different ages in an ongoing process that does not end with puberty (McCutcheon and Marinelli 2009).

Below we focus on some developmental changes that occur over this period and which are likely to affect chronic pain.

Maturation of Brainstem Descending Control Systems

It has been known for some time from the study of young rats that there is little descending inhibitory tone from higher CNS centres in the first weeks of life and that no analgesia is produced from brainstem stimulation until post-natal day

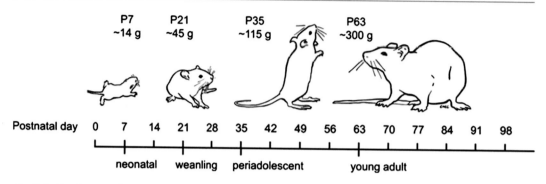

Fig. 2.4 Developmental stages of a laboratory rat (From McCutcheon and Marinelli 2009)

21 (P21) (van Praag and Frenk 1991; Fitzgerald and Koltzenburg 1986). Recent research has shown that the rostroventral medulla (RVM), which is the main output nucleus for brainstem descending control, undergoes a remarkable maturational switch after P2 (Hathway et al. 2009). Both lesioning and electrical stimulation of RVM at different post-natal ages reveal that RVM control over spinal nociceptive circuits switches from being entirely facilitatory before P21 to inhibitory at older ages. Between P25 and P35, descending inhibition begins to dominate but it is not as powerful as in the adult until P40. This gradual change is observed in the changing influence of the RVM over spinal nociceptive reflexes and dorsal horn neuronal activity over this critical periadolescent developmental period.

Childhood may therefore represent a time when the normal balance, rather than the absolute onset, of descending brainstem controls are established. A lack of balance or stability between inhibitory and excitatory supraspinal controls in early life may mean that young children are less able to mount effective endogenous control over noxious inputs compared to adults (Fig. 2.5).

Maturation of Neuroimmune Interactions

While microglia in the dorsal horn of adult animals contribute to the generation of neuropathic pain, through processes that involve their recruitment, proliferation and activation, laboratory data show that in the dorsal horn of young rats, the

microglial response to peripheral nerve injury is considerably less than that in adults (Moss et al. 2007; Vega-Avelaira et al. 2007). This may contribute to differences in pain-like hypersensitivity in young and adult animals (Moss et al. 2007; Vega-Avelaira et al. 2007). The absence of a strong neuroimmune response in young animals is not due to a general inability of immature dorsal horn neurons to respond to immune activation. Microglial activation and significant allodynia can be evoked by spinal injections of lipopolysaccharide, glutamate receptor agonists or the intrathecal application of exogenous ATP stimulated microglia at young ages when peripheral nerve injury has no effect (Moss et al. 2007). These data suggest that the resident immune system in young animals is capable of activation but fails to do so in response to peripheral nerve injury. Neuropathic pain does appear to be less prevalent in young children compared to adults (Howard 2003; Howard et al. 2005) and this could be one reason why. The differing status of the immune system and its interactions with CNS neurons in the face of peripheral injury is likely to be an area of important research in children's chronic pain in the future (Fig. 2.6).

Maturation of Cortical Pain Processing

Pain is processed at the level of the cortex at a very young age. Specific cortical haemodynamic and electrical EEG responses can be recorded from pre-term and term infants in response to noxious heel lance suggesting that nociceptive connections

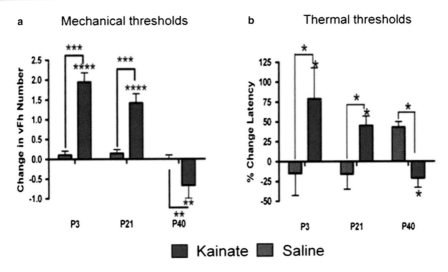

Fig. 2.5 Descending inhibition from the brainstem to the spinal cord. Excitotoxic lesioning of the rostroventral medulla (RVM) with kainate increases hindpaw mechanical and thermal thresholds in P3 and P21 rats but significantly decreases them in adult animals (P40). *Bars* indicate mean values ± s.e.m. *P<0.05, **P<0.01, ***P<0.001 and ****P<0.0001, n=6–12 in each group. *Asterisks* immediately above bars indicate significant change from baseline whilst those between bars indicate differences between open bars saline-treated and between filled bars kainate-treated animals within an age group (**a**) Mechanical thresholds, (**b**) Thermal thresholds (From Hathway et al. 2009)

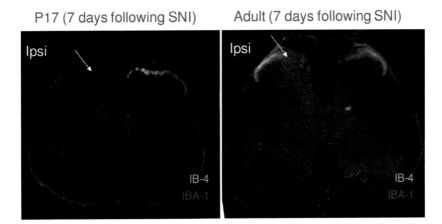

Fig. 2.6 Sections of rat lumbar spinal cord immunostained for microglia with IBA-1 (*red*) and C fibre terminals with IB-4 (*green*). In both cases the sciatic nerve on the left was cut 7 days earlier. *Left*: the nerve section was performed when the rat was 10 days old (P10). *Right*: the same lesion was performed in the adult rat. Note the great increase in microglia on the operated side in the adult but not the P10 rat (From Moss et al. 2007)

are formed with cortical neurons at an early stage (Slater et al. 2006, 2010). Nothing is known about the maturation of the pain matrix over infancy and childhood and it is not known whether chronic pain is processed centrally in young children in the same way that it is in adults.

There is evidence, however, that the presence of chronic pain does alter central processing in children as well as in adults. Two studies of cortical processing in children aged 10–15 years, one with migraine (Zohsel et al. 2008) and one with recurrent abdominal pain (Hermann et al. 2008) show evidence of an automatic attentional bias towards painful and potentially painful somatosensory stimuli. Such an attentional bias could constitute an important mechanism for these pains becoming a chronic problem. Another study of paediatric patients with complex regional pain syndrome (CRPS) suggested significant changes in CNS circuitry had taken place. CNS activation in response to mechanical (brush) and thermal (cold) stimulation during an active period of pain (CRPS(+)) and after symptomatic recovery (CRPS(−)) was evaluated using fMRI. Stimuli were applied to the affected region of the involved limb and the corresponding mirror region of the unaffected limb. The data suggest pain-induced activation of endogenous pain modulatory systems in the children's brains which persist even after nearly complete elimination of evoked pain. In addition, the 'CRPS brain' responded differently to normal stimuli applied to unaffected regions (Lebel et al. 2008). Future fMRI studies in children with chronic pain will tell us more about cortical plasticity in response to acute and chronic pain in the developing brain and how it differs from the adult, although there are specific concerns related to the imaging of pain in children (Sava et al. 2009).

The Long Term Effects of Early Pain

One possible factor in the development of chronic pain is that there is already a 'memory trace' of pain, laid down perhaps at a younger age. While this is speculation at this stage, there is some epidemiological evidence to support it (Jones et al. 2009). What is becoming increasingly clear is that early pain experience does alter mechanical and thermal nociceptive pain thresholds and acute pain sensitivity in children when they have grown up (Hermann et al. 2006; Zohsel et al. 2006; Walker et al. 2009). A feature of the immature somatosensory and nociceptive system, in both animals and man, is that it is vulnerable to excessive noxious stimulation in early life (Fitzgerald 2005; Fitzgerald and Walker 2009; Schmelzle-Lubiecki et al. 2007). Exposure to pain early in life significantly impacts upon pain experience in childhood (Grunau et al. 2006). In animal models, long after an initial tissue damaging insult to cutaneous, subcutaneous or visceral tissue has healed, animals display a widespread reduction in their baseline noxious and innocu-

ous sensitivity across the body combined with an enhanced hyperalgesia to repeat damage at the original site (Ren et al. 2004). The injury must be performed within the first weeks of life in order for this to occur. These data are supported by follow-up studies in children that have undergone intensive care procedures or surgery as neonates, who also display widespread hyposensitivity to noxious and innocuous stimuli accompanied by enhanced hyperalgesia and sensitization to inflammatory or surgical injury (Walker et al. 2009; Peters et al. 2005). The local hyperalgesia may arise from local peripheral or central sensitization, but the global threshold changes are likely to be centrally mediated. While the local hyperalgesia to repeat injury appears soon after the initial injury is performed, the global hyposensitivity is apparent only after the animal has reached its second month – which, interestingly, is exactly the time when the RVM switches its influence over the dorsal horn (Fig. 2.7).

Many of the post-natal developmental changes in nociceptive processing are dependent upon a normal balance of neural sensory activity and fail to occur if the patterns of activity are disrupted. In rat pups where spinal NMDA receptors are chronically blocked and in mutant mice where the CaMkIIα enzyme does not autophosphorylate, nociceptive processes remain immature (Beggs et al. 2002; Pattinson et al. 2006). Furthermore, maturation is delayed by blockade of low-threshold sensory afferents by peripheral anaesthetic (Waldenstrom et al. 2003) and is altered by tissue injury (Torsney and Fitzgerald 2003; Li et al. 2009). Thus dorsal horn nociceptive circuits are not fixed or preset at birth, but are in a plastic or transitory stage, responsive to the sensory experience (Granmo et al. 2008). In this way, early tissue injury may lead to changes in somatosensory processing, pain signalling and hence future analgesic responsiveness.

Both clinical and pre-clinical studies demonstrate the complexity and diversity of persistent changes in pain responses. It is too simplistic at this stage to expect that early pain experience will reliably increase the chance of developing chronic pain in childhood as multiple contributory factors may interact to influence nociceptive processing and/or the behavioural response to

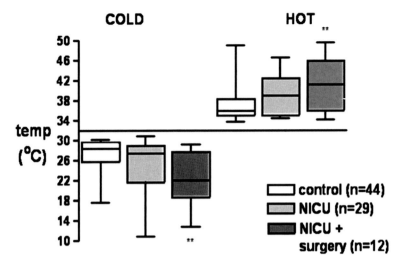

Fig. 2.7 Effect of neonatal surgery on the baseline thermal thresholds measured on the thenar eminence of 9–12-year-old children. The temperature at which the sensations of cold and hot (0 C) were perceived on the thenar eminence of the non-dominant hand are plotted for full-term control (n=44), extremely preterm children requiring neonatal intensive care (NICU) treatment (n=29) and extremely premature children who also underwent surgical operations in the neonatal period (NICU+surgery, n=12). $^{**}P<0.01$ one way ANOVA with Tukey's post hoc comparison (From Walker et al. 2009)

pain. Nevertheless, future neurobiological and clinical research into the relationship between past history and current pain in children will provide important insight into the long term plasticity that underlies chronic pain.

References

Apkarian, A. V. (2008). Pain perception in relation to emotional learning. *Current Opinion in Neurobiology, 18*, 464–468.

Beggs, S., Torsney, C., Drew, L. J., & Fitzgerald, M. (2002). The postnatal reorganization of primary afferent input and dorsal horn cell receptive fields in the rat spinal cord is an activity-dependent process. *The European Journal of Neuroscience, 16*, 1249–1258.

Bingel, U., & Tracey, I. (2008). Imaging CNS modulation of pain in humans. *Physiology (Bethesda), 23*, 371–380.

Costigan, M., Scholz, J., & Woolf, C. J. (2009). Neuropathic pain: A maladaptive response of the nervous system to damage. *Annual Review of Neuroscience, 32*, 1–32.

Craig, A. D. (2009). A rat is not a monkey is not a human: Comment on Mogil (Nature Rev. Neurosci. 10, 283–294 (2009)). *Nature Reviews Neuroscience, 10*, 466.

DeLeo, J. A., & Yezierski, R. P. (2001). The role of neuroinflammation and neuroimmune activation in persistent pain. *Pain, 90*, 1–6.

DeLeo, J. A., Tanga, F. Y., & Tawfik, V. L. (2004). Neuroimmune activation and neuroinflammation in chronic pain and opioid tolerance/hyperalgesia. *The Neuroscientist, 10*, 40–52.

Fairhurst, M., Wiech, K., Dunckley, P., & Tracey, I. (2007). Anticipatory brainstem activity predicts neural processing of pain in humans. *Pain, 128*, 101–110.

Fitzgerald, M. (2005). The development of nociceptive circuits. *Nature Reviews. Neuroscience, 6*, 507–520.

Fitzgerald, M., & Koltzenburg, M. (1986). The functional development of descending inhibitory pathways in the dorsolateral funiculus of the newborn rat spinal cord. *Brain Research, 389*, 261–270.

Fitzgerald, M., & Walker, S. (2009). Infant pain management: A developmental neurobiological approach. *Nature Clinical Practice. Neurology, 5*, 35–50.

Gebhart, G. F. (2004). Descending modulation of pain. *Neuroscience and Biobehavioral Reviews, 27*, 729–737.

Granmo, M., Petersson, P., & Schouenborg, J. (2008). Action-based body maps in the spinal cord emerge from a transitory floating organization. *The Journal of Neuroscience, 28*, 5494–5503.

Griffin, R. S., et al. (2007). Complement induction in spinal cord microglia results in anaphylatoxin C5a-mediated pain hypersensitivity. *The Journal of Neuroscience, 27*, 8699–8708.

Grunau, R. E., Holsti, L., & Peters, J. W. (2006). Long-term consequences of pain in human neonates. *Seminars in Fetal & Neonatal Medicine, 11*, 268–275.

Hathway, G., Koch, S., Low, L., & Fitzgerald, M. (2009). The changing balance of brainstem-spinal cord modulation of pain processing over the first weeks of rat postnatal life. *Journal of Physiology, 587*, 2927–2935.

Heinricher, M. M., Tavares, I., Leith, J. L., & Lumb, B. M. (2009). Descending control of nociception: Specificity, recruitment and plasticity. *Brain Research Reviews, 60*, 214–225.

Hermann, C., Hohmeister, J., Demirakca, S., Zohsel, K., & Flor, H. (2006). Long-term alteration of pain sensitivity in school-aged children with early pain experiences. *Pain, 125*, 278–285.

Hermann, C., Zohsel, K., Hohmeister, J., & Flor, H. (2008). Cortical correlates of an attentional bias to painful and innocuous somatic stimuli in children with recurrent abdominal pain. *Pain, 136*, 397–406.

Howard, R. F. (2003). Current status of pain management in children. *Journal of the American Medical Association, 290*, 2464–2469.

Howard, R., Walker, S., Mota, P., & Fitzgerald, M. (2005). The ontogeny of neuropathic pain: Postnatal onset of mechanical allodynia in rat spared nerve injury (SNI) and chronic constriction injury (CCI) models. *Pain, 115*, 382–389.

Jones, G. T., Power, C., & Macfarlane, G. J. (2009). Adverse events in childhood and chronic widespread pain in adult life: Results from the 1958 British Birth Cohort Study. *Pain, 143*, 92–96.

Kehlet, H., Jensen, T. S., & Woolf, C. J. (2006). Persistent postsurgical pain: Risk factors and prevention. *Lancet, 367*, 1618–1625.

Lacroix-Fralish, M. L., & Mogil, J. S. (2009). Progress in genetic studies of pain and analgesia. *Annual Review of Pharmacology and Toxicology, 49*, 97–121.

Latremoliere, A., & Woolf, C. J. (2009). Central sensitization: A generator of pain hypersensitivity by central neural plasticity. *The Journal of Pain, 10*, 895–926.

Lebel, A., et al. (2008). fMRI reveals distinct CNS processing during symptomatic and recovered complex regional pain syndrome in children. *Brain, 131*, 1854–1879.

Li, J., Walker, S. M., Fitzgerald, M., & Baccei, M. L. (2009). Activity-dependent modulation of glutamatergic signaling in the developing rat dorsal horn by early tissue injury. *Journal of Neurophysiology, 102*(4), 2208–2219.

McCutcheon, J. E., & Marinelli, M. (2009). Age matters. *The European Journal of Neuroscience, 29*, 997–1014.

Milligan, E. D., & Watkins, L. R. (2009). Pathological and protective roles of glia in chronic pain. *Nature Reviews. Neuroscience, 10*, 23–36.

Mogil, J. S. (2009). Animal models of pain: Progress and challenges. *Nature Reviews. Neuroscience, 10*, 283–294.

Moss, A., et al. (2007). Spinal microglia and neuropathic pain in young rats. *Pain, 128*, 215–224.

Pattinson, D., et al. (2006). Aberrant dendritic branching and sensory inputs in the superficial dorsal horn of mice lacking CaMKIIalpha autophosphorylation. *Molecular and Cellular Neurosciences, 33*, 88–95.

Peters, J. W., et al. (2005). Does neonatal surgery lead to increased pain sensitivity in later childhood? *Pain, 114*, 444–454.

Porreca, F., Ossipov, M. H., & Gebhart, G. F. (2002). Chronic pain and medullary descending facilitation. *Trends in Neurosciences, 25*, 319–325.

Ren, K., et al. (2004). Characterization of basal and re-inflammation-associated long-term alteration in pain responsivity following short-lasting neonatal local inflammatory insult. *Pain, 110*, 588–596.

Sandkuhler, J. (2009). Models and mechanisms of hyperalgesia and allodynia. *Physiological Reviews, 89*, 707–758.

Sava, S., et al. (2009). Challenges of functional imaging research of pain in children. *Molecular Pain, 5*, 30.

Schmelzle-Lubiecki, B. M., Campbell, K. A., Howard, R. H., Franck, L., & Fitzgerald, M. (2007). Long-term consequences of early infant injury and trauma upon somatosensory processing. *European Journal of Pain, 11*, 799–809.

Scholz, J., & Woolf, C. J. (2007). The neuropathic pain triad: Neurons, immune cells and glia. *Nature Neuroscience, 10*, 1361–1368.

Seifert, F., & Maihofner, C. (2009). Central mechanisms of experimental and chronic neuropathic pain: Findings from functional imaging studies. *Cellular and Molecular Life Sciences, 66*, 375–390.

Slater, R., et al. (2006). Cortical pain responses in human infants. *The Journal of Neuroscience, 26*, 3662–3666.

Slater, R., Worley, A., Fabrizi, L., Roberts, S., Meek, J., Boyd, S., & Fitzgerald, M. (2010). Evoked potentials generated by noxious stimulation in the human infant brain. *European Journal of Pain, 14*(3), 321–326.

Suzuki, R., Rygh, L. J., & Dickenson, A. H. (2004). Bad news from the brain: Descending 5-HT pathways that control spinal pain processing. *Trends in Pharmacological Sciences, 25*, 613–617.

Torsney, C., & Fitzgerald, M. (2003). Spinal dorsal horn cell receptive field size is increased in adult rats following neonatal hindpaw skin injury. *Journal de Physiologie, 550*, 255–261.

Tsuda, M., Inoue, K., & Salter, M. W. (2005). Neuropathic pain and spinal microglia: A big problem from molecules in "small" glia. *Trends in Neurosciences, 28*, 101–107.

van Praag, H., & Frenk, H. (1991). The development of stimulation-produced analgesia (SPA) in the rat. *Brain Research. Developmental Brain Research, 64*, 71–76.

Vanegas, H., & Schaible, H. G. (2004). Descending control of persistent pain: Inhibitory or facilitatory? *Brain Research. Brain Research Reviews, 46*, 295–309.

Vega-Avelaira, D., Moss, A., & Fitzgerald, M. (2007). Age-related changes in the spinal cord microglial and astrocytic response profile to nerve injury. *Brain, Behavior, and Immunity, 21*, 617–623.

Waldenstrom, A., Thelin, J., Thimansson, E., Levinsson, A., & Schouenborg, J. (2003). Developmental learning in a pain-related system: Evidence for a cross-modality mechanism. *The Journal of Neuroscience, 23*, 7719–7725.

Walker, S., Franck, L., Fitzgerald, M., Myles, J., Stocks, J., & Marlow, N. (2009). Long-term impact of neonatal intensive care and surgery on somatosensory perception in children born extremely preterm. *Pain, 141*, 79–87.

Watkins, L. R., Milligan, E. D., & Maier, S. F. (2001). Glial activation: A driving force for pathological pain. *Trends in Neurosciences, 24*, 450–455.

Wei, F., Guo, W., Zou, S., Ren, K., & Dubner, R. (2008). Supraspinal glial-neuronal interactions contribute to descending pain facilitation. *The Journal of Neuroscience, 28*, 10482–10495.

Woolf, C. J. (2004). Pain: Moving from symptom control toward mechanism-specific pharmacologic management. *Annals of Internal Medicine, 140*, 441–451.

Zhuo, M. (2008). Cortical excitation and chronic pain. *Trends in Neurosciences, 31*, 199–207.

Zohsel, K., Hohmeister, J., Oelkers-Ax, R., Flor, H., & Hermann, C. (2006). Quantitative sensory testing in children with migraine: Preliminary evidence for enhanced sensitivity to painful stimuli especially in girls. *Pain, 123*, 10–18.

Zohsel, K., Hohmeister, J., Flor, H., & Hermann, C. (2008). Altered pain processing in children with migraine: An evoked potential study. *European Journal of Pain, 12*, 1090–1101.

Theories on Common Adolescent Pain Syndromes

Jill MacLaren Chorney, Kathryn Crofton, and Brenda C. McClain

Keywords

Chronic pain- effects on families • School absenteeism • Comorbidity and pain • Psychological interventions • Coping strategies

Theories on Common Adolescent Pain Syndromes

Pain is a prevalent condition among adolescents. In fact, 30–40% of children and adolescents report experiencing pain at least once a week (Palermo 2000), and 5–25% of adolescents report some form of recurrent or chronic pain (Perquin et al. 2000; Goodman and McGrath 1991). Of those reporting recurrent pain, 30–40% of children report pain episodes at least once a week (Kristjansdottir 1997). In terms of specific pain conditions, data indicate that the most common chronic pain conditions among adolescents are headaches, abdominal pain, back pain, and musculoskeletal pain (Goodman and McGrath 1991; Morsy 2006).

Data also suggest that pain can be a long-term condition for children. In community samples, El-Metwally and colleagues (2004) found that 54% of children reporting musculoskeletal pain continued to experience pain at a 1-year follow-up. Not surprisingly, pain is also a long-term condition in clinic-referred samples. Martin and colleagues (2007) found that the majority (62%) of children who presented for treatment at a multidisciplinary clinic continued to report pain from 1 to 6 years later.

It is interesting to note that reports of chronic and recurrent pain tend to differ between sexes and across development. Prevalence data consistently suggest that reports of pain are more common in girls than boys (McGrath et al. 2000; Viry et al. 1999), a pattern that is fairly consistent across pain conditions and nationalities (Haugland et al. 2001).

Outcomes

As chronic pain among adolescents is such a prevalent issue, it is important to note the impact of such conditions on the lives of these individuals. The daily lives of adolescents living with chronic pain are permeated by their conditions. Not only are these individuals' physical capabilities impacted, so too are their familial relationships, social development, education, perception of academic ability, and sleep.

J.M. Chorney (✉)
Pediatric Anesthesia, IWK Health Centre,
Halifax, Nova Scotia, Canada
and
Department of Anesthesiology and Psychology,
Dalhousie University, Halifax, Nova Scotia, Canada
email: jill.chorney@dal.ca

B.C. McClain and S. Suresh (eds.), *Handbook of Pediatric Chronic Pain:
Current Science and Integrative Practice*, DOI 10.1007/978-1-4419-0350-1_3,
© Springer Science+Business Media, LLC 2011

Not surprisingly, the families of adolescents with a chronic pain condition are greatly affected. Caring for an adolescent with chronic pain requires a great deal of time, energy, and emotional attention. The constant demands placed upon family members, especially parents, can be draining for some. The effects on families of chronic pain patients have been greatly studied among patients with sickle cell disease (SCD) and various rheumatological conditions. Midence and colleagues (1993) administered a survey to mothers of adolescents with sickle cell disease and found that these mothers felt hopeless and frustrated when their child was experiencing a pain episode. Families with an adolescent musculoskeletal pain patient have also been found to experience a great deal of family distress (Aasland et al. 1997). In addition to the emotional burden placed on these families, they often experience financial difficulties, resulting from associated health-care costs as well as the missed days of work when caring for the ill child (Palermo 2000).

Chronic pain can also impact an adolescent's social involvement. Adolescence is typically a period of increased social involvement; however, for those afflicted by chronic pain, it may be a time of social withdrawal. Langeveld and colleagues (1997) found that adolescents with chronic headaches experienced a decrease in the amount of time spent with their peers. Similarly, adolescents with SCD experience a decrease in the amount of time spent socializing with peers, as well as time spent in activities with peers (Fuggle et al. 1996; Langeveld et al. 1997).

The impact on an adolescent's school attendance and performance has been well-studied. In fact, chronic pain conditions are responsible for more school absences than any other chronic condition (Palermo 2000). Among chronic pain conditions, headache and arthritis account for the majority of school absences (Newacheck and Taylor 1992). SCD also contributes to the high absenteeism rate among chronic pain patients, with an absenteeism rate of 21% (Shapiro et al. 1995). In addition to increased school absenteeism, chronic pain can impact an adolescent's perception of his/her academic abilities, as well as

school-related stress. One study by Walker and colleagues (1998) found that adolescents with irritable bowel syndrome (IBS) and other chronic abdominal pain experience lower perceptions of academic ability. Flato and colleagues (1998) studied adolescents with juvenile rheumatoid arthritis (JRA) and discovered that half of these adolescents reported feeling as though their pain conditions impacted their schoolwork.

Sleep is critically important to an individual's health and well-being, especially during childhood and adolescence, when a great deal of growth and development occurs. Sleep deprivation impacts many areas of an adult's life, and this is also true for adolescents. Unfortunately, chronic pain appears to interfere with adolescents meeting duration and quality of sleep requirements. In terms of specific conditions, adolescents with chronic or recurring headaches or migraines experience disturbances in their sleep (Bruni et al. 1997), as do those with JRA. In a literature review by Palermo (2000), adolescents with JRA are reportedly prone to waking during the night and to parasomnia. Adolescents with SCD are also at an increased risk for experiencing sleep deprivation, leading to fatigue, increased pain, and higher rates of school absences (Palermo 2000).

Theories on Adolescent Pain

Introduction to the Biopsychosocial Model

From the time of Descartes, pain has traditionally been discussed within a biomedical model. This model operates within a nociceptive framework, suggesting a one-to-one correspondence between nociceptive input and pain sensation. In the context of chronic pain, the biomedical model maintains that psychological or behavioral concerns may result from pain but do not influence the pain itself (MacLaren et al. 2007).

Despite the assertion of the biomedical model that pain is directly related to physiology, it is notable that a number of chronic pain conditions have little overt evidence of pathophysiology and there is wide variability in individuals' responses to the same potentially painful stimulus. As early as the 1960s, researchers began to acknowledge the contribution of more than just nociceptive input to the pain experience. The Gate Control Theory (GTC); (Melzack and Wall 1965) was the first model to recognize the contribution of central mechanisms in the pain response. Offering an alternative to the Cartesian concept of pain, the GTC posited that peripheral afferent stimulation could be modulated by descending neural impulses and that the experience of pain resulted from a balance between these sensory and central inputs. Melzack and Casey (1968) went on to describe these central processes as cognitive-evaluative (i.e., thoughts) and affective-motivational (i.e., mood and anxiety), and identified the interaction between these processes and the sensory-discriminative process (i.e., nociception) as central to the pain experience. The most recent iteration of the GTC moves beyond a simple gating mechanism to a more complex set of neural networks, referred to by Melzack as the Neuromatrix (Melzack 1999). This new "Neuromatrix Theory" of pain extends Melzack and colleagues original conceptualization by introducing the roles of genetic and immunological influences on pain.

Moving from pain-specific to more general models, the biopsychosocial framework has emerged as a guiding conceptualization for the contributors to and impacts of chronic illnesses. In line with components discussed in the Gate Control and Neuromatrix theories, the biopsychosocial model highlights the important interactions between physiological, psychological, and sociocultural influences on medical conditions. The following sections provide a discussion of the contributors to pain within a biopsychosocial framework (Fig. 3.1). Biological factors are discussed within other chapters of this book, thus psychological and social influences are highlighted here. Following the presentation of influences on pain, the implications of the biopsychosocial model on treatment of pain are discussed and data are presented on the efficacy of psychological and multimodal interventions for chronic pain.

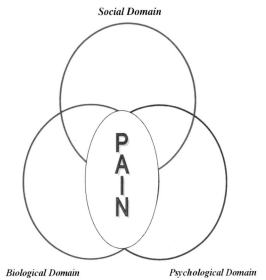

Fig. 3.1 The Pain Biopsychosocial Model. In the tripartite biopsychosocial model, one domain may play a greater role than another. The weight of each domain will depend on various factors within said domain

Psychological Influences

Affective Factors

Pain is, by definition, a sensory and emotional experience (IASP); thus it is not surprising that affective factors have been closely linked with chronic pain. In adults, comorbidity of chronic pain with anxiety and depression is well-established (Gatchel and Dersh 2002), and data in adolescents support similar relations. For example, children with recurrent abdominal pain have been found to have significantly higher incidences of depression and anxiety than children without pain (Campo et al. 2004).

Notably, the pattern of relations among anxiety, depression, and pain appear to be somewhat different in children and adolescents than in adults. Whereas depression is most commonly comorbid with pain in adults (Gatchel and Dersh 2002), anxiety appears to be the most common comorbid condition with pain in children and adolescents. In fact, Lipsitz and colleagues (2005) found that while 56% of children with non-cardiac chest pain met criteria for anxiety disorders, only 4% of children met criteria for depression. Campo et al. (2004) found a higher incidence of depression in children with recurrent abdominal pain (46%) than in the general population, but it was notable that all but one of the children with depression also met criteria for an anxiety disorder. The prevalence of anxiety disorders in this study was 76%.

Whether anxiety and depression precede pain or are consequences of pain in adolescents is difficult to determine given the lack of prospective premorbid data available in this population. In adults, depression appears to be more of a consequence than an antecedent of the onset of chronic pain. Banks and Kerns (1996) offer a stress-diathesis model to explain the relationship between depression and pain in adults. In this model, preexisting risk factors for depression (e.g., negative schemas, attributions) may be dormant until triggered by the stress of chronic pain. Once triggered, activation of risk factors results in depression in vulnerable individuals (Gatchel and Dersh 2002). Although fairly well-established in adults, the diathesis-stress conceptualization of depression and pain has not yet been confirmed in adolescents and warrants further study.

The relation of anxiety to chronic pain has also been extensively studied in adults and has received increasing attention in adolescents. In regard to the nature of this relation, some authors suggest that it is not anxiety per se that influences pain, but rather how sensitive an individual is to the physiological sensations of anxiety – a characteristic known as "anxiety sensitivity" (Norton and Asmundson 2004). Individuals who are high in anxiety sensitivity tend to interpret physiological sensations (e.g., heart palpitations) as more physically, emotionally, or socially threatening than individuals who are low in anxiety sensitivity (Reiss et al. 1986). For example, a highly anxiety-sensitive person may interpret heart palpitations as a heart attack, while a lowly anxiety sensitive person may dismiss these sensations as harmless. In adults, anxiety sensitivity is a risk factor for anxiety disorders and has been linked to pain (Stewart et al. 2006). In adolescents with

chronic pain, anxiety sensitivity has been found to be significantly related to health-related quality of life, particularly self-esteem, behavior problems, and social functioning (Tsao et al. 2007).

Closely related to anxiety sensitivity is the specific fear of pain (Muris et al. 2007). Similar to general anxiety sensitivity, injury sensitivity is the worry about painful sensations and the attribution of pain sensations as harmful (Vlaeyen and Linton 2000). Injury sensitivity is a stronger predictor of pain catastrophizing and fear of pain than anxiety sensitivity (Vancleef et al. 2006).

A discussion of fear of pain would be remiss without noting that fear of pain is an adaptive response in acute pain situations. In these situations, fear is protective and serves as a motivator to avoid potentially dangerous situations (e.g., placing a hand on a hot stove). Fear of pain becomes maladaptive, however, in chronic pain conditions. In these cases, fear of pain generalizes beyond objectively dangerous situations to any activity that an individual perceives may be related to pain (e.g., walking, school attendance); this fear then results in avoidance of an increasingly large number of activities and transitions quickly to disability (Waddell et al. 1993). Kinesiophobia, the fear of movement due to pain or (re)injury, has emerged as a significant predictor of pain-related disability and distress across several painful conditions. (Pells et al. 2007; Roelofs et al. 2004). This fear of movement can be more disabling than the pain itself (Crombez et al. 1999). The degree of kinesiophobia positively correlates with pain severity and is estimated to be a better predictor of physical disability in patients with chronic pain than many previous indices (Pells et al. 2007).

It is possible that attentional mechanisms may mediate the relations among anxiety, anxiety sensitivity, fear of pain, and pain. An intriguing study by Boyer and colleagues (2006) demonstrated that children with RAP unconsciously attended to pain-related words (e.g., ouch) more than neutral (e.g., piano) or socially threatening words (e.g., bullied). At a conscious level however, children attended significantly *less* to pain-related words than neutral words. The authors interpreted these results in a two-stage attentional process by which children with RAP are selectively hypervigalent to pain-related information but make conscious attempts to avoid or disengage from this information. Notably, children with higher anxiety demonstrated more of these attentional biases than children with lower anxiety.

Temperament and Personality Factors

Personality is generally defined as characteristic patterns of behavior, thoughts, and feelings that originate within an individual and influence how an individual responds to the environment (Carver and Scheier 2000). Early work in psychosomatic medicine attempted to reveal personality typologies associated with specific chronic pain conditions (i.e., headache personality), but this work has been challenged (Turk and Monarch 2002). Instead, current research focuses on how personality and early encounters interact with the pain experience. For example, similar to anxiety sensitivity, Conrad and colleagues (2007) found that patients with chronic pain scored significantly higher on Harm Avoidance temperament than individuals without pain. Data from this study also indicated that patients with chronic pain scored significantly lower on personality dimensions of self-directedness and cooperativeness. Interestingly, the link between personality and pain may be bidirectional. Fishbain and colleagues (2006) conducted a meta-analysis of interactions between measures of pain and personality and found that measures of personality (e.g., Minnesota Multiphasic Personality Inventory scores) were significantly affected by improvements in pain following treatment. Thus, it appears in adults that personality may not only affect pain, but may also change as a result of pain experience.

Given the developmental changes that occur in personality during childhood and adolescence, research with these groups has focused on temperament – the childhood precursor to personality. Like personality, temperament is a consistent pattern of responding to the environment, and because it is evident from minutes after birth, is generally thought to be genetic in nature. A fair amount of work has been dedicated to exploring the interaction between pain and temperament, especially in the acute pain context (Broome et al. 1998). Recently, Rocha et al. (2003) found that temperamental characteristics, including negative mood, difficulty adapting to new situations, and withdrawal, were related to higher pain sensitivity to immunization in kindergarten children. In a follow-up study, this "pain sensitive" temperament predicted children's health-care usage 7 years after the original assessment (Rocha et al. 2007). Several other studies have supported the role of children's temperament in their responses to lumbar punctures (Chen et al. 2000) and postoperative pain (Kleiber et al. 2007). It is notable that although this work has identified temperamental types that appear to be "pain sensitive," it is currently unknown whether these temperament types are reflective of a selective sensitivity to pain or an overall sensitivity to stimulation.

In terms of chronic pain, we are aware of only one study that has closely examined temperament in children and adolescents with these conditions. Conte and colleagues (2003) compared temperament in children with juvenile primary fibromyalgia syndrome (JPFS), arthritis, and no pain condition. Findings indicated that children with JPFS had significantly more temperamental instability than children with arthritis and those without pain. Although further research in temperamental influences on children's chronic pain is required, it appears that temperamental characteristics that are related to acute pain sensitivity may also be related to adolescents' chronic pain.

Coping

There is little question that living with a chronic pain condition is stressful for adolescents. Over time, adolescents develop patterns of thoughts, behaviors, and emotions that they use to cope with this stress, and a great deal of literature has been devoted to the study of these coping strategies. Coping has been defined as any "conscious volitional efforts to regulate emotion, cognition, behavior, physiology, and the environment in response to stressful events or circumstances"

(Compas et al. 2001, pp. 88). Coping strategies are acquired over time in a developmental process that is affected by cognitive and social maturation and experience interacting with the environment (Fields and Prinz 1997). By adolescence, coping styles begin to stabilize, and may continue regardless of their degree of effectiveness (Compas et al. 2001).

A wide variety of cognitive and behavioral coping strategies have been identified. Cognitive strategies include distraction, wishful thinking, problem solving, and negative thinking, while behavioral strategies include decreasing physical and social activity, seeking emotional support, and information-seeking. Although a thorough review of the coping literature is beyond the scope of this chapter, it is important to note that authors have offered a host of theoretical conceptualizations of coping behavior. Lazarus and Folkman's (1984) emotion- versus problem-focused conceptualization classifies strategies based on whether they function to modify the environment (problem-focused) or the self (emotion-focused). Other authors conceptualize coping on an approach-avoidance dimension (Roth and Cohen 1986), with approach strategies directed toward the stressful stimulus (e.g., problem solving) and avoidance strategies directed away from the stimulus (e.g., distraction). Although many conceptualizations are two-factor in nature, three-factor models have also been presented. In a study of pain-specific coping based in the approach/avoidance conceptualization, Reid and colleagues (1998) identified two subtypes of avoidant coping: problem-focused avoidance and emotion-focused avoidance. Emotion-focused avoidance strategies are those that attempt to avoid potentially negative feelings (e.g., internalizing, catastrophizing) whereas problem-focused avoidant strategies attempt to direct attention away from the stressful stimulus (e.g., distraction, positive self-talk).

Despite a wide array of conceptualizations, there is consistent evidence that some coping strategies are more adaptive than others in particular situations. For example, problem-focused or approach coping is most adaptive in situations where individuals have control over situations, whereas emotion-focused coping strategies are most adaptive in uncontrollable situations (Compas et al. 2001). In the context of pain, Reid and colleagues (1998) report that approach strategies (e.g., information seeking, problem solving) were related to decreased disability in children with rheumatoid arthritis, whereas emotion-focused avoidance strategies such as externalizing (e.g., yelling at others) were related to higher pain. Although approach strategies have received support for their efficacy, some authors argue that the uncontrollable nature of chronic pain lends itself more appropriately to the use of emotion-focused strategies (McCracken et al. 2007). In this framework, attempting to control an uncontrollable situation (i.e., pain) may be counterproductive. Alternatively, acceptance-based coping strategies focus on function in the presence of pain rather than attempts to eliminate pain (McCracken et al. 2007).

A particularly strong finding in the coping literature is the maladaptive nature of catastrophizing coping strategies. Catastrophizing coping involves exaggerated negative responses to actual or expected stress (Drahovzal et al. 2006) and was categorized by Reid and colleagues (1998) as an emotion-focused avoidance strategy. In cases of high catastrophizing, individuals expect future pain episodes and their consequences to be extremely severe (Sullivan et al. 2001) and thus experience increased distress and sensitivity to pain (Eccleston and Crombez 1999). Catastrophic thinking has been found to be related to increased pain intensity, increased disability, and lower pain tolerance (Vowles et al. 2007).

Trauma History

Experience with trauma in childhood has been associated with a variety of negative outcomes. In addition to an array of psychological effects, experience with early traumatic events has been associated with increased physical complaints. In a population based study, Chartier and colleagues (2007) found that a history of abuse was related to increased health-care usage, poorer self-reported health, more diagnosed health conditions, and pain that interfered with activity.

Of traumatic events in childhood, experience with abuse has received the most extensive study in chronic pain populations. Definitions of abuse vary based on assessment methods, but for the purposes of this section we will use those provided by Goldberg and colleagues (1999). These authors define physical abuse as physical acts of punishment that leave physical evidence (i.e., bruises and welts) and that are perpetrated by an adult in a position of authority on a child under the age of 18. Sexual abuse is defined as any sexual act performed by an adult on a child under the age of 18 (Goldberg et al. 1999). Verbal abuse is defined as "any pattern of consistent denigration, humiliation, and condemnation performed by a more powerful individual to a person under the age of 18 resulting in feelings of inferiority, lowered self-esteem, lowered self-worth, and stunted goals and ambitions."

Most of the data on links between childhood abuse and traumatic experience have been in adults and most have used retrospective reports of history of trauma in patients with chronic pain. For example, Balousek et al. (2007) examined self-reported history of abuse in a large sample ($n = 1,009$) of adults who were prescribed opioids to manage noncancer-related chronic pain. Prevalence of lifetime history of physical abuse was 47% for women and 22% of men. A similar gender distribution of history of sexual abuse was reported, with 35% of women and 10% of men reporting abuse. Comparisons trauma histories in community samples of individuals with and without chronic pain support the assertion that experience with abuse is a risk factor for chronic pain (Brown et al. 2005). There also appears to be variability across chronic pain conditions in trauma history. Goldberg et al. (1999) investigated the abuse and/or traumatic event history of 91 patients with four chronic pain conditions: facial pain, myofascial pain, fibromyalgia, and other pain. Of these 91 participants, there was a significant history of childhood verbal abuse (38%), physical abuse (>32%), and sexual abuse (22%) in the development of a chronic pain condition. Interestingly, the four pain groups were varyingly impacted by these different events. Of those participants with fibromyalgia, 25–47% experienced sexual abuse as a child.

Traumatic events other than abuse in childhood may also contribute to the development of chronic pain. Traumatic events within the family may include familial violence, parental alcoholism, parental drug abuse, divorce, or death. Goldberg and colleagues reported that more than 38% of their sample of adults with chronic pain had a family history of alcohol abuse and 15.3% had a family history of drug abuse. A family history of alcohol abuse was found to be most significant among participants with myofascial and facial pain.

Unfortunately, despite the preponderance of evidence for abuse and trauma history as a risk factor for chronic pain in adults, little is known about traumatic histories in adolescents with pain. Of the host of studies that have evaluated psychological and social correlates of pain in adolescents, to our knowledge, no study has evaluated trauma and abuse history. This appears to be the same case in the trauma literature, as studies of childhood and adolescent outcomes of trauma do not generally assess for chronic pain. However, the trauma literature does refer to chronic pain as "the next frontier" (Kendall-Tackett and Kendall-Tackett 2001).

Social Influences

Parental Influences

There is little question that chronic pain in adolescents occurs within a family context and thus is both influenced by and serves as an influence on the family system. In fact, the family context is so important in chronic pain that some authors have argued that effective interventions must be directed toward both the adolescent and the family (Kazak et al. 2002).

The most general evidence for parental influences on children's pain is in the form of family aggregation of pain. Early studies support the hypothesis that pain aggregates in families by demonstrating higher percentages of reports of pain in family members of chronic pain patients than in patients with non-chronic pain-related medical conditions (Violon and Giurgea 1984). In terms of the parent–child dyad, studies have shown that pain complaints are more likely in children of parents who also report pain (Levy et al. 2004; Mikail and von Baeyer 1990). Parents' and children's ratings of their own pain are also significantly correlated, as are the number of chronic pain conditions in the family and children's ratings of their current pain (Schanberg et al. 2001).

One potential mechanism for the clustering of pain in families is parental modeling of pain behavior. Children of parents with pain are more likely to have pain than children with parents who do not have pain, and children appear to be particularly influenced by mothers with pain (Evans and Keenan 2007). Children of parents with pain also tend to report similar pain sites as their parent (Osborne et al. 1989; Evans and Keenan 2007). Evidence from laboratory-based studies supports the importance of modeling in children's response to pain. Goodman and McGrath (1991) found that children of mothers who exaggerated their response during an experimental pain task later showed significantly lower pain thresholds during the same task than children whose mothers minimized their pain response. In other words, children's pain thresholds were influenced by the way their mothers reacted to the same circumstances.

Children learn not just from their parents' responses to pain, but also from the consequences of their parent's pain. Walker and colleagues found that children with RAP and peptic disease who had family members with *frequent illness* believed that they, such as their ill relatives, would receive sympathy and fewer responsibilities as a result of chronic pain (Walker et al. 1993).

A second potential mechanism for parents' impacts on adolescent's chronic pain is via family relationships, or interaction patterns among parents and adolescents with pain. Parents of children with pain have been found to be more anxious than parents of children without pain (Ramchandani et al. 2006), and parents' anxiety about their children's pain influences the way in which parents interact with their children (van Tilburg et al. 2006). For example, in an attempt to protect the adolescent in pain, parents may allow children to escape from chores, limit family activities, or keep children home from school (Lipani et al. 2006). Parents may also provide additional attention, reassurance, or special privileges in an attempt to soothe adolescents when in pain. Although well-intentioned, these responses serve to reinforce pain behaviors in children and can lead to increased disability (Walker et al. 1993; Peterson and Palermo 2004).

In terms of adaptive responses, there are several parent behaviors that are related to decreased disability and pain. Sanders and colleagues (1996) found that particular parent behaviors were a significant predictor of improvement in children's recurrent abdominal pain. Specifically, mothers' use of adaptive caregiving strategies (e.g., encouraging active coping, ignoring pain complaints) was found to be a significant predictor of children's pain improvements. Supporting the importance of parental behaviors, this study found that the effect of maternal caregiving was still evident after controlling for child age and child-coping behaviors.

School Influences

Adolescents spend a significant amount of their time in school and school-related activities. Unfortunately, pain often interferes with school and is related to increased school absences, missed schoolwork, and lost opportunities for social interactions. In fact, chronic and recurrent pain accounts for more absences than any other chronic illness (Palermo 2000).

An adolescent's chronic pain condition can be impacted, in part, by their academic performance, perceived social support, and responses from teachers and peers. Generally, teachers may have difficulty understanding and knowing how to react to their students with chronic pain. Unlike physical disabilities or other chronic conditions with clear explanations, teachers may find it difficult to differentiate between acceptable and unacceptable behavior in children with chronic pain. A child's academic performance and functioning can be directly affected by the way in which a teacher responds to the child (Logan et al. 2007). For example, if the teacher often allows a child to skip assignments or does not require the child's participation, the child will likely be less motivated to perform well.

Peer Influences

Just as teachers' perceptions and reactions to children with chronic pain impact the child, so too do the perceptions and reactions of peers. Nishina and colleagues (2005) suggest the possibility that peers view children with chronic pain as "sickly, timid, or weakly," especially if the child is male (Midence et al. 1993; Nishina and Juvonen 2005). The authors further suggest that these perceptions may lead to bullying. In addition to appearing sick or weak, children's frequent school absences result in fewer opportunities for social interactions with peers. Greco and colleagues (2007) found that the poor social skills of a child with chronic pain increase the likelihood that he or she will experience problems with his or her peers. These social problems were found to increase the anxiety of these children which, in turn, can lead to exacerbated pain episodes and further perpetuate the cycle.

Considerations in Treatment

The biopsychosocial model has important implications for the treatment of chronic pain in adolescents. This model highlights the importance of targeting multiple determinants of adolescents' pain, namely those that are biological, psychological, and social in nature. A general introduction to psychological interventions is provided below, followed by a review of efficacy data on these interventions and a discussion of intervention delivery considerations.

Overview of Psychological Interventions

There is a range of psychological treatments available for chronic pain in adolescents. While there is some variability in the specific procedures, most interventions that have received empirical attention are cognitive and/or behavioral in nature and many involve family components. Although a thorough presentation of the nuances of cognitive, behavioral, cognitive–behavioral, and family systems orientations are beyond the scope of this chapter, general discussions of these concepts are helpful in understanding the components of interventions that have been evaluated for adolescent chronic pain.

In general, cognitive interventions are directed toward identifying and modifying maladaptive thoughts, beliefs, or expectations. In the context of chronic pain, cognitive treatments are based on evidence that certain patterns of cognitions (e.g., catastrophizing) are associated with increased pain, as discussed earlier in this chapter. In this vein, cognitive interventions help adolescents to identify links between thoughts and pain and to generate alternative thought patterns. Specific strategies to accomplish these goals include self-monitoring to identify maladaptive thoughts, evaluating and challenging negative cognitions, thought-stopping, and positive self-talk (Hicks et al. 2006; Robins et al. 2005). Cognitive pain control strategies are also available. Imagery, distraction, and hypnosis, all work via cognitive mechanisms to focus attentional resources away from pain. The use of interactive technology for distraction in pain management is gaining recognition. Videogames, virtual reality (VR) with and without display helmets and augmented reality (AR) have affected pain threshold and pain tolerance (Dahlquist et al. 2008; Mott et al. 2008). While the predominance of pediatric VR pain literature addresses acute, procedural pain (e.g., intravenous placement, burn dressing changes), there are some case reports of efficacy in chronic pain. Immersive virtual reality as a treatment for phantom limb pain resulted in decreased phantom pain during at least one session (Murray et al. 2007). Oneal reported on a 6-month trial of VR consisting of 33 sessions for a patient with neuropathic pain previously unresponsive to pharmacological therapy. Pain intensity decreased by one-third and lasted approximately 12 h after completion of a session (Oneal et al. 2008). Cognitive strategies have added benefits of inducing positive emotions that, according to GTC, can activate descending inhibitory pain control pathways (Melzack and Wall 1965). These findings are further supported by fMRI which has shown modulation in pain-related regions of the brain in response to cognitive interventions (Hoffman et al. 2004).

In concert with cognitive interventions, behavioral strategies are generally directed toward identifying and modifying antecedents (i.e., triggers) of pain and consequences that maintain pain and disability. In terms of antecedents, behavioral strategies such as relaxation and biofeedback target muscle tension as a potential trigger of pain. Relaxation strategies such as progressive muscle relaxation have a long history of effective use in the treatment of anxiety and have been applied to the treatment of chronic pain. Biofeedback is a mechanism by which relaxation can be taught and has the added advantage of providing adolescents with objective feedback about relaxation levels via physiological measures (e.g., EMG, galvanic skin response, finger temperature).

Activity pacing is another behavioral technique that targets common triggers of pain in adolescents: overexertion or avoidance of activity. Fear of pain and subsequent avoidance of activity is common in adult chronic pain populations (Bousema et al. 2007) and recent evidence suggests that activity limitations are also common in adolescents (Long et al. 2008). Alternatively, overexertion can also be related to pain. To address both over- and under-exertion, activity-pacing interventions teach adolescents how to set attainable goals and plan steps to attain these goals within moderate activity levels.

Other behavioral strategies address social contributors to children's pain by targeting interventions toward individuals who interact with adolescents, rather than adolescents themselves. In most cases, these other individuals are family members and are usually parents. As discussed previously, family systems frameworks recognize that children's pain occurs within a complex system of interactions; thus, behavioral interventions target the way in which family members interact with adolescents in pain. In older treatments, parents were trained as administrators of simple operant interventions such as time-out for pain behavior (Miller and Kratochwill 1979). More recently, simple operant procedures have been replaced with more complex conceptualizations of parental influences on pain that highlight the pattern of interactions between parents and adolescents with pain. Interventions based on this conceptualization target the ways by which families respond to both pain and well behavior in their adolescents. For example, parental roles in the management of adolescent pain are reframed from that of protector to that of coach (Robins et al. 2005). Under this conceptualization, parents are taught to coach their children in the use of coping skills rather than attending to pain behavior. Parents are taught to encourage coping by reinforcing well behaviors (e.g., school attendance, practicing coping skills) with attention or praise, and to minimize attention to pain behaviors. Minimizing attention to pain behavior requires parents to refrain from asking questions about pain and to refrain from "protecting" their adolescent by allowing escape from chores, school, or other activities.

Efficacy of Psychological Interventions

Evidence for the efficacy of psychological interventions in the treatment of adolescent chronic pain is accumulating. Indeed, the state of the science has warranted at least two meta-analyses (Hermann et al. 1995; Eccleston et al. 2002) and a series of review articles (Janicke et al. 1999; Chen et al. 2004). Most psychological treatment studies of pain in adolescents have used combinations of cognitive and behavioral techniques, typically referred to as cognitive behavioral therapy (CBT). The exact components sometimes vary, but CBT generally involves a combination of behavioral coping skills training (e.g., relaxation, activity pacing) and cognitive strategies (e.g., identifying and modifying maladaptive cognitions). Family interventions are often included as an additional component of CBT. Although the majority of studies evaluating psychological interventions for pain have been multicomponent CBT interventions, there have been a few studies that have evaluated behavioral interventions alone (e.g., biofeedback, relaxation).

In general, evidence suggests that psychological interventions are effective in the management of chronic pain in adolescents and are not associated with adverse outcomes (McGrath and Holahan 2003; Sanders et al. 1994). The strength of evidence for the efficacy of interventions differs across pain conditions, however. Thus, studies evaluating efficacy of psychological interventions are discussed below by pain condition.

Headache

The majority of evidence for the efficacy of psychological interventions has been in the treatment of pediatric headache. In a systematic review of randomized controlled trial (RCT) of psychological interventions for chronic pain, Eccleston and colleagues (2002) identified 18 trials meeting RCT criteria, 15 of which were in pediatric headache. Another meta-analysis specific to pediatric headache included 23 studies that met RCT criteria (Trautmann et al. 2006). Interventions evaluated in studies in pediatric headache range from single-component interventions such as relaxation (McGrath et al. 1988) and biofeedback (Scharff et al. 2002) to multicomponent CBT interventions (Barry et al 1997). Results of both meta-analyses indicate that psychological interventions are effective in the management of pediatric headache. Eccleston and colleagues report a number needed to treat (NNT) for a 50% reduction in pain as 2.32 across interventions and Trautman et al. (2006) report medium effect sizes from pretreatment to posttreatment for psychological interventions.

In terms of efficacies of specific interventions, Holden and colleagues conducted a systematic review to evaluate the level of evidence of psychological treatments for pediatric recurrent headaches based on criteria established by Chambless and Hollon (1998). Briefly, these criteria were used categorize interventions into "well-established" (i.e., at least two well-designed between-groups experiments conducted by at least two separate research groups demonstrating clinical superiority to psychological placebo or alternative treatments), "probably efficacious" (i.e., two experiments showing treatment is more efficacious than wait-list control or one or more studies meeting well-established criteria but conducted by one research group), or "promising" (i.e., two or more well-controlled studies with small numbers or by the same investigator). Results of this review indicated that relaxation

therapies (relaxation training, self-hypnosis, guided imagery) qualified as well-established treatments for headache and thermal biofeedback alone was judged to be a probably efficacious treatment. However, conclusions regarding the relative efficacy of these two interventions are limited by methodological concerns. One study comparing the two indicated that relaxation and biofeedback were equally effective when compared to wait-list control (Fentress et al. 1986), while another demonstrated that autogenic training was superior to biofeedback (Labbe 1995). At the time of this review, CBT was classified as a promising intervention; however, this review was based on data available in 1999 and several well-designed studies evaluating CBT for headache have demonstrated efficacy since its publication.

Recurrent Abdominal Pain

Although not as well-studied as in treatment for headache, psychological interventions for recurrent abdominal pain (RAP) have also been evaluated. Although some early reports of case studies using operant methods were reported (Miller and Kratochwill 1979), the majority of interventions for RAP have been CBT. The systematic reviews by Eccleston et al. (2002) and Janicke and Finney (ref) identified two RAP trials, both evaluating CBT (Sanders et al. 1989,1994). In the first of these studies (Sanders et al. 1989), CBT including parent training in behavioral contingency management and child training in relaxation and cognitive strategies was compared to a wait-list control. Results indicated improvement in RAP symptoms in both groups, but a quicker improvement and a higher proportion of children who were pain-free in the CBT condition. A second study by these authors compared a similar intervention to standard pediatric care and showed significantly less pain relapse in children who received CBT. On the basis of the same Chambless recommendations used by Holden (Holden et al. 1999), Janicke and Finney (Janicke et al. 1999) judged CBT to be a "probably efficacious treatment."

Since the publication of Janicke and Finney and Eccelston and colleagues, two additional studies have been published evaluating CBT in children with RAP. One study compared CBT plus standard medical care to medical care alone (Robins et al. 2005). Results of this study indicated that children who participated in CBT had significantly less pain than those who received standard medical care alone immediately following treatment and at 1-year follow-up. Children in the CBT group also had significantly fewer school absences than children in the standard medical care group. The second study used the Internet to deliver CBT to children with RAP (Hicks et al. 2006). In an attempt to address issues with access to service, these authors developed a Web-based intervention that taught relaxation, cognitive strategies, and activity pacing, and included a relapse prevention component. Results of this study showed that significantly more children who received the intervention achieved clinically significant pain reductions than children who received standard medical care. Differences between Internet CBT and standard care groups were maintained at a 3-month follow-up. On the basis of these two additional studies, it is likely that a reexamination of evidence for CBT in the treatment of RAP would now classify this intervention as "well-established."

Disease-related pain

Psychological treatments have also been evaluated for the treatment of disease-related pain, but the data in these conditions are far less developed than in headache or RAP (Walco et al. 1999). Data on rheumatologic conditions include two small-scale trials for Juvenile Rheumatoid Arthritis (JRA) and one RCT in Juvenile Primary Fibromyalgia Syndrome (JPFS). Lavigne et al. (1992) evaluated a treatment combining relaxation, biofeedback, and parent training in contingency management for JRA. A second study in JRA by Walco et al. (1992) evaluated an intervention combining relaxation and cognitive pain control strategies (e.g., imagery, meditation) combined with parent training. Both of these studies showed efficacy of intervention from pretreatment to posttreatment, but very small sample sizes, lack of control groups, and high dropout preclude conclusions on the efficacy of CBT based on these studies. Kashikar-Zuck et al. (2005) compared children with JPFS who were

randomly assigned CBT to those who were randomly assigned to self-monitoring. Results of this study were mixed; children in both groups improved on depressive symptoms and functional measures from pretreatment to posttreatment, although children who received CBT reported significantly greater efficacy in coping with pain. There was also a trend toward children in the CBT group reporting less pain intensity than children in the self-monitoring group. It is notable that both groups in this study received an intervention that was different from standard medical care and thus it is not possible to draw conclusions about how these treatments compare to standard care. In sum, data on psychological interventions in the management of rheumatologic conditions are promising, but definitive conclusions on effectiveness of these interventions are premature.

Psychological interventions for SCD–related pain have also received empirical attention (Chen et al. 2004). In one study, Gil et al. (.Gil et al. 2001) compared a CBT intervention (relaxation, pleasant imagery, calming self-talk) to a standard care control. Results showed no difference between groups on pain and health-care usage, but children in the CBT group evidenced significantly more active coping. The authors followed-up these results and found that use of coping strategies, rather than simple group assignment, was related to pain outcomes; on the day in which children used coping strategies, they reported less pain and higher function. Several other studies of psychological interventions for SCD of differing levels of methodological rigor are available (Powers et al. 2002; Kaslow et al. 1997), but many of these interventions target outcomes in addition to pain (e.g., adherence, disease knowledge), complicating conclusions on pain management efficacy. Furthermore, some authors have argued that traditional CBT interventions may require culturally informed modifications (e.g., use of African American therapists, focus on family) to reach maximal effectiveness (Kaslow et al. 1997). Overall, however, Chen and colleagues conclude that CBT was a probably efficacious treatment based on the Chambless criteria.

Complex Regional Pain Syndrome

The role of psychological interventions in the management of CRPS is the least developed. To our knowledge, no well-controlled randomized studies have evaluated psychological interventions alone for CRPS in adolescents. Instead, evidence for the efficacy of these interventions for CRPS must be extrapolated from studies treating multiple pain conditions. For example, Eccleston and colleagues (Eccleston et al. 2003) report on the efficacy of an interdisciplinary treatment, including CBT, targeting functional gains for children with various chronic pain conditions (approximately one quarter of participants were diagnosed with CRPS). Results of this intensive residential treatment were promising, with significant improvements from pretreatment to posttreatment in measures of disability and mood. Especially notable in this study was that the CBT treatment was offered in the context of an interdisciplinary treatment in which adolescents participated in daily physical and occupational therapy. This type of treatment is in line with current recommendations for the treatment of CRPS, which stress the importance of immediate physical therapy with pharmacological and psychological interventions added in treatment refractory cases (Connelly and Schanberg 2006).

Considerations in Delivery of Psychological Interventions

Despite the mounting evidence for the efficacy of psychological and multidisciplinary treatments for pain in adolescents, there are challenges in delivering these treatments. One important consideration is how many children can be reached by an intervention. Traditional methods of delivering care require a great deal of time and resources on the part of the family. Travel to clinics for weekly appointments and the costs associated with missed work or school can serve as significant barriers to receiving treatment (Elgar and McGrath 2003). Families from low income or rural areas are at particular risk, given that they typically have access to fewer services than families in urban areas (Hunsley et al. 1997).

Advances in technology have provided unique opportunities to deliver care to adolescents who would not otherwise have access to psychological interventions. Although research on these delivery systems is still in its infancy, early work suggests that Web-based and CD-ROM administration may be effective and are not associated with more adverse effects than traditional in-person contact. For example, Connelly et al. (2006) found that a cognitive–behavioral intervention for pediatric headache delivered via CD-ROM intervention resulted in significant improvements in headache frequency, duration, and intensity when compared to standard medical care. These treatment gains were maintained at 2 and 3-month follow-up assessments. In a study of cognitive–behavioral treatment for recurrent abdominal pain delivered via the Internet, Hicks et al. (2006) found that 71% of children receiving this treatment had clinically significant improvements in their pain at 2 months, compared to only 14% of children treated with standard medical care. Taken together, early evidence for the efficacy of alternative delivery systems for cognitive–behavioral interventions appears promising, but requires further validation. Studies to date in this area have used only medical care as control conditions and have yet to compare alternative delivery systems to traditional in-person interventions.

Other studies have attempted to increase accessibility of cognitive–behavioral interventions by delivering these interventions in school settings. The most comprehensive series of studies in school settings has been conducted by Larsson and colleagues (2005, 1987). In an analysis of all adolescents treated in this series of studies, Larsson et al. (2005) concluded that school-based training in relaxation was effective in the management of tension-type headache, and to a slightly lower extent, migraine headache. These authors also examined the background of the individual providing relaxation training in schools. Results indicated that relaxation training delivered by a therapist was more effective than either self-management or relaxation training delivered by a school nurse.

The use of paraprofessionals is another means of reducing costs associated with delivering psychological interventions. Although school nurses were not as effective in delivering relaxation training as therapists in Larsson's studies, there are data to suggest that paraprofessionals can be trained to deliver some pain management interventions. Master's level paraprofessionals have been shown to be effective in the delivery of biofeedback interventions to children with headaches in primary care (Allen et al. 2002).

A final consideration in the delivery of psychological interventions for adolescents with chronic pain is the maintenance of treatment gains. Some of the studies evaluating interventions have used follow-up assessments to document the continued efficacy of their treatments, but only a few studies explicitly targeted maintenance of gain. Carson et al. (2006) evaluated the effect of adding maintenance training to traditional cognitive–behavioral interventions for rheumatoid arthritis. Maintenance training included cognitive strategies for coping with relapse, behavioral rehearsal to generalize treatment gains, and operant methods to reinforce continued use of coping skills. Contrary to hypotheses, outcomes of traditional cognitive–behavioral therapy were not significantly improved by the addition of maintenance training. High dropout rates in groups that showed initial treatment gains limited the interpretation of findings but raised an interesting question: are adolescents who improve quickly also likely to lose these gains quickly? Further research on the most effective ways to maintain treatment gains continues to be important.

In sum, the biopsychosocial model is an important framework in the treatment of chronic pain in adolescents. The recognition of psychological and social influences on pain has led to more comprehensive treatment strategies including cognitive and behavioral components. Currently, there is mounting evidence for the efficacy of psychological interventions in the treatment of chronic pain, especially in headache and recurrent abdominal pain. It is clear, however, that interdisciplinary strategies are the future of pain management and will lead to the largest treatment gains. Consideration of not only the "what" but also the "how" of delivering interventions will also continue to

be important. Alternative delivery systems, including interventions delivered via computer or paraprofessionals, hold promise in increasing accessibility to comprehensive pain management services.

References

Aasland, A., Flato, B., et al. (1997). Psychosocial outcome in juvenile chronic arthritis: A nine-year follow-up. *Clinical and Experimental Rheumatology, 15*(5), 561–568 [Journal Article. Research Support, Non-U.S. Gov't].

Allen, K. D., Elliott, A. J., et al. (2002). Behavioral pain management for pediatric headache in primary care. *Children's Health Care, 31*(3), 175–189.

Balousek, S., Plane, M. B., et al. (2007). Prevalence of interpersonal abuse in primary care patients prescribed opioids for chronic pain. *Journal of General Internal Medicine, 22*(9), 1268–1273.

Banks, S. M., & Kerns, R. D. (1996). Explaining high rates of depression in chronic pain: A diathesis stress framework. *Psychological Bulletin, 119*, 95–110.

Barry, J., von Baeyer, C. L., et al. (1997). Brief cognitive-behavioral group treatment for children's headache. *The Clinical Journal of Pain, 13*(3), 215–220.

Bousema, E. J., Verbunt, J. A., et al. (2007). Disuse and physical deconditioning in the first year after the onset of back pain. *Pain, 130*(3), 279–286.

Boyer, M., Compas, B., et al. (2006). Attentional biases to pain and social threat in children with recurrent abdominal pain. *Journal of Pediatric Psychology, 39*, 209–220.

Broome, M. E., Rehwaldt, M., et al. (1998). Relationships between cognitive behavioral techniques, temperament, observed distress, and pain reports in children and adolescents during lumbar puncture. *Journal of Pediatric Nursing, 13*(1), 48–54.

Brown, J., Berenson, K., et al. (2005). Documented and self-reported child abuse and adult pain in a community sample. *The Clinical Journal of Pain, 21*(5), 374–377.

Bruni, O., Fabrizi, P., et al. (1997). Prevalence of sleep disorders in childhood and adolescence with headache: A case-control study. (0333-1024).

Bucolo, M. J. S., Cuttle, L., Mill, J., Hilder, M., Miller, K., & Kimble, R. M. (2008). The efficacy of an augmented virtual reality system to alleviate pain in children undergoing burns dressing changes: A randomised controlled trial. *Burns, 34*(6), 803–808.

Campo, J. V., Bridge, J., et al. (2004). Recurrent abdominal pain, anxiety, and depression in primary care. *Pediatrics, 113*(4), 817–824.

Carson, J. W., Keefe, F. J., et al. (2006). A comparison of conventional pain coping skills training and pain coping skills training with a maintenance training component: A daily diary analysis of short- and long-term treatment effects. *The Journal of Pain, 7*(9), 615–625.

Carver, C. S., & Scheier, M. F. (2000). *Perspectives on personality* (4th ed.). Boston: Allyn and Bacon.

Chambless, D. L., & Hollon, S. D. (1998). Defining empirically supported therapies. *Journal of Consulting and Clinical Psychology, 66*, 7–18.

Chartier, M. J., Walker, J. R., et al. (2007). Childhood abuse, adult health, and health care utilization: Results from a representative community sample. *American Journal of Epidemiology, 165*(9), 1031–1038.

Chen, E., Craske, M. G., et al. (2000). Pain-sensitive temperament: Does it predict procedural distress and response to psychological treatment among children with cancer? *Journal of Pediatric Psychology, 25*(4), 269–278.

Chen, E., Cole, S. W., et al. (2004). A review of empirically supported psychosocial interventions for pain and adherence outcomes in sickle cell disease. *Journal of Pediatric Psychology, 29*(3), 197–209.

Compas, B. E., Connor-Smith, J. K., et al. (2001). Coping with stress during childhood and adolescence: Problems, progress, and potential in theory and research. [Review] [220 refs]. (0033-2909).

Connelly, M., & Schanberg, L. (2006). Latest developments in the assessment and management of chronic musculoskeletal pain syndromes in children. *Current Opinion in Rheumatology, 18*, 496–502.

Connelly, M., Rapoff, M. A., Thompson, N., & Connelly, W. (2006). Headstrong: A pilot study of a CDROM intervention for recurrent pediatric headache. *Journal of Pediatric Psychology, 31*, 737–747.

Conrad, R., Schilling, G., et al. (2007). Temperament and character personality profiles and personality disorders in chronic pain patients. *Pain, 133*(1–3), 197–209.

Conte, P. M., Walco, G. A., et al. (2003). Temperament and stress response in children with juvenile primary fibromyalgia syndrome. *Arthritis and Rheumatism, 48*(10), 2923–2930.

Crombez, G., Vlaeyen, J. W., Heuts, P. H., et al. (1999). Pain-related fear is more disabling than pain itself: Evidence on the role of pain-related fear in chronic back pain disability. *Pain, 80*, 329–339.

Dahlquist, L. M., Weiss, K., Clindaniel, L. D., et al. (2008). Effects of videogame distraction using a virtual reality type head-mounted display helmet on cold pressor pain in children. *Journal of Pediatric Psychology*. doi:10.1093/jpepsy/jsn023.

Drahovzal, D. N., Stewart, S. H., et al. (2006). Tendency to catastrophize somatic sensations: Pain catastrophizing and anxiety sensitivity in predicting headache. *Cognitive Behaviour Therapy, 35*(4), 226–235.

Eccleston, C., & Crombez, G. (1999). Pain demands attention: A cognitive-affective model of the interruptive function of pain. *Psychological Bulletin, 125*(3), 356–366.

Eccleston, C., Morley, S., et al. (2002). Systematic review of randomised controlled trials of psychological therapy for chronic pain in children and adolescents, with a subset meta-analysis of pain relief. *Pain, 99*(1–2), 157–165.

Eccleston, C., Malleson, P. N., Clinch, J., Connel, H., & Sourbut, C. (2003). Chronic pain in adolescents: Evaluation of a programme of interdisciplinary cognitive behaviour therapy. *Archives of Disease in childhood, 88*, 881–885.

Elgar, F. J., & McGrath, P. J. (2003). Self-administered psychosocial treatments for children and families. *Journal of Clinical Psychology, 59*(3), 321–339.

El-Metwally, A., Salminen, J. J., et al. (2004). Prognosis of non-specific musculoskeletal pain in preadolescents: A prospective 4-year follow-up study till adolescence. *Pain, 110*(3), 550–559.

Evans, S., & Keenan, T. R. (2007). Parents with chronic pain: are children equally affected by fathers as mothers in pain? A pilot study. *Journal of Child Health Care, 11*, 143–157 (1367–4935).

Fentress, D. W., Masek, B. J., et al. (1986). Biofeedback and relaxation training for pediatric headache disorders. *Developmental Medicine and Child Neurology, 28*, 139–146.

Fields, L., & Prinz, R. J. (1997). Coping and adjustment during childhood and adolescence. (0272-7358).

Fishbain, D. A., Cole, B., et al. (2006). Chronic pain and the measurement of personality: Do states influence traits? *Pain Medicine, 7*(6), 509–529 [see comment].

Flato, B., Aasland, A., et al. (1998). Outcome and predictive factors in juvenile rheumatoid arthritis and juvenile spondyloarthropathy. (0315-162X).

Fuggle, P., Shand, P. A., et al. (1996). Pain, quality of life, and coping in sickle cell disease. *Archives of Disease in Childhood, 75*(3), 199–203.

Gatchel, R. J., & Dersh, J. (2002). Psychological disorders and chronic pain: Are there cause-and-effect relationships. In D. C. Turk & R. J. Gatchel (Eds.), *Psychological approaches to pain management.* New York: Guilford.

Gil, K. M., Anthony, K. K., et al. (2001). Daily coping practice predicts treatment effects in children with sickle cell disease. *Journal of Pediatric Psychology, 26*(3), 163–173.

Goldberg, R. T., Pachas, W. N., et al. (1999). Relationship between traumatic events in childhood and chronic pain. *Disability and Rehabilitation, 21*(1), 23–30.

Goodman, J. E., & McGrath, P. J. (1991). The epidemiology of pain in children and adolescents: A review. *Pain, 46*(3), 247–264.

Greco, L. A., Freeman, K. E., et al. (2007). Overt and relational victimization among children with frequent abdominal pain: links to social skills, academic functioning, and health service use. (0146-8693): 20060713.

Haugland, S., Wold, B., et al. (2001). Subjective health complaints in adolescence. A cross-national comparison of prevalence and dimensionality. *European Journal of Public Health, 11*(1), 4–10.

Hermann, C., Kim, M., et al. (1995). Behavioral and prophylactic pharmacological intervention studies of pediatric migraine: An exploratory meta-analysis. *Pain, 60*(3), 239–255.

Hicks, C. L., von Baeyer, C. L., et al. (2006). Online psychological treatment for pediatric recurrent pain: A randomized evaluation. *Journal of Pediatric Psychology, 31*(7), 724–736.

Hoffman, H. G., Richards, T. L., Coda, B., Bills, A. R., Blough, D., Richards, A. L., & Sharar, S. R. (2004). Modulation of thermal pain-related brain activity with virtual reality: Evidence from fMRI. *NeuroReport, 15*(8), 1245–1248 [Clinical Trial. Journal Article. Randomized Controlled Trial. Research Support, Non-U.S. Gov't. Research Support, U.S. Gov't, P.H.S.].

Holden, E., Deichmann, M. M., et al. (1999). Empirically supported treatments in pediatric psychology: Recurrent pediatric headache. *Journal of Pediatric Psychology, 24*(2), 91–109.

Hunsley, J., Aubrey, T., et al. (1997). *A profile of Canadian consumers of psychological services*. Ottawa: Canadian Psychological Association.

Janicke, D. M., Finney, J. W., et al. (1999). Empirically supported treatments in pediatric psychology: Recurrent abdominal pain. *Journal of Pediatric Psychology, 24*(2), 115–127 [see comment].

Kashikar-Zuck, S., Swain, N. F., et al. (2005). Efficacy of cognitive-behavioral intervention for juvenile primary fibromyalgia syndrome. *The Journal of Rheumatology, 32*(8), 1594–1602.

Kaslow, N. J., Collins, M. H., et al. (1997). Empirically validated family interventions for pediatric psychology: Sickle cell disease as an exemplar. *Journal of Pediatric Psychology, 22*(2), 213–227.

Kazak, A. E., Simms, S., et al. (2002). Family systems practice in pediatric psychology. *Journal of Pediatric Psychology, 27*(2), 133–143.

Kendall-Tackett, K., & Kendall-Tackett, K. (2001). Chronic pain: The next frontier in child maltreatment research. *Child Abuse & Neglect, 25*(8), 997–1000 [see comment].

Kleiber, C., Suwanraj, M., et al. (2007). Pain-sensitive temperament and postoperative pain. *Journal for Specialists in Pediatric Nursing, 12*(3), 149–158.

Kristjansdottir, G. (1997). Prevalence of pain combinations and overall pain: A study of headache, stomach pain and back pain among school-children. (0300-8037).

Labbe, E. E. (1995). Treatment of childhood migraine with autogenic training and skin temperature biofeedback: A component analysis. *Developmental and Behavioral Pediatrics, 11*, 65–68.

Langeveld, J. H., Koot, H. M., et al. (1997). Headache intensity and quality of life in adolescents. How are changes in headache intensity in adolescents related to changes in experienced quality of life? *Headache, 37*(1), 37–42.

Larsson, B., Melin, L., et al. (1987). A school-based treatment of chronic headaches in adolescents. *Journal of Pediatric Psychology, 12*(4), 553–566.

Larsson, B., Carlsson, J., et al. (2005). Relaxation treatment of adolescent headache sufferers: Results from a school-based replication series. *Headache, 45*(6), 692–704.

Lavigne, J. V., Ross, C. K., et al. (1992). Evaluation of a psychological treatment package for treating pain in juvenile rheumatoid arthritis. *Arthritis Care and Research, 5*, 101–110.

Lazarus, R. S., & Folkman, S. (1984). *Stress, appraisal, and coping*. New York: Springer.

Levy, R. L., Whitehead, W. E., et al. (2004). Increasedw somatic complaints and health-care utilization in children: Effects of parent IBS status and parent response to gastrointestinal symptoms. *The American Journal of Gastroenterology, 99*(12), 2442–2451.

Lipani, T. A., Walker, L. S., et al. (2006). Children's appraisal and coping with pain: Relation to maternal ratings of worry and restriction in family activities. *Journal of Pediatric Psychology, 31*(7), 667–673.

Lipsitz, J. D., Masia, C., et al. (2005). Noncardiac chest pain and psychopathology in children and adolescents. *Journal of Psychosomatic Research, 59*(3), 185–188.

Logan, D. E., Coakley, R. M., et al. (2007). Teachers' perceptions of and responses to adolescents with chronic pain syndromes. (0146-8693): 20060412.

Long, A., Palermo, T. M., et al. (2008). Brief Report: Using actigraphy to compare physical activity levels in adolescents with chronic pain and healthy adolescents. *Journal of Pediatric Psychology, 33*(6), 660–665.

MacLaren, J. E., & Kain, Z. N. (2007). Perioperative biopsychosocial research: The future is here. (0952-8180).

Martin, A. L., McGrath, P. A., et al. (2007). Children with chronic pain: Impact of sex and age on long-term outcomes. *Pain, 128*(1–2), 13–19.

McCracken, L. M., Vowles, K. E., et al. (2007). A prospective investigation of acceptance and control-oriented coping with chronic pain. *Journal of Behavioral Medicine, 30*(4), 339–349.

McGrath, P. A., & Holahan, A. L. (2003). Psychological interventions with children and adolescents: Evidence for their effectiveness in treating chronic pain. *Seminars in Pain Medicine, 1*, 99–109.

McGrath, P., Humphreys, P., et al. (1988). Relaxation prophylaxis for childhood migraine: A randomized placebo-controlled trial. *Developmental Medicine and Child Neurology, 30*(5), 626–631.

McGrath, P. A., Speechley, K. N., et al. (2000). A survey of children's acute, recurrent, and chronic pain: Validation of the pain experience interview. *Pain, 87*(1), 59–73.

Melzack, R. (1999). From the gate to the neuromatrix. *Pain Supplement, 6*, S121–S126.

Melzack, R., & Wall, P. D. (1965). Pain mechanisms: A new theory. *Science, 150*(699), 971–979.

Melzack, R., & Casey, K. L. (1968). Sensory motivational and central control determinants of pain: A new conceptual model. In D. Kenshalo (Ed.), *The Skin Senses*, 423–443. Springfield IL: Thomas.

Midence, K., Fuggle, P., et al. (1993). Psychosocial aspects of sickle cell disease (SCD) in childhood and adolescence: A review. *The British Journal of Clinical Psychology, 32*(Pt 3), 271–280 [Review] [42 refs].

Mikail, S. F., & von Baeyer, C. L. (1990). Pain, somatic focus, and emotional adjustment in children of chronic headache sufferers and controls. *Social Science & Medicine, 31*(1), 51–59.

Miller, A. J., & Kratochwill, T. R. (1979). Reduction in frequent stomachache complaints by time out. *Behavior Therapy, 10*, 211–218.

Morsy, A. A. K. (2006). Prevalence of perceived pain and its impact on daily lives and activities of adolescents. *African Journal of Health Sciences, 13*, 18–28.

Muris, P., Meesters, C., et al. (2007). Personality and temperament correlates of pain catastrophizing in young adolescents. *Child Psychiatry and Human Development, 38*(3), 171–181.

Murray, C. D., Pettifer, S., Howard, T., Patchick, E. L., Caillette, F., Kulkarni, J., & Bamford, C. (2007). The treatment of phantom limb pain using immersive virtual reality: Three case studies. *Disability and Rehabilitation, 29*(18), 1465–1469.

Newacheck, P. W., & Taylor, W. R. (1992). Childhood chronic illness: Prevalence, severity, and impact. *American Journal of Public Health, 82*(3), 364–371.

Nishina, A., & Juvonen, J. (2005). Daily reports of witnessing and experiencing peer harassment in middle school. *Child Development, 76*(2), 435–450.

Norton, P. J., & Asmundson, G. J. (2004). Anxiety sensitivity, fear, and avoidance behavior in headache pain. *Pain, 111*(1–2), 218–223.

Oneal, B. J., Patterson, D. R., Soltani, M., Teeley, A., & Jensen, M. P. (2008). Virtual reality hypnosis in the treatment of chronic neuropathic pain: A case report. *The International Journal of Clinical and Experimental Hypnosis, 56*(4), 451–462.

Osborne, R. B., Hatcher, J. W., et al. (1989). The role of social modeling in unexplained pediatric pain. *Journal of Pediatric Psychology, 14*(1), 43–61.

Palermo, T. M. (2000). Impact of recurrent and chronic pain on child and family daily functioning: A critical review of the literature. *Journal of Developmental and Behavioral Pediatrics, 21*(1), 58–69.

Pells, J., Edwards, C. L., McDougald, C. S., Wood, M., Barksdale, C., Jonassaint, J., Leach-Beale, B., Byrd, G., Mathis, M., Harrison, M. O., Feliu, M., Edwards, L. Y., Whitfield, K. E., & Rogers, L. (2007). Fear of movement (kinesiophobia), pain, and psychopathology in patients with sickle cell disease. *The Clinical Journal of Pain, 23*(8), 707–713.

Perquin, C. W., Hazebroek-Kampschreur, A. A., et al. (2000). Pain in children and adolescents: A common experience. *Pain, 87*(1), 51–58.

Peterson, C. C., & Palermo, T. M. (2004). Parental reinforcement of recurrent pain: The moderating impact of child depression and anxiety on functional disability. *Journal of Pediatric Psychology, 29*(5), 331–341.

Powers, S. W., Mitchell, M. J., et al. (2002). Longitudinal assessment of pain, coping, and daily functioning in children with sickle cell disease receiving pain management skills training. *Journal of Clinical Psychology in Medical Settings, 9*(2), 109–119.

Ramchandani, P. G., Stein, A., et al. (2006). Early parental and child predictors of recurrent abdominal pain at school age: Results of a large population-based study. *Journal of the American Academy of Child and Adolescent Psychiatry, 45*(6), 729–736.

Reid, G. J., Gilbert, C. A., et al. (1998). The pain coping questionnaire: Preliminary validation. *Pain, 76*(1–2), 83–96.

Reiss, S., Peterson, R. A., et al. (1986). Anxiety sensitivity, anxiety frequency and the predictions of fearfulness. *Behaviour Research and Therapy, 24*(1), 1–8.

Robins, P. M., Smith, S. M., et al. (2005). A randomized controlled trial of a cognitive-behavioral family intervention for pediatric recurrent abdominal pain. *Journal of Pediatric Psychology, 30*(5), 397–408.

Rocha, E. M., Prkachin, K. M., et al. (2003). Pain reactivity and somatization in kindergarten-age children. *Journal of Pediatric Psychology, 28*(1), 47–57.

Rocha, E. M., Prkachin, K. M., et al. (2007). Temperament and pain reactivity predict health behavior seven years later. *Journal of Pediatric Psychology, 32*(4), 393–399.

Roelofs, J., Goubert, L., Peters, M. L., Vlaeyen, J. W., & Crombez, G. (2004). The Tampa Scale for Kinesiophobia: Further examination of psychometric properties in patients with chronic low back pain and fibromyalgia. *European Journal of Pain, 8*(5), 495–502.

Roth, S., & Cohen, L. J. (1986). Approach, avoidance, and coping with stress. *The American Psychologist, 41*, 813–819.

Sanders, M. R., Rebgetz, M., et al. (1989). Cognitive-behavioral treatment of recurrent nonspecific abdominal pain in children: An analysis of generalization, maintenance, and side effects. *Journal of Consulting and Clinical Psychology, 57*(2), 294–300.

Sanders, M. R., Shepherd, R. W., et al. (1994). The treatment of recurrent abdominal pain in children: A controlled comparison of cognitive-behavioral family intervention and standard pediatric care. *Journal of Consulting and Clinical Psychology, 62*(2), 306–314.

Sanders, M. R., Cleghorn, G., et al. (1996). Predictors of clinical improvement in children with recurrent abdominal pain. *Behavioural and Cognitive Psychotherapy, 24*(1), 27–38.

Schanberg, L. E., Anthony, K. K., et al. (2001). Family pain history predicts child health status in children with chronic rheumatic disease. *Pediatrics, 108*(3), E47.

Scharff, L., Marcus, D. A., et al. (2002). A controlled study of minimal-contact thermal biofeedback treatment in children with migraine. *Journal of Pediatric Psychology, 27*(2), 109–119.

Shapiro, B. S., Dinges, D. F., et al. (1995). Home management of sickle cell-related pain in children and adolescents: Natural history and impact on school attendance. *Pain, 61*(1), 139–144.

Stewart, S. H., Asmundson, G. J., et al. (2006). Anxiety sensitivity and its impact on pain experiences and conditions: A state of the art. *Cognitive Behaviour Therapy, 35*(4), 185–188.

Sullivan, M. J., Rodgers, W. M., et al. (2001). Catastrophizing, depression and expectancies for pain and emotional distress (0304-3959).

Trautmann, E., Lackschewitz, H., et al. (2006). Psychological treatment of recurrent headache in children and adolescents–a meta-analysis. *Cephalalgia, 26*(12), 1411–1426.

Tsao, J. C., Meldrum, M., et al. (2007). Anxiety sensitivity and health-related quality of life in children with chronic pain. *The Journal of Pain, 8*(10), 814–823.

Turk, D. C., & Monarch, E. S. (2002). Biopsychosocial perspective on chronic pain. In D. C. Turk & R. J. Gatchel (Eds.), *Psychological approaches to pain management*. New York: Guilford.

van Tilburg, M. A., Venepalli, N., et al. (2006). Parents' worries about recurrent abdominal pain in children. *Gastroenterology Nursing, 29*(1), 50–55. quiz 56–57.

Vancleef, L. M., Peters, M. L., Roelofs, J., & Asmundson, G. J. (2006). Do fundamental fears differentially contribute to pain-related fear and pain catastrophizing? An evaluation of the sensitivity index. *European Journal of Pain, 10*(6), 527–536.

Violon, A., & Giurgea, D. (1984). Familial models for chronic pain. *Pain, 18*(2), 199–203.

Viry, P., Creveuil, C., et al. (1999). Nonspecific back pain in children. A search for associated factors in 14-year-old schoolchildren. *Revue du Rhumatisme, 66*(7–9), 381–388. English Edition.

Vlaeyen, J. W., & Linton, S. J. (2000). Fear-avoidance and its consequences in chronic musculoskeletal pain: A state of the art. *Pain, 85*(3), 317–332.

Vowles, K. E., McCracken, L. M., et al. (2007). Processes of change in treatment for chronic pain: The contributions of pain, acceptance, and catastrophizing. *European Journal of Pain, 11*(7), 779–787.

Waddell, G., Newton, M., et al. (1993). A Fear-Avoidance Beliefs Questionnaire (FABQ) and the role of fear-avoidance beliefs in chronic low back pain and disability. *Pain, 52*(2), 157–168.

Walco, G. A., Varni, J. W., et al. (1992). Cognitive-behavioral pain management in children with juvenile rheumatoid arthritis. *Pediatrics, 89*(6 Pt 1), 1075–1079.

Walco, G. A., Sterling, C. M., et al. (1999). Empirically supported treatments in pediatric psychology: Disease-related pain. *Journal of Pediatric Psychology, 24*(2), 155–167. discussion 168–171.

Walker, L. S., Garber, J., et al. (1993). Psychosocial correlates of recurrent childhood pain: A comparison of pediatric patients with recurrent abdominal pain, organic illness, and psychiatric disorders. *Journal of Abnormal Psychology, 102*(2), 248–258.

Walker, L. S., Guite, J. W., et al. (1998). Recurrent abdominal pain: A potential precursor of irritable bowel syndrome in adolescents and young adults. *Journal of Pediatrics, 132*(6), 1010–1015.

Demographics of Chronic Pain in Children

Holly Denise Richter and Stephen Robert Hays

Keywords

Definition of chronic pain • Demographics of pediatric chronic pain • Maternal and paternal assessments of children's pain • Gender differences • Quality of life scores

Introduction

Much of what is thought to be known about chronic pain in the pediatric population has historically been extrapolated from the literature and experience in adults. Before the last several decades of the twentieth century, little research focused on pain and its management in children, and very little scientific effort addressed issues related to pediatric chronic pain. Even now, few studies describe the demographics of chronic pain in children. Investigations to date addressing incidence and prevalence, gender differences, age-dependent onset, regional findings, and other associations with chronic pain in the pediatric population exist largely in the literature of anesthesiology and various mental health disciplines, and are primarily observational in nature. Current science relating to the demographics of chronic pain in children is incomplete: a paucity of sound data continues, and much remains to be learned. (Howard 2003)

Integrative practice nonetheless demands an appreciation of demographics to the extent they are currently understood. Study of the distribution and characteristics of disease in a population enhances knowledge of how, and potentially why, disease occurs. Demographic data may assist in efforts to manage existing disease, and ideally to prevent disease in populations at risk. Particularly in the context of pediatric chronic pain, about which so much more remains to be learned, appreciation of what is currently known related to its demographics may be invaluable in identifying those children most likely affected.

Definitions

All pain is ultimately a subjective experience, and thus resistant to firm objective criteria or descriptions. A widely accepted definition of pain is that suggested by the International Association for the Study of Pain: "an unpleasant sensory and emotional experience associated with actual or potential tissue damage, or described in terms of such damage" (IASP Task Force on Taxonomy 1986). More succinctly, and relevant to pediatric patients who may be unable to verbalize their

H.D. Richter (✉)
Vanderbilt University Medical Center, 11205 W Sycamore Hills Dr Fort Wayne, IN 46814, Nashville, TN, USA 37232-9070
e-mail: holly.richter@vanderbilt.edu

B.C. McClain and S. Suresh (eds.), *Handbook of Pediatric Chronic Pain: Current Science and Integrative Practice*, DOI 10.1007/978-1-4419-0350-1_4, © Springer Science+Business Media, LLC 2011

pain experience in such terms, pain is anything children say hurts.

Definition of chronic pain is even more challenging, particularly in the pediatric population. Generally accepted timescales and frames of reference may have little meaning or relevance to children in pain, for whom chronicity may entail markedly different durations and perceptions than in adults. Nonetheless, a commonly accepted definition of chronic pain is that suggested by the International Association for the Study of Pain: "pain without apparent biological value that has persisted beyond the normal tissue healing time (usually taken to be 3 months)" (Harstall and Ospina 2003; IASP Task Force on Taxonomy 1986). Although determination of biologic value may represent a significant challenge, particularly in pediatric patients, persistent or recurrent pain lasting at least 3 months is widely accepted as a reasonable definition of chronic pain in patients of all ages including children.

For most purposes, pediatric patients are generally considered to be children less than age 18 years, although older patients with developmental delay or other significant cognitive or emotional disability may at times be appropriately considered from a pediatric perspective. Numerous specific medical diseases and diagnoses may be associated with chronic pain in children, demographics of which generally reflect those of the underlying condition. Many of these conditions are discussed in detail elsewhere, and this chapter largely explores the demographics of chronic pain in children as an independent syndrome.

Methodologic Considerations

Central to an understanding of the demographics of any disease is an understanding of the disease itself, and of the population at particular risk for developing the disease in question. Demographic data provide clues to elucidating relationships between risk factors and development of disease, and potentially between development of disease and response to therapy. In the context of ongoing and potentially debilitating disease such as chronic pain, socioeconomic impact upon patients, families, and communities may be substantial (Bursch et al. 1998), and also deserves careful consideration.

Many of the currently available demographic data on chronic pain in children derive from survey and questionnaire investigations, making objective interpretation and widespread extrapolation potentially problematic. Results from various studies are often contradictory, and the applicability of data from any one study to different patient populations or different geographic areas may be problematic. Moreover, validity and reproducibility of the survey and questionnaire tools used are frequently uncertain. Such tools are themselves frequently in need of rigorous scientific study, particularly in the pediatric population.

A comprehensive review of demographic data from studies of chronic pain in children (Goodman and McGrath 1991) explored methodologic considerations in the study of this particular disease in this particular population. Three primary areas of methodologic concern were identified: reliability and validity of pain measurement in pediatric patients; necessity but frequent absence of broad-based measurements of associated disability and chronicity of pain in children; and issues related to definition, composition, and relevance of individual study samples (Table 4.1).

Pain is a highly subjective experience varying greatly from one patient to the next and even in the same patient over time, encompassing both physical and psychological experience. Pain is thus notoriously difficult to measure objectively, and subjective patient self-report has historically been the mainstay of pain measurement. This may be particularly challenging in children, whose ability to understand and express their subjective experience may vary widely with age and developmental maturity (American Society for Pain Management Nursing: Herr et al. 2006; Stanford et al. 2006). Preschool-age children are especially likely to demonstrate a variety of response biases in evaluating their pain, even when using validated assessment tools (von Baeyer et al. 2009).

In the course of normal development, younger children tend to use a limited and fairly reproducible vocabulary in describing pain as early as toddlerhood, with emergence of more varied descriptors

Table 4.1 Methodologic concerns in tudying pediatric pain

Concern	Comments
Reliability and validity of pain measurement in pediatric patients	Effects of age, developmental maturity, parental influence, and socioeconomic status
Necessity but frequent absence of broad-based measurements of associated disability and chronicity of pain in children	Vitally important, difficult to measure, frequently not addressed, may represent greatest impact of chronic pain in children
Definition, composition, and relevance of individual study samples	Populations not always well-defined, other populations not always represented

Modified from Goodman and McGrath (1991)

including the word pain itself gradually, and frequently many years later (Stanford et al. 2005). Abnormal development poses additional challenges, as pain in children with autism and other developmental disorders may be further underappreciated and underreported (Nader et al. 2004). Differences in context and presentation of questionnaires given to pediatric patients and their families may account for some of the marked differences and contradictory results in the literature of chronic pain in children.

Numerous assessment tools are available for measurement of pain in children (Beyer, 1983; Hicks et al. 2001; McGrath et al. 1985; Merkel et al. 2002; Razmus and Wilson 2006), and are discussed in greater detail elsewhere. Accurate and valid assessment of pain in children requires selection of tools appropriate for patient age and developmental maturity, and at times relevant to underlying medical condition. Patient and caregiver reports of pain in children are not necessarily concordant, even with trained professionals using appropriate tools (Vetter and Heiner 1996).

Inconsistency and bias in studies of pediatric chronic pain may also result from discrepancies between patient and parental descriptions, and from parental influence on their children. Patients and their families do not always report similar pain scores, and do not necessarily even agree significant pain is present (Chambers et al. 1999; Chambers et al. 1998; Zuckerman et al. 1987). Maternal and paternal assessments of children's pain may also vary markedly, with complex gender interactions. Fathers often tend to report higher pain scores in daughters than in sons, but to be more accurate in their assessments; mothers often tend to rate pain similarly in daughters and

sons, but to be less accurate (Moon et al. 2008). Maternal behaviors may significantly influence reported pain scores in daughters but not in sons (Chambers et al. 2002); paternal influence on children seems to be somewhat less significant (Evans and Keenan 2007). In general, children are volitionally able to modify expression of their pain experience when asked to do so, but are better able to hide their pain than to fake its presence (Larochette et al. 2006).

Relatively few prospective data on chronic pain in children are available, although longitudinal studies have suggested associations of parental anxiety and child temperament with subsequent recurrent abdominal pain (Ramchandani et al. 2006), and of recurrent abdominal pain in childhood with enhanced somatization and greater pain associated disability in adulthood (Walker et al. 1995). Investigations of chronic pain in children to date have largely been retrospective, requiring patients and families accurately to remember and report past experience. Time frame studied may markedly affect data obtained. Data from studies of short duration may not be particularly useful or relevant to chronic pain, while data from studies involving prolonged or distant reporting may not be particularly reliable. Some prospective studies of chronic pain in children have employed diaries or other ongoing recording modalities to generate accurate long-term data, requiring considerable dedication and persistence on the part of patients and families. Interpretation of narratives generated is also labor-intensive for investigators (Meldrum et al. 2009).

Many studies report only presence of pain, without adequately or specifically addressing severity, frequency, or duration of pain experienced.

Additional difficulties may arise in interpreting studies attempting to measure pain at multiple sites or of multiple types, studies failing to address handicap and disability resulting from chronic pain, or studies neglecting to account for pain in friends or family of children with chronic pain (Goodman and McGrath 1991; Walker et al. 1991). Some studies have addressed school absenteeism, decreased social interaction, and other markers of functional impairment in children with chronic pain, but understanding of the overall disability and handicap resulting from chronic pain in children is still evolving (Hunfeld et al. 2001; Martin et al. 2007a; Mulvaney et al. 2006). In many historical studies addressing disability secondary to chronic pain in children, techniques used were not necessarily scientifically validated, although rigor of such assessment appears to have improved in recent decades (Claar and Walker 2006; Weel et al. 2005).

Applicability of results from one study population to another, or to children in general, may be particularly problematic in the context of pediatric chronic pain secondary to variability among different study samples (Goodman and McGrath 1991). Considerations of patient population, sample size, and age range of children studied may profoundly influence data obtained, as well as applicability of data to other settings. Techniques, methods, and populations studied should be considered carefully. Extrapolation of data to other potentially significantly different patient populations may be inappropriate or even misleading, contributing to the ongoing challenge of scientific study of chronic pain in children (PedIMMPACT: McGrath et al. 2008) Inquiry and education about headache symptomatology in children has been reported to increase subsequent headache complaints (Passchier et al. 1993), raising unsettling concern over potential for study of chronic pain in children to exacerbate the problem.

Although considerable attention has been directed to the staggering economic and societal burden of chronic pain in adults, remarkably little is known of the economic and societal costs of chronic pain in children. Financial consequences, loss of productivity, and health-care expenditures secondary to chronic pain have historically been thought to be of greater significance in adults than in children. It is increasingly recognized that chronic pain in children may have potentially profound effects on parental productivity, patient school performance, and even long-term health outcomes of affected children (Walker et al. 1995). The overall impact of chronic pain in children on patients, families, and communities is likely significant (Campo et al. 2007; Hotopf et al. 1998; Martin et al. 2007b; Hunfeld et al. 2001; McCaffery and Pasero 1999; Roth-Isigkeit et al. 2005), and warrants considerable further ongoing investigation (PedIMMPACT: McGrath 2008).

Incidence and Prevalence

Incidence measures the rate of occurrence of a disease or condition in a population over a specified period of time, often per year, and thus defines the number of new cases of the disease or condition in that population over that period. Prevalence measures how much of a disease or condition exists in a population at a specific point in time, and thus defines the total number of cases of the disease or condition in that population at that point. Given the inherent nature of chronic pain as an ongoing condition, as well as the overall paucity of longitudinal investigations in children allowing accurate assessment of onset, most reports of chronic pain in children describe prevalence rather than incidence. Historical estimates of the incidence and prevalence of pain of various types in children have varied widely (Goodman and McGrath 1991), with more recent reviews suggesting the prevalence of chronic pain in children to be approximately 25% (Harstall and Ospina 2003).

Results from a questionnaire survey of a representative sample of school-age children in Sweden (Brattberg 1994) indicated the prevalence of back pain and headache in this setting to be 29% and 48%, respectively. Longitudinal assessment of a subset of this study population revealed 9% and 30% of respondents still reported back pain and headache, respectively, at 2-year follow-up. No association between pain and physical factors could be identified, suggesting both types of pain reported were primarily functional.

Survey data from a representative sample of children ages 0–18 years in the Netherlands (Perquin et al. 2000) indicated 54% of respondents had experienced pain of some kind within the prior 3 months, with 25% of respondents experiencing chronic pain. These results correspond to a 3-month incidence of 54% for pain of any type, and a prevalence of 25% for chronic pain. Limb pain, headache, and abdominal pain were most commonly reported, with one half of respondents reporting pain at multiple sites and one third reporting frequent or intense pain. Pain at multiple sites and intensity of pain were strongly associated with pain chronicity.

Longitudinal assessment of a subset of this study population reporting chronic pain at baseline revealed 48% and 30% still reported chronic pain at 1- and 2-year follow-up, respectively (Perquin et al. 2003). Demographics and symptomatology were remarkably stable in those still reporting pain at 3 years (Hunfeld et al. 2002).

Survey data from a representative sample of children ages 10–18 years in Germany (Roth-Isigkeit et al. 2004) revealed even higher incidence and prevalence of pain and chronic pain in children. Over 85% of respondents had experienced pain of some kind within the prior 3 months, with over 45% of respondents experiencing chronic pain. These results correspond to a 3 month incidence of 85% for pain of any type, and a prevalence of 45% for chronic pain. Headache, abdominal pain, limb pain, and back pain were reported most commonly, and over 33% of respondents reported pain once a week or more frequently.

Subsequent evaluation of a similar population of schoolchildren elsewhere in Germany (Roth-Isigkeit et al. 2005) revealed similar results. Comparable to earlier findings, 83% of respondents had experienced pain of some kind within the prior 3 months, with over 30% of respondents experiencing chronic pain. These results correspond to a 3-month incidence of 83% for pain of any type, and a prevalence of 30% for chronic pain. Headache, abdominal pain, limb pain, and back pain were again reported most commonly.

Impairment of usual activities by pain and associated medical treatment was significant.

A recent longitudinal survey of Canadian adolescents (Stanford et al. 2008) assessed prevalence of recurrent pain at a variety of anatomic sites. Children were assessed every 2 years, for a total of up to five sequential evaluations. Weekly or more frequent headache, stomachache, and backache were reported by up to 31%, 22%, and 25% of respondents, respectively. Prevalence varied only slightly by age, with remarkably similar profiles for patients ages 12–19 years.

Despite such findings, awareness of chronic pain in children remains inadequate. A recent survey of general practitioners and specialists in chronic pain in the UK (Bhatia et al. 2008) indicated a majority of both general practitioners and specialists in chronic pain perceived chronic pain in children to be an uncommon problem, with 63% of general practitioners and 57% of specialists in chronic pain reporting the prevalence of chronic pain in children to be < 5%. Although 95% of general practitioners and 77% of specialists in chronic pain described their training in management of children with chronic pain as inadequate, only 15% of respondents overall felt children with chronic pain were best managed by specialists, and 75% of respondents overall deemed children with chronic pain to have at least a fair to good prognosis. The authors appropriately cited the ongoing need for increased education and training related to assessment and management of chronic pain in children.

Gender Differences

Gender differences in chronic pain in children are complex and incompletely understood. Although it has long been recognized, chronic pain in children appears to be more common in girls than in boys (Walco and Dampier 1987); explanations for this persistent observation are elusive. Societal roles and familial expectations may affect how children express their pain, but it is increasingly recognized that the underlying psychobiological mechanisms of pain in boys and girls may be quite different. Gender differences in parental influence on the pain experience of their children are even more complex and even less well-understood. Mothers and fathers may perceive and influence pain in their children quite differently, and such differences in both perception and influence are in turn affected by gender of the child.

Girls may experience and express pain differently than boys (Goodman and McGrath 1991). Pain scores provided by girls and boys in similar clinical settings are frequently discordant, with girls generally reporting higher pain scores than boys despite objective assessment of similar pain (Chambers et al. 1999). Girls also seem more likely than boys to report frequent, recurrent, or severe pain (Martin et al. 2007b). The extent to which such variations are secondary to differences in pain thresholds, to differences in pain descriptions, or to some combination of both, is unclear.

Maternal and paternal assessments of children's pain may also vary markedly, with complex gender interactions. Fathers frequently report higher pain scores in daughters than in sons, but their assessment tends to be more concordant with the subjective reports of both daughters and sons; mothers frequently rate pain similarly in daughters and sons, but their assessment tends to be less concordant with the subjective reports of their children (Moon et al. 2008). The reasons for such variations in parental perception of children's pain are not well-understood, although gender differences in pain experience likely persist into adulthood.

Although mothers may generally be somewhat less accurate in assessing pain in their children, they seem more able than fathers to influence their children's pain. Historical observations often described a perceived causal association between pain-promoting behaviors in mothers and chronic pain in their daughters (Walco and Dampier 1987), while more recent investigations have described associations between functional abdominal pain in children and a variety of maternal diagnoses, in particular maternal anxiety and depression (Campo et al. 2007). Maternal behaviors may significantly influence reported pain scores in daughters but not in sons (Chambers et al. 2002); paternal influence on children seems

to be somewhat less significant (Evans and Keenan 2007). An association between paternal anxiety and subsequent recurrent abdominal pain in children has been described, although odds ratios were somewhat less than for maternal anxiety (Ramchandani et al. 2006). Such differences may be secondary to the unique emotional bond between mothers and their children, given the strong likelihood of a significant biopsychosocial component to pediatric chronic pain (Merlijn et al. 2003; Palermo and Chambers 2005; Varni et al. 1989; Zeltzer et al. 1997).

Results from a questionnaire survey of a representative sample of school-age children in Sweden (Brattberg 1994) indicated back pain and headache to be more common in girls than in boys at all ages studied. Girls were also more likely than boys to report more frequent pain. Longitudinal assessment of a subset of this study population revealed persistence of similar findings at 2-year follow-up, with statistically significant associations between pain and a variety of social, psychological, and emotional factors generally thought to be more common in girls than in boys.

Survey data from a representative sample of children ages 0–18 years in the Netherlands (Perquin et al. 2000) indicated both incidence of pain of any type and prevalence of chronic pain were greater in girls than in boys at all ages studied. Girls were also significantly more likely than boys to report pain at multiple sites and more intense pain. Pain at multiple sites and intensity of pain were strongly associated with pain chronicity, all of which were more pronounced in girls than in boys.

Longitudinal assessment of a subset of this study population reporting chronic pain at baseline revealed similar findings at 1- and 2-year follow-up (Perquin et al. 2003), while demographics and symptomatology were remarkably stable in those still reporting pain at 3 years (Hunfeld et al. 2002). Prospective analysis of a subgroup of patients reporting chronic pain using 3-week patient pain diaries and a summary questionnaire (Hunfeld et al. 2001) confirmed girls were more likely than boys to experience pain, and were more likely to experience more intense and more frequent pain. Higher intensity and greater frequency of pain were correlated with lower quality-of-life scores, in particular psychological function and overall physical and functional status. Negative impact on family was noted, and stress secondary to chronic pain was significant.

Survey data from a representative sample of children ages 10–18 years in Germany (Roth-Isigkeit et al. 2004) revealed both higher incidence of pain of any type and higher prevalence of chronic pain in girls than in boys, although magnitude of difference varied by age and was not statistically significant in children younger than age 12 years. Similarly, girls tended to report overall higher visual analog scores than did boys, although magnitude of difference varied by age and was likewise not statistically significant in children younger than age 12 years.

Subsequent evaluation of a similar population of schoolchildren elsewhere in Germany (Roth-Isigkeit et al. 2005) revealed similar demographics, but also highlighted several gender differences in patient response to chronic pain. Girls over age 10 years reported significantly more limitations and restrictions of daily living secondary to their pain than did boys, and were also more likely to use medications for their pain. Girls were more likely than boys to describe their pain as being triggered by weather, medical illness, emotion, and psychosocial stress, while boys were more likely than girls to describe their pain as being triggered by physical exertion. These observations all suggest chronic pain in children frequently evolves in a highly biopsychosocial context, particularly in adolescent girls.

A recent longitudinal survey of Canadian adolescents (Stanford et al. 2008) assessed prevalence of recurrent pain at a variety of anatomic sites. Children were assessed every 2 years, for a total of up to five sequential evaluations. Girls were more likely than boys to report frequent headache, stomachache, and backache at all ages studied. Girls were also more likely to develop pain trajectories with high levels of pain across time, or with increasing pain over time, for all three types of pain. Anxiety and depression, generally thought to be more common in girls than in

boys, were also significantly correlated with such pain trajectories.

Gender differences in chronic pain in children have recently been validated in a cohort study of patients referred to an anesthesiology-based pediatric chronic pain program in the Midwestern USA (Vetter 2008). Virtually, all patients had previously been evaluated by at least one other specialist for their pain, representing a very different study sample than in other survey and questionnaire investigations of more general populations. Girls accounted for 73% of patients with chronic pain, although making up only 48% of the local population. Chronic pain was frequently associated with both anxiety and depression, both of which are generally thought to be more common in girls than in boys. Quality-of-life scores were consistently lower than generally observed in pediatric rheumatology patients, pediatric migraine patients, and even pediatric cancer patients, suggesting the overall burden of chronic pain in children may be profound. The author appropriately cited ongoing need for increased assessment of pain-associated disability in pediatric chronic patients and their families, with ongoing efforts to address underlying mechanisms and promote functional recovery.

Age-Dependent Onset

Although chronic pain in children is increasingly thought to be significantly more common than previously acknowledged (Howard 2003), it is also increasingly recognized that chronic pain in children generally displays age-dependent onset. Numerous specific medical diseases and diagnoses may be associated with chronic pain in children, demographics including age, characteristics of which generally reflect those of the underlying condition. Many of these conditions are discussed in detail elsewhere. Chronic pain in children as an independent syndrome also manifests certain specific patterns of age-dependent onset, explanations for which are incompletely understood.

Results from a questionnaire survey of a representative sample of school-age children in Sweden (Brattberg 1994) indicated the prevalence of back pain and headache in this setting to increase progressively with age, with emergence of particularly significant gender differences in adolescence. Children ages 8, 11, 13, and 17 years were asked about the presence of back pain and headache. At age 8 years, only 7% of boys and 8% of girls reported back pain, but by age 17 years 39% of boys and 58% of girls reported back pain. Similarly, at age 8 years 27% of boys and 42% of girls reported headache or neck pain, but by age 17 years 35% of boys and 71% of girls reported such pain. Prevalence increased steadily with increasing age. Although prevalence was higher for girls than for boys for both types of pain at all ages studied, gender differences increased significantly at ages 13 and 17 years, particularly for headache. Longitudinal assessment of a subset of this study population revealed similar demographics at 2-year follow-up. No association between pain and physical factors could be identified, suggesting both types of pain reported were primarily functional.

Survey data from a representative sample of children ages 0–18 years in the Netherlands (Perquin et al. 2000) indicated consistent age-dependent onset of chronic pain. Children ages 0–3 years were assessed by parental questionnaire, while children ages 4–18 years filled out questionnaires at school. Overall prevalence of chronic pain increased steadily with age, although abdominal pain was most common in children ages 4–7 years, consistent with widely recognized demographics of recurrent abdominal pain syndrome in younger school-age children (McOmber and Shulman 2008). Although girls overall were more likely to report pain of any type, chronic pain, pain at multiple sites, and frequent or severe pain, a marked increase in prevalence of chronic pain was noted between ages 12–14 years for girls but not for boys.

Longitudinal assessment of a subset of this study population reporting chronic pain at baseline revealed similar findings at 1- and 2-year follow-up, and overall pain severity remained essentially unchanged (Perquin et al. 2003). Demographics and symptomatology were remarkably stable in those still reporting pain at 3 years (Hunfeld et al. 2002). Although incidence and prevalence of chronic pain in children increased with age, symptomatology once established appeared to remain very much the same over time in children who continued to report chronic pain.

Survey data from a representative sample of children ages 10–18 years in Germany (Roth-Isigkeit et al. 2004) revealed similar age-dependent onset of pain including chronic pain in children. Children ages 10–18 years completed a previously developed survey questionnaire regarding presence of pain of any type, pain at various anatomic locations, and pain lasting more than 3 months. Data analysis included stratification by ages 10–12, 13–15, and 16–18 years, demonstrating overall increases in incidence and prevalence of pain including chronic pain with age. Although incidence of pain of any type was highest for children ages 13–15 years, prevalence of chronic pain increased steadily with age and was highest for children ages 16–18 years.

Subsequent evaluation of a similar population of schoolchildren elsewhere in Germany (Roth-Isigkeit et al. 2005) revealed similar results, but also highlighted several age differences in pain-associated disability. Prevalence of pain including chronic pain increased with age, as did both prevalence and severity of restriction of daily living attributed to pain. Overall 50% of children reported seeking professional attention for their pain, and 51% reported using pain medications. Prevalence of both doctor visits and use of pain medication increased with age. Girls over age 10 years in particular reported significantly more limitations and restrictions of daily living secondary to their pain than did boys, and were also more likely to use pain medication. In general, gender differences emerged at around age 10 years and subsequently became more significant with increasing age.

In contrast, a recent longitudinal survey of Canadian adolescents (Stanford et al. 2008) assessing prevalence of recurrent pain at a variety of anatomic sites suggested very little variation with age. Children ages 10–11 years were assessed every 2 years, for a total of up to five sequential evaluations, for presence of weekly or more frequent headache, stomachache, and backache. Prevalence varied only slightly by age, with remarkably similar profiles for patients ages 12–19 years. Discrepancies between results of this study and those of multiple other investigations may have arisen not only from differences in study populations, but from differences in types of pain studied. The Canadian study was quite specific in assessing recurrent pain, defined as pain occurring weekly or more frequently, at three specific anatomic sites. Other studies more generally assessed chronic pain, defined as pain greater than 3 months in duration, at any site reported.

Age distribution of chronic pain in children has recently been validated in a cohort study of patients referred to an anesthesiology-based pediatric chronic pain program in the Midwestern USA (Vetter 2008). Virtually, all patients had previously been evaluated by at least one other specialist for their pain, representing a very different study sample than in other survey and questionnaire investigations of more general populations. Although patients ranged in age from 2 to 21 years, the average age of patients in this cohort was 14.0 years, and the majority of patients were adolescent girls. Chronic pain in these children was frequently associated with clinically significant anxiety and depression, and overall quality-of-life scores were consistently lower than generally observed in other pediatric chronic disease populations.

Regional Findings

Rigorous assessment of regional findings pertaining to chronic pain in children is hampered by lack of broad-based data (Goodman and McGrath 1991; Harstall and Ospina 2003; Howard 2003). Individual investigations provide informative demographic descriptions of particular study samples, but allow only limited extrapolation to other populations. Numerous specific medical diseases and diagnoses may be associated with chronic pain in children, demographics including regional findings of which generally reflect those of the underlying condition. Many of these conditions are discussed in detail elsewhere. Regional findings pertaining to chronic pain in children as an independent syndrome appear largely to reflect

variations in incidence and prevalence, with symptomatology and associated disability remaining constant. Available data derive almost exclusively from Northern European and North American populations, and demographics of chronic pain in children elsewhere are largely unknown.

Results from a questionnaire survey of a representative sample of school-age children in Sweden (Brattberg 1994) indicated the prevalence of back pain and headache in this setting to be 29% and 48%, respectively, with 9% and 30% of respondents still reporting back pain and headache, respectively, at 2-year follow-up. Prevalence increased progressively with age, with emergence of particularly significant gender differences in adolescence. Although prevalence was higher for girls than for boys for both types of pain at all ages studied, gender differences increased significantly at ages 13 and 17 years, particularly for headache. Girls were also more likely than boys to report more frequent pain, with statistically significant associations between pain and a variety of social, psychological, and emotional factors generally thought to be more common in girls than in boys. No association between pain and physical factors could be identified, suggesting both types of pain reported were primarily functional.

Similar findings have been reported in several other Northern European populations. Survey data from a representative sample of children ages 0–18 years in the Netherlands (Perquin et al. 2000) indicated a 3-month incidence of 54% for pain of any type, and a prevalence of 25% for chronic pain. Limb pain, headache, and abdominal pain were most commonly reported, with one half of respondents reporting pain at multiple sites and one-third reporting frequent or intense pain. Overall prevalence of chronic pain increased steadily with age. Incidence of pain of any type and prevalence of chronic pain were greater in girls than in boys at all ages studied. Girls overall were also more likely to report pain of any type, chronic pain, pain at multiple sites, and frequent or severe pain, with a marked increase in prevalence of chronic pain noted between ages 12 and 14 years for girls but not for boys. Pain at multiple sites and intensity of pain were strongly associated with pain chronicity, all of which were more pronounced in girls than in boys.

Longitudinal assessment of a subset of this study population reporting chronic pain at baseline revealed similar demographics at 1- and 2-year follow-up, and overall pain severity remained essentially unchanged (Perquin et al. 2003). Demographics and symptomatology were again remarkably stable in those still reporting pain at 3 years (Hunfeld et al. 2002). Prospective analysis of a subgroup of patients reporting chronic pain using 3-week patient pain diaries and a summary questionnaire (Hunfeld et al. 2001) confirmed that girls were more likely than boys to experience pain, and were more likely to experience more intense and more frequent pain. Higher intensity and greater frequency of pain were correlated with lower quality-of-life scores, in particular psychological function and overall physical and functional status. Negative impact on family was noted, and stress secondary to chronic pain was significant.

Investigations in Germany have described similar overall symptomatology related to chronic pain in children, but have also reported significantly greater incidence and prevalence and somewhat more subtle gender differences. Survey data from a representative sample of children ages 10–18 years in Germany (Roth-Isigkeit et al. 2004) indicated a 3-month incidence of 85% for pain of any type, and a prevalence of 45% for chronic pain. Headache, abdominal pain, limb pain, and back pain were reported most commonly, and over 33% of respondents reported pain once a week or more frequently. Although incidence of pain of any type was highest for children ages 13–15 years, prevalence of chronic pain increased steadily with age and was highest for children ages 16–18 years. Incidence of pain of any type and prevalence of chronic pain were both generally higher in girls than in boys, although magnitude of difference varied by age and was not statistically significant in children younger than age 12 years. Similarly, girls tended to report overall higher visual analog scores than did boys, although magnitude of difference varied by age and was likewise not statistically significant in children younger than age 12 years.

Subsequent evaluation of a similar population of schoolchildren elsewhere in Germany (Roth-Isigkeit et al. 2005) revealed similar incidence and prevalence, but also highlighted several gender- and age-dependent differences in pain-associated disability and pain treatment. Similar to earlier findings, results indicated a 3-month incidence of 83% for pain of any type, and a prevalence of 30% for chronic pain. Headache, abdominal pain, limb pain, and back pain were again reported most commonly. Incidence of pain of any type and prevalence of chronic pain increased with age, as did prevalence and severity of restriction of daily living attributed to pain. Prevalence of doctor visits and use of pain medication also increased with age. Girls overall reported significantly more limitations and restrictions of daily living secondary to their pain than did boys, and were also more likely to use pain medication. In general, significant gender differences emerged at around age 10 years, and subsequently became more significant with increasing age. Overall disability associated with chronic pain in children was significant.

In contrast, a recent longitudinal survey of Canadian adolescents (Stanford et al. 2008) assessing weekly or more frequent headache, stomachache, and backache suggested incidence and prevalence similar to that in Swedish and Dutch populations, but indicated very little variation with age. Weekly or more frequent headache, stomachache, and backache were reported by up to 31%, 22%, and 25% of respondents, respectively. Prevalence varied only slightly by age, with remarkably similar profiles for patients ages 12–19 years. Gender differences were similar to those observed in other populations, with girls being were more likely than boys to report frequent headache, stomachache, and backache at all ages studied. Girls were also more likely to develop pain trajectories with high levels of pain across time, or with increasing pain over time, for all three types of pain, although considerable variation was observed when individual pain trajectories were analyzed separately. Anxiety and depression, generally thought to be more common in girls than in boys, were also significantly correlated with such pain trajectories.

A recent cohort study of patients referred to an anesthesiology-based pediatric chronic pain program in the Midwestern USA (Vetter 2008) provides demographic description of children with chronic pain referred for subspecialty management of their condition. Virtually all patients had previously been evaluated by at least one other specialist for their pain, representing a very different study sample than in other survey and questionnaire investigations of more general populations. Incidence and prevalence could not be addressed, owing to the nature of the study sample, but gender and age profiles reflected those described in European populations. Patients ranged in age from 2 to 21 years, with an average age of 14.0 years, and the majority of patients were adolescent girls. Girls accounted for 73% of patients, although making up only 48% of the local population. Chronic pain was frequently associated with both anxiety and depression. Quality-of-life scores were consistently lower than generally observed in pediatric rheumatology patients, pediatric migraine patients, and even pediatric cancer patients, suggesting the overall burden of chronic pain in children may be profound.

Other Associations

Pain is frequently a multifactorial process, particularly when chronic. Perhaps unsurprisingly, numerous associations have been described with regard to chronic pain in children pertaining both to patients and their families. Investigations have suggested a predisposition to chronic pain in children with mental health disorders, especially anxiety and depression. An association between sleep disorders and chronic pain in children has also been described. Parental diagnoses may influence likelihood of chronic pain in children, particularly maternal mental health disorders. The impact of chronic pain in children on subsequent physical and mental health has also been examined, with evidence suggesting an association between chronic pain in children

and subsequent mental but not physical health disorders.

Anxiety, Depression, and Sleep Disorders

It has long been recognized children with chronic pain frequently exhibit behavioral patterns suggestive of underlying mental health disorders (Zuckerman et al. 1987). Children with recurrent abdominal pain demonstrate high levels of somatization (Walker et al. 1991), consistent with underlying disturbances of affect and mood. Psychosocial factors have been demonstrated to exert a profound influence on quality of life in children with chronic pain, particularly adolescents (Merlijn et al. 2006), and children with chronic pain have shown promising response to cognitive–behavioral interventions (Merlijn et al. 2005). Early evidence of potentially abnormal temperament in children has been shown to be associated with subsequent recurrent abdominal pain (Ramchandani et al. 2006), while presence of anxiety or depression in adolescents at ages 10–11 years has been shown to be predictive of persistent or worsening chronic pain as adolescence progresses (Stanford et al. 2008). The association between mental health and chronic pain in children, as in adults, is likely significant.

In a blinded evaluation of patients in a primary care setting in the Eastern USA (Campo et al. 2004), children ages 8–15 years presenting with recurrent abdominal pain were significantly more likely than control patients presenting for routine care to have formal psychiatric diagnoses. Of children with recurrent abdominal pain, 79% met criteria for categorical anxiety disorder, and 53% met criteria for depressive disorder. Onset of anxiety disorder generally preceded onset of recurrent abdominal pain by several years, suggesting a possible causal association. The authors appropriately cited the need for ongoing longitudinal study of the interplay between anxiety, depression, and chronic pain in children.

These results were confirmed with questionnaire and blinded evaluations of children ages 8–15 years presenting to several primary care practices in the Midwestern USA with functional abdominal pain (Campo et al. 2007). Children with functional abdominal pain were significantly more likely than control patients presenting for routine care to have current anxiety, depression, and somatic symptoms, and were more likely to report poorer overall quality of life. Children with functional abdominal pain demonstrated greater use than control patients of ambulatory health services but not greater use of mental health services, suggesting failure to accept a primarily biopsychosocial model of their pain.

Comprehensive evaluation of children in the Eastern USA with anxiety or recurrent abdominal pain (Dorn et al. 2003) revealed remarkable psychologic and physiologic similarities among children with these diagnoses. Children with anxiety disorder or recurrent abdominal pain underwent extensive psychometric testing, as well as physiologic evaluation of stress response including vital signs and salivary cortisol levels. Scores on most psychometric measures were comparable between children with anxiety and children with recurrent abdominal pain, and were significantly higher than scores in control children. Children with anxiety and children with recurrent abdominal pain also demonstrated remarkably similar physiologic stress responses, again greater than observed in control children. The authors appropriately underscored the apparent congruity between anxiety disorder and recurrent abdominal pain in children, suggesting therapy effective in pediatric anxiety disorder might be efficacious for children with recurrent abdominal pain.

The strong association between anxiety, depression, and chronic pain in children, and the profound impact these comorbid conditions have on quality of life of children with chronic pain, have been validated in a cohort study of patients referred to an anesthesiology-based pediatric chronic pain program in the Midwestern USA (Vetter 2008). Chronic pain was frequently associated with both anxiety and depression, regardless of underlying medical diagnosis. Compared to expected regional and national norms, patients were also significantly more likely to have a non-intact family, not to attend school full-time, and to be intentionally home-schooled, all suggestive of

greater psychosocial stress in children with chronic pain. Quality-of-life scores were consistently lower than generally observed in pediatric rheumatology patients, pediatric migraine patients, and even pediatric cancer patients, suggesting the overall burden of chronic pain in children may be profound.

It has recently been recognized that sleep disorders are associated with chronic pain in children (Palermo et al. 2007). Assessment of children ages 8–15 years with or without functional abdominal pain revealed children with functional abdominal pain experienced more nightmares, increased daytime tiredness, and greater symptoms of various behavioral sleep disorders than healthy control children, although total sleep time was similar (Huntley et al. 2007). Sleep disturbance with impaired daytime function and decreased overall health-related quality-of-life has also been described in children with chronic pain secondary to juvenile idiopathic arthritis, sickle cell disease, and headache (Long et al. 2008). Several authors have appropriately called for increased awareness of the association between sleep disorders and chronic pain in children, with ongoing study of this association (Chambers et al. 2008). The extent to which sleep disorders and chronic pain in children are causally related is unknown.

Parental Mental Health

It has long been recognized that maternal depression is associated with chronic pain in children, even after controlling for other maternal medical illness (Zuckerman et al. 1987). Parental dysfunction, particularly in mothers, has also been thought to promote, maintain, and even exacerbate chronic pain in children (Walco and Dampier 1987). Parents of children with recurrent abdominal pain themselves demonstrate high levels of somatization (Walker et al. 1991), consistent with underlying disturbance of affect and mood. Mothers of children with chronic pain in turn frequently report greater signs of emotional distress than mothers of healthy children (Walker et al. 1995). Although parental influence has generally been thought to reinforce pain behaviors in children, some investigations have, to the contrary, suggested children with chronic pain actually receive less reinforcement for their pain behaviors than control children without chronic pain (Merlijn et al. 2003).

In a blinded evaluation (Campo et al. 2007), mothers of children ages 8–15 years presenting to several primary care practices in the Midwestern USA with functional abdominal pain were significantly more likely than mothers of control patients presenting for routine care to have a variety of diagnoses including formal psychiatric disorders. Specific maternal diagnoses included irritable bowel syndrome, migraine, anxiety disorder depressive disorder, and somatoform disorder. Multivariate logistical regression indicated functional abdominal pain in children to be most closely associated with maternal anxiety and maternal depression.

An association between paternal anxiety and subsequent recurrent abdominal pain in children has been described, although odds ratios were somewhat less than for maternal anxiety (Ramchandani et al. 2006). Children of mothers with chronic pain demonstrated higher rates of both physical and psychological problems than did children of fathers with chronic pain, who in turn demonstrated higher rates of both physical and psychological problems than did children of parents without chronic pain (Evans and Keenan 2007). Reasons for differing maternal and paternal influence on the chronic pain experience of children are incompletely understood and likely highly complex (Hotopf et al. 1998).

Long-Term Outcomes

Although a majority of general practitioners and specialists in chronic pain alike imagine children with chronic pain to have a fair to good prognosis (Bhatia et al. 2008), considerable evidence suggests that chronic pain in children is frequently associated with unfavorable long-term outcomes. Adults with histories of chronic pain in childhood have been found to have higher levels of pain, increased somatic complaints, and greater functional disability than control patients without histories of chronic pain in childhood (Walker et al. 1995). Unfavorable outcomes seem particularly likely in patients with primarily functional pain for which no specific underlying diagnosis is made.

Reevaluation of young adult patients first studied in a questionnaire survey of a representative sample of school-age children in Sweden 13-years later (Brattberg 2004) indicated that chronic pain in children is predictive of chronic pain in young adulthood. Back pain in childhood, weekly or more frequent headache in childhood, and often feeling nervous in childhood were all specifically and significantly associated with presence of pain in young adulthood. In contrast, self-perceived stress in childhood predicted neither stress nor pain in young adulthood.

Assessment of a sample of young adults in the Eastern USA first evaluated for recurrent abdominal pain between ages 6–17 years revealed a strong and specific association with anxiety disorder in young adulthood (Campo et al. 1999; Campo et al. 2001). Young adults with histories of recurrent abdominal pain in childhood were also more likely than control patients to perceive greater susceptibility to physical impairment and to report poorer social functioning. Trends suggestive of associations between recurrent abdominal pain in childhood and lifetime psychiatric disorder including depression were not statistically significant.

Assessment of adults identified through a national health-care database in the UK as having had persistent abdominal pain in childhood similarly revealed an association with subsequent psychiatric but not physical medical diagnoses in adulthood (Hotopf et al. 1998). Curiously, persistent abdominal pain in childhood was not associated with increased pain in adulthood, but only with increased risk for psychiatric disorders.

Reevaluation of a cohort of patients first seen in a pediatric chronic pain clinic in Eastern Canada, a mean of 3 years after their last clinic visit, revealed persistence of chronic pain in a majority of patients, with age- and gender-related patterns (Martin et al. 2007b). Over 62% of patients overall reported continuing pain. Females were significantly more likely than males to report continuing pain, particularly when their pain had recognized associated psychosocial factors. Females were also more likely than males to report using health care, medications, and non-pharmacologic interventions for pain control. Among all patients with persistent pain, pain frequency increased significantly with age. The authors appropriately noted persistence of pain, ongoing utilization of health-care resources, and worsening of symptomatology with age, all occurred despite prior treatment in a specialized pediatric chronic pain clinic.

Risk for persistent pain in some children with functional abdominal pain has been confirmed in a longitudinal analysis of pain and symptom trajectories (Mulvaney et al. 2006). Children seen in a pediatric gastroenterology clinic in the Southeastern USA for functional abdominal pain were assessed four times over 5 years. Overall pain and symptom trajectories were analyzed and found to conform to a three-trajectory model. Two trajectories were associated with relative long-term improvement, and one trajectory was associated with ongoing pain and disability. Although patients ultimately found to have persistent pain did not have the most severe pain initially, such patients did have significantly more anxiety, depression, lower perceived self-worth, and negative life events.

Ominously, the overall burden of chronic pain in children may be increasing. Longitudinal anal-ysis of demographic data in Finland suggest the prevalence of weekly or more frequent pain in the back and neck, neck and shoulder, and lower back has increased dramatically in recent decades (Hakala et al. 2002). Consistent with other investigations, pain at all sites was more common in girls, and with increasing age. Between 1985 and 2001, however, pain at each site became significantly more common in both girls and boys of all ages. The authors appropriately cautioned of unfavorable long-term outcomes as increasing numbers of children with chronic pain enter adulthood.

Conclusion

Although the methodologic considerations are considerable, current knowledge of the demographics of chronic pain in children is evolving rapidly (Table 4.2). Incidence of pain of any type in children may be as high as 50–75%, while prevalence of chronic pain in children is likely 25–50%. Chronic pain in children is generally more common in girls than in boys, particularly in adolescence. Chronic pain in children at most sites tends to become significantly more common in early adolescence, and to increase in prevalence over time thereafter. Recurrent abdominal pain is typically more common in younger school-age children. Regional differences largely reflect variations in incidence and prevalence,

Table 4.2 Summary of demographics of chronic pain in children

Parameter	Comments
Incidence, pain	~50–75%
Prevalence, chronic pain	~25–50%
Gender differences	More common in girls, particularly in adolescence; Preadolescent gender differences generally less significant
Age-dependent onset	Dramatic increase in early adolescence, then increases with age; Recurrent abdominal pain more common in early school ages
Regional differences	Largely reflect variations in incidence and prevalence; Symptomatology and associated disability relatively constant
Other associations	Mental health disorders and sleep disorders; Parental mental health disorders, particularly maternal; Increased risk of long-term pain and associated disability; Increased risk of mental health disorders

Chronic pain in children secondary to a specific disease or diagnosis will generally reflect the demographics of the underlying condition; these parameters largely pertain to chronic pain in children as an independent syndrome with symptomatology and associated disability remaining relatively constant. Chronic pain in children is associated with mental health disorders, particularly anxiety and depression, and with sleep disorders. Chronic pain in children is also associated with parental mental health disorders, particularly anxiety and depression, especially in mothers. Long-term outcomes in children with chronic pain include increased risk for persistent pain and for mental health disorders, particularly anxiety and depression. The disability and dysfunction associated with chronic pain in children may be significant. Ongoing investigations should attempt to enhance identification of children at greatest risk of chronic pain, to validate response to interventions, and to develop effective new therapies (Hicks et al. 2006).

References

American Society for Pain Management Nursing, Herr, K., Coyne, P. J., Key, T., Manworren, R., McCaffery, M., Merkel, S., Pelosi-Kelly, J., & Wild, L. (2006). Pain assessment in the nonverbal patient: Position statement with clinical practice recommendations. *Pain Management Nursing, 7*(2), 44–52.

Beyer, J.E. (1983). The Oucher: A user's manual and technical report. © 1983, J.E. Beyer. Image available online: http://www.oucher.org/the_scales.html.

Bhatia, A., Brennan, L., Abrahams, M., & Gilder, F. (2008). Chronic pain in children in the UK: A survey of pain clinicians and general practitioners. *Paediatric Anaesthesia, 18*(10), 957–966.

Brattberg, G. (1994). The incidence of back pain and headache among Swedish school children. *Quality of Life Research, 3*(Suppl 1), S27–S31.

Brattberg, G. (2004). Do pain problems in young school children persist into early adulthood? A 13-year follow-up. *European Journal of Pain, 8*(3), 187–199.

Bursch, B., Walco, G. A., & Zeltzer, L. (1998). Clinical assessment and management of chronic pain and pain-associated disability syndrome. *Journal of Developmental and Behavioral Pediatrics, 19*(1), 45–53.

Campo, J. V., Di Lorenzo, C., Bridge, J., Chiappetta, L., Colborn, D. K., Gartner, J. C., Gaffney, P., Kocoshis, S., & Brent, D. (1999). *Adult outcomes of recurrent abdominal pain: Preliminary results*. Orlando: American Gastroenterological Association.

Campo, J. V., Di Lorenzo, C., Chiappetta, L., Bridge, J., Colborn, D.K., Gartner, J.C., Jr., Gaffney, P., Kocoshis, S., & Brent, D. (2001). Adult outcomes of pediatric recurrent abdominal pain: Do they just grow out of it? *Pediatrics, 108*(1), E1.

Campo, J. V., Bridge, J., Ehmann, M., Altman, S., Lucas, A., Birmaher, B., Di Lorenzo, C., Iyengar, S., & Brent, D. A. (2004). Recurrent abdominal pain, anxiety, and depression in primary care. *Pediatrics, 113*(4), 817–824.

Campo, J. V., Bridge, J., Lucas, A., Savorelli, S., Walker, L., Di Lorenzo, C., Iyengar, S., & Brent, D. A. (2007). Physical and emotional health of mothers of youth with functional abdominal pain. *Archives of Pediatric and Adolescent Medicine, 161*(2), 131–137.

Chambers, C. T., Reid, G. J., Craig, K. D., McGrath, P. J., & Finley, G. A. (1998). Agreement between child and parent reports of pain. *The Clinical Journal of Pain, 14*(4), 336–342.

Chambers, C. T., Giesbrecht, K., Craig, K. D., Bennett, S. M., & Huntsman, E. (1999). A comparison of faces scales for the measurement of pediatric pain: Children's and parents' ratings. *Pain, 83*(1), 25–35.

Chambers, C. T., Craig, K. D., & Bennett, S. M. (2002). The impact of maternal behavior on children's pain experiences: An experimental analysis. *Journal of Pediatric Psychology, 27*(3), 293–301.

Chambers, C. T., Corkum, P. V., & Rusak, B. (2008). The importance of sleep in pediatric chronic pain–a wake-up call for pediatric psychologists. *Journal of Pediatric Psychology, 33*(3), 333–334.

Claar, R. L., & Walker, L. S. (2006). Functional assessment of pediatric pain patients: Psychometric properties of the functional disability inventory. *Pain, 121*(1–2), 77–84.

Dorn, L. D., Campo, J. C., Thato, S., Dahl, R. E., Lewin, D., Chandra, R., & Di Lorenzo, C. (2003). Psychological comorbidity and stress reactivity in children and adolescents with recurrent abdominal pain and anxiety disorders. *Journal of the American Academy of Child and Adolescent Psychiatry, 42*(1), 66–75.

Evans, S., & Keenan, T. R. (2007). Parents with chronic pain: Are children equally affected by fathers as mothers in pain? A pilot study. *Journal of Child Health Care, 11*(2), 143–157.

Goodman, J. E., & McGrath, P. J. (1991). The epidemiology of pain in children and adolescents: A review. *Pain, 46*(3), 247–264.

Hakala, P., Rimpelä, A., Salminen, J. J., Virtanen, S. M., & Rimpelä, M. (2002). Back, neck, and shoulder pain in Finnish adolescents: National cross sectional surveys. *British Medical Journal, 325*(7367), 743.

Harstall, C., & Ospina, M. (2003). How prevalent is chronic pain? *Pain: Clinical updates*, Volume XI, No. 2, 1–4. Available online: http://www.iasp-pain.org/AM/AMTemplate.cfm?Section=Home&CONTENTID=7594&TEMPLATE=/CM/ContentDisplay.cfm.

Hicks, C. L., von Baeyer, C. L., Spafford, P. A., van Korlaar, I., & Goodenough, B. (2001). The faces pain scale-revised: Toward a common metric in pediatric pain measurement. *Pain, 93*(2), 173–183.

Hicks, C. L., von Baeyer, C. L., & McGrath, P. J. (2006). Online psychological treatment for pediatric recurrent pain: A randomized evaluation. *Journal of Pediatric Psychology, 31*(7), 724–736.

Hotopf, M., Carr, S., Mayou, R., Wadsworth, M., & Wessely, S. (1998). Why do children have chronic abdominal pain, and what happens to them when they grow up? Population based cohort study. *British Medical Journal, 316*(7139), 1196–1200.

Howard, R. F. (2003). Current status of pain management in children. *The Journal of the American Medical Association, 290*(18), 2464–2469.

Hunfeld, J. A., Perquin, C. W., Duivenvoorden, H. J., Hazebroek-Kampschreur, A. A., Passchier, J., van Suijlekom-Smit, L. W., & van der Wouden, J. C. (2001). Chronic pain and its impact on quality of life in adolescents and their families. *Journal of Pediatric Psychology, 26*(3), 145–153.

Hunfeld, J. A., Perquin, C. W., Bertina, W., Hazebroek-Kampschreur, A. A., van Suijlekom-Smit, L. W., Koes, B. W., van der Wouden, J. C., & Passchier, J. (2002). Stability of pain parameters and pain-related quality of life in adolescents with persistent pain: A three-year follow-up. *The Clinical Journal of Pain, 18*(2), 99–106.

Huntley, E. D., Campo, J. V., Dahl, R. E., & Lewin, D. S. (2007). Sleep characteristics of youth with functional abdominal pain and a healthy comparison group. *Journal of Pediatric Psychology, 32*(8), 938–949.

IASP Task Force on Taxonomy. (1986). Part III: pain terms, a current list with definitions and notes on usage. In H. Merskey & N. Bogduk (Eds.), *Classification of chronic pain* (Second Editionth ed., pp. 209–214). Seattle: IASP Press.

Larochette, A. C., Chambers, C. T., & Craig, K. D. (2006). Genuine, suppressed and faked facial expressions of pain in children. *Pain, 126*(1–3), 64–71.

Long, A. C., Krishnamurthy, V., & Palermo, T. M. (2008). Sleep disturbances in school-age children with chronic pain. *Journal of Pediatric Psychology, 33*(3), 258–268.

Martin, A. L., McGrath, P. A., Brown, S. C., & Katz, J. (2007a). Anxiety sensitivity, fear of pain and pain-related disability in children and adolescents with chronic pain. *Pain Research and Management, 12*(4), 267–272.

Martin, A. L., McGrath, P. A., Brown, S. C., & Katz, J. (2007b). Children with chronic pain: Impact of sex and age on long-term outcomes. *Pain, 128*(1–2), 13–19.

McCaffery, M., & Pasero, C. (1999). *Pain clinical manual* (2nd ed.). St. Louis: Mosby.

McGrath, P. A., de Veber, L. L., & Hearn, M. J. (1985). Multidimensional pain assessment in children. In H. L. Fields, R. Dubner, & F. Cervero (Eds.), *Advances in pain research and therapy* (Vol. IX). New York: Raven.

McOmber, M. A., & Shulman, R. J. (2008). Pediatric functional gastrointestinal disorders. *Nutrition in Clinical Practice, 23*(3), 268–274.

Meldrum, M.L., Tsao, J.C., & Zeltzer, L.K. (2009). "I Can't Be What I Want to Be": Children's narratives of chronic pain experiences and treatment outcomes. *Pain Medicine, 10*(6), 1018–1034.

Merkel, S., Voepel-Lewis, T., & Malviya, S. (2002). Pain assessment in infants and young children: The FLACC scale. *The American Journal of Nursing, 102*(10), 55–58.

Merlijn, V. P., Hunfeld, J. A., van der Wouden, J. C., Hazebroek-Kampschreur, A. A., Koes, B. W., & Passchier, J. (2003). Psychosocial factors associated with chronic pain in adolescents. *Pain, 101*(1–2), 33–43.

Merlijn, V. P., Hunfeld, J. A., van der Wouden, J. C., Hazebroek-Kampschreur, A. A., van Suijlekom-Smit, L. W., Koes, B. W., & Passchier, J. (2005). A cognitive-behavioural program for adolescents with chronic pain-a pilot study. *Patient Education and Counseling, 59*(2), 126–134.

Merlijn, V. P., Hunfeld, J. A., van der Wouden, J. C., Hazebroek-Kampschreur, A. A., Passchier, J., & Koes, B. W. (2006). Factors related to the quality of life in adolescents with chronic pain. *The Clinical Journal of Pain, 22*(3), 306–315.

Moon, E. C., Chambers, C. T., Larochette, A. C., Hayton, K., Craig, K. D., & McGrath, P. J. (2008). Sex differences in parent and child pain ratings during an experimental child pain task. *Pain Research and Management, 13*(3), 225–230.

Mulvaney, S., Lambert, E. W., Garber, J., & Walker, L. S. (2006). Trajectories of symptoms and impairment for pediatric patients with functional abdominal pain: A 5-year longitudinal study. *Journal of the American Academy of Child and Adolescent Psychiatry, 45*(6), 737–744.

Nader, R., Oberlander, T. F., Chambers, C. T., & Craig, K. D. (2004). Expression of pain in children with autism. *The Clinical Journal of Pain, 20*(2), 88–97.

Palermo, T. M., & Chambers, C. T. (2005). Parent and family factors in pediatric chronic pain and disability: An integrative approach. *Pain, 119*(1–3), 1–4.

Palermo, T. M., Toliver-Sokol, M., Fonareva, I., & Koh, J. L. (2007). Objective and subjective assessment of sleep in adolescents with chronic pain compared to healthy adolescents. *The Clinical Journal of Pain, 23*(9), 812–820.

Passchier, J., Hunfeld, J. A., Jelicic, M., & Verhage, F. (1993). Suggestibility and headache reports in schoolchildren: A problem in epidemiology. *Headache, 33*(2), 73–75.

PedIMMPACT, McGrath, P. J., Walco, G. A., Turk, D. C., Dworkin, R. H., Brown, M. T., Davidson, K., Eccleston, C., Finley, G. A., Goldschneider, K., Haverkos, L., Hertz, S. H., Ljungman, G., Palermo, T., Rappaport, B. A., Rhodes, T., Schechter, N., Scott, J., Sethna, N., Svensson, O. K., Stinson, J., von Baeyer, C. L., Walker, L., Weisman, S., White, R. E., Zajicek, A., & Zeltzer, L. (2008). Core outcome domains and measures for pediatric acute and chronic/recurrent pain clinical trials: PedIMMPACT recommendations. *The Journal of Pain, 9*(9), 771–783.

Perquin, C. W., Hazebroek-Kampschreur, A. A., Hunfeld, J. A., Bohnen, A. M., van Suijlekom-Smit, L. W., Passchier, J., & van der Wouden, J. C. (2000). Pain in children and adolescents: A common experience. *Pain, 87*(1), 51–58.

Perquin, C. W., Hunfeld, J. A., Hazebroek-Kampschreur, A. A., van Suijlekom-Smit, L. W., Passchier, J., Koes, B. W., & van der Wouden, J. C. (2003). The natural course of chronic benign pain in childhood and adolescence: A two-year population-based follow-up study. *European Journal of Pain, 7*(6), 551–559.

Ramchandani, P.G., Stein, A., Hotopf, M., & Wiles, N.J.: ALSPAC STUDY TEAM. (2006). Early parental and child predictors of recurrent abdominal pain at school age: Results of a large population-based study. *Journal of the American Academy of Child and Adolescent Psychiatry, 45*(6), 729–736.

Razmus, I., & Wilson, D. (2006). Current trends in the development of sedation/ analgesia scales for the pediatric critical care patient. *Pediatric Nursing, 32*(5), 435–441.

Roth-Isigkeit, A., Thyen, U., Raspe, H. H., Stöven, H., & Schmucker, P. (2004). Reports of pain among German children and adolescents: An epidemiological study. *Acta Paediatrica, 93*(2), 258–263.

Roth-Isigkeit, A., Thyen, U., Stöven, H., Schwarzenberger, J., & Schmucker, P. (2005). Pain among children and adolescents: Restrictions in daily living and triggering factors. *Pediatrics, 115*(2), e152–e162.

Stanford, E. A., Chambers, C. T., & Craig, K. D. (2005). A normative analysis of the development of pain-related vocabulary in children. *Pain, 114*(1–2), 278–284.

Stanford, E. A., Chambers, C. T., & Craig, K. D. (2006). The role of developmental factors in predicting young children's use of a self-report scale for pain. *Pain, 120*(1–2), 16–23.

Stanford, E. A., Chambers, C. T., Biesanz, J. C., & Chen, E. (2008). The frequency, trajectories and predictors of adolescent recurrent pain: A population-based approach. *Pain, 138*(1), 11–21.

Varni, J. W., Walco, G. A., & Katz, E. R. (1989). A cognitive-behavioral approach to pain associated with pediatric chronic diseases. *Journal of Pain and Symptom Management, 4*(4), 238–241.

Vetter, T. R. (2008). A clinical profile of a cohort of patients referred to an anesthesiology-based pediatric chronic pain medicine program. *Anesthesia & Analgesia, 106*(3), 786–794.

Vetter, T. R., & Heiner, E. J. (1996). Discordance between patient self-reported visual analog scale pain scores and observed pain-related behavior in older children after surgery. *Journal of Clinical Anesthesia, 8*(5), 371–375.

von Baeyer, C. L., Forsyth, S. J., Stanford, E. A., Watson, M., & Chambers, C. T. (2009). Response biases in preschool children's ratings of pain in hypothetical situations. *European Journal of Pain, 13*(2), 209–213.

Walco, G. A., & Dampier, C. D. (1987). Chronic pain in adolescent patients. *Journal of Pediatric Psychology, 12*(2), 215–225.

Walker, L. S., Garber, J., & Greene, J. W. (1991). Somatization symptoms in pediatric abdominal pain patients: Relation to chronicity of abdominal pain and parent somatization. *Journal of Abnormal Child Psychology, 19*(4), 379–394.

Walker, L. S., Garber, J., Van Slyke, D. A., & Greene, J. W. (1995). Long-term health outcomes in patients with recurrent abdominal pain. *Journal of Pediatric Psychology, 20*(2), 233–245.

Weel, S., Merlijn, V., Passchier, J., Koes, B., van der Wouden, J., van Suijlekom-Smit, L., & Hunfeld, J. (2005). Development and psychometric properties of a pain-related problem list for adolescents (PPL). *Patient Education and Counseling, 58*(2), 209–215.

Zeltzer, L., Bursch, B., & Walco, G. (1997). Pain responsiveness and chronic pain: A psychobiological perspective. *Journal of Developmental and Behavioral Pediatrics, 18*(6), 413–422.

Zuckerman, B., Stevenson, J., & Bailey, V. (1987). Stomachaches and headaches in a community sample of preschool children. *Pediatrics, 79*(5), 677–682.

Assessment Tools in Pediatric Chronic Pain: Reliability and Validity

Thomas R. Vetter

Keywords

Pain intensity scales • Perioperative and procedure-related • Pediatric health-related quality of life (pHRQOL) • (QOL) • Measurement of pediatric pain

---

Introduction

Pediatric chronic pain is a very individual and diverse human experience (Graumlich et al. 2001; Malaty et al. 2005; Schechter et al. 2003). Chronic pain has a substantial and broad adverse impact on the daily lives of children and adolescents, resulting in significantly worse physical functioning, psychological functioning, social functioning, as well as lower satisfaction with life and decreased self-perceived health status (Merlijn et al. 2006; Palermo 2000). These detrimental effects of pediatric chronic pain frequently also adversely impact parents and other family members (Eccleston et al. 2004; Jordan 2005; Palermo 2000).

The management of the multitude of chronic pain conditions that afflict children and adolescents is a complex clinical endeavor (Zeltzer et al. 1997a, b). The assessment and treatment of pediatric chronic pain and its attendant patient disability and family dysfunction ideally involves a multidimensional and thus multidisciplinary approach that is specifically tailored to the identified biomedical, psychological, and social needs of each patient and family (Bennett et al. 2000; Bursch et al. 1998; Schechter et al. 2003).

This chapter provides an overview of the specificity and validity (Table 5.1) of presently available tools for assessing the pediatric chronic pain experience. Attention will initially be focused on the applicability of acute perioperative and procedure-related pain intensity scales in pediatric chronic pain. The significance of patient function and activities of daily living in the face of pediatric chronic pain will then be discussed, which will segue into the present major emphasis on generic measures of pediatric health-related quality of life. In contrast to such generic health status measures, condition-specific pain assessment tools, particularly for neuropathic pain and headache, will in turn be reviewed. Finally, the importance of assessing a pediatric patient's pain-coping mechanisms, self-efficacy, and family dynamics will be highlighted. This review includes pertinent theoretical underpinnings in addition to practical guidelines, so as to provide the reader with insight into both the science and application of chronic pain-related assessment tools.

T.R. Vetter (✉)
Department of Anesthesiology, University of Alabama School of Medicine, Jefferson Tower 865, 619 19th Street South, Birmingham, AL 35249-6810, USA
and
Department of Health Policy and Organization, University of Alabama at Birmingham School of Public Health, Birmingham, AL, USA
e-mail: tvetter@uab.edu

B.C. McClain and S. Suresh (eds.), *Handbook of Pediatric Chronic Pain:* *Current Science and Integrative Practice*, DOI 10.1007/978-1-4419-0350-1_5, © Springer Science+Business Media, LLC 2011

Table 5.1 Operational definition of terms (Reproduced from Stinson et al. (2006). With permission from Springer)

Term	Operational definition
Reliability	The reproducibility of a measure over different occasions and is concerned with minimizing sources of random error so that measures are reproducible (Streiner and Norman 2005). In general, acceptable reliability coefficients for research and clinical purposes are ≥0.7 and ≥0.9, respectively (Portney and Watkins 2000; Streiner and Norman 2005).
(a) Inter-rater (inter-observer) reliability	The agreement between different raters/observers of an observational measure of pain (Streiner and Norman 2005).
(b) Test–retest reliability	The agreement between observations with the same individuals on at least two occasions(Streiner and Norman 2005).
(c) Internal consistency	A type of reliability that includes the average of the correlation of scores from a measure with the scores of all of the items in the measure (Streiner and Norman 2005).
Validity	Used to assess whether the scale is measuring what it is intending to measure (Streiner and Norman 2005).
(a) Face validity	Whether the pain scale includes appropriate items that appear to measure what it is proposing to measure (Streiner and Norman 2005).
(b) Content validity	The assessment of whether the items in the pain measure include the appropriate information and content (Streiner and Norman 2005).
(c) Criterion	Includes concurrent validity and predictive validity. In concurrent validity, a new pain measure is correlated with a gold standard measure which is administered at the same time. In general, correlations between the new measure and the gold standard should be at least $r \geq 0.3$–0.5. The magnitude of the coefficients is hypothesis-dependent but should not be too high as to make the new measure redundant. In predictive validity, the correlation of the measure to the criterion variable is determined at a later time (Streiner and Norman 2005).
(d) Construct	Determines the validity of abstract variables that cannot be directly observed, such as pain. These constructs are assessed by their relationships with other variables (Streiner and Norman 2005) (Fitzpatrick et al. 1998; Streiner and Norman 2005).
1. Convergent validity	Evaluates how well items on a pain scale correlate with other measures of the same construct or related variables. In general, correlations between the measure and another measure of the same construct should be $r \geq 0.3$–0.5; however, the magnitude of the coefficients is hypothesis-dependent (Streiner and Norman 2005).
2. Discriminant validity	Evaluates how items on a pain scale correlate with other measures that are unrelated. In general, correlations between the measure and another unrelated measure should be $r < 0.3$; however, the magnitude of the coefficients is hypothesis-dependent (Streiner and Norman 2005).
Responsivity	Measures whether the measure is able to identify changes in pain over time that is clinically important to patients. An acceptable effect size should be ≥0.5; however, the effect size is hypothesis-dependent (Guyatt et al. 1989; Liang 2000).
Interpretability	The meaningfulness of the scores obtained from a pain measure (Fitzpatrick et al. 1998).
Feasibility	How easily a pain measure can be scored and interpreted (Stevens and Gibbins 2002).

Unidimensional Acute Perioperative and Procedure-Related Pain Intensity Scales

The measurement of pediatric pain conventionally falls into three basic categories: (1) patient self-report; (2) health-care provider or parent observational; and (3) physiological (Stinson et al. 2006; von Baeyer and Spagrud 2007; Walco et al. 2005). Each of these three approaches measures a different basic construct or aspect of pain – namely, the personal pain experience, outward behavioral distress, and associated sympathetic arousal, respectively – thus often resulting in discordant values (von Baeyer and Spagrud 2007; Walco et al. 2005). A unidimensional scale is innately intended to measure only one clinical element or variable.

It has been further proposed that the ideal pain scale is one that is both designed and demonstrated to be a unidimensional measure only of pain intensity (von Baeyer and Spagrud 2007).

However, pediatric chronic pain is frequently difficult for patients and their parents to describe adequately using simply a self-report or an observational unidimensional pain intensity scale (Gaffney et al. 2003; Stevens 1994). Nevertheless, as with adult chronic pain, given their ease of use and clinicians' widespread familiarity with them, acute perioperative and procedure-related unidimensional pain intensity scales (e.g., a 0–10 numerical rating scale) are often applied clinically in pediatric chronic pain conditions. The fundamental question is whether any such unidimensional pain intensity scales have demonstrated adequate validity, reliability, and responsivity (Table 5.1) in pediatric chronic pain patients. This key question has been specifically addressed by the Pediatric Initiative on Methods, Measurement, and Pain Assessment in Clinical Trials (Ped-IMMPACT) working group (http://www.immpact.org), in their process of formulating recommendations for core outcome domains and measures that should be considered by investigators conducting clinical trials for pediatric acute and chronic pain (Stinson et al. 2006; von Baeyer and Spagrud 2007).

On the basis of available evidence and the Society of Pediatric Psychology Assessment Task Force criteria for a "well-established assessment" (Table 5.2) (Cohen et al. 2006), the commissioned Ped-IMMPACT survey made no recommendations regarding the relative merits of *observational* pain measurement instruments for pediatric chronic pain lasting weeks, months, or years (von Baeyer and Spagrud 2007). This was reportedly primarily because the overt behavioral signs of pain that tend to habituate or dissipate over time, despite continued self-reported pain (von Baeyer and Spagrud 2007).

Of the total of 34 single-item, patient *self-report* measures of pain intensity that were identified by a second commissioned Ped-IMMPACT survey (Stinson et al. 2006), only the Faces Pain Scale (Bieri et al. 1990), Faces Pain Scale-Revised (Hicks et al. 2001), Oucher–Photographic (Beyer and Aradine 1986), Oucher-NRS (Beyer and Aradine 1986), Wong–Baker FACES Pain Scale (Wong and Baker 1988), and Visual Analogue Scale (Scott et al. 1977) had sufficient evidence of validity and reliability (Table 5.1) to be deemed a "well-established assessment" (Table 5.2) (Cohen et al. 2006) for both acute and chronic pediatric pain. These authors specifically recommended (1) the Faces Pain Scale-Revised for disease-related chronic pain in children between

Table 5.2 Society of Pediatric Psychology Assessment Task Force criteria for evidence-based assessment (Reproduced from Cohen et al. (2006). With permission from Oxford University Press)

Category	Criteria
Well-established assessment	The measure must have been presented in at least two peer-reviewed articles by different investigators or investigatory teams
	Sufficient detail about the measure to allow critical evaluation and replication (e.g., measure and manual provided or available upon request)
	Detailed (e.g., statistics presented) information indicating good validity and reliability in at least one peer-reviewed article
Approaching well-established	The measure must have been presented in at least two peer-reviewed articles, which might be by assessment the same investigator or investigatory team
	Sufficient detail about the measure to allow critical evaluation and replication (e.g., measure and manual provided or available upon request)
	Validity and reliability information presented in either vague terms (e.g., no statistics presented) or moderate values
Promising assessment	The measure must have been presented in at least one peer-reviewed article
	Sufficient detail about the measure to allow critical evaluation and replication (e.g., measure and manual provided or available upon request)
	Validity and reliability information presented in either vague terms (e.g., no statistics presented) or moderate values

4 and 12 years of age and (2) a 100 mm visual analogue scale for disease-related chronic pain in children over 8 years of age and in adolescents (Stinson et al. 2006).

A concomitantly published review applied a similar evidence-based framework for evaluating a diverse collection of acute and chronic pain assessment tools that are commonly used by pediatric psychologists not only for clinical trials but also in clinical practice (Cohen et al. 2008). Relying upon a somewhat different combination of systematic (objective) and expert opinion (subjective) methods in their selection and evaluation process, these authors included a number of measures that were omitted by the Ped-IMMPACT authors (Cohen et al. 2008). Of the 17 pediatric pain measures that were examined, 11 met the same Society of Pediatric Psychology Assessment Task Force criteria for a "well-established assessment" (Table 5.2) (Cohen et al. 2006) – with the Varni–Thompson Pediatric Pain Questionnaire being the only such instrument intended specifically for chronic pain (Cohen et al. 2008).

The Varni–Thompson Pediatric Pain Questionnaire

Initially, the Varni–Thompson Pediatric Pain Questionnaire (Varni et al. 1987), the current Pediatric Pain Questionnaire (PPQ) is a patient self-report instrument that is age-specific for a young child (5–7 years), child (8–12 years), or adolescent (13–18 years). Patterned after the McGill Pain Questionnaire (Melzack 1975), the PPQ assesses the intensity, location(s), and other more subjective characteristics of a patient's pain. The PPQ includes a 100 mm horizontal line (visual analogue scale) that is without numbers but ranges from a value of 0 (anchored either by a smiling carton face and "no hurt at all" or by "no pain, not hurting, no discomfort") to a value of 100 (anchored either by a sad cartoon face and "hurting a whole lot" or by "severe pain, hurting a whole lot, very uncomfortable").

The PPQ has been shown to be a valid and reliable tool for measuring pediatric self-reported chronic pain intensity in children as young as 5 years old (Varni et al. 1996a; Walco et al. 1999). The validity and reliability (Table 5.1) of the PPQ

was evaluated in a study of 100 children and adolescents with chronic musculoskeletal pain associated with rheumatologic disease (Gragg et al. 1996). The PPQ demonstrated a high correlation ($p < 0.01$) among parents, physicians, and patients. Parent and physician ratings of pain intensity also correlated well in this cohort with all measures of disease activity and functional status ($p < 0.001$) (Gragg et al. 1996). The PPQ has also been successfully used in 5–16-year-old inpatients and outpatients with sickle cell disease (Walco and Dampier 1990). The PPQ has historically been the most widely used comprehensive chronic pain questionnaire for children and adolescents (Rapoff 2003), especially those with musculoskeletal disorders (Schanberg and Sandstrom 1999). While it is a self-contained tool, the PPQ is intended to supplement the PedsQL Generic Core Scales that are discussed in detail below.

Even though the Pediatric Pain Questionnaire is now two decades old, it remains a very viable and applicable comprehensive chronic pain assessment tool (Vetter 2008). However, as with the visual Oucher pain scale (Beyer et al. 1992), the use of a smiling cartoon face to help anchor the left-side (no pain) of the young child and child versions of the PPQ may be problematic, given that the scale may actually measure pain affect rather than true pain intensity (Chambers and Craig 1998; McGrath et al. 1996; Schanberg and Sandstrom 1999). More recently developed unidimensional pediatric pain assessment tools have instead used a neutral face for this scale anchor (Bieri et al. 1990; Hicks et al. 2001).

Patient Function and Activities of Daily Living

Recurring episodic or persistent chronic pain frequently has a major adverse impact on the daily lives of children and adolescents (Palermo 2000; Roth-Isigkeit et al. 2005). The ultimate clinical goal of a pediatric chronic pain medicine program is the complete elimination of a patient's presenting pain. This clinical goal is unfortunately often unobtainable, with upward of 50% and 30% of pediatric chronic pain patients reporting persistent pain at 1-year and 2-year follow-up, respectively (Perquin et al. 2003). Therefore, the more pragmatic goal of a pediatric chronic pain medicine program is the prompt return of a patient to as normal and *functional* a life as possible – with an associated improvement in health-related quality of life – while at the same time reducing the attendant burden on and resulting dysfunction within the family unit (Hunfeld et al. 2002; Palermo 2000). "Most studies evaluating recurrent or chronic pain conditions among children, however, have been limited to descriptions of pain intensity and pain duration. The resulting effects of pain states and their impact on daily living have been studied only rarely" (Roth-Isigkeit et al. 2005, p. e153).

The widely recognized primary clinical goal of contemporary chronic pain management is to re-assimilate the patient as soon and as much as possible into his or her previously productive and meaningful societal role (American Medical Association 2007). For children and adolescents, this role includes not only consistent school attendance but also participation in extracurricular social and athletic activities and interaction with their family (Hunfeld et al. 2001b; Palermo 2000).

A more holistic approach to adult chronic pain management recognizes the importance of assessing and treating not only the biological but also the psychological and social factors contributing to a patient's chronic pain condition (Turk and Flor 1999). This biopsychosocial pain management model emphasizes that the "diversity in illness expression (which includes its severity, duration, and consequences for the individual) is accountable for by the interrelationships among biological changes, psychological status, and the social and cultural contexts. All of these variables shape the person's perception and response and response to illness" (Turk and Monarch 2002, p. 7).

A Multidimensional Biobehavioral Model of Pediatric Pain

A multidimensional Biobehavioral Model of Pediatric Pain (Fig. 5.1) has been developed in an attempt to account for the similar observed variability pediatric pain perception, pain behavior, and functional status (Varni 1995; Varni et al. 1996b). This multidimensional biobehavioral model was predicated on there being a number of potentially modifiable precipitants

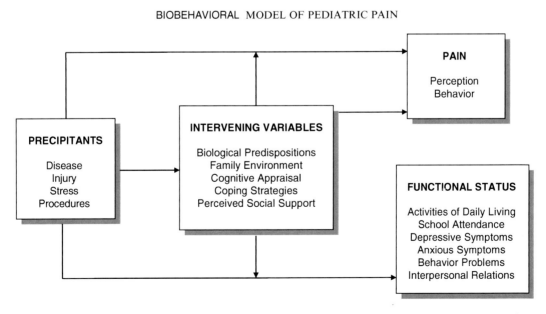

Fig. 5.1 The Biobehavioral Model of Pediatric Pain (Reproduced from Varni et al. (1996b). (With permission from Springer)

and intervening factors that contribute to pediatric pain perception and a child's associated functional status and health-related quality of life (Varni et al. 1995). It was likewise hypothesized that a bidirectional relationship and effect exist between pain perception/pain behavior and functional status. As Varni et al. (1996b) moreover noted:

> This theoretical framework is further delineated into pain antecedents, which have a causal role in pain onset or exacerbate pain intensity, pain concomitants (e.g., depression, anxiety), which occur only during a painful episode and which may be reciprocal, and pain consequences, which persist beyond pain relief and include long-term psychological, social, and physical disability. (p. 516)

The validity of this multidimensional Biobehavioral Model of Pediatric Pain was examined in a group of 8–18-year-old patients with symptomatic juvenile rheumatoid arthritis (Sawyer et al. 2005). A strong negative relationship was observed between the children's personal experience of pain (i.e., their self-reported pain intensity) and their self-reported health-related quality of life, including various aspects of functional status.

Assessing Pediatric Activities of Daily Living with Chronic Pain

In contrast to the adult population, a paucity of empirical research and clinical attention has been focused on the measurement of functional impairment vis-à-vis activities of daily living (ADLs) in children and adolescents with chronic or recurrent pain (Palermo 2000; Palermo et al. 2004). However, the valid measurement of pediatric functional impairment is crucial for better understanding the impact of pain on children's daily lives, identifying appropriate interventions, and measuring response to such interventions. Consequently, there is a clear need to assess not only a pediatric patient's chronic pain relief but also his/her ability to perform important childhood and adolescent ADLs during and following treatment (Palermo 2000; Palermo et al. 2004). Though not yet widely applied in clinical practice, at least three pediatric ADLs assessment tools have been reported in the research literature.

Functional Disability Inventory

The Functional Disability Inventory (FDI) was originally developed by Walker and Greene (1991) to assess illness-related activity limitations in children and adolescents with a variety of chronic medical conditions. The patient self-report FDI consists of 15 items addressing physical and psychosocial functioning (e.g., walking up stairs, playing with friends, and doing activities in gym) during the previous 2 weeks. For each item, the five response options range from "No Trouble" (0) to "Impossible" (4). The total FDI score is computed by summing the ratings for each item and ranges from 0 to 60. Higher scores on the FDI indicate greater disability. A parent proxy–report version of the FDI is also available, allowing parents to rate the extent of their children's disability during the past 2 weeks (Walker and Greene 1991; Walker et al. 2007).

The FDI has subsequently been widely applied in assessing functional impairment in pediatric patients suffering from chronic pain (Claar and Walker 2006; Eccleston et al. 2004), including those with headache (Lewandowski et al. 2006; Palermo et al. 2005), fibromyalgia (Kashikar-Zuck et al. 2002), juvenile rheumatoid arthritis (Reid et al. 2005), sickle cell disease (Peterson and Palermo 2004), recurrent abdominal pain (Robins et al. 2002; Walker et al. 2005), irritable bowel syndrome (Claar et al. 1999; Walker et al. 1998), and inflammatory bowel disease (Tojek et al. 2002). The FDI reportedly has well-demonstrated validity and reliability (Table 5.1) in the pediatric chronic pain population (Claar and Walker 2006).

Despite its widespread historical use as a pediatric outcomes measure, the FDI is not without limitations (Palermo et al. 2004). The FDI may not be valid in an ethnically and socioeconomically diverse pediatric population. Second, the FDI was not intended to be used as a daily report or diary instrument and thus may have more limited applicability in longitudinal pain treatment outcome research. Third, the FDI was developed based upon existing adult functional impairment measures, and it remains unclear whether these items are developmentally appropriate for children and adolescents (Palermo et al. 2004).

Child Activity Limitations Interview

Given the above purported limitations of the FDI, an apparent need existed for an additional subjective, patient self-report measure of functional impairment that would (1) contain items (questions) reflecting the specific areas of functioning of particular importance to children and adolescents with recurrent and chronic pain; (2) be valid and reliable; (3) be appropriate for use in prospective, sequential data collection (i.e., daily pain diaries) in studies of recurrent and chronic pain; and (4) be responsive to change in children's pain symptoms over time (Palermo et al. 2004). While beyond the scope of the present discussion, the robust methodology applied in designing and testing the resulting Child Activity Limitations Interview (CALI) has been well-described (Palermo et al. 2004). The CALI demonstrated face, construct, and concurrent validity (Table 5.1). Scores on the CALI were significantly related to pain symptom intensity, frequency, duration, and associated emotional upset. The CALI scores also correlated well with physician ratings of expected functional limitations and illness severity. Concurrent validity was supported by significant correlations between CALI scores and simultaneous scores on the FDI (Palermo et al. 2004).

Of note, Palermo and her colleagues (2004) insightfully sought to ensure that their questionnaire items were specific and relevant to the activities important in a given child's daily life. In the evaluation process, activities are thus eliminated that may be inapplicable and possibly inappropriate to that patient (e.g., all children may not play sports). Recognizing the wide variability among patients in their underlying interests and capabilities increased the responsivity (Table 5.1) of the CALI to a change in a patient's most pertinent activities due to pain symptom-related impairment. Using the CALI, an 8–17 year old and his/her parent are asked by a trained interviewer: (1) to choose 8 of 21 possible activities that during the previous 4 weeks were "most difficult or bothersome because of pain" and then (2) to rate each of the 8 chosen activities on a 0 ("not very difficult") to 4 ("extremely difficult") 5-point scale as to their being difficult to perform because of pain and on a 0 ("not very important") to 4 ("extremely important") 5-point scale as to their importance. The difficulty and importance ratings are summed yielding a total score ranging from 0 to 64, with higher scores indicating greater levels of activity limitation.

Child Activity Limitations Questionnaire

A paper-and-pencil version of the CALI, the Child Activity Limitations Questionnaire (CALQ), has been subsequently developed, with preliminary validity and reliability data provided by its authors (Hainsworth et al. 2007). The likely potential benefits of the CALQ include a reduction in demands on clinicians and clinical investigators, faster administration time, and greater administrative flexibility. The CALQ would appear more apropos when a clinician wants to assess quickly and serially the impact of pain on a child's day-to-day activities, without the need for trained personnel or a private meeting place for an interview. In contrast, the CALI appears more clinically applicable in serving as an introductory interaction to obtain more extensive clinical information and to allow for dialogue regarding the specifics of the child's and/or the family's expressed unique circumstances (Hainsworth et al. 2007).

Health-Related Quality of Life

In contrast to the more objective and conventional physiologic, laboratory, and radiological assessments of disease, the measurement of health-related quality of life provides more subjective but equally important information regarding the adverse effects of a chronic disease, especially one associated with pain and disability (Carr et al. 2001; Guyatt et al. 1993; Nelson and Berwick 1989). The metric of health-related quality of life can also provide clinicians with additional practical information that can be incorporated into the chronic pain treatment options presented to patients and their families (Owens 1998; Vetter 2007). Finally, despite the attendant methodological challenges, the assessment of health-related quality of life represents a vital element of pediatric outcomes research (Parsons and Mayer 2004).

However, health-related quality of life is an unfamiliar and often initially enigmatic term to many clinicians and patients (Patrick and Chiang 2000). Health-related quality of life can be better understood by examining its conceptual basis.

The Concept of Health

Health is an essential yet often difficult concept to define. Sixty years ago, the World Health Organization (WHO) classically defined health to be a state of compete physical, mental, and social well-being, and not merely the absence of disease or infirmity (World Health Organization 1948). Needless to say, such a state of complete well-being is seldom sustainable and consequently an uncommon human experience. When their health or state of complete well-being invariably gives way to illness, due to either disease, injury, genetics, personal lifestyle, socioeconomic factors or other reasons, individuals seek out health care (Patrick and Erickson 1993). Such illnesses, diseases, and injuries in children and adolescents are commonly accompanied by chronic pain that prompts medical treatment (Perquin et al. 2000a, b, 2001; Roth-Isigkeit et al. 2004).

The Concept of Quality of Life

Patients and their parents by and large seek out health care because of a perception that an affliction or malady has resulted in pain and suffering, and thus a reduction in not only health status but also attendant quality of life. Quality of life is another fundamental, albeit very subjective, concept. Quality of life intuitively conjures up happiness and satisfaction with one's life (Fayers and Machin 2000, 2007). However differently it may be defined by an individual or a group at a given point in time, quality of life also carries with it the notion of *value*, with one state of existence perceived as being if not objectively then certainly subjectively superior to another (Patrick and Erickson 1993).

The Concept of Health-Related Quality of Life

An individual's health status and quality of life are innately interconnected, thus logically giving rise to the third cardinal concept of health-related quality of life (Patrick 1998; Vetter 2007). Health-related quality of life represents the tangible application of the more general concept of quality of life in the strictly health-focused realm of clinical medicine and clinical research (Fayers and Machin 2000, 2007). Health-related quality of life concerns those attributes valued by patients, including their resultant comfort or sense of well-being; the extent to which they are able to maintain reasonable physical, emotional, and intellectual function; and the degree to which they retain their ability to participate in valued activities within the family, in the workplace, and in the community (Wenger and Furberg 1990, p. 336).

Health-related quality of life has explicitly been defined as "the value assigned to the duration of life as modified by its impairments, functional states, perceptions, and social opportunities that are influenced by disease, injury, treatment, or policy" (Patrick and Erickson 1993, p. 22).

Transforming the concept or construct of health-related quality of life into a practical and clinically applicable measurement tool requires initially identifying the various elements, formally referred to as the domains or dimensions of an individual's existence, that constitute health-related quality of life (Frytak and Kane 2006; Naughton and Shumaker 2003). The Ped-IMMPACT once again has recommended a set of core outcome domains that should be considered when designing pain clinical trials for acute pain and recurrent/chronic pain (Stinson et al. 2006; von Baeyer and Spagrud 2007). The six Ped-IMMPACT core outcome domains for acute pain include pain; global judgment of satisfaction with treatment; symptoms and adverse events; physical recovery; emotional recovery; and economic factors. The eight Ped-IMMPACT core outcomes for recurrent/chronic pain include pain; physical functioning; emotional functioning; role functioning; symptoms and adverse events; global judgment of satisfaction; sleep; and economic factors.

Health-related quality-of-life instruments are categorized as generic measures, condition-specific measures, and preference-based measures (Vetter 2007). Generic health-related quality-of-life instruments provide an overall, comprehensive perspective and thus have the ability to assess the complex continuum between well-being, disability, and death (Maciejewski 2004; McHorney 1997). Generic measures emphasize breadth over specificity by focusing on the common elements of health that transcend any one disease (Maciejewski 2006). This breadth allows generic measures to be used both in *and* across a variety of medical conditions and their related treatments.

Pediatric Health-Related Quality of Life

A growing amount of attention has been focused on the measurement of health-related quality of life in children and adolescents (Clarke and Eiser 2004; Cremeens et al. 2006; Davis et al. 2006; Eiser and Morse 2001b; Matza et al. 2004; Rajmil et al. 2004; Schmidt et al. 2002). Just as in adults, routinely assessing pediatric health-related quality of life can facilitate patient–physician communication, improve patient and parent satisfaction, identify hidden physical and psychosocial functional morbidities, and assist in point-of-service clinical decision making (Drotar 2004a; Varni et al. 2005; Vetter 2007). The measurement of health-related quality of life in pediatric clinical trials and clinical practice nevertheless remains limited as compared to the adult population (Clarke and Eiser 2004; Varni et al. 2005). "Despite considerable interest among pediatric health services researchers and their clinical colleagues, the field of HRQL research in pediatrics remains – relative to its adult counterpart – in its nascence because it has had to grapple" with identifying the best strategies to access information about children's health-related quality of life (Parsons and Mayer 2004, p. 1237).

Unique conceptual and methodological issues have impeded the standardized assessment of health-related quality of life in chronically ill children and adolescents, including those suffering from chronic pain (De Civita et al. 2005; Drotar 2004a; Matza et al. 2004). A fundamental challenge in assessing pediatric health-related quality of life is the central and complex role of child development and the associated dynamic social and psychological contexts in which a child or adolescent perceives health versus disease (Forrest et al. 2003). Parents, siblings and peers, as well as the classroom setting and the community can all play an important role in the self-perceived health-related quality of life of a child or adolescent (Matza et al. 2004). However, this methodological challenge can be overcome if sufficient consideration is given to the choice of an age-appropriate pediatric health-related quality-of-life instrument (Drotar 2004b; Eiser and Morse 2001b; Landgraf and Abetz 1996).

The use of an adult generic health-related quality-of-life measure (e.g., the 36-Item Short-Form Health Survey or SF-36) should be avoided in chronic diseases of childhood due to its likely failure to tap important pediatric health domains and its response burden (Eiser and Morse 2001c). A parental proxy assessment of a younger child's health-related quality of life is a viable alternative. However, children 8–11 years of age appear to self-report significantly lower health-related quality of life than their parents by proxy (Theunissen et al. 1998). In both, clinical research and practice, obtaining data from only either the parent or the child inherently provides a limited and potentially biased perspective (Drotar 2004b). Therefore, whenever possible the pediatric patient's own health perceptions in addition to those of a parent proxy should be elicited (Eiser and Morse 2001a). To this end, if the health survey instrument is appropriately structured, a child as young as 4 years of age can provide meaningful, even if only concrete insight into their self-perceived health-status (Riley 2004). More subjective or abstract health domains can be self-reported by subjects 8 years of age and older (Eiser et al. 2000; Matza et al. 2004).

Pediatric Generic Health-Related Quality-of-Life Measures

Based upon the three criteria of previously documented instrument validity and reliability (Table 5.1), the existence of age group–specific versions, and the availability of both a patient self-report and parent proxy–report form (Parsons and Mayer 2004), as well as the results of a recent methodical literature search (Vetter 2007), four pediatric generic health-related quality-of-life measures appear to warrant consideration in pediatric chronic pain medicine (Table 5.3).

Child Health and Illness Profile

The Child Health and Illness Profile (CHIP) (http://www.chip.jhu.edu/) has been primarily applied as a population-based measure of the effects of specific pediatric health service interventions on health status and behavior (Riley et al. 1998, 2004a, b; Starfield et al. 1995). The CHIP has also more recently been used to assess the relationship between future health-care use and a child's sense of well-being, and thus perceived health-care needs (Forrest et al. 2004). The CHIP is available in English and Spanish. The CHIP requires a minimum of 20 min to complete, making it less convenient for frequent serial administration. While the CHIP includes the health-related quality-of-life domain of physical comfort, it does not directly assess pain. In keeping with its school of public health origin, the CHIP would appear more applicable in the study of child health-care policy and the effects of not only medical but also public health and other community interventions on children's long-term health trajectories (Forrest 2004).

Child Health Questionnaire

The Child Health Questionnaire (CHQ) (http://healthactchq.com/) examines a wide array of physical and psychosocial domains, including bodily pain and discomfort (Landgraf et al. 1999). Since its inception the CHQ has been intended to be a widely applicable and multicultural instrument. Accordingly, the CHQ is available in a multitude of languages and dialects (Landgraf and Abetz 1997; Landgraf et al. 1999).

Table 5.3 Overview of pediatric generic health-related quality-of-life measurement instruments (Reproduced from Vetter (2007). With permission from Lippincott Williams Wilkins)

Instrument	Health dimensions or domains assessed	Applicable age range	Translations	Completion time	Material cost
CHIP	Satisfaction, comfort, resilience, risk avoidance, achievement	6–18 years (patient) 6–11 years (parental proxy)	Spanish	20 min (self) 20 min (parent)	Free[a,b]
CHQ	General health, change in health, physical functioning, bodily pain and discomfort, limitations in school, work, and activities with friends, behavior, mental health, and self-esteem	10–17 years (patient) 5–17 years (parental proxy)	Numerous	15–30 min (self) 7–30 min (parent)	$250[a,c]
KINDL	Physical well-being, emotional well-being, self-esteem, family, friends, and everyday functioning	4–16 years (patient) 4–16 years (parental proxy)	European	10–15 min (self) 10 min (parent)	Free[d]
PedsQL	Physical functioning, emotional functioning, social functioning, and school functioning	5–18 years (patient) 2–18 years (parental proxy)	Numerous	<5 min (self) <5 min (parent)	Free[e]

CHIP Child Health and Illness Profile, *CHQ* Child Health Questionnaire, *PedsQL* Pediatric Quality-of-Life Inventory
[a]US dollars
[b]Free only for student research project (otherwise US $250/academic study and US $1,500/commercial study)
[c]Minimum (total licensing fee based upon study design)
[d]Free only for noncommercial studies (otherwise either €200 or €400 depending on study sample size)
[e]Free only for non-funded academic study (otherwise varies from US $600/study to US $5,600/year/institution)

The CHQ has been shown to be a valid health-related quality-of-life tool in children with sickle cell disease, from both the patient and parental perspectives (Panepinto et al. 2005; Panepinto et al. 2004). However, given its substantial length and attendant respondent burden with serial administration, the CHQ is more appropriately used as a population-based pediatric health screening survey (Waters et al. 2001).

KINDL

The KINDL (http://www.kindl.org/) is based upon a conceptual model that encompasses psychological well-being, social relationships, physical function, and everyday life activities (Ravens-Sieberer and Bullinger 1998). In addition to conventional paper-and-pencil versions, two very appealing, computer-assisted, animated renditions of the KINDL known as the CAT-Screen are available (http://www.catscreen.de/). Currently maintained by the Child and Adolescent Health Group at the Robert Koch Institute in Berlin, the KINDL questionnaires are available in German, English, and nine other European languages. Only one item on the KINDL instruments directly assesses pain (Ravens-Sieberer and Bullinger 2000). To date, the KINDL has been applied in population-based, epidemiological studies of child and adolescent health, in clinical trials involving acutely and chronically ill children, and in a pediatric inpatient rehabilitation program setting (Ravens-Sieberer and Bullinger 2000).

Pediatric Quality-of-Life Inventory

The Pediatric Quality of Life Inventory (PedsQL™) (http://www.pedsql.org/) comprises a series of tools designed to measure the four primary clinical outcomes of pain intensity, generic health-related quality of life, the family impact of a chronic health condition, and parental satisfaction with medical care. The PedsQL Generic Core Scales (Version 4.0) are the principal component of the PedsQL (Varni et al. 2003). The PedsQL 4.0 Generic Core Scales are available in English, US Spanish, and a number of European languages. In a clinical research or practice setting, the PedsQL is a user-friendly instrument

that can readily be serially administered (Vetter 2008). Pain is specifically addressed within the physical function domain of the PedsQL Generic Core Scales. A 0–100 subscore can be generated for each of the four domains on the PedsQL Generic Core Scales. The Physical Functioning subscale score is conventionally reported as the PedsQL Physical Health Summary Score. The often reported PedsQL Psychosocial Health Summary Score equals the sum of the items divided by the number of items answered on the Emotional, Social, and School Functioning subscales (Varni et al. 2001).

The PedsQL has been successfully applied in a survey of health-related quality of life in childhood migraine (Powers et al. 2004) and a prospective analysis of pediatric cancer-related pain and emotional distress (Varni et al. 2004a). The PedsQL have also been effectively used to demonstrate a longitudinal relationship among health-related quality of life, pain, and coping strategies in a cohort of 8–18 year olds with juvenile idiopathic arthritis (Sawyer et al. 2004). The PedsQL has furthermore been successfully incorporated into clinical decision making in cardiology, orthopedic, and rheumatology outpatient settings (Varni et al. 2002). Like the other pediatric generic health-related quality-of-life tools, the PedsQL can be applied as school population health measure (Varni et al. 2006). Of note, the PedsQL was the most widely applied pediatric health-related quality-of-life measurement instrument in the MEDLINE database from 1966 to 2006 (Vetter 2007).

Condition-Specific Chronic Pain Assessment Tools

In contrast to the above generic health status measures, condition-specific health-related quality-of-life instruments are designed to assess specific diagnostic groups, usually with the goal of determining clinically significant responsiveness to treatment or disease progression (Patrick and Deyo 1989). Condition-specific measures are formulated to identify small incremental changes in the most relevant domains or dimensions of a particular disease (Hays 2005). This sensitivity makes condition-specific measures particularly attractive to clinicians and health outcomes researchers seeking to identify tangible interventional benefits (Atherly 2006). Depending on their design and thus targeted dimensions or domains, such chronic pain condition-specific assessment tools can generate either objective physiologic data or subjective patient-reported outcomes data. While a discussion of their individual properties and applicability is beyond the scope of this discussion, there are an ever-growing number of chronic pain condition-specific assessment tools. Representative examples for neuropathic pain (including complex regional pain syndrome) and headache will be presented here.

Neuropathic Pain and Complex Regional Pain Syndrome

Neuropathic pain is unique among chronic pain conditions in that both subjective patient-reported outcome data and more objective physiologic data from, for example, quantitative sensory testing and quantitative sudomotor axon reflex test, can be generated for its assessment (Benzon 2005; Horowitz 2007; Konen 2000; Low et al. 2006).

Complex regional pain syndrome (CRPS) is a neuropathic pain disorder of major interest to both the adult and the pediatric pain medicine community (Grabow et al. 2004; Low et al. 2007; Rho et al. 2002; Wilder 2006). Despite well over 20 years of focused research and a well-evolved treatment paradigm, the exact mechanism of CRPS remains elusive; however, peripheral sensitization of small diameter C and A delta afferent fibers to noxious stimuli appears to be the basis for the CRPS-associated hyperalgesia (Stanton-Hicks 2000, 2003). While there is no specific diagnostic laboratory test for CRPS, it has been posited that enough is now known about its pathophysiology to recommend specifically quantitative sensory testing and autonomic nervous system testing such as quantitative sudomotor axon reflex test for sweating abnormalities (Stanton-Hicks 2003).

Neuropathic Pain Intensity and Quality Scales

A series of patient-report neuropathic pain intensity and quality scales have been developed, including the Neuropathic Pain Scale (NPS) (Galer and Jensen 1997; Jensen et al. 2005, 2006; Rog et al. 2007); the Neuropathic Pain Symptoms Inventory (NPSI) (Bouhassira et al. 2004); the Leeds Assessment of Neuropathic Symptoms and Signs (LANSS) (Bennett 2001; Bennett et al. 2005; Weingarten et al. 2007); the Neuropathic Pain Questionnaire (NPQ) (Backonja and Krause 2003; Krause and Backonja 2003); and the Douleur Neuropathique 4 Questionnaire (DN4) (Bouhassira et al. 2005; Perez et al. 2007). Benzon (2005) has opportunely and succinctly stratified this constellation of neuropathic scales: (1) the NPS and NPSI evaluate the symptoms of patients with neuropathic pain, determine the efficacy of different treatments, and help elucidate the mechanism(s) of action of such treatments, whereas (2) the LANSS, NPQ, and DN4 differentiate patients with neuropathic pain from patients with non-neuropathic pain. While none of these patient-report neuropathic pain assessment tools have been formally validated in the pediatric population, it stands to reason that they can appropriately be used in symptomatic adolescent patients with normal cognitive function.

Quantitative Sensory Testing

Quantitative sudomotor axon reflex test (QST) is essentially a noninvasive computer-based method to assess thermal sensations transmitted by thinly myelinated A-delta fibers and unmyelinated C fibers, as well as vibration sensation transmitted by large myelinated A-beta fibers (Chong and Cros 2004; Meier et al. 2001). Historically, QST has had a rather broad definition, along with different commercially available QST instruments with varying specifications (e.g., thermode size and stimulus characteristics), testing protocols, algorithms, and normal values (Chong and Cros 2004). A comprehensive yet reportedly efficient QST battery and protocol have been assembled (primarily for clinical research purposes) from the wide array of published but more abbreviated quantitative sensory tests, so as to encompass measures of all the relevant sub-modalities of the somatosensory system (Rolke et al. 2006). This proposed QST battery includes cold and warm detection thresholds; number of paradoxical heat sensations during the thermal sensory limen procedure; cold and heat pain thresholds; mechanical detection threshold; mechanical pain threshold and mechanical pain sensitivity; dynamic mechanical allodynia; temporal pain summation ("wind-up"); vibration detection threshold; and pressure pain threshold (Rolke et al. 2006).

In a small-scale study of adult patients with CRPS Type 1 of a limb, quantitative mechanical and thermal sensory testing QST revealed mechanical allodynia ($p < 0.03$) and heat-pain hyperalgesia ($p < 0.04$) at their CRPS-affected site as compared to matching contralateral limb control sites (Oaklander et al. 2006). When QST values obtained in a group of 42 pediatric patients with unilateral lower extremity CRPS were compared to values previously derived from age- and sex-matched pediatric healthy controls (Sethna et al. 2007), the QST values in general did not differ significantly between the CRPS study patients and the normal reference values, except for cold and heat pain detection thresholds. Allodynia to cold and/or heat ($p < 0.001$) occurred in 50% of the pediatric CRPS patients, and cold allodynia was the most commonly observed QST abnormality (Sethna et al. 2007). Other previous QST-based studies of CRPS Type I patients have identified similar varying abnormalities (Kemler et al. 2000; Sieweke et al. 1999).

QST is a subjective and laborious process, which requires study subject/patient cooperation and thus is felt by some to yield subjective data (Oaklander et al. 2006). "QST is highly dependent on the full cooperation of the patient and may be falsely abnormal if the patient is biased toward an abnormal result or is cognitively impaired. No algorithm can reliably distinguish between psychogenic and organic abnormality" (Chong and Cros 2004, p. 744). For example, QST did not permit discrimination among subjects simulating sensory loss, subjects with normal responses, and subjects with peripheral neuropathy (Freeman et al. 2003). Therefore, despite its widespread use in neuropathic pain research, QST does not appear promising or applicable for routine clinical diagnosis (Oaklander et al. 2006), especially given that no diagnostically useful pattern has emerged from larger studies of CRPS patients (Birklein et al. 2000).

Quantitative Sudomotor Axon Reflex Test

Quantitative sudomotor axon reflex test (QSART) was developed to detect in humans, with high sensitivity, autonomic postganglionic sudomotor abnormalities by quantifying postganglionic sweat output resulting from axon reflex stimulation using acetylcholine electrophoresis (Low et al. 1983). QSART is one of a number of published quantitative autonomic tests of sudomotor, baroreceptor, vasomotor, and cardiovagal function (Hilz and Dutsch 2006; Horowitz 2007; Low and Mathias 2005). Along with resting sweat output and resting skin temperature, QSART has historically been used to diagnose reflex sympathetic dystrophy and to determine the factors predictive of a positive response to a sympathetic block (Chelimsky et al. 1995). Of note, on sudomotor testing, approximately 80% of patients with "burning feet" syndrome, the most common presentation of small-fiber neuropathy (DSFN), also have abnormal QSART responses (Low et al. 2006; Stewart et al. 1992). More recently, QSART has been employed in human research on the presumed in part sudomotor mechanism of CRPS (Birklein et al. 1997, 1998; Chemali et al. 2001; Sandroni et al. 1998). However, a positive result on QSART is not a sine qua non for a diagnosis of CRPS (Horowitz 2007; Wasner et al. 2003).

Headache

A tangible amount of research attention has been focused on health-related quality-of-life issues in pediatric and adolescent patients suffering from headaches (Bandell-Hoekstra et al. 2000, 2001). This is not surprising in light of the high prevalence of headache in this age group (Perquin et al. 2000a). Hunfeld et al. (2001a) compared a group of adolescents suffering from chronic headaches with a similar group of adolescents suffering from either chronic abdominal pain, back pain, or limb pain. They observed that the adolescent headache patients reported the poorest quality of life, as measured by the Quality of Life Pain-Youth Questionnaire. The headache patients also exhibited the greatest amount of school absenteeism. A subsequent study of children with chronic headaches reinforced the previously proposed complex relationship between pediatric headaches, patient quality of life, coping strategies, and both personal and situational factors (Frare et al. 2002). Affecting between 5% and 7% of adolescents, migraine headaches are especially problematic in the 12–17-year-old age group, due to an even greater reduction in quality of life and attendant patient disability (Tkachuk et al. 2003).

Headache Impact Test

Developed by a panel of headache clinicians and the psychometric team that developed the SF-36, the Headache Impact Test (HIT-6) (http://www. headachetest.com/) measures the impact of headaches on a patient's ability to function on the job, at home, at school, and in social situations (Bayliss and Batenhorst 2002). The HIT-6 was developed using the more contemporary Item Response Theory (IRT) (Bjorner et al. 2003a, b, c). IRT allowed for the systematic selection of only six items (i.e., headache-related questions) from an existing pool of 54 questionnaire items and 35 other items proposed by a panel of headache clinicians. The resulting condition-specific health-related quality-of-life measure is intended for both screening and monitoring of headache patients in clinical research and practice (Kosinski et al. 2003a, b).

Each of the six headache-specific questions on the HIT-6 is answered on a 5-point Likert scale (never, rarely, sometimes, very often, and always). The total score on the HIT-6 ranges from 36 ("never" an adverse headache impact on all six questions) to 78 ("always" an adverse headache impact on all six questions). The six questions on the HIT-6 are cognitively appropriate for an early adolescent. The HIT-6 can be completed in 2–3 min and thus poses minimal respondent burden. The HIT-6 is available in 28 languages and dialects. In a neurology-based headache clinic setting, the HIT-6 has exhibited satisfactory internal consistency and construct validity comparable to the gold-standard SF-36 (Kawata et al. 2005).

Pediatric Pain Coping Mechanisms, Self-Efficacy, and Family Dynamics

There is an increasing recognition of the importance of assessing pain-coping mechanisms, self-efficacy, and family dynamics in children and adolescents suffering from chronic pain conditions (Anthony and Schanberg 2007; Bursch et al. 2006; Eccleston et al. 2002; Palermo 2000). Family and situational factors in particular can play a major role in the natural history of pediatric chronic illness and chronic pain (Chambers 2003; McGrath and Hillier 2003). Greater clinical attention therefore needs to be focused on consistently determining and in turn longitudinally addressing the strength of a pediatric patient's pain-coping mechanisms, self-efficacy, the presence of pain-promoting versus pain-reducing parental behaviors (i.e., family "sickness model"), and preexisting parental pain and disability, all of which appear to be valid prognosticators of eventual patient outcome (Brace et al. 2000; Chambers et al. 2002; Crushell et al. 2003; Frare et al. 2002; Kashikar-Zuck et al. 2001; Lynch et al. 2006; Peterson and Palermo 2004).

Contending with a child who is suffering from a chronic medical condition, especially one that is associated with chronic pain and disability, is also a potent parental and family stressor (Eccleston et al. 2004; Jordan 2005). Consequently, effective pediatric pain management is one of the cornerstones of the family-centered philosophy and health-care model traditionally embraced by the pediatric health-care community (Johnson et al. 1992).

Child Self-Efficacy Scale

The Child Self-Efficacy Scale has been preliminarily shown to be a valid and reliable instrument (Table 5.1) for measuring self-efficacy related to a child functioning normally when in pain (Bursch et al. 2006). The seven-item Child Self-Efficacy Scale assesses perceived ability to perform seven basic functions (e.g., make it through a day of school, do house chores, do homework) when being in pain. There are parallel content, patient self-report and parent proxy–report versions of the paper and pencil survey. The items on the Child Self-Efficacy Scale are answered/scored on a 1 ("very sure") to 5 ("very unsure") Likert scale, with a lower total score indicating greater self-efficacy.

In a cohort of 67 9–18 year olds, with predominantly abdominal pain, headaches, and back pain (Bursch et al. 2006), the Child Self-Efficacy Scale demonstrated excellent reliability (Cronbach's coefficient $\alpha = 0.89$ for the final child version and Cronbach's coefficient $\alpha = 0.90$ for the final parent version). Strong evidence for construct validity was supported by 23 of 27 hypothesized correlations with benchmark values from the simultaneous administered Children's Health Questionnaire (Landgraf et al. 1999), Children's Somatization Inventory (Walker et al. 1991), and Pediatric Symptom Checklist (Jellinek et al. 1986).

PedsQL Family Impact Module

The PedsQL Family Impact Module has been preliminarily shown to be a valid and reliable instrument (Table 5.1) for measuring the effects of a complex chronic pediatric health condition on the parents and family (Varni et al. 2004b). The 36-item PedsQL Family Impact Module assesses the parent's own self-reported physical, emotional, social, and cognitive functioning, communication, and worry, in addition to the parent's perspective on family daily activities and family relationships. The items on the PedsQL Family Impact Module are reverse-scored and linearly transformed to a 0–100 scale, so that higher scores indicate better functioning (less negative family impact) (Varni et al. 2004b).

When administered to 23 families of children with complex chronic health conditions, internal consistency reliability was observed for the PedsQL Family Impact Module Total Scale Score (Cronbach's coefficient $\alpha = 0.97$), Parent HRQOL Summary Score (Cronbach's coefficient $\alpha = 0.96$), and Family Functioning Summary Score (Cronbach's coefficient $\alpha = 0.90$) (Varni et al. 2004b).

Conclusions

Pediatric chronic pain is both an individual and a public health concern (Vetter 2008). The clinical services and expertise exist to address the range of biomedical, psychological, and social aspects of pediatric chronic pain. The issue often at hand is how best to allocate finite institutional and societal resources so as to bridge the gap between the present reality and ideal clinical management.

Like any clinical endeavor, in order for a pediatric chronic pain medicine program to succeed, sufficient patient care resources need to be allocated by health-care organizations. This allocation of health-care resources must be diligently examined and justified. While this allocation of resources can at least initially be justified intuitively or via a survey or needs assessment of the targeted patient population, a longitudinal positive impact on the targeted patient population must also be demonstrated via formal health program evaluation. Such population-based health services research require the timely and sequential collection of relevant and valid patient self-reported *and* parent proxy–reported clinical outcomes data.

Measuring chronic pain intensity is no longer simply enough. There is a need to measure multiple domains of functioning, even if the connections between pain intensity, physical disability, and adaptive functioning are not as strong or consistent as might be expected (Gauntlett-Gilbert and Eccleston 2007). Pediatric chronic pain patients exhibit a significant degree of pain-related disability that is correlated not only with pain intensity, but also with comorbid patient depression and a dysfunctional parental relationship. The intuitive linear relationship that pain leads to functional disability, which in turn leads to diminished social and adaptive functioning, however, appears to be only partially true (Gauntlett-Gilbert and Eccleston 2007). The exact relationship between pain and psychosocial factors such as depression and parent–child interactions remains enigmatic (Gauntlett-Gilbert and Eccleston 2007). Nonetheless, it is clear that these psychosocial factors nevertheless play an important clinical role in the disability associated with and, thus, the optimal treatment of pediatric chronic pain.

References

American Medical Association (2007). *Assessing & treating persistent nonmalignant pain: An overview.* Retrieved December 25, 2007, from http://www.ama-cmeonline.com/pain_mgmt/module07/index.htm.

Anthony, K. K., & Schanberg, L. E. (2007). Assessment and management of pain syndromes and arthritis pain in children and adolescents. *Rheumatic Diseases Clinics of North America, 33*(3), 625–660.

Atherly, A. (2006). Condition-specific measures. In R. L. Kane (Ed.), *Understanding health care outcomes research* (2nd ed., pp. 165–183). Boston: Jones and Bartlett.

Backonja, M. M., & Krause, S. J. (2003). Neuropathic pain questionnaire – short form. *Clinical Journal of Pain, 19*(5), 315–316.

Bandell-Hoekstra, I. E., Abu-Saad, H. H., Passchier, J., & Knipschild, P. (2000). Recurrent headache, coping, and quality of life in children: A review. *Headache, 40*(5), 357–370.

Bandell-Hoekstra, I. E., Abu-Saad, H. H., Passchier, J., Frederiks, C. M., Feron, F. J., & Knipschild, P. (2001). Prevalence and characteristics of headache in Dutch schoolchildren. *European Journal of Pain, 5*(2), 145–153.

Bayliss, M. S., & Batenhorst, A. S. (2002). *The HIT-6: A user's guide.* Lincoln: QualityMetric.

Bennett, M. I. (2001). The LANSS Pain Scale: The Leeds assessment of neuropathic symptoms and signs. *Pain, 92*(1–2), 147–157.

Bennett, S. M., Huntsman, E., & Lilley, C. M. (2000). Parent perceptions of the impact of chronic pain in children and adolescents. *Children's Health Care, 29*(3), 174–159.

Bennett, M. I., Smith, B. H., Torrance, N., & Potter, J. (2005). The S-LANSS score for identifying pain of predominantly neuropathic origin: Validation for use in clinical and postal research. *Journal of Pain, 6*(3), 149–158.

Benzon, H. T. (2005). The neuropathic pain scales. *Regional Anesthesia and Pain Medicine, 30*(5), 417–421.

Beyer, J. E., & Aradine, C. R. (1986). Content validity of an instrument to measure young children's perceptions of the intensity of their pain. *Journal of Pediatric Nursing, 1*(6), 386–395.

Beyer, J. E., Denyes, M. J., & Villarruel, A. M. (1992). The creation, validation, and continuing development of the Oucher: A measure of pain intensity in children. *Journal of Pediatric Nursing, 7*(5), 335–346.

Bieri, D., Reeve, R. A., Champion, G. D., Addicoat, L., & Ziegler, J. B. (1990). The Faces Pain Scale for the self-assessment of the severity of pain experienced by children: Development, initial validation, and preliminary investigation for ratio scale properties. *Pain, 41*(2), 139–150.

Birklein, F., Sittl, R., Spitzer, A., Claus, D., Neundorfer, B., & Handwerker, H. O. (1997). Sudomotor function in sympathetic reflex dystrophy. *Pain, 69*(1–2), 49–54.

Birklein, F., Riedl, B., Claus, D., & Neundorfer, B. (1998). Pattern of autonomic dysfunction in time course of complex regional pain syndrome. *Clinical Autonomic Research, 8*(2), 79–85.

Birklein, F., Riedl, B., Sieweke, N., Weber, M., & Neundorfer, B. (2000). Neurological findings in complex regional pain syndromes–analysis of 145 cases. *Acta Neurologica Scandinavica, 101*(4), 262–269.

Bjorner, J. B., Kosinski, M., & Ware, J. E., Jr. (2003a). Calibration of an item pool for assessing the burden of headaches: An application of item response theory to the headache impact test (HIT). *Quality of Life Research, 12*(8), 913–933.

Bjorner, J. B., Kosinski, M., & Ware, J. E., Jr. (2003b). The feasibility of applying item response theory to measures of migraine impact: A re-analysis of three clinical studies. *Quality of Life Research, 12*(8), 887–902.

Bjorner, J. B., Kosinski, M., & Ware, J. E., Jr. (2003c). Using item response theory to calibrate the Headache Impact Test (HIT) to the metric of traditional headache scales. *Quality of Life Research, 12*(8), 981–1002.

Bouhassira, D., Attal, N., Fermanian, J., Alchaar, H., Gautron, M., Masquelier, E., Rostaing, S., Lanteri-Minet, M., Collin, E., Grisart, J., & Boureau, F. (2004). Development and validation of the Neuropathic Pain Symptom Inventory. *Pain, 108*(3), 248–257.

Bouhassira, D., Attal, N., Alchaar, H., Boureau, F., Brochet, B., Bruxelle, J., Cunin, G., Fermanian, J., Ginies, P., Grun-Overdyking, A., Jafari-Schluep, H., Lanteri-Minet, M., Laurent, B., Mick, G., Serrie, A., Valade, D., & Vicaut, E. (2005). Comparison of pain syndromes associated with nervous or somatic lesions and development of a new neuropathic pain diagnostic questionnaire (DN4). *Pain, 114*(1–2), 29–36.

Brace, M. J., Scott Smith, M., McCauley, E., & Sherry, D. D. (2000). Family reinforcement of illness behavior: A comparison of adolescents with chronic fatigue syndrome, juvenile arthritis, and healthy controls. *Journal of Developmental and Behavioral Pediatrics, 21*(5), 332–339.

Bursch, B., Walco, G. A., & Zeltzer, L. (1998). Clinical assessment and management of chronic pain and pain-associated disability syndrome. *Journal of Developmental and Behavioral Pediatrics, 19*(1), 45–53.

Bursch, B., Tsao, J. C., Meldrum, M., & Zeltzer, L. K. (2006). Preliminary validation of a self-efficacy scale for child functioning despite chronic pain (child and parent versions). *Pain, 125*(1–2), 35–42.

Carr, A. J., Gibson, B., & Robinson, P. G. (2001). Measuring quality of life: is quality of life determined by expectations or experience? *British Medical Journal (Clinical Research Ed.), 322*(7296), 1240–1243.

Chambers, C. T. (2003). The role of family factors in pediatric pain. In P. J. McGrath & G. A. Finley (Eds.), *Pediatric pain: Biological and social context* (pp. 99–103). Seattle: IASP Press.

Chambers, C. T., & Craig, K. D. (1998). An intrusive impact of anchors in children's faces pain scales. *Pain, 78*(1), 27–37.

Chambers, C. T., Craig, K. D., & Bennett, S. M. (2002). The impact of maternal behavior on children's pain experiences: An experimental analysis. *Journal of Pediatric Psychology, 27*(3), 293–301.

Chelimsky, T. C., Low, P. A., Naessens, J. M., Wilson, P. R., Amadio, P. C., & O'Brien, P. C. (1995). Value of autonomic testing in reflex sympathetic dystrophy. *Mayo Clinic Proceedings, 70*(11), 1029–1040.

Chemali, K. R., Gorodeski, R., & Chelimsky, T. C. (2001). Alpha-adrenergic supersensitivity of the sudomotor nerve in complex regional pain syndrome. *Annals of Neurology, 49*(4), 453–459.

Chong, P. S., & Cros, D. P. (2004). Technology literature review: Quantitative sensory testing. *Muscle and Nerve, 29*(5), 734–747.

Claar, R. L., & Walker, L. S. (2006). Functional assessment of pediatric pain patients: Psychometric properties of the functional disability inventory. *Pain, 121*(1–2), 77–84.

Claar, R. L., Walker, L. S., & Smith, C. A. (1999). Functional disability in adolescents and young adults with symptoms of irritable bowel syndrome: The role of academic, social, and athletic competence. *Journal of Pediatric Psychology, 24*(3), 271–280.

Clarke, S. A., & Eiser, C. (2004). The measurement of health-related quality of life (QOL) in paediatric clinical trials: A systematic review. *Health and Quality of Life Outcomes, 2*, 66.

Cohen, L. L., La Greca, A. M., Blount, R. L., Kazak, A. E., Holmbeck, G. N., & Lemanek, K. L. (2006). Introduction to special issue: Evidence-based assessment in pediatric psychology. *Journal of Pediatric Psychology, 33*(9), 911–915.

Cohen, L. L., Lemanek, K., Blount, R. L., Dahlquist, L. M., Lim, C. S., Palermo, T. M., McKenna, K. D., & Weiss, K. E. (2008). Evidence-based assessment of pediatric pain. *Journal of Pediatric Psychology, 33*, 939–955.

Cremeens, J., Eiser, C., & Blades, M. (2006). Characteristics of health-related self-report measures for children aged three to eight years: A review of the literature. *Quality of Life Research, 15*(4), 739–754.

Crushell, E., Rowland, M., Doherty, M., Gormally, S., Harty, S., Bourke, B., & Drumm, B. (2003). Importance of parental conceptual model of illness in severe recurrent abdominal pain. *Pediatrics, 112*(6 Pt 1), 1368–1372.

Davis, E., Waters, E., Mackinnon, A., Reddihough, D., Graham, H. K., Mehmet-Radji, O., & Boyd, R. (2006). Paediatric quality of life instruments: A review of the impact of the conceptual framework on outcomes. *Developmental Medicine and Child Neurology, 48*(4), 311–318.

De Civita, M., Regier, D., Alamgir, A. H., Anis, A. H., Fitzgerald, M. J., & Marra, C. A. (2005). Evaluating health-related quality-of-life studies in paediatric populations: Some conceptual, methodological and developmental considerations and recent applications. *Pharmacoeconomics, 23*(7), 659–685.

Drotar, D. (2004a). Measuring child health: Scientific questions, challenges, and recommendations. *Ambulatory Pediatrics, 4*(4 Suppl), 353–357.

Drotar, D. (2004b). Validating measures of pediatric health status, functional status, and health-related quality of life: Key methodological challenges and strategies. *Ambulatory Pediatrics, 4*(4 Suppl), 358–364.

Eccleston, C., Morley, S., Williams, A., Yorke, L., & Mastroyannopoulou, K. (2002). Systematic review of randomised controlled trials of psychological therapy for chronic pain in children and adolescents, with a subset meta-analysis of pain relief. *Pain, 99*(1–2), 157–165.

Eccleston, C., Crombez, G., Scotford, A., Clinch, J., & Connell, H. (2004). Adolescent chronic pain: Patterns and predictors of emotional distress in adolescents with chronic pain and their parents. *Pain, 108*(3), 221–229.

Eiser, C., & Morse, R. (2001a). Can parents rate their child's health-related quality of life? Results of a systematic review. *Quality of Life Research, 10*(4), 347–357.

Eiser, C., & Morse, R. (2001b). The measurement of quality of life in children: Past and future perspectives. *Journal of Developmental and Behavioral Pediatrics, 22*(4), 248–256.

Eiser, C., & Morse, R. (2001c). Quality-of-life measures in chronic diseases of childhood. *Health Technology Assessment, 5*(4), 1–157.

Eiser, C., Mohay, H., & Morse, R. (2000). The measurement of quality of life in young children. *Child: Care, Health and Development, 26*(5), 401–414.

Fayers, P. M., & Machin, D. (2000). *Quality of life: Assessment, analysis, and interpretation.* West Essex: Wiley.

Fayers, P. M., & Machin, D. (2007). *Quality of life: Assessment, analysis, and interpretation of patient-reported outcomes.* Hoboken: Wiley.

Fitzpatrick, R., Davey, C., Buxton, M. J., & Jones, D. R. (1998). Evaluating patient-based outcome measures for use in clinical trials. *Health Technology Assessment, 2*(14), 1–74. i–iv.

Forrest, C. B. (2004). Outcomes research on children, adolescents, and their families: Directions for future inquiry. *Medical Care, 42*(4 Suppl), 19–23. III.

Forrest, C. B., Shipman, S. A., Dougherty, D., & Miller, M. R. (2003). Outcomes research in pediatric settings: Recent trends and future directions. *Pediatrics, 111*(1), 171–178.

Forrest, C. B., Riley, A. W., Vivier, P. M., Gordon, N. P., & Starfield, B. (2004). Predictors of children's healthcare use: The value of child versus parental perspectives on healthcare needs. *Medical Care, 42*(3), 232–238.

Frare, M., Axia, G., & Battistella, P. A. (2002). Quality of life, coping strategies, and family routines in children with headache. *Headache, 42*(10), 953–962.

Freeman, R., Chase, K. P., & Risk, M. R. (2003). Quantitative sensory testing cannot differentiate simulated sensory loss from sensory neuropathy. *Neurology, 60*(3), 465–470.

Frytak, J. R., & Kane, R. L. (2006). Measurement. In R. L. Kane (Ed.), *Understanding health care outcomes research* (2nd ed., pp. 83–120). Boston: Jones and Bartlett.

Gaffney, A., McGrath, P. A., & Dick, B. (2003). Measuring pain in children: Developmental and instrument issues. In N. L. Schechter, C. B. Berde, & M. Yaster (Eds.), *Pain in infants, children, and adolescents* (2nd ed., pp. 128–141). Philadelphia: Lippincott Williams & Wilkins.

Galer, B. S., & Jensen, M. P. (1997). Development and preliminary validation of a pain measure specific to neuropathic pain: The Neuropathic Pain Scale. *Neurology, 48*(2), 332–338.

Gauntlett-Gilbert, J., & Eccleston, C. (2007). Disability in adolescents with chronic pain: Patterns and predictors across different domains of functioning. *Pain, 131*(1–2), 132–141.

Grabow, T. S., Christo, P. J., & Raja, S. N. (2004). Complex regional pain syndrome: Diagnostic controversies, psychological dysfunction, and emerging concepts. *Advances in Psychosomatic Medicine, 25*, 89–101.

Gragg, R. A., Rapoff, M. A., Danovsky, M. B., Lindsley, C. B., Varni, J. W., Waldron, S. A., & Bernstein, B. H. (1996). Assessing chronic musculoskeletal pain associated with rheumatic disease: Further validation of the pediatric pain questionnaire. *Journal of Pediatric Psychology, 21*(2), 237–250.

Graumlich, S. E., Powers, S. W., Byars, K. C., Schwarber, L. A., Mitchell, M. J., & Kalinyak, K. A. (2001). Multidimensional assessment of pain in pediatric sickle cell disease. *Journal of Pediatric Psychology, 26*(4), 203–214.

Guyatt, G. H., Deyo, R. A., Charlson, M., Levine, M. N., & Mitchell, A. (1989). Responsiveness and validity in health status measurement: A clarification. *Journal of Clinical Epidemiology, 42*(5), 403–408.

Guyatt, G. H., Feeny, D. H., & Patrick, D. L. (1993). Measuring health-related quality of life. *Annals of Internal Medicine, 118*(8), 622–629.

Hainsworth, K. R., Davies, W. H., Khan, K. A., & Weisman, S. J. (2007). Development and preliminary validation of the child activity limitations questionnaire: Flexible and efficient assessment of pain-related functional disability. *Journal of Pain, 8*(9), 746–752.

Hays, R. D. (2005). Generic versus disease-targeted instruments. In P. Fayers & R. Hays (Eds.), *Assessing quality of life in clinical trials* (2nd ed., pp. 3–8). New York: Oxford University Press.

Hicks, C. L., von Baeyer, C. L., Spafford, P. A., van Korlaar, I., & Goodenough, B. (2001). The Faces Pain Scale-Revised: Toward a common metric in pediatric pain measurement. *Pain, 93*(2), 173–183.

Hilz, M. J., & Dutsch, M. (2006). Quantitative studies of autonomic function. *Muscle and Nerve, 33*(1), 6–20.

Horowitz, S. H. (2007). The diagnostic workup of patients with neuropathic pain. *Medical Clinics of North America, 91*(1), 21–30.

Hunfeld, J. A., Passchier, J., Perquin, C. W., Hazebroek-Kampschreur, A. A., van Suijlekom-Smit, L. W., & van der Wouden, J. C. (2001a). Quality of life in adolescents with chronic pain in the head or at other locations. *Cephalalgia, 21*(3), 201–206.

Hunfeld, J. A., Perquin, C. W., Duivenvoorden, H. J., Hazebroek-Kampschreur, A. A., Passchier, J., van Suijlekom-Smit, L. W., & van der Wouden, J. C. (2001b). Chronic pain and its impact on quality of life in adolescents and their families. *Journal of Pediatric Psychology, 26*(3), 145–153.

Hunfeld, J. A., Perquin, C. W., Bertina, W., Hazebroek-Kampschreur, A. J. M., van Suijlekom-Smit, L. W. A., Koes, B. W., van der Wouden, J. C., & Passchier, J. (2002). Stability of pain parameters and pain-related quality of life in adolescents with persistent pain: A three-year follow-up. *The Clinical Journal of Pain, 18*(2), 99–106.

Jellinek, M. S., Murphy, J. M., & Burns, B. J. (1986). Brief psychosocial screening in outpatient pediatric practice. *Journal of Pediatrics, 109*(2), 371–378.

Jensen, M. P., Dworkin, R. H., Gammaitoni, A. R., Olaleye, D. O., Oleka, N., & Galer, B. S. (2005). Assessment of pain quality in chronic neuropathic and nociceptive pain clinical trials with the Neuropathic Pain Scale. *Journal of Pain, 6*(2), 98–106.

Jensen, M. P., Friedman, M., Bonzo, D., & Richards, P. (2006). The validity of the neuropathic pain scale for assessing diabetic neuropathic pain in a clinical trial. *Clinical Journal of Pain, 22*(1), 97–103.

Johnson, B. H., Jeppson, E. S., & Redburn, L. (1992). *Caring for children and families: Guidelines for hospitals.* Bethesda: Association for the Care of Children's Health.

Jordan, A. (2005). The impact of pediatric chronic pain on the family. *Pediatric pain letter: Commentaries on pain in infants, children, and adolescents.* Retrieved December 17, 2006, from http://pediatric-pain.ca/ppl/issues/v7n1_2005/v7n1_jordan.pdf.

Kashikar-Zuck, S., Goldschneider, K. R., Powers, S. W., Vaught, M. H., & Hershey, A. D. (2001). Depression and functional disability in chronic pediatric pain. *Clinical Journal of Pain, 17*(4), 341–349.

Kashikar-Zuck, S., Vaught, M. H., Goldschneider, K. R., Graham, T. B., & Miller, J. C. (2002). Depression, coping, and functional disability in juvenile primary fibromyalgia syndrome. *Journal of Pain, 3*(5), 412–419.

Kawata, A. K., Coeytaux, R. R., Devellis, R. F., Finkel, A. G., Mann, J. D., & Kahn, K. (2005). Psychometric properties of the HIT-6 among patients in a headache-specialty practice. *Headache, 45*(6), 638–643.

Kemler, M. A., Reulen, J. P., van Kleef, M., Barendse, G. A., van den Wildenberg, F. A., & Spaans, F. (2000). Thermal thresholds in complex regional pain syndrome type I: Sensitivity and repeatability of the methods of limits and levels. *Clinical Neurophysiology, 111*(9), 1561–1568.

Konen, A. (2000). Measurement of nerve dysfunction in neuropathic pain. *Current Review of Pain, 4*(5), 388–394.

Kosinski, M., Bayliss, M. S., Bjorner, J. B., Ware, J. E., Jr., Garber, W. H., Batenhorst, A., Cady, R., Dahlof, C. G., Dowson, A., & Tepper, S. (2003a). A six-item short-form survey for measuring headache impact: The HIT-6. *Quality of Life Research, 12*(8), 963–974.

Kosinski, M., Bjorner, J. B., Ware, J. E., Jr., Batenhorst, A., & Cady, R. K. (2003b). The responsiveness of headache impact scales scored using 'classical' and 'modern' psychometric methods: A re-analysis of three clinical trials. *Quality of Life Research, 12*(8), 903–912.

Krause, S. J., & Backonja, M. M. (2003). Development of a neuropathic pain questionnaire. *Clinical Journal of Pain, 19*(5), 306–314.

Landgraf, J. M., & Abetz, L. (1996). Measuring health outcomes in pediatric populations: Issues in psychometrics and application. In B. Spilker (Ed.), *Quality of life and pharmacoeconomics in clinical trials* (2nd ed., pp. 793–802). Philadelphia: Lippincott-Raven.

Landgraf, J. M., & Abetz, L. (1997). Functional status and well-being of children representing three cultural groups: Initial self-reports using the CHQ-CF-87. *Psychology and Health, 12*, 839–854.

Landgraf, J. M., Abetz, L., & Ware, J. E. (1999). *The CHQ: A user's manual.* Boston: HealthAct.

Lewandowski, A. S., Palermo, T. M., & Peterson, C. C. (2006). Age-dependent relationships among pain, depressive symptoms, and functional disability in youth with recurrent headaches. *Headache, 46*(4), 656–662.

Liang, M. H. (2000). Longitudinal construct validity: Establishment of clinical meaning in patient evaluative instruments. *Medical Care, 38*(9 Suppl), II84–90.

Low, P. A., & Mathias, C. J. (2005). Quantitation of autonomic impairment. In P. J. Dyck & P. K. Thomas (Eds.), *Peripheral neuropathy* (4th ed., pp. 1103–1133). Philadelphia: Elsevier Saunders.

Low, P. A., Caskey, P. E., Tuck, R. R., Fealey, R. D., & Dyck, P. J. (1983). Quantitative sudomotor axon reflex test in normal and neuropathic subjects. *Annals of Neurology, 14*(5), 573–580.

Low, V. A., Sandroni, P., Fealey, R. D., & Low, P. A. (2006). Detection of small-fiber neuropathy by sudomotor testing. *Muscle and Nerve, 34*(1), 57–61.

Low, A. K., Ward, K., & Wines, A. P. (2007). Pediatric complex regional pain syndrome. *Journal of Pediatric Orthopedics, 27*(5), 567–572.

Lynch, A. M., Kashikar-Zuck, S., Goldschneider, K. R., & Jones, B. A. (2006). Psychosocial risks for disability in children with chronic back pain. *Journal of Pain, 7*(4), 244–251.

Maciejewski, M. (2004). Generic measures. In R. L. Kane (Ed.), *Understanding health care outcomes research* (1st ed., pp. 19–52). Sudbury: Jones and Bartlett.

Maciejewski, M. (2006). Generic measures. In R. L. Kane (Ed.), *Understanding health care outcomes research* (2nd ed., pp. 123–164). Boston: Jones and Bartlett.

Malaty, H. M., Abudayyeh, S., O'Malley, K. J., Wilsey, M. J., Fraley, K., Gilger, M. A., Hollier, D., Graham, D. Y., & Rabeneck, L. (2005). Development of a multidimensional measure for recurrent abdominal pain in children: Population-based studies in three settings. *Pediatrics, 115*(2), 210–215.

Matza, L. S., Swensen, A. R., Flood, E. M., Secnik, K., & Leidy, N. K. (2004). Assessment of health-related quality of life in children: A review of conceptual, methodological, and regulatory issues. *Value in Health, 7*(1), 79–92.

McGrath, P. A., & Hillier, L. M. (2003). Modifying the psychological factors that intensify chidren's pain and prolong disability. In N. L. Schechter, C. B. Berde, & M. Yaster (Eds.), *Pain in infants, children, and adolescents* (2nd ed., pp. 85–104). Philadelphia: Lippincott Williams & Wilkins.

McGrath, P. A., Seifert, C. E., Speechley, K. N., Booth, J. C., Stitt, L., & Gibson, M. C. (1996). A new analogue scale for assessing children's pain: An initial validation study. *Pain, 64*(3), 435–443.

McHorney, C. A. (1997). Generic health measurement: past accomplishments and a measurement paradigm for the 21st century. *Annals of Internal Medicine, 127*(8 Pt 2), 743–750.

Meier, P. M., Berde, C. B., DiCanzio, J., Zurakowski, D., & Sethna, N. F. (2001). Quantitative assessment of cutaneous thermal and vibration sensation and thermal pain detection thresholds in healthy children and adolescents. *Muscle and Nerve, 24*(10), 1339–1345.

Melzack, R. (1975). The McGill Pain Questionnaire: Major properties and scoring methods. *Pain, 1*(3), 277–299.

Merlijn, V. P. B. M., Hunfeld, J. A. M., van der Wouden, J. C., Hazebroek-Kampschreur, A. A. J. M., Passchier, J., & Koes, B. W. (2006). Factors related to the quality of life in adolescents with chronic pain. *Clinical Journal of Pain, 22*(3), 306–315.

Naughton, M. J., & Shumaker, S. A. (2003). The case for domains of function in quality of life assessment. *Quality of Life Research, 12*(Suppl 1), 73–80.

Nelson, E. C., & Berwick, D. M. (1989). The measurement of health status in clinical practice. *Medical Care, 27*(3 Suppl), S77–90.

Oaklander, A. L., Rissmiller, J. G., Gelman, L. B., Zheng, L., Chang, Y., & Gott, R. (2006). Evidence of focal small-fiber axonal degeneration in complex regional pain syndrome-I (reflex sympathetic dystrophy). *Pain, 120*(3), 235–243.

Owens, D. K. (1998). Spine update. Patient preferences and the development of practice guidelines. *Spine, 23*(9), 1073–1079.

Palermo, T. M. (2000). Impact of recurrent and chronic pain on child and family daily functioning: A critical review of the literature. *Journal of Developmental and Behavioral Pediatrics, 21*(1), 58–69.

Palermo, T. M., Witherspoon, D., Valenzuela, D., & Drotar, D. D. (2004). Development and validation of the Child Activity Limitations Interview: A measure of pain-related functional impairment in school-age children and adolescents. *Pain, 109*(3), 461–470.

Palermo, T. M., Platt-Houston, C., Kiska, R. E., & Berman, B. (2005). Headache symptoms in pediatric sickle cell patients. *Journal of Pediatric Hematology and Oncology, 27*(8), 420–424.

Panepinto, J. A., O'Mahar, K. M., DeBaun, M. R., Rennie, K. M., & Scott, J. P. (2004). Validity of the child health questionnaire for use in children with sickle cell disease. *Journal of Pediatric Hematology/Oncology, 26*(9), 574–578.

Panepinto, J. A., O'Mahar, K. M., DeBaun, M. R., Loberiza, F. R., & Scott, J. P. (2005). Health-related quality of life in children with sickle cell disease: Child and parent perception. *British Journal of Haematology, 130*(3), 437–444.

Parsons, S. K., & Mayer, D. K. (2004). Health-related quality of life assessment in hematologic disease. *Hematology and Oncology Clinics of North America, 18*(6), 1235–1248.

Patrick, D. L. (1998). Quality of life and health status: Concepts and types of measures. In P. Armitage (Ed.), *Encyclopedia of biostatistics* (Vol. 5, pp. 3609–3613). West Sussex: Wiley.

Patrick, D. L., & Chiang, Y. P. (2000). Measurement of health outcomes in treatment effectiveness evaluations: Conceptual and methodological challenges. *Medical Care, 38*(Suppl), II14–25.

Patrick, D. L., & Deyo, R. A. (1989). Generic and disease-specific measures in assessing health status and quality of life. *Medical Care, 27*(3 Suppl), S217–232.

Patrick, D. L., & Erickson, P. (1993). *Health status and health policy: Quality of life in health care evaluation and resource allocation.* New York: Oxford Press.

Perez, C., Galvez, R., Huelbes, S., Insausti, J., Bouhassira, D., Diaz, S., & Rejas, J. (2007). Validity and reliability of the Spanish version of the DN4 (Douleur Neuropathique 4 questions) questionnaire for differential diagnosis of pain syndromes associated to a neuropathic or somatic component. *Health and Quality of Life Outcomes, 5*(1), 66.

Perquin, C. W., Hazebroek-Kampschreur, A. A., Hunfeld, J. A., Bohnen, A. M., van Suijlekom-Smit, L. W., Passchier, J., & van der Wouden, J. C. (2000a). Pain in children and adolescents: A common experience. *Pain, 87*(1), 51–58.

Perquin, C. W., Hazebroek-Kampschreur, A. A., Hunfeld, J. A., van Suijlekom-Smit, L. W., Passchier, J., & van der Wouden, J. C. (2000b). Chronic pain among children and adolescents: Physician consultation and medication use. *Clinical Journal of Pain, 16*(3), 229–235.

Perquin, C. W., Hunfeld, J. A., Hazebroek-Kampschreur, A. A., van Suijlekom-Smit, L. W., Passchier, J., Koes, B. W., & van der Wouden, J. C. (2001). Insights in the use of health care services in chronic benign pain in childhood and adolescence. *Pain, 94*(2), 205–213.

Perquin, C. W., Hunfeld, J. A., Hazebroek-Kampschreur, A. A., van Suijlekom-Smit, L. A., Passchier, J., Koes, B. W., & van der Wouden, J. C. (2003). The natural course of chronic benign pain in childhood and adolescence: A two-year population-based follow-up study. *European Journal of Pain, 7*(6), 551–559.

Peterson, C. C., & Palermo, T. M. (2004). Parental reinforcement of recurrent pain: The moderating impact of child depression and anxiety on functional disability. *Journal of Pediatric Psychology, 29*(5), 331–341.

Portney, L. G., & Watkins, M. P. (2000). Statistical measures of reliability. In W. M. Portney LG (Ed.), *Foundation of clinical research: Applications to practice* (2nd ed., pp. 570–586). Upper Saddle River: Prentice-Hall.

Powers, S. W., Patton, S. R., Hommel, K. A., & Hershey, A. D. (2004). Quality of life in paediatric migraine: Characterization of age-related effects using PedsQL 4.0. *Cephalalgia, 24*(2), 120–127.

Rajmil, L., Herdman, M., Fernandez de Sanmamed, M. J., Detmar, S., Bruil, J., Ravens-Sieberer, U., Bullinger, M., Simeoni, M. C., & Auquier, P. (2004). Generic health-related quality of life instruments in children and adolescents: A qualitative analysis of content. *Journal of Adolescent Health, 34*(1), 37–45.

Rapoff, M. A. (2003). Pediatric measures of pain: The pain behavior observation method, Pain Coping Questionnaire (PCQ), and Pediatric Pain Questionnaire. *Arthritis and Rheumatism, 49*(5S), S90–S95.

Ravens-Sieberer, U., & Bullinger, M. (1998). Assessing health-related quality of life in chronically ill children with the German KINDL: First psychometric and content analytical results. *Quality of Life Research, 7*(5), 399–407.

Ravens-Sieberer, U., & Bullinger, M. (2000). *KINDLQuestionnaire for measuring health-related quality of life in children and adolescents revised version (english manual).* Berlin: Robert Koch Institute.

Reid, G. J., McGrath, P. J., & Lang, B. A. (2005). Parent-child interactions among children with juvenile fibromyalgia, arthritis, and healthy controls. *Pain, 113*(1–2), 201–210.

Rho, R. H., Brewer, R. P., Lamer, T. J., & Wilson, P. R. (2002). Complex regional pain syndrome. *Mayo Clinic Proceedings, 77*(2), 174–180.

Riley, A. W. (2004). Evidence that school-age children can self-report on their health. *Ambulatory Pediatrics, 4*(Suppl(4)), 371–376.

Riley, A. W., Forrest, C. B., Starfield, B., Green, B., Kang, M., & Ensminger, M. (1998). Reliability and validity of the adolescent health profile-types. *Medical Care, 36*(8 (Print)), 1237–1248.

Riley, A. W., Forrest, C. B., Rebok, G. W., Starfield, B., Green, B. F., Robertson, J. A., & Friello, P. (2004a). The child report form of the CHIP-child edition: Reliability and validity. *Medical Care, 42*(3), 221–231.

Riley, A. W., Forrest, C. B., Starfield, B., Rebok, G. W., Robertson, J. A., & Green, B. F. (2004b). The parent report form of the CHIP-child edition: Reliability and validity. *Medical Care, 42*(3), 210–220.

Robins, P. M., Smith, S. M., & Proujansky, R. (2002). Children with recurrent abdominal pain: Comparison of community and tertiary care samples. *Childrens Health Care, 31*, 93–106.

Rog, D. J., Nurmikko, T. J., Friede, T., & Young, C. A. (2007). Validation and reliability of the Neuropathic Pain Scale (NPS) in multiple sclerosis. *Clinical Journal of Pain, 23*(6), 473–481.

Rolke, R., Magerl, W., Campbell, K. A., Schalber, C., Caspari, S., Birklein, F., & Treede, R. D. (2006). Quantitative sensory testing: A comprehensive protocol for clinical trials. *European Journal of Pain, 10*(1), 77–88.

Roth-Isigkeit, A., Thyen, U., Raspe, H. H., Stoven, H., & Schmucker, P. (2004). Reports of pain among German children and adolescents: An epidemiological study. *Acta Paediatrica, 93*(2), 258–263.

Roth-Isigkeit, A., Thyen, U., Stoven, H., Schwarzenberger, J., & Schmucker, P. (2005). Pain among children and adolescents: Restrictions in daily living and triggering factors. *Pediatrics, 115*(2), e152–162.

Sandroni, P., Low, P. A., Ferrer, T., Opfer-Gehrking, T. L., Willner, C. L., & Wilson, P. R. (1998). Complex regional pain syndrome I (CRPS I): Prospective study and laboratory evaluation. *Clinical Journal of Pain, 14*(4), 282–289.

Sawyer, M. G., Whitham, J. N., Roberton, D. M., Taplin, J. E., Varni, J. W., & Baghurst, P. A. (2004). The relationship between health-related quality of life, pain and coping strategies in juvenile idiopathic arthritis. *Rheumatology, 43*(3), 325–330.

Sawyer, M. G., Carbone, J. A., Whitham, J. N., Roberton, D. M., Taplin, J. E., Varni, J. W., & Baghurst, P. A. (2005). The relationship between health-related quality of life, pain, and coping strategies in juvenile arthritis–a one year prospective study. *Quality of Life Research, 14*(6), 1585–1598.

Schanberg, L. E., & Sandstrom, M. J. (1999). Causes of pain in children with arthritis. *Rheumatic Diseases Clinics of North America, 25*(1), 31–53. vi.

Schechter, N. L., Berde, C. B., & Yaster, M. (2003). Pain in infants, children, and adolescents: An overview. In N. L. Schechter, C. B. Berde, & M. Yaster (Eds.), *Pain in infants, children, and adolescents* (2nd ed., pp. 3–18). Philadelphia: Lippincott Williams & Wilkins.

Schmidt, L. J., Garratt, A. M., & Fitzpatrick, R. (2002). Child/parent-assessed population health outcome measures: A structured review. *Child: Care, Health and Development, 28*(3), 227–237.

Scott, P. J., Ansell, B. M., & Huskisson, E. C. (1977). Measurement of pain in juvenile chronic polyarthritis. *Annals of the Rheumatic Diseases, 36*(2), 186–187.

Sethna, N. F., Meier, P. M., Zurakowski, D., & Berde, C. B. (2007). Cutaneous sensory abnormalities in children and adolescents with complex regional pain syndromes. *Pain, 131*(1–2), 153–161.

Sieweke, N., Birklein, F., Riedl, B., Neundorfer, B., & Handwerker, H. O. (1999). Patterns of hyperalgesia in complex regional pain syndrome. *Pain, 80*(1–2), 171–177.

Stanton-Hicks, M. (2000). Complex regional pain syndrome (type I, RSD; type II, causalgia): Controversies. *Clinical Journal of Pain, 16*(2 Suppl), S33–40.

Stanton-Hicks, M. (2003). Complex regional pain syndrome. *Anesthesiology Clinics of North America, 21*(4), 733–744.

Starfield, B., Riley, A. W., Green, B. F., Ensminger, M. E., Ryan, S. A., Kelleher, K., Kim-Harris, S., Johnston, D., & Vogel, K. (1995). The adolescent child health and illness profile. A population-based measure of health. *Medical Care, 33*(5), 553–566.

Stevens, B. (1994). Pain assessment in children: Birth through adolescence. *Child and Adolescent Clinics of North America, 6*, 725–743.

Stevens, B., & Gibbins, S. (2002). Clinical utility and clinical significance in the assessment and management of pain in vulnerable infants. *Clinics in Perinatology, 29*(3), 459–468.

Stewart, J. D., Low, P. A., & Fealey, R. D. (1992). Distal small fiber neuropathy: Results of tests of sweating and autonomic cardiovascular reflexes. *Muscle and Nerve, 15*(6), 661–665.

Stinson, J. N., Kavanagh, T., Yamada, J., Gill, N., & Stevens, B. (2006). Systematic review of the psychometric properties, interpretability and feasibility of self-report pain intensity measures for use in clinical trials in children and adolescents. *Pain, 125*(1–2), 143–157.

Streiner, D. L., & Norman, G. R. (2005). *Health measurement scales: A practical guide to their development and use* (3rd ed.). Oxford: Oxford University Press.

Theunissen, N. C., Vogels, T. G., Koopman, H. M., Verrips, G. H., Zwinderman, K. A., Verloove-Vanhorick, S. P., & Wit, J. M. (1998). The proxy problem: Child report versus parent report in health-related quality of life research. *Quality of Life Research, 7*(5), 387–397.

Tkachuk, G. A., Cottrell, C. K., Gibson, J. S., O'Donnell, F. J., & Holroyd, K. A. (2003). Factors associated with migraine-related quality of life and disability in adolescents: A preliminary investigation. *Headache, 43*(9), 950–955.

Tojek, T. M., Lumley, M. A., Corlis, M., Ondersma, S., & Tolia, V. (2002). Maternal correlates of health status in adolescents with inflammatory bowel disease. *Journal of Psychosomatic Research, 52*(3), 173–179.

Turk, D. C., & Flor, H. (1999). Chronic pain: A biobehavioral perspective. In R. J. Gatchel & D. C. Turk (Eds.), *Psychosocial factors in pain: Critical perspectives* (pp. 18–34). New York: The Guilford Press.

Turk, D. C., & Monarch, E. S. (2002). Chronic biopsychosocial perspective on chronic pain. In D. C. Turk & R. J. Gatchel (Eds.), *Psychological approaches to pain management: A practitioner's handbook* (2nd ed., pp. 3–29). New York: Guilford Press.

Varni, J. W. (1995). Pediatric pain: A decade biobehavioral perspective. *Behavioral Therapist, 18*, 65–70.

Varni, J. W., Thompson, K. L., & Hanson, V. (1987). The Varni/Thompson Pediatric Pain Questionnaire. I. Chronic musculoskeletal pain in juvenile rheumatoid arthritis. *Pain, 28*(1), 27–38.

Varni, J. W., Blount, R. L., Waldron, S. A., & Smith, A. J. (1995). Management of pain and distress. In M. C. Roberts (Ed.), *Handbook of pediatric psychology* (2nd ed., pp. 105–123). New York: Guilford Press.

Varni, J. W., Rapoff, M. A., Waldron, S. A., Gragg, R. A., Bernstein, B. H., & Lindsley, C. B. (1996a). Chronic pain and emotional distress in children and adolescents. *Journal of Developmental and Behavioral Pediatrics, 17*(3), 154–161.

Varni, J. W., Rapoff, M. A., Waldron, S. A., Gragg, R. A., Bernstein, B. H., & Lindsley, C. B. (1996b). Effects of perceived stress on pediatric chronic pain. *Journal of Behavioral Medicine, 19*(6), 515–528.

Varni, J. W., Seid, M., & Kurtin, P. S. (2001). PedsQL 4.0: Reliability and validity of the Pediatric Quality of Life Inventory version 4.0 generic core scales in healthy and patient populations. *Medical Care, 39*(8), 800–812.

Varni, J. W., Seid, M., Knight, T. S., Uzark, K., & Szer, I. S. (2002). The PedsQL 4.0 Generic Core Scales: Sensitivity, responsiveness, and impact on clinical decision-making. *Journal of Behavioral Medicine, 25*(2), 175–193.

Varni, J. W., Burwinkle, T. M., Seid, M., & Skarr, D. (2003). The PedsQL 4.0 as a pediatric population health measure: Feasibility, reliability, and validity. *Ambulatory Pediatrics, 3*(6), 329–341.

Varni, J. W., Burwinkle, T. M., & Katz, E. R. (2004a). The PedsQL in pediatric cancer pain: A prospective longitudinal analysis of pain and emotional distress. *Journal of Developmental and Behavioral Pediatrics, 25*(4), 239–246.

Varni, J. W., Sherman, S. A., Burwinkle, T. M., Dickinson, P. E., & Dixon, P. (2004b). The PedsQL Family Impact Module: Preliminary reliability and validity. *Health and Quality of Life Outcomes, 2*, 55.

Varni, J. W., Burwinkle, T. M., & Lane, M. M. (2005). Health-related quality of life measurement in pediatric clinical practice: An appraisal and precept for future research and application. *Health and Quality of Life Outcomes, 3*, 34.

Varni, J. W., Burwinkle, T. M., & Seid, M. (2006). The PedsQL 4.0 as a school population health measure: Feasibility, reliability, and validity. *Quality of Life Research, 15*(2), 203–215.

Vetter, T. R. (2007). A primer on health-related quality of life in chronic pain medicine. *Anesthesia and Analgesia, 104*(3), 703–718.

Vetter, T. R. (2008). A clinical profile of a cohort of patients referred to an anesthesiology-based pediatric chronic pain medicine program. *Anesthesia and Analgesia, 106*(3), 786–794.

von Baeyer, C. L., & Spagrud, L. J. (2007). Systematic review of observational (behavioral) measures of pain for children and adolescents aged 3 to 18 years. *Pain, 127*(1–2), 140–150.

Walco, G. A., & Dampier, C. D. (1990). Pain in children and adolescents with sickle cell disease: A descriptive study. *Journal of Pediatric Psychology, 15*(5), 643–658.

Walco, G. A., Sterling, C. M., Conte, P. M., & Engel, R. G. (1999). Empirically supported treatments in pediatric psychology: Disease-related pain. *Journal of Pediatric Psychology, 24*(2), 155–167. discussion 168–171.

Walco, G. A., Conte, P. M., Labay, L. E., Engel, R., & Zeltzer, L. K. (2005). Procedural distress in children with cancer: Self-report, behavioral observations, and physiological parameters. *Clinical Journal of Pain, 21*(6), 484–490.

Walker, L. S., & Greene, J. W. (1991). The functional disability inventory: Measuring a neglected dimension of child health status. *Journal of Pediatric Psychology, 16*(1), 39–58.

Walker, L. S., Garber, J., & Greene, J. W. (1991). Somatization symptoms in pediatric abdominal pain patients: Relation to chronicity of abdominal pain and parent somatization. *Journal of Abnormal Child Psychology, 19*(4), 379–394.

Walker, L. S., Guite, J. W., Duke, M., Barnard, J. A., & Greene, J. W. (1998). Recurrent abdominal pain: A potential precursor of irritable bowel syndrome in adolescents and young adults. *Journal of Pediatrics, 132*(6), 1010–1015.

Walker, L. S., Smith, C. A., Garber, J., & Claar, R. L. (2005). Testing a model of pain appraisal and coping in children with chronic abdominal pain. *Health Psychology, 24*(4), 364–374.

Walker, L. S., Smith, C. A., Garber, J., & Claar, R. L. (2007). Appraisal and coping with daily stressors by pediatric patients with chronic abdominal pain. *Journal of Pediatric Psychology, 32*(2), 206–216.

Wasner, G., Schattschneider, J., Binder, A., & Baron, R. (2003). Complex regional pain syndrome–diagnostic, mechanisms, CNS involvement and therapy. *Spinal Cord, 41*(2), 61–75.

Waters, E. B., Salmon, L. A., Wake, M., Wright, M., & Hesketh, K. D. (2001). The health and well-being of adolescents: A school-based population study of the self-report Child Health Questionnaire. *Journal of Adolescent Health, 29*(2), 140–149.

Weingarten, T. N., Watson, J. C., Hooten, W. M., Wollan, P. C., Melton, L. J., 3rd, Locketz, A. J., Wong, G. Y., & Yawn, B. P. (2007). Validation of the S-LANSS in the community setting. *Pain, 132*(1–2), 189–194.

Wenger, N. K., & Furberg, C. D. (1990). Cardiovascular disorders. In B. Spilker (Ed.), *Quality of life assessment in clinical trials* (pp. 335–345). New York: Raven.

Wilder, R. T. (2006). Management of pediatric patients with complex regional pain syndrome. *Clinical Journal of Pain, 22*(5), 443–448.

Wong, D. L., & Baker, C. M. (1988). Pain in children: Comparison of assessment scales. *Pediatric Nursing, 14*(1), 9–17.

World Health Organization. (1948). *Constitution of the World Health Organization. Basic documents*. Geneva: World Health Organization.

Zeltzer, L. K., Bush, J. P., Chen, E., & Riveral, A. (1997a). A psychobiologic approach to pediatric pain: Part I. History, physiology, and assessment strategies. *Current Problems in Pediatrics, 27*(6), 225–253.

Zeltzer, L. K., Bush, J. P., Chen, E., & Riveral, A. (1997b). A psychobiologic approach to pediatric pain: Part II. Prevention and treatment. *Current Problems in Pediatrics, 27*(7), 264–284.

Psychiatric Considerations in Pediatric Chronic Pain

6

Mi-Young Ryee

Keywords

Anxiety and chronic pain • Somatoform Disorders • Factitious Disorder • Sick role

Introduction

The International Association for the Study of Pain defines pain as "an unpleasant sensory and emotional experience," which recognizes both the physiological and psychological aspects of pain. According to the Biobehavioral Model of Pediatric Pain (Varni 1989), biological factors (e.g., temperament, age, gender, cognitive development), family factors, cognitive perceptions, coping styles, and perception of social support work together to influence the experience of pain. Each of these cognitive, emotional, and physiological variables can have an exacerbating or ameliorating effect on pain management; therefore, each is a potential target for intervention. The psychological aspects of chronic pain have received increased attention due to concerns about the many potentially negative consequences related to pediatric chronic pain such as missed school, restrictions in daily activities and

emotional and behavioral problems (Varni 1989). In pediatric populations, the impact of chronic pain is not limited to the patient, but also affects, and is affected by, the family as well. Parents, especially, play an important role in how children and adolescents cope with pain.

The purpose of this chapter is to provide an overview of psychiatric considerations in pediatric chronic pain including the psychological factors that influence perceptions and management of chronic pain in children and adolescents, and associated psychiatric problems. In particular, there will be an exploration of the cognitive and behavioral aspects that mediate the pain experience and coping, review of psychiatric problems such as anxiety, depression, and somatoform disorders as they relate to pediatric pain, and the impact of chronic pain on school functioning.

Psychological Factors that Influence Pain Perception and Maintenance

Psychological aspects of chronic pain such as cognitive and environmental variables can shape perception and maintenance of pain-related behaviors in children and adolescents. Cognitive components include what children

Mi-Y. Ryee (✉)
Department of Psychiatry and Behavioral Sciences, Psychology, Northwestern University's Feinberg School of Medicine, Chicago, IL, USA
and
Children's Memorial Hospital, Department of Psychiatry, and Behavioral Sciences, Chicago, IL, USA
email: mryee@childrensmemorial.org

B.C. McClain and S. Suresh (eds.), *Handbook of Pediatric Chronic Pain: Current Science and Integrative Practice*, DOI 10.1007/978-1-4419-0350-1_6, © Springer Science+Business Media, LLC 2011

87

and adolescents pay attention to, and how they interpret information. Environmental aspects include how external factors including parental behavior and changes in day-to-day functioning impact children and adolescents dealing with chronic pain.

Cognitive Aspects of Pain Perception and Maintenance in Pediatric Populations

Attention

Several models have considered the role of attention on pain perception and management (Compas and Boyer 2001; Walker 1999; Zeltzer et al. 1997). Zeltzer et al. (1997) proposed that difficulty shifting attention away from pain may be an important component for children with chronic pain. Walker (1999) suggested that children's greater attention to pain exacerbates their anxiety and fear, which then intensifies their perception of pain. Some children with chronic pain exhibit other attentional patterns as well. Boyer et al. (2006) found that children with abdominal pain in their study showed attentional biases for words (presented at a subliminal level) related to social threat as well as pain. In addition to exacerbating the perception of pain, greater attention to pain-related stimuli may also take away from learning and utilizing more constructive strategies for coping with pain (Compas and Boyer 2001).

Cognitive Appraisals

The accuracy of pain-related perceptions is another important cognitive aspect of pain. More "catastrophic thinking about pain" (Vlaeyen and Linton 2000) has been associated with children's perceptions of greater pain intensity, reduced pain tolerance (Piira et al. 2002), and increased impairment of functioning (Crombez et al. 2003; Vervoort et al. 2006; Lynch et al. 2006). Catastrophizing has also been shown to affect emotional functioning, with increased catastrophic thinking linked with greater anxiety and depression (Eccleston et al. 2004).

For children with chronic pain, negative thinking overall is associated with psychological distress (Gil et al. 1991, 2001), as well as, greater report of pain intensity (Thomsen et al. 2002). Children's negative appraisals of their coping (e.g., confidence

in ability to change or adapt to stress) has also been linked to decreased likelihood of utilizing more adaptive coping strategies (Walker et al. 2007).

Environmental Aspects of Chronic Pain in Pediatric Populations

Parental Attention

Attention related to pain can be a powerful source of reinforcement (Fordyce 1989). For all children and adolescents, including those struggling with chronic pain, parental attention is an important force that helps shape behaviors. Parents can have a positive influence when they encourage adaptive coping and functional behaviors (Chambers et al. 2002). However, research has shown that greater parental attention to pain, especially solicitous attention, is associated with maintenance of pain in pediatric patients (Gidron et al. 1995). Parental reinforcement of children's pain has also been associated with greater functional disability independent of other factors contributing to pain coping including reports of stress (Whitehead et al. 1994) and perceptions of pain severity (Gidron et al. 1995). Even negative reinforcement from parents (e.g., parental frustration) has been shown to help prolong somatic symptoms in children with recurrent abdominal pain (Walker et al. 2002).

Reduction in Daily Demands

In addition to attention, changes in daily responsibilities can also impact children and adolescents' pain-related behaviors. The pain relief associated with behaviors, such as lying down, taking medication, and missing school, can reinforce these behaviors. Respite from daily tasks that may be a potential source of distress or dislike, such as schoolwork or chores, can also inadvertently reinforce pain behaviors (Allen and Mathews 1998).

Walker et al. (2002) provided a developmental perspective to the reduction in daily demands related to chronic pain and symptom maintenance in children with recurrent abdominal pain. The researchers found that limitations in daily activities and responsibilities predicted symptom maintenance in children with lower reported global self-worth and academic competence (Walker et al. 2002).

Psychiatric Comorbidity and Pediatric Chronic Pain

Research has shown the interplay between chronic pain in children and adolescents and psychiatric disorder (Konijnenberg et al. 2006; Vaalamo et al. 2002). In particular, anxiety and depression are two common psychiatric problems seen in pediatric chronic pain populations (Campo et al. 2004; Dorn et al. 2003; Martin-Herz et al. 1999). In a study of children and adolescents with abdominal pain, Mulvaney et al. (2006) found that patients who had long-term problems with pain (no symptom improvement at 5-year follow up) had greater reports of anxiety and depressive symptoms at baseline. Depression and anxiety can impact the onset and maintenance of pain in children (Martin-Herz et al. 1999) and, conversely, chronic pain can also lead to emotional distress in the form of anxiety and depression. Varni et al. (1996) identified perception of pain intensity, in particular, was associated with depressive and anxiety symptoms in their study of children and adolescents with rheumatologic diseases.

Anxiety

The association between anxiety and chronic pain has been seen in clinical (Garber et al. 1990; Hodges et al. 1985) and community-based (Egger et al. 1999; Hyams et al. 1996) samples of children and adolescents. Hodges et al. (1985) found children with recurrent abdominal pain endorsed similar levels of anxiety as children with psychiatric diagnoses. Dorn et al. (2003) found that children with recurrent abdominal pain exhibited physiological markers of stress that were more similar to a cohort of children diagnosed with an anxiety disorder than healthy controls. In children and adolescents with noncardiac chest pain, Lipsitz et al. (2004) found that youth with noncardiac chest pain exhibited higher levels of anxiety sensitivity compared to their cohorts with benign heart murmurs (Lipsitz, Masia-Warner, Apfel, Marans, Hellstern, Forand, Levenbraun, & Fyer 2004).

While the precise mechanism of how anxiety and chronic pain are related is not yet fully understood, studies have demonstrated associations between aspects of anxiety and chronic pain. Specifically, attentional bias toward internal and/or external threats (Boyer et al. 2006) and catastrophizing (Crombez et al. 2003; Vervoort et al. 2006), which are common characteristics of anxiety, are also shown to affect pediatric chronic pain. Merikangas and Stevens (1997) proposed two ways in which the link between anxiety and pain (migraine) can be considered – unidirectional (pain causing anxiety or vice versa) or shared vulnerability (anxiety and pain share common risk factors).

Depression

Many children and adolescents with chronic pain are vulnerable to depressive symptoms (Garber et al. 1990; Kashikar-Zuck et al. 2001; Mulvaney et al. 2006; Varni et al. 1996). In a heterogeneous group of children presenting in an outpatient pain clinic with diverse pain complaints (e.g., back pain, abdominal pain, limb pain, neuropathic pain, etc.), Kashikar-Zuck et al. (2001) found that most of the children in their sample endorsed mild to moderate levels of depression, and 15% of patients endorsed severe levels of depression. Specifically, maladaptive coping such as internalizing and catastrophizing in this sample of children was associated with depression (Kashikar-Zuck et al. 2001).

Risk for depression may come both from difficulties coping adaptively with chronic pain, as well as, challenges in managing the disruptions to daily life that are a result of persistent pain. Less adaptive coping with chronic pain has been associated with greater disability in children (Schanberg et al. 1996). Also, managing the interruptions to everyday events, such as, school and social activities is a common problem for pediatric management of chronic pain (Kashikar-Zuck et al. 2001). This disturbance in daily activities has been linked to depressive symptoms (Kashikar-Zuck et al. 2001). Compared to their healthy counterparts, children with chronic abdominal pain experience greater difficulties in the areas of school, home, and social functioning (Walker and Greene 1989). Interestingly, Lewandowski et al. (2006) found that functional disability was associated with depressive symptoms in their sample of children with headaches, but not adolescents. This suggests the importance of examining developmental differences between children and adolescents in relation to chronic pain and depression.

Somatoform Disorders

Somatoform disorders are a class of diagnoses that are characterized by "the presence of physical symptoms that suggest a general medical condition … and are not fully explained by a general medical condition, by the direct effects of a substance, or by another mental disorder…" (DSM-IV-TR). Two pain-specific diagnoses within somatoform disorders include Pain Disorder Associated With Psychological Factors and Pain Disorder Associated With Both Psychological Factors and a General Medical Condition. The prominent features of pain disorders include (a) severity of pain that warrants clinical attention; (b) pain that causes significant functional distress or impairment; (c) psychological factors that contribute to the onset, severity, or maintenance of pain; (d) pain not intentionally produced to maintain a "sick role" (Factitious Disorder) or for secondary gain (Malingering); and (e) pain symptoms are not better accounted for by other psychiatric disorders (DSM-IV-TR). Pain Disorder Associated With a General Medical Condition, which is not a psychiatric disorder, describes a condition when the general medical condition is the primary component of the pain presentation, and if there are psychological factors, these factors are not deemed to have a significant role on the onset, severity, or maintenance of pain (DSM-IV-TR).

Conversion Disorder and Somatoform Disorder Not Otherwise Specified are two other somatoform disorders that may also be seen in children and teenagers with chronic pain. Pain is not a necessary component for diagnosis, but may be present along with other physical complaints. Similar to pain disorders, Conversion Disorder and Somatoform

Disorder Not Otherwise Specified, are characterized by (a) the unintentional (subconscious) manifestations of somatic symptoms without a clear medical cause (after full evaluation), not related to the effects of substances and not better accounted for as a common practice within a specific culture; (b) symptoms cause significant functional distress or impairment; and (c) psychological factors contribute to the onset, severity, or maintenance of pain symptoms (DSM-IV-TR). Conversion Disorder involves sensory or motor symptoms suggestive of a neurologic or other general medical condition (e.g., problems with walking, swallowing, seizure-like episodes, etc.) while Somatoform Disorder Not Otherwise Specified involves more general physical complaints (e.g., fatigue, gastrointestinal complaints, appetite changes, etc.).

Kozlowska et al. (2007) found that separation/loss (e.g., separation from a parent, death of a loved one) and family conflict/violence were the most commonly reported life stressors among their sample of children and adolescents with Conversion Disorder. Although there is no clear etiology for somatoform disorders, oftentimes, an emotional conflict or stressor is thought to be related to the onset and maintenance of somatic symptoms.

Given that physical complaints, and/or pain specifically, are key components of somatoform disorders, children and teenagers with somatoform disorders often present initially to their primary care physician or medical subspecialists. The complicated relationship between psychological and physical factors can make the diagnosis and treatment of somatoform disorders challenging for health professionals within and outside of mental health.

Treatment

Psychological interventions can target several different aspects of chronic pain in pediatric populations. Cognitive and behavioral skills are often used together to encourage adaptive coping with pain. Cognitive-behavioral therapies have been shown to help reduce pain in children with recurrent abdominal pain (Sanders et al. 1994), fibromyalgia (Degotardi et al. 2006), and rheumatoid arthritis (Walco et al. 1992). Distraction has many forms and can help divert attention away from pain. Children and adolescents can engage in passive (e.g., being read a book by a parent) or active distraction (e.g., playing a video game) that help take their thoughts away from pain. Guided imagery can also serve as a distraction tool that can direct attention away from pain, or channel it toward adaptive management. Walco and colleagues (Walco et al. 1992) used imagery, both thinking of pleasant scenes and images focused specifically on pain reduction or elimination (e.g., "pain switches"), which combined with progressive muscle relaxation, and meditative breathing helped with pain reduction in children with juvenile rheumatoid arthritis. Biofeedback, which encourages increased awareness and control of physiological variables (e.g., heart rate, temperature, muscle tension, etc.) can be directed toward greater relaxation (Holden et al. 1998; Lavigne et al. 1992) or targeting specific areas/functions that may be contributing to pain (Gauthier et al. 1996).

Gil and colleagues (Gil et al. 1997, 2001) found calming self-statements combined with various relaxation techniques (deep breathing, imagery, and counting relaxation), led to immediate reduction in negative thinking and pain reports in children with sickle cell disease during a laboratory pain task. Similarly, Sanders and colleagues showed that encouraging self-statements, along with relaxation and distraction were successful in pain reduction for children with recurrent abdominal pain, compared to children on a wait-list (Sanders et al. 1989) and children receiving standard pediatric care (continued follow-up with a gastroenterologist who provided reassurance of a lack of serious medical cause and encouraged parents to permit children to return to full activities) (Sanders et al. 1994).

Another focus of treatment may include addressing any underlying psychological factors contributing to the maintenance of the somatic presentation, for example, parent–child relationship, concerns about school re-entry, etc. Behavioral interventions such as differential attention and providing reinforcement of functional behaviors encourage use of adaptive coping while minimizing secondary gains.

While there are no controlled outcome studies of somatoform disorders in pediatrics, there is a literature of case reports or case series that link successful outcomes to a rehabilitative approach to treatment (Brazier and Venning 1997). Depending on the nature and severity of the pain difficulties, a combination of physical and psychological rehabilitation may be recommended. With regard to psychological interventions, behavioral techniques (Campo and Negrini 2000), relaxation skills, and family therapy (Lock and Giammona 1999) have been identified as important components of successful treatment of somatoform disorders. The level of therapy and pharmacological intervention necessary will vary according to the degree of functional impairment, parental abilities, and existence of any comorbid psychiatric diagnoses. Partial psychiatric hospitalization (day treatment) or intensive inpatient or outpatient rehabilitation programs may be recommended in cases where significant functional impairments persist beyond what can appropriately be addressed with general outpatient care.

Given the interplay between physiological and psychological symptoms, medical providers play an important role in working with families of children and adolescents with somatoform disorders. Clear feedback and recommendations with an emphasis on the link between psychological and physiological components (versus exclusive focus on one or the other) are helpful (Brazier and Venning 1997; Gooch et al. 1997; Palermo and Scher 2001). If more intensive psychiatric or rehabilitative services are necessary, the involvement of the medical clinicians in supporting the plan is beneficial in making such a recommendation more acceptable to families.

Impact of Chronic Pain on School

Difficulties managing chronic pain in pediatric populations can lead to significant impairments in school functioning. Chronic pain can be disruptive to school attendance, academic performance, and ability to cope with classroom demands (Allen et al. 1999; Palermo 2000). Children with chronic pain have been shown to experience high rates of school absences (Newacheck and Taylor 1992), especially for children with headaches (Stang and Osterhaus 1993; Carlsson et al. 1996), abdominal pain (Walker et al. 1998), and musculoskeletal pain (Mikkelsson, Salminen, & Kautiainen, 1997).

For school staff, managing a student with chronic pain can be a difficult task. One large challenge for school personnel is limited understanding of pediatric chronic pain (Power et al. 1999). Additional barriers to successful management in the classroom include collaboration between parents and school staff, and teachers' difficulties in balancing school policies and classroom requirements while accommodating students' individual needs (Logan and Curran 2005). With regard to areas of improvement, a study by Logan and Curran (2005) found that school personnel highlighted the need for more overall collaboration with medical teams, schools, and families. From the medical teams in particular, school staff wanted more information about the specific medical diagnoses and guidance on how symptoms should be managed at school (Logan and Curran 2005).

Conclusion

Chronic pain in pediatrics is multifaceted and understanding its many dimensions is essential to effective treatment. The psychological aspects of chronic pain play a critical role to the onset and maintenance in children and adolescents. Identification and effective treatment of the psychological components related to chronic pain, as well as, any possible comorbid psychiatric disorders is important as cognitive, emotional, behavioral, and social factors can facilitate adaptive management or exacerbate poor coping and functional impairments. Early intervention is also important because pediatric chronic pain increases the risk for adult chronic pain (Campo et al. *1999*; Walker et al. *1995*). Additionally, a multisystemic approach that includes collaboration with parents, medical providers, and schools is essential to target the many areas that are affected by pediatric chronic pain.

References

Allen, K. D., & Mathews, J. R. (1998). Management of recurrent pain in children. In T. S. Watson & F. Gresham (Eds.), *Handbook of child behavior therapy: Ecological considerations in assessment, treatment, and evaluation* (pp. 263–285). New York: Plenum.

Allen, K. D., Mathews, J. R., & Shriver, M. D. (1999). Children and recurrent headaches: Assessment and treatment implications for school psychologists. *School Psychology Review, 28*(2), 266–279.

American Psychiatric Association. (2000). *Diagnostic and statistical manual of mental disorders, fourth edition text revision.* Washington, DC: American Psychiatric Association.

Boyer, M. C., Compas, B. E., Stanger, C., Colletti, R. B., Konik, B. S., Morrow, S. B., & Thomsen, A. H. (2006). Attentional biases to pain and social threat in children with recurrent abdominal pain. *Journal of Pediatric Psychology, 31*(2), 209–220. 6.

Brazier, D. K., & Venning, H. E. (1997). Conversion disorders in adolescents: A practical approach to rehabilitation. *British Journal of Rheumatology, 36,* 594–598.

Campo, J. V., & Negrini, B. J. (2000). Case study: Negative reinforcement and behavioral management of conversion disorder. *Journal of the American Academy of Child and Adolescent Psychiatry, 39*(6), 787–790.

Campo, J. V., Di Lorenzo, C., Bridge, J., Chiappetta, L., Colborn, D. K., Gartner, J. C., Gaffney, P., Kocoshis, S., & Brent, D. (1999). *Adult outcomes of recurrent abdominal pain: Preliminary results.* Orlando: American Gastroenterological Association.

Campo, J. V., Bridge, J., Ehmann, M., Altman, S., Lucas, A., Birmaher, B., Di Lorenzo, C., Iyengar, S., & Brent, D. A. (2004). Recurrent abdominal pain, anxiety, and depression in primary care. *Pediatrics, 113,* 817–824.

Carlsson, J., Larsson, B., & Mark, A. (1996). Psychosocial functioning in schoolchildren with recurrent headaches. *Headache, 36,* 77–82.

Chambers, C. T., Craig, K. D., & Bennett, S. M. (2002). The impact of maternal behavior on children's pain experiences: An experimental analysis. *Journal of Pediatric Psychology, 27,* 293–301.

Compas, B. E., & Boyer, M. C. (2001). Coping and attention: Implications for child health and pediatric conditions. *Developmental and Behavioral Pediatrics, 22*(5), 323–333.

Crombez, G., Bijttebier, P., Eccleston, C., Mascagni, T., Mertens, G., Goubert, L., & Verstraeten, K. (2003). The child version of the pain catastrophizing scale (PCS-C): A preliminary validation. *Pain, 104*(3), 639–646.

Degotardi, P. J., Klass, E. S., Rosenberg, B. S., Fox, D. G., Gallelli, K. A., & Gottlieb, B. S. (2006). Development and evaluation of a cognitive-behavioral intervention for juvenile fibromyalgia. *Journal of Pediatric Psychology, 31*(7), 714–723.

Dorn, L., Campo, J., Thato, S., Dahl, R., Lewin, D., Chandra, R., & Di Lorenzo, C. (2003). Psychological comorbidity and stress reactivity in children and adolescents with recurrent abdominal pain and anxiety disorders. *Journal of the American Academy of Child and Adolescent Psychiatry, 42*(1), 66–75.

Eccleston, C., Crombez, G., Scotford, A., Clinch, J., & Connell, H. (2004). Adolescent chronic pain: Patterns and predictors of emotional distress in adolescents with chronic pain and their parents. *Pain, 108*(3), 221–229.

Egger, H., Costello, E., Erkanli, A., & Angold, A. (1999). Somatic complaints and psychopathology in children and adolescents: Stomach aches, musculoskeletal pains, and headaches. *Journal of the American Academy of Child and Adolescent Psychiatry, 38*, 852–860.

Fordyce, W. E. (1989). The cognitive/behavioral perspective on clinical pain. In J. D. Loeser & K. J. Egan (Eds.), *Managing the chronic pain patient* (pp. 51–64). New York: Raven.

Garber, J., Zeman, J., Walker, L. (1990). Recurrent abdominal pain in children: Psychiatric diagnoses and parental Psychopathology. *Journal of the American Academy of Child and Adolescent Psychiatry, 29*(4), 648–656.

Gauthier, J. G., Ivers, H., & Carrier, S. (1996). Nonpharmacological approaches in the management of recurrent headache disorders and their comparison and combination with pharmacotherapy. *Clinical Psychology Review, 16*, 543–517.

Gidron, Y., McGrath, P. J., & Goodday, R. (1995). The physical and psychosocial predictors of adolescents' recovery from oral surgery. *Journal of Behavioral Medicine, 18*, 385–399.

Gil, K. M., Williams, D. A., Thompson, R. J., & Kinney, T. R. (1991). Sickle cell disease in children and adolescents: The relation of child and parent coping strategies to adjustment. *Journal of Pediatric Psychology, 16*, 643–663.

Gil, K. M., Wilson, J. J., Edens, J. L., Workman, E., Ready, J., et al. (1997). Cognitive coping skills training in children with sickle cell disease pain. *International Journal of Behavioral Medicine, 4*, 364–377.

Gil, K. M., Anthony, K. K., Carson, J. W., Redding-Lallinger, R., Daeschner, C. W., & Ware, R. E. (2001). Daily coping practice predicts treatment effects in children with sickle cell disease. *Journal of Pediatric Psychology, 26*, 163–173.

Gooch, J. L., Wolcott, R., Speed, J., et al. (1997). Behavioral management of conversion disorder in children. *Archives of Physical Medical and Rehabilitation, 78*, 264–268.

Hodges, K., Kline, J., Barbero, G., & Woodruff, C. (1985). Anxiety in children with recurrent abdominal pain and their parents. *Psychosomatics, 26*, 859–866.

Holden, E. W., Levy, J. D., Deichmann, M. M., & Gladstein, J. (1998). Recurrent pediatric headaches: Assessment and intervention. *Journal of Developmental and Behavioral Pediatrics, 19*, 109–116.

Hyams, J., Burke, G., Davis, P., Rzepski, B., & Andrulinos, P. (1996). Abdominal pain and irritable bowel syndrome in adolescents: A community-based study. *The Journal of Pediatrics, 129*, 220–226.

Kashikar-Zuck, S., Goldschneider, K., Powers, S., Vaught, M., & Hershey, A. (2001). Depression and functional disability in chronic pediatric pain. *The Clinical Journal of Pain, 17*, 341–349.

Konijnenberg, A. Y., de Graeff-Meeder, E., van der Hoeven, J., Kimpen, J., Buitelaar, J., & Uiterwaal, C. (2006). Psychiatric morbidity in children with medically unexplained chronic pain: Diagnosis from the pediatrician's perspective. *Pediatrics, 117*, 889–897.

Kozlowska, K., Nunn, K. P., Rose, D., Anne, M., Ouvrier, R. A., & Varghese, J. (2007). Conversion disorder in Australian pediatric practice. *Journal of the American Academy of Child and Adolescent Psychiatry, 46*(1), 68–75.

Lavigne, J. V., Ross, C. K., Berry, S. L., Hayford, J. R., & Pachman, L. M. (1992). Evaluation of a psychological treatment package for treating pain in juvenile rheumatoid arthritis. *Arthritis Care and Research, 5*, 101–110.

Lewandowski, A. S., Palermo, T. M., & Peterson, C. C. (2006). Age-dependent relationships among pain, depressive symptoms, and functional disability in youth with recurrent headaches. *Headache, 46*(4), 656–662.

Lipsitz, J. D., Masia-Warner, C., Apfel, H., Marans, Z., Hellstern, B., Forand, N., Levenbraun, Y., & Fyer, A. J. (2004). Anxiety and depressive symptoms and anxiety sensitivity in youngsters with noncardiac chest pain and benign heart murmurs. *Journal of Pediatric Psychology, 29*(8), 607–612.

Lock, J., & Giammona, A. (1999). Severe somatoform disorder in adolescence: A case series using a rehabilitation model for intervention. *Clinical Child Psychology and Psychiatry, 4*, 341–351.

Logan, D. E., & Curran, J. A. (2005). Adolescent chronic pain problems in the school setting: Exploring the experiences and beliefs of selected school personnel through focus group methodology. *The Journal of Adolescent Health, 37*(4), 281–288.

Lynch, A. M., Kashikar-Zuck, S., Goldschneider, K. R., & Jones, B. A. (2006). Psychosocial risks for disability in children with chronic back pain. *The Journal of Pain, 7*(4), 244–251.

Martin-Herz, S. P., Smith, M. S., & McMahon, R. J. (1999). Psychosocial variables associated with headache in junior high school students. *Journal of Pediatric Psychology, 24*, 13–23.

Merikangas, K. R., & Stevens, D. E. (1997). Comorbidity of migraine and psychiatric disorders. *Neurologic Clinics, 15*(1), 115–123.

Mikkelsson, M., Salminen, J. J., & Kautiainen, H. (1997). Non-specific musculoskeletal pain in pre-adolescents. Prevalence and 1-year persistence. *Pain, 73*, 29–35.

Mulvaney, S. A., Lambert, W., Garber, J., & Walker, L. (2006). Trajectories of symptoms and impairment in pediatric chronic pain: A 5 year longitudinal study. *Journal of the American Academy of Child Psychiatry, 45*(6), 737–744.

Newacheck, P. W., & Taylor, W. R. (1992). Childhood chronic illness: Prevalence, severity, and impact. *American Journal of Public Health, 82*(3), 364–371.

Palermo, T. M. (2000). Impact of recurrent and chronic pain on child and family daily functioning: A critical review of the literature. *Journal of Developmental and Behavioral Pediatrics, 21*, 58–69.

Palermo, T. M., & Scher, M. S. (2001). Treatment of functional impairment in severe somatoform pain disorder: A case example. *Journal of Pediatric Psychology, 26*(7), 429–434.

Piira, T., Taplin, J. E., Goodenough, B., & von Baeyer, C. L. (2002). Cognitive-behavioral predictors of children's tolerance of laboratory –induced pain: Implications for clinical assessment and future directions. *Behaviour Research and Therapy, 40*, 571–584.

Power, T. J., Heathfield, L. T., Mcgoey, K. E., & Blum, N. J. (1999). Managing and preventing chronic health problems in children and youth: School psychology's expanded mission. *School Psychology Review, 28*, 251–263.

Sanders, M. R., Rebgetz, M., Morrison, M., Bor, W., Gordon, A., Dadds, M., & Shepherd, R. (1989). Cognitive-behavioral treatment of recurrent nonspecific abdominal pain in children: An analysis of generalization, maintenance and side effects. *Journal of Consulting and Clinical Psychology, 57*, 294–300.

Sanders, M. R., Shepherd, R. W., Cleghorn, G., & Woolford, H. (1994). The treatment of recurrent abdominal pain in children: A controlled comparison of cognitive-behavioral family intervention and standard pediatric care. *Journal of Consulting and Clinical Psychology, 62*, 306–314.

Schanberg, L. E., Keefe, F. J., Lefebvre, J. C., et al. (1996). Pain coping strategies in children with primary fibromyalgia syndrome: Correlation with pain, physical function, and psychological distress. *Arthritis Care and Research, 9*, 89–96.

Stang, P. E., & Osterhaus, J. T. (1993). Impact o f migraine in the United States: Data from the National Health Interview Survey. *Headache, 33*, 29–35.

Thomsen, A. H., Compas, B. E., Colletti, R. B., Stranger, C., Boyer, M. C., & Konik, B. S. (2002). Parent reports of coping and stress responses in children with recurrent abdominal pain. *Journal of Pediatric Psychology, 27*, 215–226.

Vaalamo, I., Pulkkinen, L., Kinnunen, T., Kaprio, J., & Rose, R. (2002). Interactive effects of internalizing and externalizing problem behaviors on recurrent pain in children. *Journal of Pediatric Psychology, 27*(3), 245–257.

Varni, J. W. (1989). *An empirical model for the biobehavioral investigation of pediatric pain*. Invited plenary address at the annual meeting of the American Pain Society, Phoenix.

Varni, J. W., Rapoff, M. A., Waldron, S. A., Gragg, R. A., Bernstein, B. H., & Lindsley, C. B. (1996). Chronic pain and emotional disorder in children and adolescents. *Journal of Developmental and Behavioral Pediatrics, 17*(3), 154–161.

Vervoort, T., Goubert, L., Eccleston, C., Bijttebier, P., & Crombez, G. (2006). Catastrophic thinking about pain is independently associated with pain severity, disability, and somatic complaints in school children and children with chronic pain. *Journal of Pediatric Psychology, 31*(7), 674–683.

Vlaeyen, J. W. S., & Linton, S. J. (2000). Fear-avoidance and its consequences in chronic musculoskeletal pain: A state of the art. *Pain, 85*, 317–332.

Walco, G. A., Varni, J. W., & Ilowite, N. T. (1992). Cognitive-behavioral pain management in children with juvenile rheumatoid arthritis. *Pediatrics, 89*, 1075–1079.

Walker, L. S. (1999). The evolution of research on recurrent abdominal pain: History, assumptions, and a conceptual model. In P. J. McGrath & G. A. Finley (Eds.), *Chronic and Recurrent Pain in Children and Adolescents* (pp.141–172). Seattle: International Association for the Study of Pain.

Walker, L. S., & Greene, J. W. (1989). Children with recurrent abdominal pain and their parents: More somatic complaints, anxiety and depression than other patient families? *Journal of Pediatric Psychology, 14*, 231–243.

Walker, L. S., Garber, J., Van Slyke, D. A., & Greene, J. W. (1995). Long-term health outcomes in patients with recurrent abdominal pain. *Journal of Pediatric Psychology, 20*, 233–245.

Walker, L. S., Guite, J. W., Duke, M., Barnard, J. A., & Greene, J. W. (1998). Recurrent abdominal pain: A potential precursor of irritable bowel syndrome in adolescents and young adults. *The Journal of Pediatrics, 132*(6), 1010–1015.

Walker, L. S., Claar, R. L., & Garber, J. (2002). Social consequences of children's pain: When do they encourage symptoms maintenance? *Journal of Pediatric Psychology, 27*(8), 689–698.

Walker, L. S., Smith, C. A., Garber, J., & Claar, R. L. (2007). Appraisal and coping with daily stressors by pediatric patients with chronic abdominal pain. *Journal of Pediatric Psychology, 32*(2), 206–216.

Whitehead, W. E., Crowell, M. D., Heller, B. R., Robinson, J. C., Schuster, M. M., & Horn, S. (1994). Modeling and reinforcement of the sick role during childhood predicts adult illness behavior. *Psychosomatic Medicine, 56*, 541–550.

Zeltzer, L. Z., Bursch, B., & Walco, G. (1997). Pain responsiveness and chronic pain: A psychobiological perspective. *Developmental and Behavioral Pediatrics, 18*(6), 413–422.

Clinical Management of Musculoskeletal Pain Syndromes

7

Lynn M. Rusy

Keywords

Musculoskeletal pain (MSP) • Myofascial pain syndromes • Overuse syndromes • Growing pains

The child presenting to the general practitioner with complaints of musculoskeletal pain is common and pediatricians need to be more knowledgeable of these conditions. It presents a challenge to make the diagnosis without invasive and expensive testing. A complete physical exam is essential. Often, simple reassurance, analgesics, physical therapy, and lifestyle changes are sufficient for most complaints. More specific knowledge of the multidisciplinary approach needed to treat fibromyalgia (FM) and myofascial pain syndrome (MFPS) can be helpful.

Muscles represent 40% of the body mass by weight. Muscles lift the corners of children's mouths so they can smile; raise the arm, and wrist so they can wave and lift the legs so they can walk. Musculoskeletal pain (MSP) has long plagued children and, although common, has received less attention than other areas of chronic pain in children, such as headache and abdominal pain. Musculoskeletal pain in children is widespread, affecting 7–15% of school-age children (Goodman and McGrath 1991). An analysis of 1,000 consecutive general pediatric visits, found MSP complaints 6.1% of the time, with complaints including knee arthralgias (33%), other joint (ankle, wrist) arthralgias (28%), soft tissue pain (18%), hip pain (6%), and back pain (6%) (de Inocencio 1998) . In addition, there were also reports of pain from repetitive sports injuries, juvenile rheumatoid arthritis, systemic lupus, fibromyalgia, myofascial pain, hip disorders, cancer, and benign growing pains. This chapter covers more benign forms of MSP in children and adolescents, namely fibromyalgia, myofascial pain, sports injuries, and growing pains. It will discuss occurrence, possible etiologies, and clinical management.

In the evaluation of a child with MSP, history and physical examination of the musculoskeletal system is important. Trauma and overuse injuries are usually self-evident on history and physical examination. The majority of MSP in children are benign, but systemic diseases such as joint infections, malignancies, or rheumatologic conditions may present initially as MSP and full evaluation is crucial.

L.M. Rusy (✉)
Jane B. Pettit Pain and Paliative Care Center,
Medical College of Wisconsin,
9000 West Wisconsin Avenue,
Milwaukee, WI 53226, USA
email: lrusy@mcw.edu

B.C. McClain and S. Suresh (eds.), *Handbook of Pediatric Chronic Pain:*
Current Science and Integrative Practice, DOI 10.1007/978-1-4419-0350-1_7,
© Springer Science+Business Media, LLC 2011

Fibromyalgia

Chronic pain syndromes, specifically fibromyalgia (FM) and myofascial pain syndrome (MFPS) can cause significant morbidity with school absence. The concept of fibrositis dates back to the early 1900s, when two French doctors, Balfeur and Valleix, described "shooting painful points" found with palpation calling them "inflammatory hyperplasia of connective tissue in patches" (Goldenberg 1987). Medical investigators at the turn of the century reported that they had seen under a microscope, inflamed areas of fibrous tissue or fascia that surrounds muscles and binds them together. The name fibrositis implied that the cause of the condition was inflammatory, but with more sophisticated microscopes and carefully designed research studies, investigators have shown that there is little inflammation in muscle or soft tissue of fibromyalgia patients. At the beginning of this period, the syndrome was considered to be a label for any poorly understood chronic pain condition. The syndrome fell out of favor because there were no objective abnormalities, i.e., no laboratory tests or x-ray findings; the opinion that there was inflammation was wrong and the medical field began calling it "psychogenic rheumatism." Many doctors thought, incorrectly that patients' symptoms were "all in their heads." Fibrositis, as it was then called, became a long-term, neglected syndrome.

Over the past decade, there has been renewed interest in studying the syndrome. The term "fibromyalgia" (fibro, fiber; my, muscle; algia, pain) has gradually replaced fibrositis as the name of choice. FM is now a well-recognized syndrome of diffuse, aching pain or stiffness in the muscles and joints accompanied by fatigue, poor sleep, and diagnostic findings on physical examination (Smythe 1989). It is now the second or third most common diagnosis made in rheumatologic offices; it affects 4–6 million adult Americans, or 4–6% of the population. There is a female preponderance of 1:6 (Pellegrino 1993). Findings in children are similar (Buskila et al. 1993; Malleson et al. 1992). An outcome study, in the Journal of Rheumatology, found the incidence in children aged 9–15 was 6.2%.

Classification

The classification criteria (Table 7.1) to make the diagnosis were set out by the American College of Rheumatology in a multicenter study of 558 patients, 293 with FM and 265 controls (Wolfe et al. 1990). The purpose was to define the syndrome by the recognition of its characteristics by interested investigators in multiple centers in the USA and Canada. The first criteria is the presence of widespread pain, identified when all of the following were present: pain on the left side of the body, pain on the right side of the body, pain above and below the waist as well as axial skeletal pain (cervical spine, thoracic spine, anterior chest, and low back). There had to be greater than three sites of pain for greater than 3 months. There was an absence of any other systemic disease to account for this. Widespread pain in the review turned out to have high sensitivity – 97.6%. Most patients have a hard time accurately pinpointing the pain and usually just say "it hurts all over." Adjectives like burning, knowing, shooting, and stabbing are often used. The second criteria are the presence of characteristic muscle tender points and these tender points were the most powerful discriminator between fibromyalgia and controls. The main findings on physical exam are the tender points in characteristic locations. Tender points are areas in soft tissue, muscles, tendons or ligaments, which are extremely tender when pressed, and may cause

Table 7.1 Fibromyalgia criteria

Major criteria	Minor criteria
Widespread pain (three locations, greater than 3 months)	Sleep disturbance
Characteristic muscle tender points (pain in 11 out of 18 points with digital palpation)	Morning stiffness Irritable stomach Dizziness Irritable bladder Irritable bowel Raynaud's phenomena Depression Anxiety Headaches TMJ syndrome Restless leg syndrome Mitral valve prolapse

the individual to flinch or jump. Pain, on digital palpation must be present in at least 11 of 18 tender point sites: occiput, low cervical, trapezius, supraspinatus, second rib, lateral epicondyle, gluteal, greater trochanter, and medial knee (Fricton 1990). Digital palpation should be performed by the pulp of the thumb with an approximate force of 4 kg (Yunas 1989). One may elicit transient dimpling or contraction, called a local twitch response. Muscles have a particular consistency that feels like nylon bands when they are rubbed deeply. Sometimes, a large area is involved that feels like a lump, called an FM nodule. The skin overlying the tender area is often hypersensitive and scratching it can leave red marks, known as dermatographia. Tenderness to palpation in FM may not be limited to these tender points, but instead extend throughout the entire body, with a possible central augmentation of pain processing, to both pressure and heat (Petzke et al. 2003).

A patient can be said to have FM if both these major criteria are satisfied. In addition to these major criteria, there is a list of minor criteria or symptoms that often accompany the condition (Bell et al. 1994). Fatigue and sleep disturbance are always found. The fatigue is present throughout the day, but especially prominent in late afternoon. They may be so exhausted that they cannot concentrate on simple cognitive activities and find that a nap is necessary. This can be very problematic for the patient when school is in session. They may not have difficulty falling asleep due to exhaustion, but there are frequent awakenings and sleep is non-restorative. Therefore, in the morning, patients with FM feel stiff and exhausted, even after 8–10 h of rest, feeling as if they have not slept at all.

Depression and anxiety are common. Feelings of low self esteem, frequent crying spells and even thoughts of suicide are common in FM. A relationship between fibromyalgia and psychiatric disorders has been suggested. Using the MMPI, there is higher rate of depression, hysteria and hypochondriasis, but the MMPI was not designed to be used when chronic conditions are present (Smythe 1984). A patient will score 40% higher on these scales if chronic illnesses are present. It is hard to separate symptoms of depression from symptoms that may be present as a manifestation of the chronic illness. Symptoms such as fatigue, sleep disturbance, and headache are present on both the depression checklist as well as fibromyalgia. Overall, there has not been a single, telltale psychological factor that is always associated with FM. FM symptoms get worse with stress and depression, but the physical symptoms may not have a psychiatric etiology. A minority of patients may have ongoing depression, but most should not be considered to have a primary psychiatric condition accounting for FM.

Irritable bowel syndrome is found in 50–80% of FM patients (Waylonis and Heck 1992). Signs and symptoms include frequent bowel cramping, abdominal pain due to food intolerances, diarrhea, and constipation. Irritable bladder can also occur which manifests as painful urination with normal urinalysis.

Tension headaches and migraines are common. Raynaud's phenomenon is seen in approximately 40% of these patients. Restless leg syndrome is common, especially at night (Felson and Goldenberg 1986). Tempero-mandibular joint syndrome and mitral valve prolapse are also common. Dizziness is a common subjective complaint, but specific balance testing with diagnostic physical exams and advanced rotary chair testing did not reveal any central or peripheral vestibular abnormalities (Rusy et al. 1999). The sternocleidomastoid muscles along with the trapezius muscles stabilize and fix the head in space. It may be that the musculoskeletal abnormalities, especially in the neck where the tender points are clustered, affect proprioception orientation, resulting in perceived dizziness.

Etiology

The cause of FM is unknown, but various etiologies have been proposed, including genetic, viral, neurotransmitter abnormalities, endocrine abnormalities, immune disorders, allergic factors, and structural muscle changes. It has been postulated to be inherited in an autosomal dominant pattern (Pellegrino et al. 1989). There is a possible gene for FM that is linked to the HLA region (Yunus et al. 1999). Viral or infectious etiologies have been proposed, as many patients will report temporally associated onset of FM symptoms with a viral illness or flu-like malady. Viral titers and markers such as Epstein Barr virus have been unsupportive of this. Immunological disorders such as rheumatoid arthritis, osteoarthritis, or Raynaud's phenomenon are found in a subset of these patients, but the significance of this is tenuous. A subset of FM symptoms posttrauma, such as whiplash, is seen (Banic et al. 2003).

Endocrine disorders such as thyroid problems and growth hormone deficiencies may occur in some FM patients. Since growth hormone is produced during sleep, the link between this and FM, with known sleep disturbances, may be key in allowing us to fully understand the condition. Due to the problems with sleep, it has been postulated that there may be a neurochemical basis for FM. There is an alpha wave intrusion of delta sleep or stage 4 sleep (Roizenblatt et al. 1997). Experiments that disturb this stage of sleep in normal subjects show that these subjects develop musculoskeletal disturbances similar to FM. A serotonin disorder was speculated to be present, as well as abnormalities in the neurochemical tryptophan. Treatment with tryptophan has not been helpful (Moldofsky and Lue 1980), however, and studies looking at substance P and other endorphins in CSF have been equally disappointing (Caruso et al. 1990). Fibromyalgia patients may also have sleep apnea, restless leg syndrome, bruxism, and sleep myoclonus. Given these sleep problems, it is easy to see why chronic fatigue occurs and can be incapacitating. The female preponderance in FM is not explained by hormonal changes since estrogen levels are normal (Bengtsson et al. 1986a).

FM has been termed the "invisible condition" because the muscles appear normal. Bengtsson et al. (1986b) studied patients with FM compared to rheumatoid arthritis, measuring specific laboratory and muscle testing. He wanted to see if there were any neurophysiologic signs of neuropathy or myopathy. He found patients with FM had normal on erythrocyte sedimentation rate (ESR), vitamin levels, myoglobin, CBC, electrolytes, liver function, hormone levels, ANA,

antinuclear antibodies against smooth muscle, and thyroid function. Electromyographic (EMG) examination signals were also essentially normal (Lund et al. 1986). The same authors (Bengtsson et al. 1986b) did, however, find a pathological distribution of muscle surface oxygenation, low levels of high-energy phosphates and discrete changes in morphology in painful muscles. They found less ATP, ADP, and phosphoric creatinine, postulating local tissue hypoxia may account for these points of tenderness. The cause was not understood; however, as normal values obtained in the forearm ischemic test indicate, the low levels of high-energy phosphates are not due to glycogenolysis. Henriksson (1989) also showed a reduction of high-energy phosphates in biopsies of individuals with FM, but a magnetic resonance spectroscopic study by de Blecourt et al. (1991) failed to confirm the presence of these high-energy abnormalities. The combination of decreased oxygen and energy causes early muscle fatigue, less efficient contractions and pain (Kalyan-Dijilani et al. 1984). It is proposed that in posttraumatic injury as seen in whiplash, plasticity changes occur in the central nervous system that result in neuronal hyperexcitability, exaggerated pain responses, and FM syndrome in the absence of tissue damage (Banic et al. 2003). Thus, FM muscle tissue appears histologically normal, yet the patients complain of significant pain.

FM is a clinical syndrome that lacks specific diagnostic tests. Patients with FM experience chronic pain that is not degenerative or deforming and really has no known impact on mortality; however, the quality of living is often impeded. Most patients have seen numerous medical specialists including GPs, pediatricians, neurologists, rheumatologists, gastroenterologists, general practitioners, psychologists, and psychiatrists. Investigations may have included x-rays, CT/MRI scans, endoscopies, EMGs, blood tests, and even nerve conduction studies, all of which have been costly and non-revealing. The diagnosis is best entertained over time and with a careful physical exam for the tender points. Children can be diagnosed with FM, but it is more commonly diagnosed between the ages of 25 and 35 years.

Treatment

Unfortunately, there is no single cure for the condition. The good news is that it is nondeforming and there are interventions that can be done to control the symptoms. FM treatment is not about addressing the pain of tender points and trigger points, but instead is directed toward the whole person and the impact of the disorder on their life. Successful management of FM involves a number of different treatment modalities. An integrated, multidisciplinary team approach, in which the patient is the team leader and is responsible for finding out the therapies that work best for him/her is essential.

Education

A stepwise program emphasizing education, medications, exercise, and cognitive behavioral therapy is indicated. Every patient should be educated about the condition, what to expect, and what they can do to alleviate the pain and fatigue. Discussion about exercise, stress reduction, and sleep are important. There is strong evidence that intensive patient education is an effective treatment for FM (Nicassio et al. 1997). Randomized and controlled trials compared patient education to wait-listed, noninformed patients, using lectures, written materials, group discussions, and demonstrations. The educational groups improved in several outcomes, including sleep, quality of life, fatigue, and self-efficacy; these changes were maintained for 3–12 months. Non-pharmacological therapy is the mainstay of treatment for FM. While many patients do need to be treated with some pharmaceutical agent, these non-pharmacological approaches may relieve the majority of the pain without the side effects often seen with chronic use of analgesic medication.

Non-Pharmacologic Therapy/Exercise

Exercise designed to relieve spasm and improve muscle blood flow is indicated on a regular basis (McCain 1986). Cardiovascular exercise on a regular basis showed significant improvement in pain, sleep, and decreased number of tender points (McCain et al. 1988). Aerobic exercises are those that increase the body's heart rate to a target range to achieve the desired conditioning of the heart, lungs, and muscles. Common aerobic exercises include walking, biking, swimming, and jogging. Muscle pain is a deterrent to starting an exercise regimen and lack of fitness may be prevalent in patients with FM. Because of deconditioning, exercise programs should begin gradually, with the goal being regular activity with increasing effort on good days. Exercise videotapes have been produced that are designed for the pediatric patient with fibromyalgia. These instructional films include a warm-up, aerobic section, and cool down, with several examples of increasing levels of effort (Rusy 1996; Oakville Trafalgar Hospital 1992). Stretching, flexibility exercises, and attention to posture are encouraged. Exercise is important and must be continued even on days when pain is elevated. It is suggested to lower the level of effort on days of high pain intensity. There is often an initial period of exercise-induced discomfort, but patients have to push through this period. Once their muscles are more fit and stronger, the muscle pain will decrease and their pain baseline will lessen. YMCA swim classes are often designed for people with FM or MPS. Exercising in warm water has many benefits, even for those who cannot swim. The body's weight is buoyed by the water, thereby reducing the stress on the muscles and joints. The water must be kept at a comfortable temperature, usually 85°F.

Benefits of exercise extend beyond cardiovascular effects and decreased pain. Regular exercise has distinct physiological benefit, providing a sense of relaxation and overall well-being (Mannerkorpi et al. 1999). A program that mother and daughter can perform together can improve bonding since it is often that both have FM. The exercise program can give patients a greater sense of participation in their treatment program and garners an internal focus of control over their condition. Typically with time, there is improvement in pain and better realization of the effort needed to stay healthy and in control of the pain.

Physical Therapy

Physical therapy modalities for musculoskeletal pain might include ultrasound treatment of sore musculature, transcutaneous electrical nerve stimulation (TENS) unit, posture training, and instruction on stretching exercises. Ultrasound improves range of motion in conjunction with stretching (Malanga and Nadler 1999). Stretching exercises decrease muscle tenderness and increase range of motion in FM (Wright and Schiffman 1995). Correction of poor posture will alleviate some of the pain symptoms of FM, as poor posture has been associated with the presence of trigger points (Fricton 1990). The application of heat or spray in combination with stretching further provides relief of pain (Sheon and the Goff group 1997). Cooling in the form of a suboccipital ice pillow may be effective in the treatment of headache, especially if applied early (Glass 1992). Alternative physical therapy modalities such as the Feldenkrais method and Alexander technique involve reeducating the body with slow, nonaerobic movement, emphasizing consciousness of movement and reduction of stress on joints and muscles (Ramsey 1997; Feldenkrais Method 2000). A physical therapy program that is modality intensive only provides short-lived relief. The patient must be encouraged to continue self-directed therapy rather than ongoing guidance since regular exercise and stretch will provide longer-lasting relief.

Needle Techniques

Trigger point injections and needling is effective in relieving the pain associated with the trigger points. Injections are commonly done with local anesthetics, corticosteroids, saline, and botulinum toxin (Travell and Simmons 1983). There is little evidence of the benefit of steroid, and repeated steroid injection may predispose the patient to myotoxicity and focal tissue loss (Rosen 1994). Saline has some anesthetic properties when injected and may be useful in patients allergic to local anesthetics. Botox theoretically should inactivate a trigger point region for longer than local anesthetic injections (Moreno-Lopez et al. 1997). The injection technique involves identifying the maximal tender point, and advancing the needle (# 30 gauge) with quick insertion through the skin into the center of the point, followed by injection of the substance chosen.

The patient often verbalizes that the pain is reproduced by the needle and there may be a local twitch response. The injections may be used singularly as a diagnostic technique or as a treatment regimen with a series of repeat injections, coupled with stretching and physical therapy. Trigger point bands shorten muscle and prevent adequate stretching, so the injection may relieve pain, restore normal muscle length, and allow for maintenance stretching and exercise. The injections may be repeated weekly, monthly, or as needed; however, it must be stressed to the patient that injections alone are not complete treatment and works best when coupled with the stretching and exercise. Complications of injections include allergic reactions to selected agents, hematoma, syncope, infection, nerve injury, penetration of an organ, or vascular injury (Gerwin 2000). As always with children, their ability to cooperate is essential. Most children will be able to tolerate injections in the teenage years without much difficulty.

Acupuncture

Acupuncture provides another needling technique for pain relief for FM. Acupuncture, a therapeutic procedure based on traditional Chinese medicine for pain relief, has been used in China for at least 2,000 years (Melzack 1989). Acupuncture is based on a theory that energy flows throughout the body along meridians, which are connected to acupuncture points (Helms 1995). When the flow of energy is "obstructed," pain results and restoration of that energy eliminates or reduces pain (Rusy and Weisman 2000). Insertion of fine needles at acupuncture points along the involved meridian restores the energy flow. According to Melzack, intense stimulation from acupuncture activates small fibers that project to the cells in the periaqueductal gray (PAG) area. Cells in PAG then activate serotonergic and noradrenergic system that modulates pain transmission through dorsal horns. PAG projections are thought to serve as descending inhibitory pathways to pain. There is evidence that acupuncture stimulates production of endorphins, serotonin, and acetylcholine within the central nervous system, which enhances analgesia (Pomeranz 1996). Numerous studies (Deluz et al. 1992; Berman et al. 1999; Sandberg et al. 1999) have reported acupuncture to be effective in treating adult FM patients. Acupuncture can be used in patients of all ages, however, when needles are employed, cooperation is needed. Generally at the age of 10, patients will adjust well to acupuncture (Rusy and Weisman 2000). A retrospective case study on pediatric patients' experience with acupuncture revealed that 67% of children 5–20 years old (median 16 years) rated their experience as "positive or pleasant" (Kemper et al. 2000). Additionally, 60% of the parents felt that the acupuncture was a positive experience.

Medications

Pharmacotherapy has been most successful with central nervous system agents such as tricyclic antidepressants (TCA), selective serotonin reuptake inhibitors (SSRI), muscle relaxants or anticonvulsants. These drugs affect a broad range of activities in the brain and spinal cord, including modulation of pain sensitivity and tolerance (Goldenberg et al. 2004). TCAs, mainly amitriptyline or nortriptyline, have strong evidence for efficacy (Carette et al. 1986). Amitriptyline, together with naproxen, was studied in a randomized fashion and shown to be effective in FM (Goldenberg et al. 1986). Amitriptyline can help with sleep, which is usually disturbed in FM, as well as overall well-being. The non-restorative sleep in children with FM should be treated with attention to sleep hygiene (time to bed, mattress quality, temperature of room), but the low dose of TCA adds to quality of restorative sleep in this population. SSRIs along with dual-reuptake inhibitors (Zijstra et al. 2002) have modest efficacy, for many of the same reasons (Arnold et al. 2002). Pregabalin, a second-generation anticonvulsant, 450 mg per day (Crofford et al. 2002), is effective and now recommended for FM by the FDA for adults. Tramadol, with or without acetaminophen, is effective in three randomized controlled studies of FM (Biasi et al. 1998; Russell et al. 2000; Bennett et al. 2003). Tramadol can,

however, lower seizure threshold in patients on TCAs and should therefore not be used more than two to three times per day when in this combination. Cyclobenzaprine (Bennett 1988), with tricyclics has been shown to be beneficial in randomized controlled studies as well. Triptan medications (oral, subcutaneous, or nasal) are useful for migraine symptoms on a PRN basis. There is no evidence that nonsteroidal antiinflammatory medications (NSAIDS) alone are efficacious, although when in combination with other agents, namely the TCAs, they have better efficacy (Goldenberg et al. 1986). Cyclooxygenase-2 (COX-2) NSAIDS, such as celecoxib, may offer benefit by being gastrointestinal sparing (Chandramouli 2002). Useful medications and doses are reviewed on Table 7.2. There is no evidence (Goldenberg et al. 2004) for the efficacy of opioids, thyroid hormone (unless existing hypothyroidism), calcitonin, guaifenesin (Bennett et al. 1996), magnesium, growth hormone, or benzodiazepines (Bennett et al. 1998). Likewise, prednisone (Clark et al. 1985) or other steroids have not been shown to be helpful or indicated.

Cognitive behavioral therapies (Singh et al. 1998), mind–body therapies such as meditation, movement therapies (Hadhazy et al. 2000), and instruction of coping strategies (Schanberg et al. 1996; Kashikar-Zuck et al. 2002) have been shown to be effective adjunct therapies for patients with FM. Behavioral interventions aimed at increasing the perception of pain control are

Table 7.2 Medications for fibromyalgia

Medication name	Dosage
Amitriptyline (Elavil)	10–50 mg QHS
Nortriptyline (Pamelor)	10–20 mg QHS
Sertraline (Zoloft)	50–100 mg daily
Pregabalin (Lyrica)	50–100 mg BID
Tramadol (Ultran)	50–100 mg QID PRN
Cyclobenzaprine (Flexeril)	10 mg Q6 h PRN
Celebrex (Celecoxib)	100–200 mg BID
Naproxyn (Aleve)	250–500 mg PO BID
Sumatiptan (Imitrex)	Oral (50–100 mg) PRN Q8, SQ (6 mg), nasal (5–20 mg)

beneficial in treating pediatric FM. Nielson et al. (2000) was able to develop an activity-pacing scale as an element of chronic pain-coping inventory of tools for children with FM to use even with variable pain intensity as does exist in FM. EMG-biofeedback training has shown benefit in patients with FM (Ferraccioli 1987). Clinical benefit was observed in 56% of patients studied, with ongoing depression suspected as the reason for those that failed to respond.

Prognosis

Outcome of FM is more favorable in children than adults (Buskila et al. 1995). Outcome studies in children have been more promising, giving children a more favorable chance to "outgrow" the condition. This outcome study looked at 338 boys and girls and discovered 15 that met criteria for FM. On second examination 30 months later, 11 of those 15 no longer met the criteria for FM. While many patients ultimately require some pharmacotherapy, however, a well-planned, multidisciplinary approach to pain management was essential. The continued adjunctive use of non-pharmacological therapies, such as regular exercise, acupuncture, massage, cognitive behavioral therapy, attention to sleep hygiene, and physical therapy modalities produces sustained results.

Myofascial Pain Syndrome (MFPS)

Fewer tender points than the number required to make a diagnosis of FM may be found on physical exam and a patient may then be said to have MFPS. This often involves trauma to an individual muscle and pain localized there. MFPS is often treated with local anesthetic sprays or injections, becoming chronic only if left untreated. One often thinks that MFPS may be the precursor to development of FM, with fulfillment of all diagnostic criteria over time. It may be that the two conditions reflect two ends of a spectrum of disease, with MFPS being a more localized form of dysfunction, and FM being a more generalized form of the same disease process (Croft et al. 1996).

Trauma, Sport Injury

Trauma and sport-related injuries are common causes of MSP in children (de Inocencio 1998). Etiologies may include overuse syndromes such as shin splints, chondromalacia patella, contusions, and boney fractures. Chondromalacia refers to a condition in which there is a pathological change in the cartilage of the patella. Osgood-Schlatter syndrome is a syndrome of normal skeletal growth variants. Overuse syndromes are repeated microtraumas that occur faster than the body can heal. Micheli noted that while overuse syndromes were once felt to be an adult phenomena, they are becoming more common in children due to their increased participation in organized, competitive sports (Micheli and Klein 1991). With histories of overuse, x-rays are usually done although a bone scan may be more specific in revealing small stress fractures. NSAIDS and rest are usually indicated. Tendonitis in the forearms and hands is common, and may be associated with excessive computer use or video games (Zapata et al. 2006).

Growing Pains

Recurrent leg pains (growing pains) in children 4–6 years of age are common, 36% in general population (Evans and Scutter 2004). The natural history is pain occurring later in the day or at night, for at least 3 months and is severe enough either to wake the child from sleep or interfere with daily activities (Naish and Apley 1950). Growing pains are usually bilateral and it is not associated swelling or tenderness. The symmetrical occurrence is usually in the thighs, knees, calves, or shins. Often, the painful episode is preceeded by a day involving increased physical activity (Abu-Arafeh and Russel 1996). They have negative laboratory or radiological findings. It is a diagnosis of exclusion. There is never morning stiffness or a limp, and pain-free intervals can be for days to months (Peterson 1986). The term growing pain is a misnomer as there is no evidence to suggest that it is caused by growth. They are typically managed with reassurance, massage, rest, icing, muscle stretching, heat, acetaminophen, or NSAIDS.

Conclusions

Chronic neuromuscular pain has an impact on patients' lives that is disproportionate to the threat it poses to health. It is rarely life-threatening, but can be debilitating and has a considerable effect on a child's overall quality of life and ability to participate in activities that nurture well-being. It presents a challenge of making the diagnosis with a minimum of invasive and expensive testing. A complete physical exam is essential as well as a fund of knowledge of these disorders so that unnecessary testing and invasive procedures are avoided. More evidence-based knowledge is needed to treat FM and MPS.

References

Abu-Arafeh, I., & Russel, G. (1996). Recurrent limb pain in schoolchildren. *Archives of Disease in Childhood, 74*, 336–339.

Arnold, L. M., Hess, E. V., Hudson, J. L., et al. (2002). Randomized, placebo controlled double blind, flexible dose study of fluoxetine in the treatment of women with fibromyalgia. *The American Journal of Medicine, 112*, 191–197.

Banic, B., Petersen-Felix, S., Andersen, O. K., et al. (2003). Evidence for spinal cord hypersensitivity in chronic pain after whiplash injury and in fibromyalgia. *Pain, 107*, 7–15.

Bell, D. S., Bell, K. M., & Cheney, P. R. (1994). Primary juvenile fibromyalgia syndrome and chronic fatigue Syndrome in adolescents. *Clinical Infectious Diseases, 1*, S21–S23.

Bengtsson, A., Henriksson, K. G., Jorfeldt, L., et al. (1986a). Primary fibromyalgia: A clinical laboratory study of 55 patients. *Scandinavian Journal of Rheumatology, 15*, 340–347.

Bengtsson, A., Henriksson, K. G., Larsson, J., et al. (1986b). Muscle biopsy in primary fibromyalgia: Light microscopical and histochemical findings. *Scandinavian Journal of Rheumatology, 15*, 1–6.

Bennett, R. M. (1988). A comparison of cyclobenzaprine and placebo in the management of fibrositis. *Arthritis and Rheumatism, 31*, 1535–1543.

Bennett, R. M., Degarmo, P., & Clark, S. R. (1996). A one year double blind placebo controlled study of guafenisin in fibromyalgia [Abstract]. *Arthritis and Rheumatism, 39*, S2–S12.

Bennett, R. M., Clark, S. C., & Walczyk, J. A. (1998). Randomized double blind placebo controlled study of growth hormone in the treatment of fibromyalgia. *The American Journal of Medicine, 104*, 227–231.

Bennett, R. M., Kamin, M., & Rosenthal, K. R. (2003). Tramadol and acetaminophen combination tablets in the treatment of fibromyalgia pain. *The American Journal of Medicine, 114*, 537–545.

Berman, B. M., Ezzo, J., Hadhazy, V., et al. (1999). Is acupuncture effective in the treatment of fibromyalgia? *The Journal of Family Practice, 48*(3), 213–218.

Biasi, G., Manca, S., Manganelli, S., et al. (1998). Tramadol in fibromyalgia syndrome: A controlled clinical trial versus placebo. *International Journal of Clinical Pharmacology Research, 18*, 13–19.

Buskila, D., Press, J., Gedalia, A., et al. (1993). Assessment of non-articular tenderness and prevalence of fibromyalgia in children. *The Journal of Rheumatology, 20*, 368–370.

Buskila, D., Neuman, L., Hershmaan, E., et al. (1995). Fibromyalgia syndrome in children – An outcome study. *The Journal of Rheumatology, 22*, 525–528.

Carette, S., McCain, G. A., Bell, D. A., et al. (1986). Evaluation of amitriptyline in primary fibrositis. *Arthritis and Rheumatism, 29*(5), 655–659.

Caruso, I., Sarzi Puttini, I., Cazzola, M., et al. (1990). Double blind study of 5-hydroxytryptophan versus placebo in the treatment of primary fibromyalgia syndrome. *The Journal of International Medical Research, 18*, 201–209.

Chandramouli, J. (2002). What is the most effective therapy for preventing NSAID-induced gastropathy? *Journal of Pain and Palliative Care Pharmacotherapy, 16*(2), 23–36.

Clark, S., Tidal, E., & Bennett, R. M. (1985). A double blind cross over trial of prednisone versus placebo in the treatment of fibrositis. *The Journal of Rheumatology, 12*, 980–983.

Crofford, L., Russell, I. J., Mease, P., et al. (2002). Pregabalin improves pain associated with fibromyalgia syndrome in a multicenter, randomized placebo controlled monotherapy trial (abstract). *Arthritis and Rheumatism, 46*, S613.

Croft, P., Burt, J., Schollum, J., et al. (1996). More pain, more tender points: Is fibromyalgia just on end of a continuous spectrum? *Annals of the Rheumatic Diseases, 55*, 482–485.

de Blecourt, A. C., Wolf, R. F., van Rijswik, M. H., et al. (1991). Invivo P magnetic resonance spectroscopy (MRS) of tender points in patients with primary fibromyalgia syndrome. *Rheumatology International, 11*, 51–54.

de Inocencio, J. (1998). Musculoskeletal pain in primary pediatric care: Analysis of 1000 consecutive general pediatric clinic visits. *Pediatrics, 102*, 63.

Deluz, C., Bosia, L., Zirbs, A., et al. (1992). Electroacupuncture in fibromyalgia: Results of a controlled trial. *British Medical Journal, 305*, 1249–1252.

Evans, A. M., & Scutter, S. D. (2004). Prevalence of growing pains in young children. *The Journal of Pediatrics, 145*, 255–258.

Feldenkrais Method. (2000). health yahoo.com/health/alternative_medicine/alternative_ther.../feldenkrais_method.

Felson, D. T., & Goldenberg, D. L. (1986). The natural history of fibromyalgia. *Arthritis and Rheumatism, 29,* 1522–1526.

Ferraccioli, G. (1987). EMG Biofeedback training in fibromyalgia syndrome. *The Journal of Rheumatology, 14,* 820–825.

Fricton, J. R. (1990). Myofascial pain syndrome: Characteristics and epidemiology. *Advances in Pain Research and Therapy., 17,* 107–127.

Gerwin, R. D. (2000). Advances in the treatment of neuromuscular pain: Trigger point injection therapy for neuromuscular pain. Continuing medical education. Johns Hopkins University, pp. 12–17.

Glass, D. E. (1992). Tension headache and some psychiatric aspects of headache. *Headache Quarterly, Current Treatment and Research, 3,* 262–269.

Goldenberg, D. L. (1987). Fibromyalgia syndrome, an emerging but controversial condition. *The Journal of American Medical Association, 257*(20), 2782–2787. May 22/29.

Goldenberg, D. L., Felson, D. T., & Dinerman, H. (1986). A randomized, controlled trial of amitriptyline and naproxen in the treatment of patients with fibromyalgia. *Arthritis and Rheumatism, 29*(11), 1371–1347.

Goldenberg, D. L., Burckhardt, C., & Crofford, L. (2004). Management of fibromyalgia syndrome. *The Journal of Ameriacan Medical Association, 292*(19), 2388–2395.

Goodman, J. E., & McGrath, P. J. (1991). The epidiology of pain in children and adolescents: A review. *Pain, 46,* 247–264.

Hadhazy, V. A., Ezzo, J., Creamer, P., et al. (2000). Mind body therapies for the treatment of fibromyalgia. a systems review. *The Journal of Rheumatology, 27*(12), 2911–2918.

Helms, J. M. (1995). *Acupuncture energetics* (pp. 19–34). Berkeley: Med Acupuncture.

Henriksson, K. G. (1989). Muscle pain in neuromuscular disorders and primary fibromyalgia. *Neurologija, 38,* 213–221.

Kalyan-Dijilani, U. P., Kalyan-Raman, K., Yunas, M. B., et al. (1984). Muscle pathology in primary fibromyalgia syndrome: A light microscopic, histochemical and ultrastructural study. *The Journal of Rheumatology, 11,* 808–813.

Kashikar-Zuck, S., Vaught, M. H., Goldschneider, K. R., et al. (2002). Depression, coping, and functional disability in juvenile primary fibromyalgia syndrome. *The Journal of Pain, 3*(5), 412–419.

Kemper, K. J., Sarah, R., Silver-Highfield, E., et al. (2000). On pins and needles? Pediatric pain patients' experience with acupuncture. *Pediatrics, 105*(4), 941–947.

Lund, N., Bengtsson, A., & Thorcorg, P. (1986). Muscle tissue oxygen pressure in patients with primary fibromyalgia. *Scandinavian Journal of Rheumatology, 15,* 165–173.

Malanga, G. A., & Nadler, S. F. (1999). Non operative treatment of low back pain (review). *Mayo Clinic Proceedings, 74,* 1135–1148.

Malleson, P. N., Al-Matar, M., & Petty, R. E. (1992). Idiopathic Musculoskeletal pain syndrome in children. *The Journal of Rheumatology, 19,* 1786–1789.

Mannerkorpi, K., Kroksmark, T., & Ekdahl, C. (1999). How patients with fibromyalgia experience their symptoms in everyday life. *Physiotherapy Research International, 4,* 100–122.

McCain, G. A. (1986). Role of physical fitness training in the fibrositis/fibromyalgia syndrome. *The American Journal of Medicine, 81,* 73–77.

McCain, G. A., Bell, D. A., Mai, F. M., et al. (1988). A controlled study of the effects of a supervised cardiovascular fitness training program on the manifestations of primary fibromyalgia. *Arthritis and Rheumatism, 31,* 1135–1141.

Melzack, R. (1989). Folk medicine and the sensory modulation of pain. In P. D. Wall & R. Melzack (Eds.), *Textbook of pain* (2nd ed., pp. 897–905). London: Churchill Livingston.

Micheli, L. J., & Klein, J. D. (1991). Sports injuries in children and adolescents. *British Journal of Sports Medicine, 25*(1), 6–9.

Moldofsky, H., & Lue, F. A. (1980). The relationship of alpha and delta EEG frequencies to pain and mood in fibrositis patients treated with chlorpromazine and L-Tryptophan. *Electroencephalography and Clinical Neurophysiology, 50,* 71–80.

Moreno-Lopez, B., Pastor, A. M., de la Cruz, R. R., et al. (1997). Dose-dependent central effects of botulinum neurotoxin type A: A pilot study in the alert behaving cat. *Neurology, 48,* 456–464.

Naish, J. M., & Apley, J. (1950). Growing pains, a clinical study of non-arthritic limb pain in children. *Archives of Disease in Childhood, 26*(126), 134–140.

Nicassio, P. M., Radojevic, V., Weisman, M. H., et al. (1997). A comparison of behavioral and educational interventions for fibromyalgia. *The Journal of Rheumatology, 24,* 2000–2007.

Nielson, W. R., Jensen, M. P., & Hill, M. L. (2000). An activity pacing scale for the chronic pain coping inventory: development in a sample of patients with fibromyalgia syndrome. *Pain, 89,* 111–115.

Oakville-Trafalger Memorial Hospital. (1992). Fibromyalgia exercise video.

Pellegrino, M. J. (1993). *Fibromyalgia-managing the pain.* Columbus: Anadem.

Pellegrino, M. J., Waylonis, G. W., & Sommer, A. (1989). Familial occurrence of primary fibromyalgia. *Archives of Physical Medicine and Rehabilitation, 70,* 61–63.

Peterson, H. (1986). Growing pains. *Pediatric Clinic of North America, 33,* 1365–1372.

Petzke, F., Clauw, D. J., Ambrose, K., et al. (2003). Increased pain sensitivity in fibromyalgia: effects of stimulus type and mode of presentation. *Pain, 105,* 403–413.

Pomeranz, B. (1996). Scientific research into acupuncture for the relief of pain. *Journal of Alternative and Complementary Medicine, 2*(1), 53–60.

Ramsey, S. M. (1997). Holistic manual therapy techniques. *Primary Care, 24,* 759–786.

Roizenblatt, S., Tufik, S., Goldenberg, J., et al. (1997). Juvenile fibromyalgia: Clinical and polysomnographic aspects. *The Journal of Rheumatology, 24*(3), 579–585.

Rosen, N. B. (1994). Physical medicine and rehabilitation in management. *Bailliere's Clinical Rheumatology, 8*(4), 907.

Russell, J., Kamin, M., Bennet, R. M., et al. (2000). Efficacy of Tramadol in treatment of pain in fibromyalgia. *Journal of Clinical Rheumatology, 6*, 250–257.

Rusy, L. M. (1996). *Low impact exercise workout.* Milwaukee: Maxishare, Children's Hospital of Wisconsin.

Rusy, L. M., & Weisman, S. J. (2000). Complementary therapies for acute pediatric pain management. *Pediatric Clinics of North America, 47*(3), 589–599.

Rusy, L. M., Harvey, S. A., & Beste, D. J. (1999). Pediatric fibromyalgia and dizziness: Evaluation of vestibular function. *Journal of Developmental and Behavioral Pediatrics, 20*(4), 211–215.

Sandberg, M., Lundeberg, T., & Gerdle, B. (1999). Manual acupuncture in fibromyalgia: A long term pilot study. *Journal of Musculoskeletal Pain., 73*(3), 39–57.

Schanberg, L. E., Keefe, F. J., Lefebvre, J. C., et al. (1996). Pain coping strategies in children with juvenile primary fibromyalgia syndrome: Correlation with pain, physical function and psychological distress. *Arthritis Care and Research, 9*(2), 89–95.

Sheon, R. P., & the Goff group. (1997). Repetitive strain injury 2: Diagnostic and treatment tips on six common problems. *Postgraduate Medicine, 102*(88), 79–85.

Singh, B. B., Berman, B. M., Hadhazy, V. A., et al. (1998). A pilot study of cognitive behavioral therapy in fibromyalgia. *Alternative Therapies in Health and Medicine, 4*(2), 67–70.

Smythe, H. A. (1984). Problems with the MMPI (editorial). *The Journal of Rheumatology, 11*, 417–418.

Smythe, H. A. (1989). Non articular rheumatism and psychogenic musculoskeletal syndromes. In D. J. McCarthy (Ed.), *Arthritis and allied conditions: A textbook of rheumatology* (pp. 1241–1254). Philadelphia: Lea & Febiger.

Travell, J. G., & Simmons, D. G. (1983). *Myofascial pain and dysfunction: The trigger point manual.* Baltimore: Williams & Wilkins.

Waylonis, G. W., & Heck, W. (1992). Fibromyalgia syndrome, new associations. *American Journal of Physical Medicine & Rehabilitation, 71*, 343–348.

Wolfe, F., Smythe, H. A., Yunus, M. B., et al. (1990). The American College of Rheumatology 1990 criteria for the classification of fibromyalgia. Report of the Multicenter Criteria Committee. *Arthritis and Rheumatism, 33*(2), 160–172.

Wright, E. F., & Schiffman, E. L. (1995). Treatment alternatives for patients with masticatory myofascial pain. *Journal of the American Dental Association, 126*, 1030–1039.

Yunas, M. B., Masi, A. T., & Aldag, J. C. (1989). Preliminary criteria for primary fibromyalgia syndrome (PFS): Multivariate analysis of consecutive series of PFS, other pain patients, and normal subjects. *Clinical and Experimental Rheumatology, 7*, 63–69.

Yunus, M. B., Khan, M. A., Rawlings, K. K., et al. (1999). Genetic linkage analysis of multicase families with fibromyalgia syndrome. *The Journal of Rheumatology, 26*(2), 408–411.

Zapata, A. L., Pantoja, A. J., Leone, C., et al. (2006). Pain and musculoskeletal pain syndromes in adolescents. *The Journal of Adolescent Health, 38*, 769–771.

Zijstra, T. R., Barendregt, P. J., & van de Laar, M. A. (2002). Venlafexedine in fibromyalgia: results of a randomized placebo controlled double blind trial [Abstract]. *Arthritis and Rheumatism, 46*, S105.

Functional Abdominal Pain in Children

8

Miguel Saps and Gati Dhroove

Keywords

Functional gastrointestinal disorders • Functional abdominal pain (FAP)
• School stress • Corticotropin-releasing factor (CRF) • Visceral
hypersensitivity • Irritable bowel syndrome (IBS)

Introduction

Approximately 50 years ago, Apley and Naish described children who presented with repeated episodes of abdominal pain for at least 3 months without any identifiable cause under the term recurrent abdominal pain (Apley and Naish 1958). Later studies showed that this term was a "waste basket" encompassing functional and organic conditions. More recent symptom-based criteria, known as Rome criteria, exclusively define those gastrointestinal conditions thought to be of functional origin and without clinical evidence of anatomical or structural abnormalities. The third edition of the Rome criteria (Rasquin 2006), classifies pain-predominant functional gastrointestinal disorders (FGIDs) in four different conditions: childhood functional abdominal pain, functional dyspepsia, irritable bowel syndrome (IBS), and abdominal migraine (Table 8.1). The criteria has established an addi-

tional subgroup (childhood functional abdominal pain syndrome), to define those children meeting criteria for childhood functional abdominal pain in association with non-GI complaints or altered daily function. In order to facilitate the reader's understanding, we refer to the group of pain-predominant FGIDs as "functional abdominal pain" (FAP), a term that is commonly used to describe these conditions. This chapter discusses the epidemiology, pathogenesis, and treatment of the most common forms of FAP. Abdominal migraine (Abu-Arafeh and Russell 1995), an uncommon condition representing only 1–2% of all children with FAP will only be described briefly.

Many diseases can cause chronic abdominal pain, but in clinical practice, most children presenting with abdominal pain have an FGID without any evidence of organic disease. They are considered to have FAP, one of the most common GI conditions. FAP is a global health problem occurring in children of different ethnicities, nationalities, and geographic locations (Saps et al. 2008a). FAP represents 2–4% of all pediatric office visits (Starfield et al. 1984) and 4% of in-home consultations (Saps et al. 2008a). Despite these impressive figures, office-based data misrepresent the totality of the problems as only

M. Saps (✉)
Divisions of Pediatric Gastroenterology, Children's
Memorial Hospital, Northwestern University's Feinberg
School of Medicine, Chicago, IL, USA
e-mail: msaps@childrensmemorial.org

B.C. McClain and S. Suresh (eds.), *Handbook of Pediatric Chronic Pain:*
Current Science and Integrative Practice, DOI 10.1007/978-1-4419-0350-1_8,
© Springer Science+Business Media, LLC 2011

Table 8.1 Classification of functional abdominal pain (FAP) disorders according to the Rome III criteria

Disorder	Symptoms
Functional dyspepsia[a]	• Persistent or recurrent pain or discomfort in the upper abdomen
	• Not relieved by defecation or associated with the onset of a change in stool frequency or form
	• No evidence of an inflammatory, anatomic, metabolic, or neoplastic process
Irritable bowel syndrome[a]	Abdominal discomfort or pain associated with two or more of the following at least 25% of the time:
	• Improved with defecation
	• Onset associated with a change in stool frequency or form
	• No evidence of an inflammatory, anatomic, metabolic, or neoplastic process
Childhood functional abdominal pain[a]	• Episodic or continuous abdominal pain
	• Insufficient criteria for other functional gastrointestinal disorder
	• No evidence of an inflammatory, anatomic, metabolic, or neoplastic process
Childhood functional abdominal pain syndrome[a]	Childhood functional abdominal pain associated with one or more of the following at least 25% of the time:
	• Interference with daily functioning or sleep
	• Additional somatic symptoms, such as headache, limb pain
Abdominal migraine	Paroxysmal, intense, periumbilical pain lasting ≥1 h Interferes with normal activities. Associated with two or more of the following:
	• Anorexia, nausea, vomiting, headache, photophobia, pallor
	• Intervening periods of health (weeks–months)
	• No evidence of an inflammatory, anatomic, metabolic, or neoplastic process

[a] Children in these groups should have at least 8 weeks of continuous or intermittent symptoms

3% of children who complain of abdominal pain at the community level seek medical attention (Saps et al. 2008b). A prospective community-based study has shown that an average of 38% of elementary school children complain of abdominal pain weekly with 90% of children reporting abdominal pain at least once during a 6-month period (Saps et al. 2008b). Symptoms consistent with IBS occur in 6% of middle school students and 14% of high school students (Hyams et al. 1996). In children, abdominal pain has been associated with worse quality of life, school absenteeism, and higher anxiety and depression scores. A long-term follow-up study has shown that adults with a history of FAP as children have higher prevalence of psychiatric disorders and often require treatment with psychoactive medications (Campo et al. 2001). The impact of abdominal pain in terms of economic costs and burden on the family life is also substantial (Saps et al. 2008b). Studies have shown that parents of children with abdominal pain are subject to significant health-care expenditure (Saps et al. 2008a) and frequently miss work to care for their sick children.

Pathogenesis

The pathogenesis of FAP remains unclear. The most accepted model (biopsychosocial model) proposes that there is no single etiology to these conditions. FAP results from the interplay of different factors including biological, psychological, and social factors. There is evidence to support that genetic factors contribute to the manifestation of FAP. Studies have shown clustering of FGIDs in families. Twin studies have shown a higher prevalence of FAP in monozygotic than dizygotic twins (Wojczynski et al. 2007). But, family dynamics and learnt behavior also play an important role in the pathogenesis of these conditions. Mothers of children with chronic abdominal pain report more somatic and depressive symptoms in their children than the children themselves (Garber et al. 1991). Walker et al.

have shown that solicitous or encouraging responses from the mother to the child's pain reinforces the child's symptoms and enhances sick role behaviors (Walker et al. 1991, 2006a). It is likely that in the setting of specific hereditary factors, environmental factors, including learnt behaviors that do not usually cause functional alterations may lead to the manifestation of FAP later in life.

In children, FAP has also been associated with poor coping skills (Walker et al. 2006b). Differences in pain- and stress-related coping abilities among children may explain variations in severity of pain and interference with daily activities. Epidemiological studies have shown that while some children with abdominal pain are barely affected in their daily activities, others are greatly affected in terms of school attendance, sleep, and social activities. Stress may also play a role in the pathogenesis of FGIDs in children and adults. Children who are bullied at school and those who are high achievers have a higher incidence of FAP than their peers (Ball and Weydert 2003; Boey and Goh 2001; Greco et al. 2007). School stress may be a contributing factor to the seasonal variation of abdominal pain as manifested by a higher frequency of abdominal pain consultations during winter months (Saps et al. 2008b, c; MacIver et al. 2007). Depression, anxiety, and stressful events predispose adult patients with acute gastroenteritis to develop postinfectious IBS. Activation of brain corticotropin-releasing factor (CRF) (also known as corticotropin-releasing hormone – CRH) pathways participate in the behavioral and visceral responses to stress. Experiments in CRF_1 knockout mice demonstrated the primary role of CRF_1 receptors in stress-related endocrine (Bale and Vale 2004), behavioral (Kehne and De Lombaert 2002), and autonomic (Yokotani et al. 2001) responses. Studies have shown that CRF_1 signaling in the brain and the gut may play a role in the comorbidity of anxiety/depression and IBS (Tache et al. 2005).

A common tool to most studies evaluating visceral hypersensitivity is the rectal balloon distention, a test that discriminates IBS from healthy controls with a sensitivity of 95% and a specificity of 72% (Bouin et al. 2002). IBS patients report that rectal balloon distention elicit symptoms similar to those felt during IBS episodes. Patients with IBS have increased visceral sensitivity, a proposed marker of IBS, to colorectal distention than healthy controls (Talley 1998). CRF modifies rectal sensation in healthy volunteers and patients with IBS. CRF and other CRF-related peptides such as urocortins interact with CRF subtype 1 and 2 receptors located in the gut. CRF gene expression is up-regulated by stress (Imaki et al. 1991) which in turn affects colonic motility (Pavcovich et al. 1998). Animal studies have shown that stress enhances abdominal contractions, a surrogate presentation of pain, in response to rectal distension via pathways involving CRF and intestinal mast cells (Gue et al. 1997). CRF release during acute stressful events increases colonic transit via neuronal pathways and stimulates colonic mucin secretion through the activation of neurons and mast cells (Castagliuolo et al. 1996).

The study of the interactions of peripheral components such as enteric receptors, afferent neurons, and cerebral networks and the different mechanisms involved in the alteration of the brain gut axis provides important insight in the understanding of the pathogenesis of FGIDs. Studies on visceral hypersensitivity, have demonstrated the involvement of peripheral and central neurons. Inflammatory processes may sensitize parietal mechanoreceptors in the gut (Delvaux 2002). Biopsies taken from patients with IBS demonstrated increased numbers of mast cells in close proximity with mucosal nerves. The severity and frequency of abdominal pain have been shown to be positively correlated with the proximity of the nerves to the mast cells and their degranulation products (Barbara et al. 2004).

It is likely that in some cases the initial trigger to the manifestation of FGIDs may occur at the gut level where local conditions affect the peripheral pathways and alter sensation at the nerve endings. In other cases, "central" triggering factors or a combination of central and peripheral factors may lead to the manifestation of an FGID.

Infectious agents affecting the GI tract may play a role in the pathogenesis of FGIDs. Studies have shown that IBS and dyspepsia can develop as a sequela of an acute gastrointestinal infection

(Gwee et al. 2003; Neal et al. 1997). Saps et al. found a higher prevalence of IBS and dyspepsia in children exposed to bacterial gastrointestinal infections years earlier as compared to controls (Saps et al. 2008d). Gut sensory and motor changes persist even after the acute inflammation has resolved (Barbara et al. 1997). Patients with postinfectious bacterial IBS have faster gut transit times and increased rectal sensitivity than controls (Gwee et al. 1999). Persistence of inflammatory cells in the intestinal mucosa, including increase in lamina propria plasma cells, mononuclear cells, and cytokines has been found in apparently normal mucosa few months after an episode of acute enteritis has resolved (Gwee et al. 2003; Collins 1992). The presence of a higher density of 5-hydroxytryptamine enteroendocrine cells suggests the participation of the neuroendocrine system. Increased numbers of T lymphocytes in rectal biopsies a year after the clinical resolution of an episode of acute bacterial gastroenteritis suggests persistent immune activation (Spiller et al. 2000). The possible effect of viral infections in the incidence of postinfectious IBS remains unclear (Saps et al. 2009). An adequate quantity and composition of the gut flora is fundamental for the correct function of the GI tract. Among the multiple functions of the gut flora that affect the GI tract are the maturation of the lymphoid tissue and the immune regulation and protection against pathogens. The gut flora influences the physiology of the gut by modifying gut sensation and motor functions. Although the role of the gut flora in the pathophysiology of symptoms in IBS remains controversial, a study found increased flora (small bowel bacterial overgrowth) in up to 80% of patients with IBS (Galatola et al. 1991; Lin 2004; Pimentel et al. 2006).

Animal models have shown that colonic irritation with daily mustard enemas leads to chronic visceral hypersensitivity (allodynia and hyperalgesia) associated with central sensitization (Kellow et al. 1991). In this experiment, neonatal but not adult rats, undergoing chemical colonic irritation exhibited chronic visceral hypersensitivity long time after the stimulus ceased and in the presence of normal biopsies.

The demonstration of a differential response to the chemical agent at different ages substantiates the role of early life events as proposed in the biopsychosocial model. Proving the effect of early life events in the pathogenesis of FGIDs in children is a difficult task. Neonates are exposed to a multitude of elements. Among all these possible contributing factors, demonstrating the effect of a specific factor that may predispose infants and toddlers to develop FGIDs several years later is methodologically complicated. However, a study has shown a possible association between early life events and functional intestinal disorders later life. In this study, neonates exposed to gastric suction at birth had a higher frequency of functional intestinal symptoms than sibling controls that were not exposed to gastric suction (Anand et al. 2004). The authors proposed that noxius stimuli at birth may predispose to the development of long-term visceral hypersensitivity and cognitive hypervigilance later in life. An animal study has demonstrated that orogastric suctioning during the neonatal period resulted in visceral hyperalgesia in adult rats (Smith et al. 2007).

Electrophysiological recordings of viscerosensitive neurons in the lumbosacral region of the spinal cord (L5–S1) showed enhanced impulse responses to colorectal distention in comparison to control animals. The rats in this study displayed hypersensitivity to cutaneous nociceptive stimulation predominantly in lumbosacral dermatomes. Studies have shown enhanced spinal cord processing with hyperexcitability of spinal nociceptive neurons in patients with IBS (Bueno et al. 2000). Similar to patients with fibromyalgia, IBS patients may develop widely distributed hyperalgesia. Secondary hyperalgesia may constitute a common mechanism involved in the pathogenesis of IBS and other conditions such as fibromyalgia and complex regional pain syndrome (CRPS).

The incorporation of PET scanning and more recently fMRI in the investigation of FGIDs led to a greater understanding of the role of the central nervous system (CNS) in the pathogenesis of this group of conditions. The CNS may affect peripheral activity through the modulation of peripheral nociceptive input. The summation of peripheral and central effects may result in visceral hypersensitivity (Kellow et al. 1991). IBS patients have detectable differences in regional cerebral blood flow in fMRI studies when compared to controls. As an in-depth analysis of all the areas involved is beyond the scope of this chapter, we briefly summarize some of these findings. Studies suggest the existence of an abnormal cerebral sensory processing in response to colonic distention in IBS patients (Silverman et al. 1997; Mertz et al. 2000; Naliboff et al. 2001; Bernstein et al. 2002). IBS patients demonstrate a decreased activation of pain inhibition circuits like cortico-pontine circuit and an increased activation of pain facilitation circuits like limbic and paralimbic circuits. Preliminary evidence suggests alterations in the activation of regions involved in the attention processes and response selection and regions involved with emotional and autonomic responses to stimuli. Some of the areas of activation are thought to be related to the amplification of threat appraisal, enhanced anxiety responses, and hypervigilance (Naliboff et al. 2001). Patients with IBS have a differential pattern of activation of the prefrontal cortex (PFC) and anterior cingulate cortex (ACC) to supraliminal and subliminal colonic stimulation. IBS patients also have a higher activation of the hippocampus in response to supraliminal stimulation in comparison with controls (Andresen et al. 2005). A common feature of various studies is the greater degree of activation of the dorsal sub region of the ACC, an area that has been shown to relate to the cognitive processing of sensory input (Mertz et al. 2000; Naliboff et al. 2001). These and other findings substantiate the proposed interactions of the brain gut axis and the integration of the various biological and psychosocial domains of the biopsychosocial model for FGIDs (Dunlop et al. 2003).

Management

Principles of Treatment

The multitude of biological, psychological, and social factors that may be involved in the pathogenesis of FGIDs and the chronic nature of these conditions make the management of this group of patients distinct and challenging. The following general principles based on research and experience may be helpful in the treatment of FAP. Establishing a therapeutic physician–patient relationship proves to be helpful in symptom reduction and adherence to treatment. The physician should take a thorough history attempting to unveil possible triggers to the symptoms. Those should be addressed during consultation and treatment. Most children will improve with reassurance and time. Community studies have shown improvement of abdominal pain in untreated children (Saps and Di Lorenzo 2007). The practitioner should assure the family that although these are chronic conditions with high impact on quality of life, they are benign in nature. Often, patients and families are afraid to ask questions on the nature and prognosis of the disease. The patients may have consulted with other practitioners who had conducted multiple tests with negative results that may have further contributed to anxiety and uncertainty in patients and families. The physician should encourage the families to ask questions. Questions should be answered demonstrating empathy and understanding and validating the symptoms. Patients are frequently afraid of being judged and labeled

Factors involved in the pathogenesis of FAP

1. Genetics and environment
   - Past and early life events
2. Psychosocial factors
   - Coping style
   - Social interactions
   - Depression/anxiety
   - Secondary gains
3. Visceral hyperalgesia secondary to
   - Inflammation and infection
     - Trauma
     - Stress
   Motility disorders

as psychiatric cases and often feel either not believed or understood. It should be clearly stated that the symptoms "are not in your head" and that the presenting symptoms are real. The role of stressors and the importance of the brain gut axis in the pathophysiology of symptoms should be explained. It is important to educate the patient and the family. Individualizing the condition and discussing the diagnosis and prognosis helps understanding, provides reassurance, and allows patients and families to conduct their own "research" and confirm the benign nature of the condition. There are no clinically available biological markers for FGIDs, hence testing should be limited. The physician should avoid extensive testing and should project a positive attitude toward the condition and its potential prognosis. Repeated and extensive testing may confuse the patient and raise questions on the ability of the doctor to diagnose and treat FAP. Negative testing should be considered as a confirmation of the functional nature of FAP and should not result in repeated or more extensive testing. The practitioner should demonstrate confidence and be available for further questions demonstrating a commitment to curing the condition. It should be made clear that the cooperation of the patient and family is necessary and that the patient should be an integral part and a protagonist of his or her own recovery. Real and achievable goals should be set. The goal of the treatment should be to decrease pain and improve quality of life. Setting the goal on abolishing pain may result in failure and loss of trust if a new episode of pain occurs. If the patient is currently missing school, returning to school should be encouraged. It should be explained that school attendance is not part of the problem and in fact is part of the solution. Children in school get more distracted and less focused on pain and their ailments. Adequate social interaction facilitates healing. Parents should be discouraged from reinforcing the symptoms and allowing secondary gains. Different approaches or a combination of strategies may be required for different patients. The treatment should be tailored to individual needs and cases. The nature

Guidelines to Establish a Therapeutic Physician–Patient Relationship

1. Conduct a patient-centered interview.
2. Obtain a thorough history and physical examination.
3. Validate the pain: reassure the child and family that the pain is not imaginary.
4. Address patient's concerns and assess patient's understanding of the nature of the disease.
5. Educate the patient on the chronic and benign nature of the disease.
6. Respond to the patient's symptoms with empathy.
7. Provide psychosocial support to the patient and the family, establishing an ongoing relationship.
8. Discuss the possible link between stressors and symptoms and help patients identify triggering factors.
9. Limit laboratory investigations.
10. Explain that the effectiveness of the treatment is based on the combined effort of physician, patients, and the family.
11. Help the child to cope with the condition.
12. Children should be encouraged to go back to the school and resume their routine activities.
13. Explain that the goal of the treatment is to decrease pain and improve the quality of life.
14. Explain to the patient about the different treatment options available and help them select the appropriate treatment.

of the condition may require a multidisciplinary and personalized approach. The use of complementary therapies may improve the outcome of FAP. However, the utilization of complementary therapies is sometimes difficult. Some patients may be reluctant to use alternative therapies while in other cases, insurance or geographical limitations and the unavailability of complementary practitioners may preclude their use.

Evidence-Based Management

Pharmacotherapy

There is a paucity of evidence-based therapies for the treatment of FAP in children. Treatment is usually based on adult data, poorly designed studies, or anecdotal experience. A technical review by the American Academy of Pediatrics and the North American Society of Gastroenterology Hepatology and Nutrition and a meta-analysis by the Cochran's group found little evidence to recommend most of the treatments that are currently used (Di Lorenzo et al. 2005). In the next few pages we discuss evidence-based therapies for the treatment of FAP in children.

H2-receptor antagonists: A double-blind, placebo- controlled crossover trial evaluated the efficacy of famotidine in the treatment of abdominal pain and dyspeptic symptoms in children (See et al. 2001). Twenty five children were enrolled and randomized to 3 weeks of famotidine or placebo followed by a crossover period. Famotidine was given at a dose of 0.5 mg/kg/dose twice daily (maximum 40 mg). Famotidine was superior to placebo (68% vs. 12%) in improving dyspeptic symptoms. However, the effect of famotidine in abdominal pain was less clear. A subcommittee of the American Academy of Pediatrics (AAP) and the North American Society for Pediatric Gastroenterology, Hematology, and Nutrition (NASPGHAN) reviewed the study and concluded that H2-receptor antagonists could be beneficial for children with severe dyspeptic symptoms (including heartburn), but found inconclusive evidence to recommend H2-receptor antagonists in the treatment of abdominal pain in children with dyspepsia (evidence quality B) (Di Lorenzo et al. 2005).

Cyproheptadine: The treatment of FAP in children was explored in a double-blind, placebo-controlled trial of cyproheptadine (Sadeghian et al. 2008). Twenty-nine children with a diagnosis of FAP, ranging in age from 4 to 12 years received cyproheptadine (0.25–0.5 mg/kg/day) in two divided doses or placebo for 2 weeks. Primary outcome measures included self-reported change in the duration and frequency of abdominal pain and parental assessment of the child's improvement. At the end of the study, 86% of children receiving cyproheptadine compared to 36% of those receiving placebo reported improvement or resolution of abdominal pain. The study also showed a significant difference in parental satisfaction between both drug and placebo, with almost all parents reporting satisfaction with the drug. The authors propose that the mechanism of action of cyproheptadine may result from its anti-serotonin or calcium-channel blocking effects.

Selective serotonin receptor agonists: Serotonin has a central role in modulating motility, visceral perception, and intraluminal secretion in the gastrointestinal tract. Tegaserod (5-hydroxytryptamine; 5-HT) is a selective serotonin receptor agonist acting at $5-HT_4$ receptors located in the gut wall. Tegaserod, which is currently not available for commercial use, has been used in the treatment of IBS with constipation in adults and children with promising results. A clinical trial on 48 adolescents with constipation-predominant IBS, randomized to an osmotic laxative alone or a combination of tegaserod and osmotic laxative showed a beneficial effect of tegaserod in improving the frequency of bowel movements and reducing pain (Khoshoo et al. 2006). Patients that were exclusively treated with laxatives had improvement in constipation but no improvement in pain. A retrospective study on the efficacy of tegaserod in improving constipation and abdominal pain found moderate or significant relief of abdominal pain and bloating in 64% of cases in children with constipation (Liem et al. 2008).

Selective serotonin reuptake inhibitors (SSRI): A preliminary open label flexible dose study was conducted to assess the efficacy of citalopram, an SSRI, in the management of recurrent abdominal pain in children (Campo et al. 2004). In this 12-week exploratory study, 25 children received an initial daily dose of 10 mg. If no clinical response was obtained, the dosage was progressively increased, with the maximum administration being 40 mg at week 4. At the end of the study 68% of all children received 40 mg of citalopram. At week 12, it was found that 50% of the children completing the study viewed their symptoms as "very much improved." Parental and child reports showed a significant improvement in abdominal pain index as well as improvement in comorbid anxiety and depression. However, the lack of blinding of both, subjects and clinicians, the absence of a placebo group, and randomization constitute important methodological limitations of this study. Therefore, we cannot definitely conclude that the observed improvement of the group of patients receiving citalopram is due to the effect of this drug.

Tricyclic antidepressants (TCA): Adult studies have shown a beneficial effect of various tricyclic antidepressants in the treatment of IBS (Drossman et al. 1997). Two recent studies evaluated their efficacy in the treatment of functional abdominal pain disorders in children. The first study included 33 adolescents 12–18 years diagnosed with IBS from a suburban pediatric gastroenterology clinic. Subjects were randomized to amitriptyline or placebo for 8 weeks at a dose of 10, 20, or 30 mg of according to their weight. End points were assessed at 4, 8, and 11 weeks. The study concluded that amitriptyline was superior to placebo in improving quality of life and pain. However, pain improved only in certain areas of the abdomen and not others and at specific times of follow-up and not in every evaluation. In addition the authors found an unusual response to placebo. While a meta-analysis of studies on IBS found an average positive placebo effect of 40%, the authors found a negative placebo effect. It is possible that this negative placebo effect may be responsible of the significant difference in pain relief between amitriptyline and placebo found in this study. Subsequently, a larger multicenter pediatric study found dissimilar results. This randomized double-blinded placebo-controlled trial evaluated the efficacy of amitriptyline in 90 children of all ages (Saps et al. 2008e) diagnosed with the three most common diagnoses included in the definition of FAP (dyspepsia, IBS, and childhood functional abdominal pain) and at six tertiary care centers geographically dispersed in the USA. The study found that amitriptyline and placebo were equally effective in improving all self report measures: pain relief, global sense of improvement, satisfaction with treatment, interference with quality of life, and psychological testing scores (depression and somatization). The study showed improvement in 59% of subjects in the amitriptyline group in intention to treat analysis and higher in the per-protocol analysis but no significant difference between amitriptyline and placebo. Children in the placebo group had an unusually high positive placebo effect that the authors explained by the achievement of an effective patient–family–doctor relation. It is possible that the very high placebo effect obtained in this study may explain the lack of difference between drug and placebo.

Peppermint oil: This is the concentrated oil of the herb "Mentha Paprika." Studies suggest that peppermint oil may have beneficial effects relieving colonic spasm (Leicester and Hunt 1982; Jarvis et al. 1992; Sparks et al. 1995; Kingham 1995) dyspeptic symptoms and flatulence (Westphal et al. 1996). Its proposed mechanism of action is as a Ca^{2+} channels blocker (Hawthorn et al. 1988; Nolon and Friend 1994). Kline et al. (2001) conducted a randomized double-blind clinical trial to evaluate the efficacy of pH-dependent enteric-coated peppermint oil capsules in treating IBS in children. Forty-two children were randomized to one (30–45 kg) or two (>45 kg) 187 mg capsules three times daily of a commercial preparation or placebo for 2 weeks. Children receiving peppermint oil had a 76% reduction of abdominal pain in comparison with 19% in those receiving placebo. No adverse events were reported. Enteric-coated peppermint oil is difficult to obtain in pharmacies, generally not on the formulary for insurance companies and relatively expensive. Non-enteric-coated preparations may lead to esophagitis and mild rectal burning probably due to the menthol component of peppermint oil. After reviewing this study, a technical report from the AAP and NASPGHAN considered that there was quality B evidence to recommend peppermint oil in the treatment of chronic abdominal pain while the Cochrane report found that there was not enough evidence to recommend it (Di Lorenzo et al. 2005).

Although the use of other drugs, such as antiemetics, simethicone, antidiarrheals, laxatives, bulking agents/fiber, or antispasmodics, are commonly used by clinicians to manage symptoms associated with chronic abdominal pain in children, no studies have been published on their efficacy for pain relief in children with FAP.

Complementary and Alternative Therapies

In line with adult data (Gonsalkorale et al. 2003), studies in children have shown a beneficial effect of complementary and alternative therapies including cognitive-behavioral therapy and hypnotherapy in the treatment of FAP. The demonstrated efficacy of these strategies provides further support to the validity of the bidirectional communication between the gut and the brain (brain gut axis) and the biopsychosocial model by achieving relief of functional gastrointestinal symptoms through interventions aimed at modifying psychological and social factors.

Cognitive behavioral therapy: Cognitive-behavioral strategies include attention, distraction, hypnosis, imagery, thought-stopping, and music therapy. Cognitive strategies are aimed at lowering attention and decreasing the perception of pain by encouraging the patient to focus on a pleasant thought or image. Although the mechanism of action of cognitive techniques is incompletely understood, it has been hypothesized that those may help reducing pain through the activation of endogenous opioid and non-opioid pain-suppressing systems (Heyneman et al. 1990). The behavioral aspects involved in this form of therapy are aimed at changing the attitudes of children toward pain. Behavioral strategies include exercise, modeling, biofeedback, operant conditioning, relaxation, art and play therapy, and desensitization. Cognitive behavioral therapy strategies can also include parents that may initiate, maintain, or exacerbate pain. A meta-analysis of studies on the treatment of recurrent abdominal pain in children through cognitive behavioral therapy has shown the beneficial effect of cognitive behavioral strategies in treating children with recurrent abdominal pain (Bursch 2008). Guided imagery therapy is a two-step cognitive-behavioral technique in which the child is first induced into a state of deep relaxation and then guided in imagining scenes that enables the improvement of symptoms, achievement of self-regulation, and behavioral adjustment. In older children and adults, guided imagery therapy can also be self-directed, where the own individual puts himself into a relaxed state and creates his own images. Three studies indicated that guided imagery may be beneficial in the treatment of FAP (Weydert et al. 2006; Youssef et al. 2004; Ball et al. 2003). The small sample size (10–20 patients) of all the studies and the lack of randomization of most of the studies does not allow to definitively concluding whether this technique is beneficial on the treatment of children with FAP.

Hypnotherapy: A clinical trial evaluated the effect of hypnotherapy in the treatment of FAP in children. Fifty three children diagnosed with IBS and FAP were randomly assigned to six sessions (over 3 months) of either hypnotherapy or supportive medical care (education, diet, proton pump inhibitors). Children were followed clinically up to 12 months. Patients in the hypnotherapy group had a significant reduction in pain intensity and frequency in comparison to the control group. The benefit of hypnotherapy was not only demonstrated during treatment but at all times even after discontinuation of therapy (Vlieger et al. 2007). At 12 months, only 5% of children in the hypnotherapy group reported no benefit in pain relief, while almost half of the children in the control group had no benefit. A Cochrane's meta-analysis and the technical report of AAP and NASPGHAN concluded that cognitive behavioral therapy may be a useful intervention for children with FAP (Di Lorenzo et al. 2005).

There is no evidence to support other forms of complementary or alternative therapy such as acupuncture or herbal-based Chinese medicine in the treatment of abdominal pain in children.

Probiotics: These are living microorganisms which when administered in adequate amounts may be beneficial to the host's health. Probiotics have multiple effects on the host including reestablishing intestinal microbial balance, immune modulation, antibacterial, and protection of mucosal barrier. The possible role of inflammatory changes and alterations in the gut flora in the pathogenesis of FGIDs has led to a surge of trials evaluating the efficacy of probiotics in the treatment of IBS. There have been several adult and three pediatric trials published on the possible benefit of probiotics in the treatment of FGIDs. Unfortunately, differences in methodologies, strains, doses, and time of follow-up among trials limit the possibility of comparing or generalizing the results (Drouault-Holowacz et al. 2008; Kim et al. 2005; O'Mahony et al. 2005). All pediatric studies have shown improvement in bloating (Drouault-Holowacz et al. 2008). However, the results of studies assessing the efficacy of probiotics in improving abdominal pain in children are less clear. While some studies have shown no clear benefit in pain relief (Nobaek et al. 2000), a recent multicenter study published in abstract form has shown a beneficial effect of VSL3, a commercial preparation of seven probiotics in the treatment of FAP in children (Guandalini et al. 2008). Despite the lack of conclusive evidence of their benefit, probiotics are frequently used in the treatment of abdominal pain due to their demonstrated safety in otherwise healthy children.

Lactose: Although many parents link the onset of symptoms to the ingestion of dairy products, studies do not conclusively show that avoiding lactose benefits children with FAP (evidence quality B) (technical report AAP) (Di Lorenzo et al. 2005). Frequently, a thorough history reveals that the ingestion of dairy products does not consistently result in abdominal pain and that abdominal pain often occurs at times of no ingestion of dairy products. The demonstration of the lack of temporal relation of the onset of abdominal pain and its relation with dairy products ingestion during the consultation usually reassures the parents.

Conclusion

Although functional abdominal pain is commonly seen in children, the treatment is multidimensional. A thorough understanding of the use of cognitive behavioral modification may be necessary to adequately treat the condition. Family therapy may be needed to reduce the enmeshment in children with the parents. A child-focused approach with the aid of alternative medicine may decrease symptoms and reduce the incidence of pain, thereby limiting the functional disability that this condition may lead to in the adolescent period.

References

Abu-Arafeh, I., & Russell, G. (1995). Prevalence and clinical features of abdominal migraine compared with those of migraine headache. *Archives of Disease in Childhood, 72*, 413–417.

Anand, K. J., Runeson, B., & Jacobson, B. (2004). Gastric suction at birth associated with long-term risk for functional intestinal disorders in later life. *Jornal de Pediatria, 144*, 449–454.

Andresen, V., Bach, D. R., Poellinger, A., Tsrouya, C., Stroh, A., Foerschler, A., Georgiewa, P., Zimmer, C., & Monnikes, H. (2005). Brain activation responses to subliminal or supraliminal rectal stimuli and to auditory stimuli in irritable bowel syndrome. *Neurogastroenterology and Motility, 17*, 827–837.

Apley, J., & Naish, N. (1958). Recurrent abdominal pains: A field survey of 1,000 school children. *Archives of Disease in Childhood, 33*, 165–170.

Bale, T. L., & Vale, W. W. (2004). CRF and CRF receptors: Role in stress responsivity and other behaviors. *Annual Review of Pharmacology and Toxicology, 44*, 525–557.

Ball, T. M., & Weydert, J. A. (2003). Methodological challenges to treatment trials for recurrent abdominal pain in children. *Archives of Pediatrics & Adolescent Medicine, 157*, 1121–1127.

Ball, T. M., Shapiro, D. E., Monheim, C. J., & Weydert, J. A. (2003). A pilot study of the use of guided imagery for the treatment of recurrent abdominal pain in children. *Clinical Pediatrics (Philadelphia), 42*, 527–532.

Barbara, G., Vallance, B. A., & Collins, S. M. (1997). Persistent intestinal neuromuscular dysfunction after acute nematode infection in mice. *Gastroenterology, 113*, 1224–1232.

Barbara, G., Stanghellini, V., De Giorgio, R., Cremon, C., Cottrell, G. S., Santini, D., Pasquinelli, G., Morselli-

Labate, A. M., Grady, E. F., Bunnett, N. W., Collins, S. M., & Corinaldesi, R. (2004). Activated mast cells in proximity to colonic nerves correlate with abdominal pain in irritable bowel syndrome. *Gastroenterology, 126*, 693–702.

Bernstein, C. N., Frankenstein, U. N., Rawsthorne, P., Pitz, M., Summers, R., & McIntyre, M. C. (2002). Cortical mapping of visceral pain in patients with GI disorders using functional magnetic resonance imaging. *The American Journal of Gastroenterology, 97*, 319–327.

Boey, C. C., & Goh, K. L. (2001). The significance of life-events as contributing factors in childhood recurrent abdominal pain in an urban community in Malaysia. *Journal of Psychosomatic Research, 51*, 559–562.

Bouin, M., Plourde, V., Boivin, M., Riberdy, M., Lupien, F., Laganiere, M., Verrier, P., & Poitras, P. (2002). Rectal distention testing in patients with irritable bowel syndrome: Sensitivity, specificity, and predictive values of pain sensory thresholds. *Gastroenterology, 122*, 1771–1777.

Bueno, L., Fioramonti, J., & Garcia-Villar, R. (2000). Pathobiology of visceral pain: molecular mechanisms and therapeutic implications. III. Visceral afferent pathways: a source of new therapeutic targets for abdominal pain. *American Journal of Physiology. Gastrointestinal and Liver Physiology, 278*, G670–G676.

Bursch, B. (2008). Psychological/cognitive behavioral treatment of childhood functional abdominal pain and irritable bowel syndrome. *Journal of Pediatric Gastroenterology and Nutrition, 47*, 706–707.

Campo, J. V., Di Lorenzo, C., Chiappetta, L., Bridge, J., Colborn, D. K., Gartner, J. C., Jr., Gaffney, P., Kocoshis, S., & Brent, D. (2001). Adult outcomes of pediatric recurrent abdominal pain: Do they just grow out of it? *Pediatrics, 108*, E1.

Campo, J. V., Dahl, R. E., Williamson, D. E., Birmaher, B., Perel, J. M., & Ryan, N. D. (2004). Recurrent abdominal pain, anxiety, and depression in primary care. *Pediatrics, 113*, 817–824.

Castagliuolo, I., Lamont, J. T., Qiu, B., Fleming, S. M., Bhaskar, K. R., Nikulasson, S. T., Kornetsky, C., & Pothoulakis, C. (1996). Acute stress causes mucin release from rat colon: Role of corticotropin releasing factor and mast cells. *The American Journal of Physiology, 271*, G884–G892.

Collins, S. M. (1992). Is the irritable gut an inflamed gut? *Scandinavian Journal of Gastroenterology Supplement, 192*, 102–105.

Delvaux, M. (2002). Role of visceral sensitivity in the pathophysiology of irritable bowel syndrome. *Gut, 51*, 67–71.

Di Lorenzo, C., Colletti, R. B., Lehmann, H. P., Boyle, J. T., Gerson, W. T., Hyams, J. S., Squires, R. H., Jr., Walker, L. S., & Kanda, P. T. (2005). Chronic abdominal pain in children: A technical report of the American academy of pediatrics and the North American society for pediatric gastroenterology, hepatology and nutrition. *Journal of Pediatric Gastroenterology and Nutrition, 40*, 249–261.

Drossman, D. A. (2006). The functional gastrointestinal disorders and the Rome III process. *Gastroenterology, 130*, 14.

Drossman, D. A., Whitehead, W. E., & Camilleri, M. (1997). Irritable bowel syndrome: A technical review for practice guideline development. *Gastroenterology, 112*, 2120–2137.

Drouault-Holowacz, S., Bieuvelet, S., Burckel, A., Cazaubiel, M., Dray, X., & Marteau, P. (2008). A double blind randomized controlled trial of a probiotic combination in 100 patients with irritable bowel syndrome. *Gastroentérologie Clinique et Biologique, 32*, 147–152.

Dunlop, S. P., Jenkins, D., & Spiller, R. C. (2003). Distinctive clinical, psychological, and histological features of postinfective irritable bowel syndrome. *The American Journal of Gastroenterology, 98*, 1578–1583.

Galatola, G., Grosso, M., Barlotta, A., Ferraris, R., Rovera, L., Ariano, M., Cottino, F., & De La Pierre, M. (1991). Diagnosis of bacterial contamination of the small intestine using the 1 g [14 C] xylose breath test in various gastrointestinal diseases. *Minerva Gastroenterologica e Dietologica, 37*, 169–175.

Garber, J., Walker, L. S., & Zeman, J. (1991). Somatization symptoms in a community sample of children and adolescents: Further validation of the children's somatization inventory. *Psychological Assessment, 3*, 588–595.

Gonsalkorale, W. M., Miller, V., Afzal, A., & Whorwell, P. J. (2003). Long term benefits of hypnotherapy for irritable bowel syndrome. *Gut, 52*, 1623–1629.

Greco, L. A., Freeman, K. E., & Dufton, L. (2007). Overt and relational victimization among children with frequent abdominal pain: Links to social skills, academic functioning, and health service use. *Journal of Pediatric Psychology, 32*, 319–329.

Guandalini, S., Chiaro, A., Labalestra, V., Gopalan, S., Romano, C., & Canani, R. B. (2008). Efficacy of the probiotic VSL#3 in children with irritable bowel syndrome: an international, randomized, placebo-controlled, double-blind, cross-over trial. *American Journal Gastroenterol, 103*.

Gue, M., Del Rio-Lacheze, C., Eutamene, H., Theodorou, V., Fioramonti, J., & Bueno, L. (1997). Stress-induced visceral hypersensitivity to rectal distension in rats: role of CRF and mast cells. *Neurogastroenterology and Motility, 9*, 271–279.

Gwee, K. A., Leong, Y. L., Graham, C., McKendrick, M. W., Collins, S. M., Walters, S. J., Underwood, J. E., & Read, N. W. (1999). The role of psychological and biological factors in postinfective gut dysfunction. *Gut, 44*, 400–406.

Gwee, K. A., Collins, S. M., Read, N. W., Rajnakova, A., Deng, Y., Graham, J. C., McKendrick, M. W., & Moochhala, S. M. (2003). Increased rectal mucosal expression of interleukin 1beta in recently acquired post-infectious irritable bowel syndrome. *Gut, 52*, 523–526.

Hawthorn, M., Ferrante, J., Luchowski, E., Rutledge, A., Wei, X. Y., & Triggle, D. J. (1988). The actions of peppermint oil and menthol on calcium channel dependent processes in intestinal, neuronal and cardiac preparations. *Alimentary Pharmacology & Therapeutics, 2,* 101–118.

Heyneman, N., Fremow, W., & Gano, D. (1990). Individual differences and effectiveness of different coping strategies for pain. *Cognitive Therapy Research, 14,* 63–77.

Hyams, J. S., Burke, G., Davis, P. M., Rzepski, B., & Andrulonis, P. A. (1996). Abdominal pain and irritable bowel syndrome in adolescents: A community-based study. *Jornal de Pediatria, 129,* 220–226.

Imaki, T., Nahan, J. L., Rivier, C., Sawchenko, P. E., & Vale, W. (1991). Differential regulation of corticotropin-releasing factor mRNA in rat brain regions by glucocorticoids and stress. *The Journal of Neuroscience, 11,* 585–599.

Jarvis, L. J., Hogg, H., & Houghton, C. D. (1992). Topical peppermint oil for the relief of colonic spasm at barium enema. *Clinical Radiology, 46,* 435.

Kehne, J., & De Lombaert, S. (2002). Non-peptidic CRF1 receptor antagonists for the treatment of anxiety, depression and stress disorders. *Current Drug Targets. CNS and Neurological Disorders, 1,* 467–493.

Kellow, J. E., Eckersley, C. M., & Jones, M. P. (1991). Enhanced perception of physiological intestinal motility in the irritable bowel syndrome. *Gastroenterology, 101,* 1621–1627.

Khoshoo, V., Armstead, C., & Landry, L. (2006). Effect of a laxative with and without tegaserod in adolescents with constipation predominant irritable bowel syndrome. *Alimentary Pharmacology & Therapeutics, 23,* 191–196.

Kim, H. J., Vazquez Roque, M. I., Camilleri, M., Stephens, D., Burton, D. D., Baxter, K., Thomforde, G., & Zinsmeister, A. R. (2005). A randomized controlled trial of a probiotic combination VSL# 3 and placebo in irritable bowel syndrome with bloating. *Neurogastroenterology and Motility, 17,* 687–696.

Kingham, J. G. (1995). Peppermint oil and colon spasm. *Lancet, 346,* 986.

Kline, R. M., Kline, J. J., Di Palma, J., & Barbero, G. J. (2001). Enteric-coated, pH-dependent peppermint oil capsules for the treatment of irritable bowel syndrome in children. *Jornal de Pediatria, 138,* 125–128.

Leicester, R. J., & Hunt, R. H. (1982). Peppermint oil to reduce colonic spasm during endoscopy. *Lancet, 2,* 989.

Liem, O., Mousa, H. M., Benninga, M. A., & Di Lorenzo, C. (2008). Tegaserod use in children: A single-center experience. *Journal of Pediatric Gastroenterology and Nutrition, 46,* 54–58.

Lin, H. C. (2004). Small intestinal bacterial overgrowth: A framework for understanding irritable bowel syndrome. *Journal of the American Medical Association, 292,* 852–858.

MacIver, R., Mears, C., Di Lorenzo, C., & Saps, M. (2007). Seasonal nurse consultations for abdominal pain in an adolescent population. *Journal of Pediatric Gastroenterology and Nutrition, 45,* E13.

Mertz, H., Morgan, V., Tanner, G., Pickens, D., Price, R., Shyr, Y., & Kessler, R. (2000). Regional cerebral activation in irritable bowel syndrome and control subjects with painful and nonpainful rectal distention. *Gastroenterology, 118,* 842–848.

Naliboff, B. D., Derbyshire, S. W., Munakata, J., Berman, S., Mandelkern, M., Chang, L., & Mayer, E. A. (2001). Cerebral activation in patients with irritable bowel syndrome and control subjects during rectosigmoid stimulation. *Psychosomatic Medicine, 63,* 365–375.

Neal, K. R., Hebden, J., & Spiller, R. (1997). Prevalence of gastrointestinal symptoms six months after bacterial gastroenteritis and risk factors for development of the irritable bowel syndrome: Postal survey of patients. *British Medical Journal, 314,* 779–782.

Nobaek, S., Johansson, M. L., Molin, G., Ahrne, S., & Jeppsson, B. (2000). Alteration of intestinal microflora is associated with reduction in abdominal bloating and pain in patients with irritable bowel syndrome. *The American Journal of Gastroenterology, 95,* 1231–1238.

Nolon, H. W., & Friend, D. R. (1994). Mental B-D-glucuronide: A potential prodrug for treatment of the irritable bowel syndrome. *Pharmaceutical Research, 2,* 1707–1711.

O'Mahony, L., McCarthy, J., Kelly, P., Hurley, G., Luo, F., Chen, K., O'Sullivan, G. C., Kiely, B., Collins, J. K., Shanahan, F., & Quigley, E. M. (2005). Lactobacillus and bifidobacterium in irritable bowel syndrome: Symptom responses and relationship to cytokine profiles. *Gastroenterology, 128,* 541–551.

Pavcovich, L. A., Yang, M., Miselis, R. R., & Valentino, R. J. (1998). Novel role for the pontine micturition center, Barrington's nucleus: Evidence for coordination of colonic and forebrain activity. *Brain Research, 784,* 355–361.

Pimentel, M., Park, S., Mirocha, J., Kane, S. V., & Kong, Y. (2006). The effect of a nonabsorbed oral antibiotic (rifaximin) on the symptoms of the irritable bowel syndrome: A randomized trial. *Annals of Internal Medicine, 145,* 557–563.

Sadeghian, M., Farahmand, F., Fallahi, G. H., & Abbasi, A. (2008). Cyproheptadine for the treatment of functional abdominal pain in childhood: A double-blinded randomized placebo-controlled trial. *Minerva Pediatrica, 60,* 1367–1374.

Saps, M., & Di Lorenzo, C. (2007). An epidemiological study of common GI symptoms in school-age children. *Gastroenterology, 132,* A-325.

Saps, M., Bolioli, P., Espana, M., Marshall, B. M., & Di Lorenzo, C. (2008a). Cost and consultation patterns of abdominal pain in Uruguayan children. *Journal of Pediatric Gastroenterology and Nutrition, 46,* 159–163.

Saps, M., Seshadri, R., Sztainberg, M., Schaffer, G., Marshall, B. M., & Di Lorenzo, C. (2008b). A prospective school-based study of abdominal pain and other common somatic complaints in children. *Jornal de Pediatria, 154,* 322–326.

Saps, M., Blank, C., Khan, S., Seshadri, R., Marshall, B., Bass, L., & Di Lorenzo, C. (2008c). Seasonal variation in the presentation of abdominal pain. *Journal of Pediatric Gastroenterology and Nutrition, 46,* 279–284.

Saps, M., Pensabene, L., Di Martino, L., Staiano, A., Wechsler, J., Zheng, X., & Di Lorenzo, C. (2008d). Post-infectious functional gastrointestinal disorders in children. *Jornal de Pediatria, 152*, 812–816, 816 e1.

Saps, M., Youssef, N. N., Miranda, A., Nurko, S., Cocjin, J., & Di Lorenzo, C. (2008e). Evaluation of the efficacy of amitriptyline in children with abdominal pain of non organic origin. *Journal of Pediatric Gastroenterology and Nutrition,* In Press.

Saps, M., Youssef, N., Miranda, A., Nurko, S., Cocjin, J., & Di Lorenzo C. (2009). Multicenter, randomized, placebo-controlled trial of amitriptyline in children with functional gastrointestinal disorders. *Gastroenterology, 137*, 1261–9.

See, M. C., Birnbaum, A. H., Schechter, C. B., Goldenberg, M. M., & Benkov, K. J. (2001). Double-blind, placebo-controlled trial of famotidine in children with abdominal pain and dyspepsia: Global and quantitative assessment. *Digestive Diseases and Sciences, 46*, 985–992.

Silverman, D. H., Munakata, J. A., Ennes, H., Mandelkern, M. A., Hoh, C. K., & Mayer, E. A. (1997). Regional cerebral activity in normal and pathological perception of visceral pain. *Gastroenterology, 112*, 64–72.

Smith, C., Nordstrom, E., Sengupta, J. N., & Miranda, A. (2007). Neonatal gastric suctioning results in chronic visceral and somatic hyperalgesia: Role of corticotropin releasing factor. *Neurogastroenterology and Motility, 19*, 692–699.

Sparks, M. J., O'Sullivan, P., Herrington, A. A., & Morcos, S. K. (1995). Does peppermint oil relieve spasm during barium enema? *The British Journal of Radiology, 68*, 841–843.

Spiller, R. C., Jenkins, D., Thornley, J. P., Hebden, J. M., Wright, T., Skinner, M., & Neal, K. R. (2000). Increased rectal mucosal enteroendocrine cells, T lymphocytes, and increased gut permeability following acute Campylobacter enteritis and in post-dysenteric irritable bowel syndrome. *Gut, 47*, 804–811.

Starfield, B., Katz, H., Gabriel, A., Livingston, G., Benson, P., Hankin, J., Horn, S., & Steinwachs, D. (1984). Morbidity in childhood – A longitudinal view. *The New England Journal of Medicine, 310*, 824–829.

Tache, Y., Million, M., Nelson, A. G., Lamy, C., & Wang, L. (2005). Role of corticotropin-releasing factor pathways in stress-related alterations of colonic motor function and viscerosensibility in female rodents. *Gender Medicine, 2*, 146–154.

Talley, N. J. (1998). Irritable bowel syndrome: disease definition and symptom description. *The European Journal of Surgery. Supplement, 1998*, 24–28.

Vlieger, A. M., Menko-Frankenhuis, C., Wolfkamp, S. C., Tromp, E., & Benninga, M. A. (2007). Hypnotherapy for children with functional abdominal pain or irritable bowel syndrome: A randomized controlled trial. *Gastroenterology, 133*, 1430–1436.

Walker, L. S., Garber, J., & Greene, J. W. (1991). Somatization symptoms in pediatric abdominal pain patients: Relation to chronicity of abdominal pain and parent somatization. *Journal of Abnormal Child Psychology, 19*, 379–394.

Walker, L. S., Williams, S. E., Smith, C. A., Garber, J., Van Slyke, D. A., & Lipani, T. A. (2006a). Parent attention versus distraction: Impact on symptom complaints by children with and without chronic functional abdominal pain. *Pain, 122*, 43–52.

Walker, L. S., Smith, C. A., Garber, J., & Claar, R. L. (2006b). Appraisal and coping with daily stressors by pediatric patients with chronic abdominal pain. *Journal of Pediatric Psychology, 32*, 206–216.

Westphal, J., Horning, M., & Leonhardt, K. (1996). Phytotherapy in functional upper abdominal complaints. *Phytomedicine, 2*, 285–291.

Weydert, J. A., Shapiro, D. E., Acra, S. A., Monheim, C. J., Chambers, A. S., & Ball, T. M. (2006). Evaluation of guided imagery as treatment for recurrent abdominal pain in children: A randomized controlled trial. *BMC Pediatrics, 6*, 29.

Wojczynski, M. K., North, K. E., Pedersen, N. L., & Sullivan, P. F. (2007). Irritable bowel syndrome: A co-twin control analysis. *The American Journal of Gastroenterology, 102*, 2220–2229.

Yokotani, K., Murakami, Y., Okada, S., & Hirata, M. (2001). Role of brain arachidonic acid cascade on central CRF1 receptor-mediated activation of sympatho-adrenomedullary outflow in rats. *European Journal of Pharmacology, 419*, 183–189.

Youssef, N. N., Rosh, J. R., Loughran, M., Schuckalo, S. G., Cotter, A. N., Verga, B. G., & Mones, R. L. (2004). Treatment of functional abdominal pain in childhood with cognitive behavioral strategies. *Journal of Pediatric Gastroenterology and Nutrition, 39*, 192–196.

Chronic and Recurrent Pelvic Pain

Lynda Wells

Keywords

Chronic and recurrent pelvic pain (CPP) • Ovarian masses • Somatization • Pelvic congestion syndrome • Abuse and CPP

Introduction

Chronic and recurrent pelvic pain (CPP) in children and adolescents has been recognized for decades. However, data on the etiology, natural history, treatment, and long-term consequences of painful pelvic conditions in these patients are lacking. The problem's prevalence remains uncertain, and the majority of therapies are extrapolated from research on adults. The normal developmental changes and coping strategies of children and adolescents and the role of the family and social environment are only now being examined and understood. The complex nature of pain and its context has led to recommendations for a multimodal and multidisciplinary approach to patient care.

On October 15, 2007, the International Association for the Study of Pain (IASP) launched the Global Year Against Pain in Women, a theme chosen because of the major humanitarian, social, and economic implications of pain in women (Collett et al. 2007). Many women's pain began at

the onset of puberty. This chapter cites literature on childhood and early adult pelvic pain because much adult pain studied started in adolescence. Women, in general, suffer more pain than men because of gender-related hormonal effects (Fillingim 2000; Greenspan et al. 2007), gynecologic and obstetric conditions (Collett et al. 2007), and longer exposure to degenerative conditions due to their longer life span. Gender-related psychologic and sociocultural factors play a key role in treatment seeking and responses. Education is vital for improving health and access to appropriate care for pain conditions, especially among women.

CPP is a significant public health problem (Tu et al. 2006), with a prevalence in developed countries of 24%, comparable to back pain. The American College of Obstetricians and Gynecologists defines it as noncyclic or cyclic pain of 3 or 6 months duration, respectively, that interferes with normal activities (Scialli et al. 2000) and is associated with significant physical and cognitive disability (Economy and Laufer 1999). The IASP defines CPP as having a gynecologic origin but no identified, definitive lesion or cause. Four criteria that focus on the behavioral components constituting CPP include pain refractory to medical management; significant impairment of physical (including sexual)

L. Wells (✉)
University of Virginia School of Medicine,
Charlottesville, VA, USA
e-mail: LTRW6R@hscmail.mcc.virginia.edu

B.C. McClain and S. Suresh (eds.), *Handbook of Pediatric Chronic Pain:*
Current Science and Integrative Practice, DOI 10.1007/978-1-4419-0350-1_9,
© Springer Science+Business Media, LLC 2011

function; vegetative signs of depression; and/or a change in the patient's role in the family due to the pain, or the family considering the pain to be its highest priority problem (Sanfilippo and Black 2003). CPP also has been described as resulting from a complex interaction among neurologic, musculoskeletal, and endocrine systems that is further influenced by behavior and psychologic factors (Wadhwa et al. 2004).

CPP can be caused by structural diseases of the pelvis or gastrointestinal tract (e.g., endometriosis, adhesions, and inflammatory bowel disease (IBD)), urologic, neurologic, or musculoskeletal disorders (Venbrux et al. 2002), peripheral or central nervous system (CNS) dysfunction, environmental or psychologic factors, or a combination thereof. Endometriosis, adhesions, irritable bowel syndrome (IBS), and interstitial cystitis (IC) are its most common causes (Thomson and Redwine 2005). Women with CPP have higher rates of undiagnosed psychologic morbidity, inappropriate health-care utilization, and long-term disability.

Somatization Versus Organic Disease

Adolescents undergo significant physical, psychologic, emotional, and social changes as they mature, and develop coping strategies for adapting to independent life. The medical practitioner's challenge is to determine whether the etiology of CPP is organic, functional, or both, in the context of this complex interplay of physical, cognitive, and environmental factors (Economy and Laufer 1999; Stones et al. 2000), and to select treatments appropriate for disease management and the patient's maturity. Thus, knowledge of the developmental stages in this population and the various etiologies of pelvic pain is required. Parental involvement in patient care raises unique issues of confidentiality in the provider–patient relationship (Song and Advincula 2005).

Nearly 3–5% of all visits to primary care providers (PCPs) in the 11–21-year age group are for abdominal pain (Song and Advincula 2005). The most common cause of cyclic abdominal pain in adolescents is dysmenorrhea (Economy and Laufer 1999). CPP prevalence in women is 10–12%, constitutes 10–15% of visits to gynecologists and PCPs, and is the indication for 30–40% of all laparoscopies (Economy and Laufer 1999).

Evaluation

Be systematic and comprehensive. CPP in adolescents usually has a multifactorial etiology (i.e., gynecologic, gastrointestinal, urologic, musculoskeletal, vascular, rheumatologic, neurologic, and psychiatric disorders), so a multidisciplinary team approach is recommended and all organ systems should be evaluated. A list of possible differential diagnoses and diagnostic tests was provided in Table 1 of Solnik (2006). A careful history is essential to guide physical examination, further investigation, additional referrals, and management. Also, pain itself has many facets and should be evaluated as physical, psychologic, social, emotional, and spiritual.

To facilitate the characterization of pain symptoms and their effect on daily life, the International Pelvic Pain Society (www.pelvicpain.org) developed a pelvic pain assessment form (Scialli et al. 2000). Also, an interview strategy called **SAFE** (**S**everity, **A**ffect, **F**amily, and **E**nvironment) has been developed to provide the clinician with a comprehensive framework to evaluate medical and psychologic components (Rickert and Kozlowski 2000). A study utilizing the **SAFE** approach to evaluate CPP in 200 girls aged 13–23 years found it to be very effective at guiding gynecologists in their evaluation of the organic and psychologic components of pelvic pain (Wadhwa et al. 2004). It allowed the early recognition of psychosocial and environmental factors and the establishment of long-term patient relationships to prevent symptom recurrence and future disability. Attention to organic and other causative factors from the start of therapy was more likely to result in a reduction in pelvic pain than the standard approach (assess and rule out organic disease before evaluating for psychosocial or psychosexual involvement).

History

This should include a description of the pain's onset, location, severity, duration, relationship to the menstrual cycle, and exacerbating and relieving factors. Accompanying symptoms (e.g., fever, nausea, vomiting, diarrhea, dysuria, abnormal vaginal bleeding, or dizziness) should be identified. CPP is localized to the pelvis, anterior abdominal wall at or below the umbilicus, lower back, and buttocks. Cyclic pain is almost always of gynecologic origin (Hewitt and Brown 2000). Pelvic pain of nonorganic origin is almost never acute and nonrecurrent.

Menstrual, sexual, contraceptive, bowel, urinary, general health, family, and sexual/physical abuse histories should be elicited, along with previous medical and surgical treatments and the patient's response to each. Sleep pattern, nutrition, diet, and exercise habits should be assessed for general physical well-being; disturbed sleep may be a sign of depression. Changes in general health (e.g., weight change, fever, fatigue, joint pain, headaches, mood change) and habits (e.g., smoking, alcohol, and drug use) should be noted, along with the overall impact of the pain on lifestyle including work, school, exercise, family life, and mood. The possibility of secondary gain for the patient or their family should be explored. A symptom diary may be very helpful in elucidating the etiology of pelvic pain. It is important to monitor the efficacy of therapeutic interventions and long-term management.

Standardized, self-reported review of symptoms checklists to assess somatization and global symptomatology are recommended. Ideally, information should be obtained from the patient and family separately (Taylor et al. 1996). Emotional and psychologic factors may contribute significantly to pain symptoms and affect treatment response. Patients should be screened for depression and anxiety; the West Haven-Yale

Multidimensional Pain Inventory, Minnesota Multiphasic Personality Inventory, and Beck Depression Inventory quantify the impact of pain on the adolescent's life and identify depressive symptoms such as suicidal ideation (Economy and Laufer 1999).

Physical Examination

General appearance, including posture and affect, should be noted; tall, slender physique is associated with endometriosis (Hediger et al. 2005). Abdominal examination should assess rigidity, peritoneal irritation, ascitic fluid, palpable masses, and bowel sounds. Areas of maximal tenderness and trigger points – i.e., areas of increased irritability and sensitivity that are locally tender when compressed and elicit referred pain/tenderness when stimulated – should be identified; local anesthetic infiltration of these points can be diagnostic and therapeutic (Economy and Laufer 1999).

Pelvic examination is extensive. To improve yield, ensure good communication with full explanations before starting the examination and give constant reassurance. Inspect the external genitalia, use a "pediatric" speculum, and one finger instead of two for vaginoabdominal or rectoabdominal examination. An obstructive müllerian anomaly should be considered if the pain is atypical or severe or an abdominal mass is present on examination; introduction of a cotton-tipped swab into the vagina can identify these abnormalities in virgins. Palpate external structures to elicit muscular pain. Cervical motion tenderness; uterine size, tenderness, and mobility; adnexal masses and mobility; uterosacral, posterior cul-de-sac, and rectovaginal nodularity; and urethral, trigone, and vaginal fornices tenderness should be noted. Analyze specimens of any discharge. A speculum examination should include taking specimens for Neisseria gonorrhea (NG) and Chlamydia trachomatis, and a Papanicolaou smear.

Pelvic inflammatory disease (PID) should be ruled out in all sexually active adolescents regardless of physical findings.

Psychologic Examination

All disease is experienced in a cultural, social, and psychologic context (Stones et al. 2000). An abundance of literature links CPP in adults to adverse life events such as childhood sex abuse and mood disorder. Individual psychologic consultation can help identify and treat issues of adaptation and mood and improve coping skills, thereby enhancing functioning with respect to chronic illness and pain (Greco 2003). Depression, anxiety, and fear may perpetuate and intensify the overall pain experience. Epidemiologic studies show that the prevalence of moderate-to-severe psychiatric disorders in children is 14–20% and rising (Silber and Pao 2003).

Investigations

Investigations should be guided by findings on history and physical examination. Laboratory tests should include a pregnancy test if sexually active, stool guaiac, urinalysis, cervical culture, cytology, erythrocyte sedimentation rate (ESR) and C-reactive protein (CRP) as indicators of inflammation, and complete blood count (CBC) with white cell count differential to evaluate inflammation, ischemia, or infection (Economy and Laufer 1999).

Imaging studies may include endovaginal or abdominal ultrasound in the diagnosis of adnexal torsion, hemoperitoneum, hemorrhagic corpus luteum cyst, and severe PID; magnetic resonance imaging (MRI) in diagnosing obstructive müllerian anomalies; and spiral CT to image a large tubo-ovarian abscess (TOA) or appendicitis (Economy and Laufer 1999).

Laparoscopy is the gold standard in diagnosing endometriosis and PID, although it is not performed routinely in the latter due to the need for general anesthesia. It facilitates diagnosis of organic disease, provides histopathologic documentation, and reassures patients and their parents if the results are negative. Laparoscopy should be considered if medical treatment fails (e.g., dysmenorrhea) or if surgical treatment is indicated by the diagnosis (e.g., appendicitis, obstructive

müllerian anomaly). However, surgery should be deferred in the former until mood disturbance or somatization has been addressed and symptoms and signs reevaluated (Stones et al. 2000).

In one study of 1,194 laparotomies, 63% of patients with a normal pelvic exam had abnormal surgical findings and 17.5% of patients with an abnormal exam had normal surgical findings. In cases where pain persisted in the same location for over 6 months, positive findings on laparoscopy were 83% (Economy and Laufer 1999). Positive findings did not necessarily correspond to the cause of pain, and negative findings did not exclude the presence of a somatic cause.

Microlaparoscopy and "pain mapping" may be useful in associating pathology and symptoms (Economy and Laufer 1999). Due to limited visualization and pain tolerance, microlaparoscopy under local anesthetic has been reserved largely for diagnostic use. Extensive operations are best performed under general anesthesia in a day-surgery unit or hospital.

Laparoscopic studies in adolescent girls specifically have identified treatable pelvic disease in 91% of patients (including 52% endometriosis, 9% uterine abnormalities) and in 73% (67% visible endometriosis, 10% normal pelvis, 7% müllerian abnormalities). Other studies have shown a preponderance of PID and adnexal masses, suggesting a diversity in patient populations (Economy and Laufer 1999). One study correlating pelvic examination, ultrasound, and laparoscopic findings reported a predictive value of normal and abnormal findings at pelvic examination of 43% and 94%, respectively. Most common diagnoses were adnexal mass (31%) and endometriosis (20%). The predictive value of an abnormal ultrasound was high at 92%, whereas a normal ultrasound had a lower predictive value of 60%. It was surmised that a normal pelvic examination and ultrasound was predictive of a normal laparoscopy only 50% of the time.

In a study by Almeida and Val-Gallas (1997), 50 women aged 18–45 years (mean age 27 years) with a history of CPP of at least 6 months duration and failed medical treatment underwent conscious pain mapping via microlaparoscopy with conscious sedation. Endometriosis was identified in 42 patients (82%) although pain was not reliably reproduced by probing. Also, 31 patients (62%) had adhesions; of these, 24 reported tenderness during probing of the adhesions. Thirteen patients (26%) had an anatomically abnormal or painful appendix; subsequent appendectomy revealed abnormal pathology in 9 of the 13 appendices. Forty-five of the forty-eight women who underwent operative laparoscopy after conscious mapping had significant improvement in symptoms and physical findings. Conscious mapping had a positive impact on patient understanding of treatment regimens. Laparoscopic uterosacral nerve ablation (LUNA) was performed only in women with tenderness on probing or whose uterosacral ligaments were endometriotic. Consistent with other reports, endometriosis and adhesions were the most common causes of pelvic tenderness by probing. The relief experienced by patients was not related to the extent of their disease but to the specific site where pain could be reproduced. The appendix's role in CPP was the most significant finding in that study (Almeida and Val-Gallas 1997) and in the one by Chandler et al. (2002). This technique could focus treatment on painful lesions only with subsequent minimization of morbidity and trauma, especially when fertility preservation is desired.

Management

Treatment is aimed at improving quality of life by reducing pain, disability, and maladaptive behaviors and improving patients' function and ability to cope (Greco 2003). Concurrent treatment of organic and psychologic morbidity is achieved using gynecologists, pediatricians, gastroenterologists, psychiatrists/health psychologists, nurses trained in chronic pain evaluation and management, anesthesiologists, surgeons, interventional radiologists, behavioral medicine specialists, social workers, and physical therapists (Venbrux et al. 2002). Continued participation in school or work and age-appropriate activities is essential and may require coordinated efforts between the school/employer and a psychologist (Greco 2003).

If no specific etiology is found, management should include cognitive-behavioral therapy (CBT) (Economy and Laufer 1999). Some consider cognitive and behavioral strategies (e.g., guided imagery, progressive muscle relaxation, biofeedback, and self-hypnosis) to be integral components of a multidisciplinary approach to CPP management (Greco 2003).

First-line pharmacotherapy includes oral analgesics (primarily nonsteroidal anti-inflammatory drugs (NSAIDs)) scheduled and not "as needed." Generally, narcotic analgesics are not needed and should be avoided because of increased gut dysmotility and possible increased pain.

Antidepressants should be prescribed to treat depressive symptoms and restore normal sleep. Antidepressants' neuromodulatory and analgesic properties also can be useful in relieving the pain (Greco 2003). Tricyclic antidepressants are most appropriate in patients with sleep disorders because of their sedative properties, but less useful in constipation where the cholinergic slowing of the gut can exacerbate symptoms. Because of the risk of dysrhythmias, a baseline ECG should be obtained prior to commencing therapy. This class of drug should not be used with tramadol because of the increased risk of seizures. Serotonin reuptake inhibitors may be most useful in patients with chronic pain and depressed mood.

Education might be necessary to clarify that the effectiveness of psychologic therapy does not imply a psychologic origin to pain (Greco 2003).

Somatization

Emotional and psychologic stress can be experienced as a physical condition (e.g., "butterflies" in one's stomach before a test). This is not considered pathologic. However, extremes of this behavior can be debilitating and result in frequent contact with health-care providers and significant cost to the patient and society. Importantly, these symptoms are spontaneous and not feigned, distinguishing them from malingering and factitious disorder (Silber and Pao 2003).

The American Psychiatric Association's *Diagnostic and Statistical Manual of Mental Disorders* (DSM-IV) defines somatoform disorder as the presence of physical symptoms that are not fully explainable by a medical condition or by the effects of any substance or mental disorder (American Psychiatric Association 1994). It has been described as the presence of physical symptoms suggesting an underlying medical condition that either is not found or does not fully account for the level of functional impairment (Fritz et al. 1997). Diagnosable somatoform disorders represent the severe end of a continuum that includes unexplained "functional" symptoms in the middle and transient, everyday aches and pains at the other end. Diagnostic criteria for somatoform disorders have been established in adults but are only now being developed in children (Silber and Pao 2003). Currently, somatoform disorders are classified as

- Somatic Complaint Variation: the universally experienced discomforts and complaints that do not interfere with daily functioning. This is not considered pathologic.
- Somatic Complaint Problem: one or more physical complaints that cause sufficient distress and impairment (physical, social, or school) to be problematic. With the onset of adolescence, somatic complaints are joined by more emotional distress, social withdrawal, and academic difficulties. More severe complaints may result in school refusal, aggressive behavior, and recurrent pain syndromes.
- Undifferentiated Somatoform Disorder: emerges during adolescence. Multiple severe symptoms are manifest for at least 6 months and are significantly disabling.
- Somatoform Disorder, Not Otherwise Specified: encompasses adolescents with somatoform symptoms but who do not meet criteria for any specific somatoform disorder.

Pain disorder is a new classification in DSM-IV (Fritz et al. 1997). Its essential characteristics are as follows: the patient experiences clinically significant pain that causes distress and/or functional impairment; psychologic factors are judged to play a major role in the pain's onset, severity, or maintenance; and the pain is neither feigned nor part of a mood, anxiety, or psychotic disorder. It is known that recurring pain or other physical symptoms can lower a child's organically based threshold to pain. Stress exacerbates physical symptoms in children with and without somatization problems.

Clinical Characteristics of Somatization

Somatization starts in childhood and adolescence and continues into adulthood. The assumption is that there is some basis for a child's physical complaints and that the intensity of the meaningfulness of the symptoms has become exaggerated. There is no difference in the frequency of somatic complaints between pre-pubertal girls and boys. More girls than boys report somatic complaints after puberty and during adolescence. Characteristics of children more likely to somatize are conscientious, sensitive, insecure, and anxious. They are described as good children who strive for high achievement in school and other activities.

The prevalence of somatic symptoms in the pediatric population is high at 10–15% (Terre and Ghiselli 1997). Young children experience affective distress in the form of somatic sensations. Initially, these are monosymptomatic (e.g., abdominal pain or headache). Recurrent abdominal pain accounts for 5% of doctor's visits, and 20–50% of children report headaches. As the child ages, limb pain, neurologic symptoms, insomnia, and fatigue emerge; 10% of teenagers report recurrent headaches, chest pain, nausea, and fatigue. In a sample of 12–16 year olds, distressing somatic symptoms were identified in 11% of girls and 4% of boys; the gender disparity persists into adulthood. A higher rate of somatization was found in lower socioeconomic groups (Silber and Pao 2003).

Several studies have looked at the incidence of somatic conditions in healthy individuals and have attempted to characterize the natural history in the community. Lieb et al. (2002) found that German adolescents and young adults (14–24 years) studied over a 4-year period had a lifetime prevalence of any specific somatoform disorder of 2.6%, with pain disorder being the highest at 1.7%. Being female, preexisting substance use, affective and anxiety disorders, and experiencing physical threats increased the risk of somatoform conditions in adolescents and young adults. Among females, rape or sexual abuse was found to be a predictor for the new onset of somatoform disorders and syndromes. High social class and higher educational level were negatively associated with new onset of somatoform disorders. This is supported by Taylor et al. (1996), who found somatization disorder to be more common in females and those who failed to graduate from high school. All persons with somatization disorder also had another psychiatric illness, most commonly simple phobia, affective disorder, and panic disorder. Fifty-five percent of adults reported their first somatic symptom before the age of 15 years, and remission of symptoms was rare.

A similar study of children aged 4–15 years in pediatric primary care found that somatization increased with age (0.99% in 4–5 year olds; 1.7% in 6–10 year olds; 2.5% in 11–15 year olds) (Campo et al. 1999). Somatization was associated with lower levels of parental education, urban residence, Medicaid receipt, and non-intact or dysfunctional family status. Somatizing children were more fearful of novelty, prone to separation concerns and worry, and more likely to miss school. Adolescents with somatizing tendencies reported lower self-esteem, lower perception of parental affection, and more depressive symptoms (Rhee et al. 2005). Depression is an antecedent to somatic symptoms. The younger the patient, the more likely somatization will develop.

School refusers who endorsed severe gastrointestinal symptoms were over eight times more likely to have separation anxiety disorder than those without gastrointestinal symptoms (Bernstein et al. 1997). This is in keeping with data that childhood anxiety disorders frequently take the course of somatoform disorders. Trait anxiety (i.e., the chronic tendency to respond anxiously to stress and psychologic threat), anxiety sensitivity (i.e., specific tendency to react anxiously to one's own anxiety and anxiety-related sensations), and parents' anxiety-encouraging behaviors have been shown to be significantly positively associated with somatization symptoms in children (Muris and Meesters 2004). This suggests common vulnerability factors in childhood to anxiety and somatization.

Among healthy adolescents aged 11–15 years, girls showed higher levels of anxiety sensitivity, cognitive anxiety symptoms, pain and other somatization complaints, trait anxiety, and panic symptoms than boys (Muris et al. 2001). Anxiety sensitivity was significantly related to pain anxiety symptoms. Fear of pain is one factor thought to mediate the development of chronic pain complaints in adults. Altered perceptions of bodily sensations in the direction of catastrophic misinterpretations may lead to fear of such sensations.

Hostility, depression, and somatization were found to be the most common psychiatric symptoms in 154 males and 136 females aged 13–17 years admitted to a psychiatric unit for evaluation (Kişlal et al. 2005). Female adolescents showed significantly higher scores for anxiety, depression, somatization, and global severity index variables than males, and 67% females and 73% males with anxiety disorder had physical complaints; 2–10% was diagnosed with functional pain. Somatoform disorders are more common in adolescents than in children or adults because adolescents are much more concerned with their bodily changes and development and are experiencing peak emotional lability. Adolescents with psychiatric problems report significantly more symptoms such as loss of appetite, fatigue, headache, back pain, tachycardia, dizziness, nausea, weight loss, anemia, tingling sensations, blushing, and speech disorders. Patients with high psychometric scores should have a psychiatric evaluation.

Onset of Somatization

Somatization is considered to be a learned behavior. Children who fit the diagnosis of pain disorder have more family members as "pain models" than children whose pain is related solely to an organic cause (Silber and Pao 2003; Terre and Ghiselli 1997). In a study of the 4–8-year-old children of women with somatization disorders, women with chronic pain of organic origin, and healthy women, only women with somatization disorders caused somatization behavior in their children (Craig et al. 2002). Their health anxieties were reflected by their children, who were more likely to have emotional and behavioral problems, greater concerns about their own health and the health of others, and higher consultation rates for symptoms that are commonly considered functional. Mothers discouraged coping with pain and attributed more symptom-related disability to their offspring. Frequent visits to health-care providers also reinforced illness beliefs. Somatizing mothers were more likely to have received poor quality parenting and to have witnessed chronic physical illness from an early age.

A child may learn through direct experience or by observation that sickness brings more attention. A number of pain reduction measures, such as taking medicine, staying in bed, or missing school, reinforced by the reduction of pain, lead to increased use of pain-reduction behaviors. Sick behaviors can be positively reinforced by parents especially when this facilitates family functioning by diverting attention away from parental or parent–child conflict, bringing the parents closer together to attend to the illness, or allowing the family to receive a variety of medical and family support services. The role of the family in the development or maintenance of somatic symptoms can be seen in the associations between physical problems of parents and children within the same family. One study showed an incidence of 54% of the child mimicking the parent. Conversely, parents were shown to increase somatic and pain symptoms after their child was diagnosed with recurrent abdominal pain.

Maltreated children who are suddenly living in a new environment, who are neglected or rejected by their peers, or who have few cognitive and social skills (e.g., those from families of low intellectual-cultural orientation) may be very susceptible to the attention received from adults when they are sick or have physical complaints. Additionally, some children have a history of being abused less frequently when they are sick.

Alternatively, somatization may arise when a child's somatic complaints are more acceptable than the expression of strong feelings. They gain attention for physical symptoms but not emotional distress; this reinforcement is known as the "psychosomatic pathway" (Silber and Pao 2003).

Children with severe somatic complaints perceive greater parental encouragement of illness behavior than children with emotional complaints or controls (Muris and Meesters 2004). Parents particularly responded to symptoms with increased attention and special privileges. Girls are more prone to internalize problems leading to somatization, and to perceive their health status in terms of their socioemotional needs. Boys tend to externalize and act out and have fewer somatic symptoms. Additionally, girls receive more encouragement for illness behavior than boys, and mothers encourage illness behavior more than fathers (Terre and Ghiselli 1997). Adolescents with pain syndromes leading to school absences may experience more maternal reinforcement of illness behavior than matched controls with pain who attend school.

Terre and Ghiselli (1997) confirmed that adequate structure and support are central family tasks, the absence of which may seriously compromise healthy development, especially in early adolescence when youngsters begin to gain greater access to influences outside the family. Family organization may confer particular advantages for managing diverse stressors (e.g., the numerous biopsychosocial changes associated with early adolescence). Absence of family nurturance, predictable standards, and appropriate structure makes youth more likely to develop psychologic maladaption (e.g., low self-esteem, self-regulation disorders) and may heighten risk for a variety of problem behaviors. Enmeshed, overprotective, rigid families are associated with the development and maintenance of psychosomatic symptoms in children. A marked degree of closeness or togetherness between family members is a risk factor for chronic pain. Supportive and caring peer relationships protect youngsters from physical symptoms.

Coping Styles

Coping styles in adults with chronic pain showed that somatization and denial were modal defense strategies (Monsen and Havik 2001), indicating a tendency to deny psychologic distress and to transform personal conflicts into more socially acceptable problems, such as somatic complaints or pain. Elevated somatization, depression, anxiety, and obsession scores suggested that subjects were characterized by worry, resignation, and rigidity. This manifested itself in interpersonal relationships as trying too hard to please, having difficulty in feeling and expressing anger toward others, having difficulty being assertive, and experiencing social anxiety and embarrassment. Overall, the modal characteristics of this group of pain patients could be characterized as conventional and submissive, with high degrees of psychologic distress and few significant bodily findings.

Hastie et al. (2005), in a study of pain-relieving coping behaviors in healthy undergraduates by ethnic group, found that African Americans use more passive strategies and prayer, and employ a wider breadth of coping strategies when faced with threat, including pain. Hispanics show increased use of spirituality and support seeking within their own ethnic and religious communities as a way to manage pain and chronic illness and utilize more nontraditional therapies than Caucasians. Emotional factors contribute more to pain in Hispanics than African Americans or whites. Whites report more active pain-coping strategies and utilize more traditional health care than African Americans, Hispanics, and other racial groups.

In whites, pain-reducing behaviors were instigated by severity and level of interference. African Americans reacted to total number of pain sites, level of interference, and frustration. Hispanics were motivated by level of interference, worry, and frustration. The extent to which these contributed to pain was predictive of the total number of pain-reducing behaviors.

It is not known whether using multiple types of pain-reducing behaviors is adaptive or maladaptive. As ethnic differences in behavioral responses to pain are present before the development of a clinical pain condition, it suggests that these responses are acquired early in life based on cultural, economic, or other environmental factors. The number and types of pain coping behaviors should be assessed and their impact on treatment acknowledged.

Similarly, culture played no role in pain perception among 16- and 17-year-old Israeli Arab girls of Muslim, Druze, and Christian ethnicity (Goldstein-Ferber and Granot 2006). Rather, somatization, genetic neural sensitivities, and individual personality traits determined the severity of pain.

Diagnosis

Establishing a diagnosis of somatoform illness evolves over time along three simultaneous tracks: (i) ruling out organic disease as the cause of symptoms, (ii) identifying psychosocial dysfunction, and (iii) containing and alleviating stressors (Silber and Pao 2003). Evidence supporting significant psychologic factors in the etiology of pain may include onset of pain after specific trauma or stress; disability or handicap out of proportion to reported pain; clear secondary gain from the pain, and exacerbations predictably linked to stressful events. The cause of the pain, affective suffering, disability, and handicap are all components of pain and are best evaluated independently, so that organically caused pain but psychologically determined handicap can be identified.

A thorough biopsychosocial assessment is essential and may be therapeutic in itself. Findings highly suggestive of somatization disorder are a history of multiple somatic complaints, multiple physician visits and specialty consultations, a family member who has chronic and recurrent symptoms, and dysfunction in the primary areas of life (family, peers, school). A detailed school history showing the number of days missed each year is essential (Silber and Pao 2003). Concurrent depression and anxiety rates are high, especially in girls. Lower socioeconomic level and non-intact families are associated with increased incidence of psychiatric disorders (Campo et al. 1999).

Stress has been implicated as a triggering factor for somatization and is often attached to parental anxiety. The most common cause of stress is pressure on the child to perform (Silber and Pao 2003). Intrafamilial competition and hostility can create high levels of "background" stress. The critical role of family stress on health across the life span raises the possibility of distinct family risk factors for somatization at different developmental levels.

When evaluating somatic complaints, it is important to avoid unnecessary, repetitive, or extensive testing as this may serve to reinforce somatic complaints. It is important to know what the patient and their family fear or believe about their disease. A thorough medical workup should be performed, but only once. Investigations should be guided by history and physical examination only as indicated and in a systematic fashion. If evidence suggests somatization, a screening baseline of CBC, urinalysis, ESR or CRP, and occasionally stool guaiac and blood chemistry should suffice (Silber and Pao 2003). Benign, face-saving remedies (e.g., lotions, vitamins, heating pads) should be used during the acute phase. Physician contact should not be contingent on escalating sick role behavior.

Explicitly including psychosomatic etiologies in the initial patient assessment makes it easier to present this as a diagnosis and for the patient and family to accept behavioral and psychologic interventions.

Treatment

Acknowledging the child's suffering and the parents' difficulties in caring for the child is immensely important. Treatment is multifaceted and focused on reducing dysfunction rather than identifying a final diagnosis. Constant motivation of the patient and family to work together in dealing with their symptoms and complaints is required. Physical and psychologic treatments must be provided simultaneously to demonstrate

that the problem has physical and psychologic components. Indeed, until comorbid psychiatric conditions (e.g., depression, anxiety disorder, substance abuse) are addressed an improvement in somatization is unlikely. Realistic expectations for how long symptom resolution and psychosocial function improvement will take are important. Psychotherapeutic interventions focus on education, changes in reinforcement, and developing coping skills. Self-monitoring techniques such as hypnosis, relaxation, and biofeedback have proven successful. Operant conditioning is often used to increase the reinforcement that a child receives for healthy behavior and to reduce the reinforcement received for complaints about symptoms. Family CBT has demonstrated decreased pain, increased function, and lower relapse rates compared to a standard psychiatric consultation intervention (Allen et al. 2006). CBT for somatization disorder is focused on stress management, activity regulation, emotional awareness, cognitive restructuring, and interpersonal communication.

Working with parents on their own concerns and behaviors related to their child is often essential. Providing insight into the long-term effects of their short-term interventions helps. Whenever possible, the clinician, child, school personnel, and parents should meet to decide on a plan of cooperation to help the child reduce his or her somatic symptoms when at school (Haugaard 2004; Silber and Pao 2003).

Psychopharmacology is appropriate to treat comorbidities or if somatic symptoms have led to significant impairment of greater than 3 months duration (Silber and Pao 2003). Fears of abandonment after a diagnosis of somatization can be dispelled by arranging frequent follow-up visits to preempt the family's needs and to minimize the appearance of new symptoms. This also reduces emergency room visits and makes overall management easier.

Even if somatization disorder is diagnosed, it is necessary to reassess the course of the illness at intervals as other psychiatric disorders may emerge. Those associated most commonly with somatic complaints in pediatric patients are anxiety disorder, depression, attention-deficit/hyperactivity disorder, substance use disorder, and conduct disorder (Silber and Pao 2003). Any new symptoms should be assessed on their merits because somatization does not preclude the onset of organic conditions.

Unfortunately, the current medical infrastructure conspires against the optimal management of these patients. With appropriate interventions, the prognosis for children and adolescents with somatization disorders is very good. Only those patients who have the severe, undifferentiated form of somatoform disorder, which is closely related to personality disorder, have a long and persistent course continuing into adulthood (Silber and Pao 2003).

A study of the association between social environments (school, family, friends, neighborhood) and general well-being, health, and psychologic adjustment reported that improved family environment and fewer stressful life events were associated with lower levels of psychologic distress, which in turn correlated with fewer somatic complaints. A causal association between life events and somatic complaints was weakly statistically significant. It is important to consider the environmental context when attempting to intervene with somatizing youth. Incorporating neighborhood influences into a practitioner's assessment may lead to systems level interventions, such as problem-solving for physical safety by creating linkages with neighbors, or simply allowing teens to acknowledge and process the impact of living in difficult environments. However, the clinical focus should remain on optimizing functioning rather than problem-solving within the context of their communities.

Diagnoses of Organic Disease – Gynecologic Origin

Common gynecologic causes of pelvic pain in adolescents include dysmenorrhea, endometriosis, PID, pelvic adhesions, pregnancy (intrauterine or ectopic), adnexal torsion, hemorrhage, and rupture.

Dysmenorrhea

Dysmenorrhea is the most common cause of pelvic pain in adolescent girls, with a prevalence of 40–90% (Tu et al. 2007). It is described as primary when associated with menses in the absence of pelvic pathology, and secondary when associated with underlying pathology. Secondary dysmenorrhea commonly extends beyond the duration of the menstrual period. Dysmenorrhea is often associated with changes in mood (e.g., premenstrual syndrome and premenstrual dysphoric disorder) and interferes with daily living as evidenced by the majority of sufferers reporting missing work or school as a consequence. A typical history in functional dysmenorrhea is cramping, dull, midline, or generalized abdominal pain beginning within 1–24 h of the onset of menstruation and continuing for 24–48 h. Frequently occurring somatic comorbidities include backache, nausea, vomiting, diarrhea, headache, and thigh pain. Physical findings in primary dysmenorrhea are a normal pelvic and abdominal examination except for uterine tenderness during menses. In secondary dysmenorrhea, uterine tenderness may be present independent of menses and other signs pertinent to the underlying pathology may be elicited.

Risk factors include younger age, low body mass index, smoking, alcohol use, early menarche, prolonged or aberrant menstrual flow, related perimenstrual somatic complaints, pelvic infections, previous sterilization, somatization, psychologic disturbance, and a history of sexual assault. Higher parity, a stable relationship, physical exercise, fish intake, and oral contraceptives are protective (Tu et al. 2007). Pain intensity increases with increasing severity of depression, anxiety, and somatic complaints.

Elevated levels of eicosanoids (biologically active lipids) are a key cause of dysmenorrhea. They mediate hyperalgesia and inflammatory pain while lowering the pain threshold during menstruation (Tu et al. 2007). Levels decrease in response to NSAIDs, which explains their analgesic efficacy in this population.

NSAIDs and combined oral contraceptive pills (COCPs) are first-line treatment for dysmenorrhea. Ideally, NSAIDs should be commenced 24–48 h before the anticipated onset of menses to inhibit prostaglandin synthesis and continued until the third to fifth day of menstruation. NSAIDs provide effective relief in 80% of women with dysmenorrhea, and, if they do not, induction of anovulation using COCPs might help. COCPs attenuate hyperactive myometrial activity, reduce menstrual fluid volume, lower endometrial COX-2 levels throughout menstruation, and keep prostaglandin production in check.

COCPs and NSAIDs are considered first-line treatment for dysmenorrhea. Progestins alone can induce anovulation, although caution must be used to prevent estrogen deficiencies and loss of bone mineral density. Progestins can be administered orally (e.g., medroxyprogesterone acetate, norethindrone), by depot injection (medroxyprogesterone acetate), and via intrauterine systems (e.g., levonorgestrel intrauterine system, which releases 20 µg/day of a progestin derivative directly on the endometrium).

When medical treatments fail, laparoscopy may be indicated to confirm the diagnosis and provide treatment. The prevalence of endometriosis is high in adolescents with dysmenorrhea who do not respond to NSAIDs and COCPs. Early surgical intervention has been shown to improve symptoms and function and maintain future fertility (see "Endometriosis" below).

"Natural" remedies that may have utility include magnesium and vitamin B1 through possible interference with prostaglandin production, although evidence of efficacy from randomized controlled trials is lacking (Tu et al. 2007). Omega-3 fatty acids from fish oil decrease menstrual pain intensity but can cause nausea and exacerbate acne. Transcutaneous electrical nerve stimulation (TENS) and acupuncture may be of benefit. TENS is thought to work by increasing uterine blood flow and reducing myometrial ischemia. Acupuncture appears to work in concert with serotonin and endorphin mediators to inhibit pain sensitivity and is considered effective for the treatment of dysmenorrhea by a National Institutes of Health consensus conference (Greco 2003).

Behavioral interventions have been shown to be helpful. Their usefulness is based upon recognition of central sensitization to pain perception in dysmenorrhea sufferers. These strategies include relaxation, biofeedback, CBT, pain management counseling, and lifestyle changes (e.g., quitting smoking and alcohol use and maintaining an optimal body mass index).

Endometriosis

Endometriosis is the presence of endometrial stroma and glands in aberrant locations outside the endometrial cavity. Its prevalence is 69.6–73% in adolescents who suffer persistent pelvic pain or dysmenorrhea refractory to first-line medical therapy. The diagnosis is made by laparoscopy and histologic confirmation. Approximately 70% of adolescent patients with CPP have endometriosis (Greco 2003; Propst and Laufer 1999). Its incidence increases from 12% in 11–13 year olds to 54% in 20–21 year olds. There also may be a genetic predisposition. Of women with endometriosis, 6.9% report a first-degree relative with the same condition vs. 1% of women without endometriosis. Inheritance is probably polygenic and multifactorial. Endometriosis should be suspected in those with a family history and is more likely to occur in patients with reproductive tract anomalies associated with retrograde flow. Although these patients tend to present at a younger age and with more severe pain, endometriosis resolves once a patent outflow tract is established.

Five theories regarding the pathogenesis of endometriosis have been proposed: the genetic theory, theory of embryonic müllerian rests, retrograde menstruation and implantation, coelomic metaplasia, and unintentional surgical transplantation (Batt and Mitwally 2003).

Adolescents with endometriosis can have cyclic (64%) and/or acyclic (36%) pain. Unlike functional dysmenorrhea, endometriosis-related pain tends to increase in severity over time and may occur throughout the month. Pain is the most frequent presenting complaint, infertility being rare in this age group. Physical signs suggestive of endometriosis include fixed, retroverted uterus; uterosacral ligament abnormalities; lateral displacement of the cervix; cervical stenosis; cul-de-sac tenderness, and nodularity. Endometriomas are rare in adolescents (Economy and Laufer 1999).

The definitive diagnosis of endometriosis is by laparoscopy and biopsy of lesions. Endometriosis is staged using the revised criteria of the American Society for Reproductive Medicine point-based classification system (American Society for Reproductive Medicine 1997). There is a natural progression from "clear" and "red" atypical lesions to classic "black" lesions over about a 10-year period. In the study by Propst and Laufer (1999), 77.4% of subjects with endometriosis had stage I disease and 22.6% had stage II disease. No subject had stage III–IV disease. This compares with 27% of women who presented with stage III–IV disease in the study by Hornstein et al. (1995).

Interestingly, pain severity is not always related to the extent of disease. Women with severe disease may be asymptomatic, and those with minimal observable disease may suffer debilitating pain. Based on this observation, Momoeda et al. (2002) studied whether pain was associated with the pathophysiology of endometriosis per se. Dysmenorrhea's severity was linked to the progression of endometriosis in patients whose primary complaint was infertility but not pain. Furthermore, dysmenorrhea was significantly associated with invasive cul-de-sac lesions but not ovarian endometrial cysts and peritoneal implants. Finally, endometriosis-related pain symptoms were all correlated with stage of endometriosis.

It is hypothesized that pain arises from peritoneal inflammation, prostaglandin release, swelling of endometriotic implants or adhesion, and scar formation (Economy and Laufer 1999). Some evidence suggests that black, brown, or gray implants (uncommon in adolescence) are more frequently associated with deep dyspareunia and that depth and volume of these implants may be related to severity of pelvic pain, particularly

lesions in the rectovaginal septum (Economy and Laufer 1999).

Management is based on pain severity, previous treatment response, and fertility preservation and is tailored to each patient's symptoms. Adolescents may be less compliant, so frequent appointments to reinforce the treatment plan with them and their families will improve communication and increase compliance (Economy and Laufer 1999). A multimodal approach is recommended incorporating selected medication trials, surgery, physical therapy, biobehavioral therapy, and complementary/alternative therapies (American College of Obstetricians and Gynecologists 2005; Greco 2003; Highfield et al. 2006; Solnik 2006). The American College of Obstetricians and Gynecologists Committee on Adolescent Health published a protocol to guide the evaluation and treatment of adolescent pelvic pain and endometriosis (American College of Obstetricians and Gynecologists 2005).

Surgical treatment consists of resection or fulguration of all visible lesions at the time of diagnosis, lysis or resection of adhesions, and restoration of normal pelvic anatomy. Ideally, a surgeon who can identify early endometriotic lesions should do the procedure. Surgical success rates at reducing pain are high; adult studies report 70–100% improvement immediately post-surgery, 82% improvement at 1 year, and 66% at 5 years. Implants and adhesions can reform, the incidence being 40% by 9 years for the former and 40–50% for the latter (Propst and Laufer 1999). Another study reported 62.5% resolution of symptoms after 6 months in patients with stage I–III disease. The greatest benefit was observed in those with the severest disease (Economy and Laufer 1999).

LUNA has been suggested to treat midline pelvic pain associated with endometriosis. It involves resection or ablation of the sensory nerve fibers to the cervix at their attachment point, thus interrupting the sympathetic fibers from the superior hypogastric plexus and the parasympathetic fibers from S2–4. In a small study of 21 adults with primary dysmenorrhea, 81% experienced immediate benefit, which fell to 50% at 1 year. LUNA has not been studied in adolescents.

Reports of uterine prolapse as a consequence of LUNA suggest that this should be avoided in adolescents until data supporting its safety and efficacy are available.

After surgical treatment has eradicated visible endometriosis, medical treatment is reinstated to treat microscopic disease, control pain, and minimize disease progression. As ectopic endometrial tissue is hormonally responsive (Economy and Laufer 1999), hormonal suppression with estrogens, progestins, and androgens is used depending on the patient's age, severity of symptoms, duration of symptoms, and extent of disease. The goal is to create a state of chronic anovulation, either pseudopregnancy or pseudomenopause. Combined progestin-dominant oral contraceptive pills are the mainstay of treatment and are preferred in girls under 16 years. About 50–80% experience reduced pain and dysmenorrhea on this treatment. Triphasic pills are ineffective because of the smaller doses of progestins. High doses of progestins alone are required for pain relief (e.g., medroxyprogesterone acetate 30–50 mg/day orally or 150 mg intramuscularly (IM) every 1–3 months). At these doses, the side effects of weight gain, bloating, acne, headaches, fluid retention, emotional lability, and irregular bleeding can limit their usefulness. Progestins act by creating an antiestrogenic environment that inhibits endometriotic implant growth.

Danazol, a 17 α-ethinyl testosterone derivative, is highly efficacious in controlling pain by causing endometrial atrophy. Unfortunately, its masculinizing side effects make it unsuitable for adolescent use.

The current and most widely used first-line treatment is gonadotrophin-releasing hormone agonists (GnRH-a). The acyclic, low-estrogen environment suppresses endometrial growth and bleeding in endometrial implants and prevents further seeding. GnRH-a can be administered as a nasal spray or as subcutaneous or IM injections. Pelvic pain is reduced by 30–80%. The most important side effect is bone mineral density loss. For this reason, it is not recommended in girls less than 16 years of age and is not used for greater than 6 months. One study reported a 5.9–13.8% decrease in vertebral bone mass over a 6-month period. The rate of bone loss can be slowed but not prevented by prescribing "add back" therapy with estrogen and/or progestins. Use of continuous COCPs and then cyclic COCPs is recommended after the 6-month treatment phase with GnRH-a and "add back" therapy in older adolescents (Economy and Laufer 1999).

Acupuncture to treat endometriosis was deemed beneficial in 70% of patients and by 59% of parents (Greco 2003). Case reports support acupuncture use in endometriosis when other interventions fail (Highfield et al. 2006).

IC often coexists with endometriosis (see below). It should be evaluated in all patients who fail to respond to treatment for endometriosis alone.

Pelvic Inflammatory Disease

PID represents infection in the upper genital tract, presenting as a spectrum of inflammatory disorders within the upper genital tract of women that include any combination of endometritis, salpingitis, TOA, and pelvic peritonitis (Newkirk 1996). PID is a syndrome with a broad clinical spectrum and multiple etiologies (Igra 1998). No laboratory tests can diagnose it. Nearly 18% of women with laparoscopically documented salpingitis develop PID (Haggerty et al. (2005).

PID most frequently arises from NG or Chlamydia infections (25–40%). These infections are reportable diseases in most states. Organisms from the lower genital tract then gain ascent, leading to a polymicrobial infection. Cultures reveal mixed aerobic and anaerobic infections in 25–60% of cases. PID occurring within a week of menses is suggestive of NG or Chlamydia. Symptoms occurring 2 weeks after menses are associated with non-gonococcal and non-chlamydial organisms 66% of the time (Braverman 2000).

One in five PID cases occurs in women less than 19 years old. A sexually active 15 year old has a 1:8 chance of developing PID as compared with 1:80 for a 24 year old (Braverman 2000). Thus adolescents have the highest PID rate among sexually experienced women.

The higher relative risk for PID in younger women is attributed to physiologic (low levels of protective antibodies, columnar epithelium on the ectocervix, and greater penetration of cervical mucus), behavioral, and cognitive risk factors (Champion et al. 2005). The latter include age of first coitus, numbers of sex partners, recurrence of sexually transmitted disease (STD), and health-seeking behaviors. Adolescents seek treatment 2 days later than adults on average, making them more vulnerable to PID complications (e.g., infertility, TOA, perihepatitis, CPP, ectopic pregnancy).

Diagnosis relies on clinical judgment coupled with empiric therapeutic intervention and careful follow-up. For patients with mild symptoms, the Centers for Disease Control and Prevention (CDC) recommends that lower abdominal, adnexal, and cervical motion tenderness be sufficient evidence for initiating broad-spectrum antibiotics before culture results are available, provided that competing diagnoses are adequately excluded (e.g., appendicitis, ectopic pregnancy) (Newkirk 1996).

The majority of patients are treated as outpatients who must receive close follow-up and be reevaluated 48–72 h after starting therapy. Patients who have an unclear diagnosis, cannot tolerate oral medication, are pregnant, have severe illness including TOA, have failed outpatient therapy, or are noncompliant should be hospitalized for initial treatment. Oral therapy is usually started within 24 h of clinical improvement.

Risk factors for development of CPP in women with PID include nonblack race/ethnicity, being married, a low score on mental health assessment, smoking, two or more prior episodes of PID, douching, nonelevated white cell count, and not having endometriosis or endometrial gonorrhea or Chlamydia (Ness et al. 2002).

Pelvic Adhesions

Pelvic adhesions can arise after surgery, endometriosis, and acute/chronic infections. Evidence regarding the role of adhesions in CPP and the benefits of adhesiolysis is conflicting. Ostensibly, only adhesions restricting movement or distensibility of pelvic or gastrointestinal organs cause pain. There is little correlation between the extent of adhesions and reported pain. In one study, 89% of adolescents who underwent adhesiolysis for pelvic pain reported symptom improvement. In long-term follow-up of 48 patients 2–5 years after adhesiolysis, 37% reported complete/near-complete pain relief while 30% reported significant pain relief. The high rate of adhesion reformation should be balanced against the benefits of adhesiolysis.

Pregnancy

Pelvic pain can occur in intrauterine and ectopic pregnancies. It is prudent to perform pregnancy tests in all sexually active adolescents.

Adnexal Torsion

Although uncommon, torsion of a fallopian tube or ovary may be the cause of right-sided pelvic pain. It is frequently acute in onset and can be recurrent. Ovarian cysts or masses without torsion are usually painless (Rickert and Kozlowski 2000).

Ovarian Abnormalities

Asymptomatic, spontaneously regressing functional ovarian cysts are the most common ovarian abnormality in adolescents (Song and Advincula 2005). They typically regress over 2–3 cycles and are managed conservatively. Occasionally they cause lower abdominal pain associated with ovulation, rupture, or torsion. The former usually lasts for 48 h and responds to NSAIDs or COCPs. Rupture is associated with pain, lack of fever, normal peripheral white cell count, free fluid in the posterior cul-de-sac, and resolution within 72 h. Torsion typically presents as unilateral, colicky, lower abdominal pain with fever and elevated white cell count (Hewitt and Brown 2000).

Ovarian masses more often associated with CPP include hemorrhagic corpus luteal cysts, mature cystic teratomas, serous or mucinous cytoadenomas, and endometriomas. Ovarian cystectomy with preservation of normal ovarian tissue may be indicated (Brown and Hewitt 2004).

Obstructive Malformations of the Reproductive Tract

Obstructive malformation of the reproductive tract should be considered in all types of CPP in adolescents. Anomalies arise from abnormalities of agenesis, vertical fusion, lateral fusion, or resorption during development (Economy and Laufer 1999). Laparoscopies for failure of medical therapy document the incidence of müllerian abnormalities at 6–9%. Evaluation includes physical examination, ultrasound, and MRI. Multiplanar MRI, which provides excellent visualization of subperitoneal structures, is being used increasingly for surgical planning and more precise delineation of anomalies. Surgical correction, the treatment of choice, should be performed in a timely fashion to prevent development of endometriosis as a consequence of retrograde menstruation or to resolve endometriosis when already present.

Individuals with vaginal agenesis and obstructed uterine horns can be managed with menstrual suppression using continuous COCPs until fertility is desired (Economy and Laufer 1999).

Diagnoses of Organic Disease – Non-gynecologic Origin

Gastrointestinal Etiologies (Brown and Hewitt 2004)

Organic causes of CPP include IBD and lactose intolerance. Constipation, the most common cause of non-gynecologic CPP in children, can be organic or functional in origin (Hewitt and Brown 2000). IBS, childhood functional abdominal pain (FAP), and childhood FAP syndrome

(FAPS) are functional gastrointestinal disorders (FGIDs). By definition, they cannot be explained by structural or biochemical abnormalities. Criteria for the diagnosis of functional abdominal disorders in children and adolescents are outlined in the Rome III classifications (Rasquin et al. 2006). Organic and FGIDs can coexist (e.g., IBS and Crohn's disease).

Crohn's disease has an insidious onset and can present with CPP. Failure to thrive, arthralgias, recurrent aphthous ulcers, and an elevated ESR suggest the diagnosis. Ulcerative colitis (UC) can be associated with CPP but is rarely the presenting complaint. UC is usually accompanied by tenesmus and explosive diarrhea. Both conditions are diagnosed using imaging studies and histologic methods.

Lactose intolerance can be diagnosed on history and negative abdominal examination. Susceptible populations include African Americans and persons of Middle Eastern and Mediterranean ethnicity. Dietary modification relieves the symptoms.

Constipation is defined as chronic retention of stool regardless of the stooling pattern. Chronic accumulation of stool leads to indistinct periumbilical pain. Constipation is diagnosed by abdominal palpation of a fecal mass, rectal examination, and plain abdominal radiographs. When associated with an organic disorder, treatment of the primary disease and symptom relief are the therapeutic goals.

Functional constipation has a peak incidence at 2–4 years, with increased prevalence in males. The longer functional constipation goes on the less successful the treatment. Up to 84% of children with functional constipation present with fecal incontinence. Painful bowel movements can lead to retentive behavior. This is a vicious cycle because the passage of a large fecal load is uncomfortable, reinforcing the fear of pain; thus the child continues to avoid defecation. Urinary problems are common in these children. Patients with functional constipation have a lower quality of life and exhibit poorer self-esteem, more social withdrawal, more anxiety related to toilet training, and a coping style based on denial (Rasquin et al. 2006). Treatment is based on addressing the fears and concerns of the patient and family.

Fecal impaction can be treated with 1–1.5 g/kg/day of polyethylene glycol for 3 days. Stool softeners, dietary changes, and positive reinforcement of good toileting constitute the mainstay of therapy.

About 15–20% of adolescents have symptoms consistent with IBS (Song and Advincula 2005). Physical examination and growth curves are normal, and there are no symptoms of significant organic disease. FAP may reflect visceral (intestinal or uterine) hypersensitivity (Brown and Hewitt 2004; Rasquin et al. 2006). Neural impulses between the enteric nervous system and CNS lead to altered pain perceptions. It may be related to infection, inflammation, intestinal trauma, or allergy and may be associated with disordered gut motility. A genetic predisposition and psychosocial factors (e.g., early life experiences, conditioning factors, physical stress, personal or social coping systems, and psychologic stress) influence the expression of symptoms and illness behavior (Baccini et al. 2003; Rasquin et al. 2006; Song and Advincula 2005). A high prevalence of prior physical and sexual abuse has been reported in women with IBS compared with women with organic disorders (Baccini et al. 2003). The history of abuse sets the stage for the clinical expression of symptoms. Anxiety, depression, and impaired psychosocial adjustment are more prevalent in patients with IBS than controls.

Treatment is aimed at reassurance and symptom relief. Reviewing the role of stress and anxiety in IBS will help the family understand why the pain occurs as well as its triggers. IBS can be managed but not cured. Pharmacologic therapies include antispasmodics, peppermint oil (children only), tricyclic antidepressants, and selective serotonin reuptake inhibitors for the symptomatic treatment of pain (severe/refractory cases), fiber bulking agents in cases with constipation, and antidiarrheals (e.g., loperamide) in cases with diarrhea. Antidepressants and serotonin reuptake inhibitors are less effective in children than in adults. The selective partial 5-HT$_4$ agonist, tegaserod, has been approved for IBS with constipation although its utility in the pediatric population has not been determined.

Psychologic and behavioral therapies include CBT, psychotherapy, hypnosis, relaxation training, and family/group therapy. The patient and family may be resistant to engaging in these therapies. Therefore, the initial approach is to involve dietary, educational, and pharmacologic measures. If these fail, patients should be referred to a psychologist or psychiatrist.

The diagnosis of childhood FAP includes all of the following: episodic or continuous abdominal pain, insufficient criteria for other FGIDs, and no evidence of inflammatory, anatomic, metabolic, or neoplastic causes for the pain. The pain must be present at least once a week for at least 2 months. When loss of daily functioning or additional somatic symptoms are also present for at least 25% of the time, FAP is known as FAPS. These conditions are associated with high levels of anxiety, depression, and somatization. A biopsychosocial treatment approach is recommended (Rasquin et al. 2006).

Interstitial Cystitis and Urologic Causes

IC, or pelvic pain of bladder origin, is a common cause of CPP in adults (Chung et al. 2005). The etiology of IC is unknown although it is thought to be multifactorial and progressive, involving bladder epithelial dysfunction, mast cell activation, and bladder sensory nerve upregulation. Its estimated prevalence in the USA is 10–510 per 100,000 cases. IC is characterized by urinary urgency and frequency and by pelvic, perineal, and/or abdominal pain in the absence of a urinary tract infection. It occurs predominantly in females and is associated with dyspareunia and cyclic pain from menses. About 15% of patients with IC present with CPP alone and report no urologic symptoms. Findings on physical examination include tenderness of the bladder base, anterior vaginal wall, and/or uterus.

Diagnostic criteria for IC have been defined by the National Institutes of Health-National Institute of Diabetes and Digestive and Kidney Diseases (NIH-NIDDK), including the presence of ten glomerulations per quadrant in 3 of 4 quadrants of the bladder cavity and terminal hematuria

(Hanno et al. 1999). The potassium sensitivity test (PST) to evaluate bladder epithelial dysfunction is both sensitive and specific. Up to 81% of patients with IC have endometriosis (Chung et al. 2005). A comorbid relationship with fibromyalgia and IBS also has been described (Powell-Boone et al. 2005).

One hundred seventy-eight adult women (aged 18–60 years) with CPP were studied prospectively using the PST, cystoscopy, hydrodistension, and laparoscopy to determine the prevalence of IC and endometriosis. Cystoscopic findings that met NIH-NIDDK criteria for IC were present in 89% of patients. Seventy-five percent had histologic evidence of endometriosis, and 65% had both. Of the 82% of patients with a positive PST, 78% had irritative voiding symptoms and 96% had cystoscopic evidence of IC; 12% of patients with a negative PST had IC on cystoscopy, and 72% had endometriosis on laparoscopy. Of the 134 patients diagnosed with endometriosis, 86% also had IC. Conversely, of the 159 patients with IC, 72% also had endometriosis. If cystoscopy alone had been used to diagnose IC, 20% of cases would have been missed. As IC and endometriosis frequently exist concomitantly in patients with CPP who present with uterine and bladder tenderness, both conditions should be evaluated even when the diagnosis of one has been confirmed. Whenever possible, cystoscopy with hydrodistension should be performed concurrently with laparoscopy to avoid the need for a second procedure under general anesthesia and to facilitate more timely diagnosis and treatment. A positive PST may be considered sufficient to diagnose IC. A negative test should be followed up by cystoscopy. In CPP, consider the bladder as a cause early in the diagnostic workup. A possible pathophysiologic basis for the increased risk of one condition with the other is altered immune function.

IC is usually treated with simple, conservative methods including diet, pelvic floor physical therapy, and medications such as hydroxyzine and pentosan polysulfate sodium. The recently noted efficacy of COCPs in the treatment of IC supports the role of the gonadal hormones estrogen and progesterone in the etiopathogenesis of IC. Estradiol may influence pathophysiologic responses via bladder mast cells expressing high-affinity estrogen receptors found in patients with IC. Gonadal hormonal activity can influence pain responses by peripheral actions on bladder-related, primary afferent neuronal responses, similar to actions on uterine afferents. Centrally, endogenous opioid and gonadal hormone systems interact reciprocally, supporting hormonal therapy to modulate pain sensation selectively.

Urolithiasis should be ruled out in patients with hematuria but no pyuria or bacteria. Plain radiographs, cystoscopy, and high urine calcium/creatinine ratio facilitate diagnosis (Hewitt and Brown 2000).

Pain of Musculoskeletal Origin

Pelvic musculoskeletal tension is thought to be responsible for about 8% of CPP in North American adults. Pain arises from excessive physical activity (Hewitt and Brown 2000), abnormal posture, sacro-iliac dysfunction, and shortening and spasm of the psoas, abdominal, levator ani, and piriformis muscles (Song and Advincula 2005; Tu et al. 2006). Pelvic muscular dysfunction is also thought to contribute to the etiology of other CPP conditions such as chronic prostatitis and IC (Tu et al. 2006) and can arise consequent to functional and organic pain conditions (Solnik 2006). As pain increases, patients develop splinting and limit physical activities and exercise. Musculoskeletal dysfunction may induce tissue damage, resulting in the development of trigger points, which were found in 75% of 177 patients referred to a pelvic pain clinic (Song and Advincula 2005).

Myofascial trigger points (myofascial pain syndromes) occur within taut bands of skeletal muscle. Subsequent referred pain may be visceral and can present as dysmenorrhea, dyspareunia, or bladder or gastrointestinal symptoms. Abdominal examination focuses on deep and superficial palpation to distinguish trigger points from primary visceral pain. Single-finger palpation is used to locate trigger points, starting closest to the area of pain. When pain is reproduced, the rectus abdominis muscle should be flexed by elevating the leg. Visceral pain is not reproduced in this way. Trigger points in piriformis and levator ani can be palpated via the lateral wall of the vagina and lateral fornices.

In the study by Tu et al. (2006) of 955 patients presenting at a gynecologic CPP clinic, 22% had piriformis pain and 14% had levator ani pain. Both subgroups had pain on defecation and multiple additional abdominopelvic pain sites. However, there was no association with prior sexual abuse or dyspareunia. The prevalence of non-musculoskeletal causes of CPP (e.g., endometriosis, IBS) was unchanged in this population. Patients with levator ani pain reported more surgeries for pain than patients with other types of pain. As in other causes of CPP, psychologic impairment was associated with increased pain intensity and surgical interventions.

Trigger point injections (3–5 ml of 0.25% bupivacaine into each trigger point) can be diagnostic and therapeutic. Resolution or improvement in pain, lasting weeks to months, has been reported in up to 89% of patients. Physical therapy, massage, biofeedback, NSAIDs, and muscle relaxants, including botulinum toxin A, constitute the remainder of therapy.

Autoimmune Inflammation

Startseva (1980) first postulated that painful endometriosis was associated with humoral and cell-mediated immunity. Since then, the presence of chronic inflammation of the pelvic peritoneum in the absence of endometriosis has been sited as a cause of CPP, with an estimated prevalence of 14.6%. Over one third of cases are associated with autoimmune disease, suggesting an etiologic systemic disorder of immunity.

In a study of 40 women with CPP (Thomson and Redwine 2005) and histologic findings of chronic inflammation of the peritoneum and elevated concentrations of cytokines and prostaglandins in the peritoneal fluid, 30% reported 80–100% resolution of pain on a regimen of hydroxychloroquine 200 mg b.i.d. and methotrexate 10 mg weekly. Pain was characteristically sharp, stabbing, accentuated mid-cycle, and prior to periods, and accompanied by lower abdominal and sometimes rebound tenderness. Skin hypersensitivity of the anterior abdominal wall over the area of pain was present, indicative of an inflammatory origin of pain. Most had cervical excitation tenderness. Chronic inflammatory changes with tenderness in the vagina were associated with dyspareunia and/or vaginal discharge. Clinically, the pain and tenderness were out of proportion to the degree of inflammation, probably secondary to hyperalgesia.

Chronic systemic inflammation may represent a persistent, unrecognized infection; dysregulation of elements of the immune system in which there is failure of the inflammatory switch-off mechanism; or true autoimmunity in which tissue damage/immune activation is self-perpetuating because of continued presence of self-antigen. Genetic, dietary, and environmental factors may be involved in development of the systemic inflammatory state.

Based on these data, the authors recommended that peritoneal membrane and fluid should be sampled and examined histologically whenever laparoscopy is performed for CPP. If chronic inflammation is detected, these patients may respond to disease-modifying anti-rheumatic drugs.

Vascular Etiologies

CPP arising from ovarian and pelvic varices is variously known as pelvic congestion syndrome, pelvic pain syndrome, or pelvic venous incompetence. It was first reported in adult women in the 1950s. Diagnostic features are pelvic pain in the upright position, during or after intercourse, and the presence of other varicosities in the thigh, buttocks, perineum, vulva, or vagina. Generally, pain is relieved in the supine position. Symptoms may increase in the postpartum interval. An MRI scan acquired in the coronal, axial, and sagittal projections is the preferred imaging study for diagnosis. Patients with a negative scan but a strong clinical history should undergo selective ovarian and internal iliac contrast venography; laparoscopy may miss varices. Treatment involves bilateral venography and embolization of the ovarian and internal iliac veins to reduce the theoretical chance of recurrence. In one study of 56 adult women (Venbrux et al. 2002), average pain scores fell from 7.8 (baseline) to 4.2 at 3 months, 3.8 at 6 months, and 2.7 at 12 months post-embolization. Other studies have shown a reduction in CPP of 50–80%. Embolization had no effect on menstrual cycle interval or length. Sclerosing agents cause significant discomfort, and overnight admission for pain control is warranted.

A study to delineate the psychosocial characteristics associated specifically with CPP caused by pelvic venous congestion (PVC) in 164 subjects (Fry et al. 1997) revealed higher paternal overprotection, less outwardly directed hostility, and more inwardly directed hostility than in CPP controls without PVC. Overprotection was inversely related to poor-quality parental care. In patients with CPP secondary to PVC, paternal overprotection may be an index of more extensive disturbance in the father–daughter dyad and in childhood and the family in general. These factors may predispose to the later development of personality traits and patterns of social interactions that contribute to the development of PVC, perhaps via the medium of the hypothalamic–pituitary–ovarian axis, and the perception of the sensations generated as painful.

Trauma-Related Pain

Substantial research supports a link between CPP, somatization, symptom load, and abuse in women. Abused adolescents report more pathologic symptoms than their non-abused peers despite similar disease severity (Champion et al. 2005). Thus, victims of sexual or physical abuse may express medically unexplained physical symptoms as part of a long-term adaptation to their traumatic experience. Sexual or physical abuse occurring in females during childhood and again in adulthood has been found to be strongly associated with pelvic pain complaints. Recurrent STD or PID may explain previously documented relationships between sexual abuse and subsequent development of CPP in women

(Champion et al. 2005). The sex partners of abused adolescents tend to have a higher number of sex partners. Thus, they are exposed to an even higher risk of recurrent STD, greater symptomatology, and development of PID, regardless of their own sexual activity.

Interpersonal childhood trauma (i.e., sexual abuse, physical abuse, emotional abuse, neglect) has been linked to somatization in adults (Waldinger et al. 2006). The risk for trauma exposure peaks among females in adolescence (16–20-year age range) (Seng et al. 2005). Posttraumatic stress disorder (PTSD) has twice the prevalence in girls than in boys aged 12–24 years. Depression occurs in the aftermath of PTSD in 25–70% of children and adolescents and is associated with poor health. Poor maternal physical health and a child's level of traumatic stress symptoms are the strongest predictors of poor child health. Dissociative and borderline personality diagnoses occur among young women disproportionately; these comorbid conditions are associated with somatization.

A descriptive epidemiologic case-control analysis of 1,672 females aged 0–17 years with PTSD (Seng et al. 2005) confirmed its association with adverse health outcomes. The pattern in adolescents resembles that of adult women in that the odds for physical comorbidity increased when PTSD was complicated by depression, dissociation, or borderline personality disorder. The latter conditions are related to early and repeated interpersonal trauma. The most common diagnoses in children with PTSD were chronic fatigue, fibromyalgia, IBS, CPP, and dysmenorrhea. A traumatic stress-related origin should be considered in pediatric and adolescent patients who present with multiple idiopathic physical symptoms. Interdisciplinary collaboration or integrated primary mental health care may improve well-being in the short term and over the life span.

PTSD conveys a risk for health problems above and beyond that associated with poverty (Seng et al. 2005). Establish when physical symptoms developed in childhood trauma survivors (Farley and Keaney 1997).

When 426 healthy male and female college students were questioned about abuse history, recent pain, health-care utilization, perceived health and psychologic variables, females had significantly higher rates for all types of abuse except physical abuse during childhood (43.3% vs. 23.8% in males) (Fillingim et al. 1999). Abused subjects reported significantly greater pain and health-care utilization. They perceived their health as poor and complained of more headaches and back and muscular pain. Sex abuse was associated with increased abdominal pain in females only. Abused subjects reported greater somatization, depression, negative emotionality, disinhibition, and use of catastrophizing as a pain-coping strategy.

The mechanisms whereby traumatic experiences lead to increased negative affectivity, which increases awareness of negative physical and psychologic experiences, are unclear. Reduced hippocampal volume has been reported in traumatized persons. Maladaptive coping patterns may covary with depression and somatization in abused individuals and could explain their increased pain complaints. In general, females employed catastrophizing, praying, and hoping as coping styles whereas males tended to reinterpret or ignore pain sensations.

Studies of the relationship between sexual abuse, somatization, and dissociation found that sexual abuse survivors had significantly higher dissociative experience scale scores and significantly more chronic physical symptoms than non-abused women (Badura et al. 1997; Farley and Keaney 1997). Somatization can be viewed as an extreme point on a continuum of dissociative behaviors. In the past, these behaviors were diagnosed as conversion disorder. In sexual abuse, the number of perpetrators was the most potent factor determining severity and number of symptoms in adulthood. When sexual trauma occurred around the time of puberty, childbirth itself became traumatic, with subjects reporting more pregnancy and childbirth complications, caesarian sections, and hysterectomies. This suggests that the developmental stage at which abuse occurs is important.

Women with CPP were considerably more likely to have experienced severe childhood sexual abuse and to use dissociation as a coping

mechanism compared with non-sexually-abused controls. The high rate of somatization in dissociative disorders suggests that when the mind cannot remember traumatic events (dissociation), somatization is the body's way of remembering. It is an indicator of psychologic conflict. Somatization in abused women frequently meets the DSM-IV definition of undifferentiated somatoform disorder (Samelius et al. 2007).

A similar study in 46 patients, ages 18–47, referred to a CPP clinic investigated adaptive and maladaptive coping styles in relation to a history of sexual or physical abuse and dissociation, somatization, and substance abuse compared with non-abused controls (Badura et al. 1997). Abused subjects had significantly higher dissociation, somatization, and substance abuse scores than non-abused controls. There were no significant differences between groups for adaptive and maladaptive coping. Significant positive correlations were identified between dissociation and somatization, between substance abuse and maladaptive coping, between somatization and substance abuse, and between somatization and maladaptive coping.

Survivors of abuse often have low self-esteem, self-efficacy, and self-worth. Stressful events, such as abuse, undermine personal coping strategies and result in avoidance-based coping. Self-abusive behavior such as substance abuse is a pervasive, avoidance-based coping response.

Higher rates of medical attention seeking apparently unrelated to CPP suggest that women with CPP may "convert" psychologic difficulties into physical symptoms and favor a somatic over a psychologic representation of distress. By converting their issues, problems are not dealt with directly, and somatization becomes an avoidant coping strategy. Childhood physical abuse was associated more strongly with later somatization, depression, and anxiety. History of sexual abuse is a significant predisposing risk for somatization and nonsomatic CPP. Thus, both sexual abuse and physical abuse have important links to somatization.

There is a clear relationship between childhood sexual abuse and later alcohol and substance abuse. In one crisis clinic, abused people were ten times more likely than non-abused people to have a substance abuse history and twice as likely to abuse alcohol. Chemical abuse may be an avoidance behavior to separate from their environment and emotional distress.

Treatment for women with comorbid dissociation and somatization should focus on developing more adaptive ways of coping.

Another study (Samelius et al. 2007) investigating the relationship between somatization and lifetime exposure to physical, sexual, and psychologic abuse in 800 women found that psychologic abuse, regardless of duration, was associated with somatization but not physical abuse. Sexual abuse with penetration was not associated with somatization, but sexual contact abuse was. Dissociation was found to serve as a mediator in the link between sexual abuse and somatization. Factors other than severity of abuse, such as whether the abused woman perceived her experience as abuse, appear to be more decisive for developing somatization in abused women. Abuse should be taken into account in patients with somatization symptoms. In contrast to other studies, being abused as a child/teenager only was not associated with somatization whereas abuse as an adult or as both a child and adult were.

Childhood trauma fosters the development of insecure and fearful attachment, including the expectation that others will not meet one's emotional needs. This expectation in turn promotes increased emphasis on and reporting of somatic concerns as a way to seek help from those who are expected to be unresponsive to emotional distress (Waldinger et al. 2006). From a caregiver's perspective, these patients appear fragile, needy, and difficult to reassure. This may create a dyadic feedback pattern that results in mutual misunderstanding and frustration, poor doctor–patient relationships, and suboptimal care (Stones et al. 2000). Insecure attachment did not mediate a link to somatization in men. Both childhood trauma and insecure attachment make independent contributions to the prediction of somatic symptoms. Screening patients for histories of childhood trauma can help clinicians be sensitive to many abuse survivors' fears about physical examination, medical procedures, and boundaries in the doctor–patient relationship.

A history of physical or sexual abuse independently predicts greater health-care utilization in both men and women (Fillingim and Edwards 2005; Salmon and Calderbank 1996). It is associated with more frequent PCP visits, increased numbers of hospital admissions and operations, and more hypochondriasis, disease conviction, and somatization compared with non-abused controls (Salmon and Calderbank 1996). Women with CPP have a high rate of psychologic dysfunction, including depression and somatic symptoms. In general population studies, a history of physical or sexual abuse is associated with greater reporting of pelvic pain, dyspareunia, and dysmenorrhea. However, the above symptoms are not manifested equally in all patients with CPP. Studies show that patients with cyclic pain have less psychologic distress and abuse than those with continuous chronic pain. People with diffuse pain report more depression, anxiety, and severe pain than those with more focused pain. Leserman et al. (2006) studied 289 women aged 18–66 years referred to a pelvic pain clinic to determine which types of CPP were associated with abuse. Forty-eight percent of subjects reported a lifetime history of sexual and/or physical abuse. Patients with diffuse pain had the worst health status, with worse physical functioning, more pain, more non-pelvic medical symptoms, more days in bed because of illness, more lifetime surgeries, and more trauma compared with women with other CPP subtypes. Women with vulvovaginal pain reported the best mental and physical health and the least trauma. The presence of endometriosis was not significantly related to any measure of mental or physical health status. Disease type did not predict physical or mental health status as accurately as type and site of pain. The authors propose that CPP be evaluated as seven subtypes predictive of health status. These are as follows:

1. Diffuse abdominal/pelvic pain – i.e., pain elicited during examination that was not localized and was without a single reproducible point or tender palpable spot; 39.3% of subjects in this study had a secondary or tertiary diagnosis of another musculoskeletal type disorder (e.g., levator spasm, piriformis/SI joint pain, fibromyalgia)

2. Vulvovaginal pain – symptoms in the vulvar region; focal and reproducible on physical exam

3. Cyclic pain – at least 2 weeks of a pain-free interval each month with clear cyclic exacerbation; usually pain occurred during the luteal menstrual phase; 37.9% of subjects had uterine tenderness on examination

4. Neuropathic pain – pain disorders initiated after surgery

5. Nonlocal pain – unable to reproduce the pain on physical exam

6. Trigger points – focal single point tenderness on abdominal exam that reproduced more than 50% of their chief complaints; 29.4% had other musculoskeletal disorders

7. Fibroid tumor pain – pain on palpation of the uterus or menorrhagia with daily pressure and/or pain with menstrual exacerbation

Children with histories of physical or sexual abuse often manifest somatic complaints and somatization disorder, and score higher on measures of somatization than controls.

Conversion disorder, a form of somatoform disorder, is accompanied by an attitude of disinterest despite serious symptoms. Hypochondrias (preoccupation with the idea of having a serious disease) and body dysmorphic disorder (preoccupation with an imagined or exaggerated defect in physical appearance) also are listed under somatoform disorders in the DSM-IV (Silber and Pao 2003).

Pudendal Neuralgia

Pudendal neuralgia typically presents as burning pain in the penis, scrotum, labia, perineum, or anorectal region (Antolak et al. 2002; Society for Pudendal Neuralgia 2008). It is aggravated by sitting, relieved by standing, and absent when recumbent or sitting on a toilet seat. The diagnosis is based on a typical history and exclusion of other diagnoses. Prostatitis-like urogenital pain and voiding and sexual dysfunction are the hallmarks of pudendal neuropathy in males. Altered skin sensation in the pudendal distribution and reproduction of the pain with pressure on the pudendal trunk (transvaginally or transrectally) are present on examination.

The etiology is thought to arise from compression or inflammation of the S2, 3, 4 nerve roots, compression or entrapment of the nerve along its course, or tension injuries (Society for Pudendal Neuralgia 2008). Compression or entrapment of the nerve along its course is associated with hypertrophy of the pelvic floor muscles. Bony remodeling of the ischial spine resulting from activity of the pelvic floor muscles leads to juxtaposition of the sacrotuberous (ST) and sacrospinous (SSp) ligaments, which compress the pudendal nerve in the narrowed interligamentous space. Elongation of the ischial spine in response to the same muscular forces presents an additional site for repetitive microtrauma of the pudendal nerve.

The pudendal nerve exits the pelvis with piriformis via the greater sciatic notch. Abduction and flexion of the thigh cause hypertrophy of piriformis. If the sciatic notch is narrowed because of posterior orientation of the ischial spine and piriformis hypertrophy, the pudendal nerve can be compressed against the posterior edge of the SSp ligament. The ischial spines develop from a separate ossification center that arises between 13 and 15 years of age. Ossification is complete by 23–25 years. This interval of development is when youth engage in athletic pursuits that induce hypertrophy of the pelvic floor muscles and the extensors and rotators of the hip. Thus, in young athletes, anatomic changes are established for future CPP.

Tension causing excessive stretching of the nerve associated with straining in chronic constipation, vaginal delivery, and squatting with heavy weights causes inflammation. Tension is aggravated by pelvic floor dysfunction, genital prolapse, and descending perineum syndrome (Society for Pudendal Neuralgia 2008). It is surmised that the gluteus muscle exerts a shearing effect as it extends the hip, while the pelvic floor is forced inferiorly during the Valsalva maneuver (Antolak et al. 2002).

The mechanism of neural injury depends upon its etiology. Entrapment and compression cause inflammation, ischemia, demyelination, and scarring. The latter are associated with permanent nerve damage. Stretching is less damaging and does not usually result in demyelination. However, function can be just as impaired.

Pudendal nerve block may be diagnostic and therapeutic. Electrophysiologic studies can identify the site and type of damage. Three-dimensional imaging techniques can identify anatomic distortion at sites associated with nerve entrapment (Antolak et al. 2002).

Treatment is multimodal including pharmacologic, behavioral, and surgical interventions. Physical therapy is the mainstay of treatment because of the close etiology between musculoskeletal and neuronal dysfunction. The goals of therapy are to restore normal length to the pelvic floor and pelvic floor relaxation techniques. It should incorporate connective tissue mobilization, neural mobilization, and a home exercise program. Antidepressant and anticonvulsant drugs are prescribed to alleviate neuropathic pain. Nerve blocks, singly or repeated, are said to benefit 15–60% of patients (Society for Pudendal Neuralgia 2008). Activities that aggravate the pain must be avoided (e.g., cycling, sitting). Doughnut cushions are helpful in relieving pressure on the perineum. Where nerve entrapment is identified, surgical release may be indicated. Physical therapy as an adjunct to surgery is important as pain can persist postoperatively if musculoskeletal dysfunction continues.

Vulvodynia, defined by the International Society for the Study of Vulvar Disease as burning, stinging, irritation, or rawness at the introitus of at least 3 months duration, may be related to neuralgia (Reed et al. 2000). On examination, the pain is reproducible with pressure. Dermatologic and infectious etiologies are absent. It is not more likely in patients with psychologic distress. Most sufferers continue to participate in an active sex life despite discomforts.

Conclusion

The diagnosis and treatment of CPP requires an understanding of the complex interactions between organic and psychologic factors. Individual patient and family characteristics, including an appreciation of their health and functional expectations, personality traits, coping styles, and cognitive, intellectual, economic, emotional, and social resources, are essential to successful management. Functional, psychiatric, and organic disorders must be treated concurrently. Treatment should be provided as indicated in an honest, open, supportive, and nonthreatening environment. Multidisciplinary teams should be engaged and a long-term approach to therapy adopted.

References

Allen, L. A., Woolfolk, R. L., Escobar, J. I., Gara, M. A., & Hamer, R. M. (2006). Cognitive-behavioral therapy for somatization disorder: A randomized controlled trial. *Archives of Internal Medicine, 166*, 1512–1518.

Almeida, O. D., Jr., & Val-Gallas, J. M. (1997). Conscious pain mapping. *The Journal of the American Association of Gynecologic Laparoscopists, 4*, 587–590.

American College of Obstetricians and Gynecologists. (2005). ACOG committee opinion. Number 310, April 2005. Endometriosis in adolescents. *Obstetrics and Gynecology, 105*, 921–927.

American Psychiatric Association. (1994). *Diagnostic and statistical manual of mental disorders* (4th ed.). Washington DC: American Psychiatric Association.

American Society for Reproductive Medicine. (1997). Revised American Society for Reproductive Medicine classification of endometriosis: 1996. *Fertility and Sterility, 67*, 817–821.

Antolak, S. J., Jr., Hough, D. M., Pawlina, W., & Spinner, R. J. (2002). Anatomical basis of chronic pelvic pain syndrome: The ischial spine and pudendal nerve entrapment. *Medical Hypotheses, 59*, 349–353.

Baccini, F., Pallotta, N., Calabrese, E., Pezzotti, P., & Corazziari, E. (2003). Prevalence of sexual and physical abuse and its relationship with symptom manifestations in patients with chronic organic and functional gastrointestinal disorders. *Digestive and Liver Disease, 35*, 256–261.

Badura, A. S., Reiter, R. C., Altmaier, E. M., Rhomberg, A., & Elas, D. (1997). Dissociation, somatization, substance abuse, and coping in women with chronic pelvic pain. *Obstetrics and Gynecology, 90*, 405–410.

Batt, R. E., & Mitwally, M. F. (2003). Endometriosis from thelarche to midteens: Pathogenesis and prognosis, prevention and pedagogy. *Journal of Pediatric and Adolescent Gynecology, 16*, 337–347.

Bernstein, G. A., Massie, E. D., Thuras, P. D., Perwien, A. R., Borchardt, C. M., & Crosby, R. D. (1997). Somatic symptoms in anxious-depressed school refusers. *Journal of the American Academy of Child and Adolescent Psychiatry, 36*, 661–668.

Braverman, P. K. (2000). Sexually transmitted diseases in adolescents. *The Medical Clinics of North America, 84*, 869–889.

Brown, R. T., & Hewitt, G. D. (2004). Chronic pelvic pain and recurrent abdominal pain in female adolescents. *Endocrine Development, 7*, 213–224.

Campo, J. V., Jansen-McWilliams, L., Comer, D. M., & Kelleher, K. J. (1999). Somatization in pediatric primary care: Association with psychopathology, functional impairment, and use of services. *Journal of the American Academy of Child and Adolescent Psychiatry, 38*, 1093–1101.

Champion, J. D., Piper, J. M., Holden, A. E., Shain, R. N., Perdue, S., & Korte, J. E. (2005). Relationship of abuse and pelvic inflammatory disease risk behavior in minority adolescents. *Journal of the American Academy of Nurse Practitioners, 17*, 234–241.

Chandler, B., Beegle, M., Elfrink, R. J., & Smith, W. J. (2002). To leave or not to leave? A retrospective review of appendectomy during diagnostic laparoscopy for chronic pelvic pain. *Missouri Medicine, 99*, 502–504.

Cheong, Y., & Stones, R. W. (2006). Chronic pelvic pain: Aetiology and therapy. *Best Practice & Research. Clinical Obstetrics & Gynaecology, 20*, 695–711.

Chung, M. K., Chung, R. P., & Gordon, D. (2005). Interstitial cystitis and endometriosis in patients with chronic pelvic pain: The "Evil Twins" syndrome. *Journal of the Society of Laparoendoscopic Surgeons, 9*, 25–29.

Collett, B. J., Berkley, K., & Task Force on Fact Sheets for the Global Year Against Pain 'Pain in Women' 2007/8. (2007). The IASP Global Year against pain in women. *Pain, 132*(Suppl 1), S1–S2.

Craig, T. K., Cox, A. D., & Klein, K. (2002). Intergenerational transmission of somatization behaviour: A study of chronic somatizers and their children. *Psychological Medicine, 32*, 805–816.

Economy, K. E., & Laufer, M. R. (1999). Pelvic pain. *Adolescent Medicine, 10*, 291–304.

Farley, M., & Keaney, J. C. (1997). Physical symptoms, somatization, and dissociation in women survivors of childhood sexual assault. *Women & Health, 25*, 33–45.

Fillingim, R. B. (2000). Sex, gender and pain: Women and men really are different. *Current Review of Pain, 4*, 24–30.

Fillingim, R. B., & Edwards, R. R. (2005). Is self-reported childhood abuse history associated with pain perception among healthy young women and men? *The Clinical Journal of Pain, 21*, 387–397.

Fillingim, R. B., Wilkinson, C. S., & Powell, T. (1999). Self-reported abuse history and pain complaints among young adults. *The Clinical Journal of Pain, 15*, 85–91.

Fritz, G. K., Fritsch, S., & Hagino, O. (1997). Somatoform disorders in children and adolescents: A review of the past 10 years. *Journal of the American Academy of Child and Adolescent Psychiatry, 36*, 1329–1338.

Fry, R. P., Beard, R. W., Crisp, A. H., & McGuigan, S. (1997). Sociopsychological factors in women with chronic pelvic pain with and without pelvic venous congestion. *Journal of Psychosomatic Research, 42*, 71–85.

Goldstein-Ferber, S., & Granot, M. (2006). The association between somatization and perceived ability: Roles in dysmenorrhea among Israeli Arab adolescents. *Psychosomatic Medicine, 68*, 136–142.

Greco, C. D. (2003). Management of adolescent chronic pelvic pain from endometriosis: A pain center perspective. *Journal of Pediatric and Adolescent Gynecology, 16*(3 Suppl), S17–S19.

Greenspan, J. D., Craft, R. M., LeResche, L., Arendt-Nielsen, L., Berkley, K. J., Fillingim, R. B., Gold, M. S., Holdcroft, A., Lautenbacher, S., Mayer, E. A., Mogil, J. S., Murphy, A. Z., Traub, R. J., & Consensus Working Group of the Sex, Gender, and Pain SIG of the IASP. (2007). Studying sex and gender differences in pain and analgesia: A consensus report. *Pain, 132*(Suppl 1), S26–S45.

Haggerty, C. L., Peipert, J. F., Weitzen, S., Hendrix, S. L., Holley, R. L., Nelson, D. B., Randall, H., Soper, D. E., Wiesenfeld, H. C., Ness, R. B., & PID Evaluation and Clinical Health (PEACH) Study Investigators. (2005). Predictors of chronic pelvic pain in an urban population of women with symptoms and signs of pelvic inflammatory disease. *Sexually Transmitted Diseases, 32*, 293–299.

Hanno, P. M., Landis, J. R., Matthews-Cook, Y., Kuşek, J., Nyberg, L., Jr., & The Interstitial Cystitis Database Study Group. (1999). The diagnosis of interstitial cystitis revisited: Lessons learned from the National Institutes of Health Interstitial Cystitis Database study. *The Journal of Urology, 161*, 553–557.

Hastie, B. A., Riley, J. L., & Fillingim, R. B. (2005). Ethnic differences and responses to pain in healthy young adults. *Pain Medicine, 6*, 61–71.

Haugaard, J. J. (2004). Recognizing and treating uncommon behavioral and emotional disorders in children and adolescents who have been severely maltreated: Somatization and other somatoform disorders. *Child Maltreatment, 9*, 169–176.

Hediger, M. L., Hartnett, H. J., & Louis, G. M. (2005). Association of endometriosis and body size and figure. *Fertility and Sterility, 84*, 1366–1374.

Hewitt, G. D., & Brown, R. T. (2000). Acute and chronic pelvic pain in female adolescents. *The Medical Clinics of North America, 84*, 1009–1025.

Highfield, E. S., Laufer, M. R., Schnyer, R. N., Kerr, C. E., Thomas, P., & Wayne, P. M. (2006). Adolescent endometriosis-related pelvic pain treated with acupuncture: Two case reports. *Journal of Alternative and Complementary Medicine, 12*, 317–322.

Hornstein, M. D., Harlow, B. L., Thomas, P. P., & Check, J. L. (1995). Use of a new CA 125 assay in the diagnosis of endometriosis. *Human Reproduction, 10*, 932–934.

Igra, V. (1998). Pelvic inflammatory disease in adolescents. *AIDS Patient Care and STDs, 12*, 109–124.

Kişlal, F. M., Kutluk, T., Çetin, F. C., Derman, O., & Kanbur, N. Ö. (2005). Psychiatric symptoms of adolescents with physical complaints admitted to an adolescence unit. *Clinical Pediatrics, 44*, 121–130.

Leserman, J., Zolnoun, D., Meltzer-Brody, S., Lamvu, G., & Steege, G. F. (2006). Identification of diagnostic subtypes of chronic pelvic pain and how subtypes differ in health status and trauma history. *American Journal of Obstetrics and Gynecology, 195*, 554–561.

Lieb, R., Zimmermann, P., Friis, R. H., Höfler, M., Tholen, S., & Wittchen, H.-U. (2002). The natural course of DSM-IV somatoform disorders and syndromes among adolescents and young adults: A prospective-longitudinal community study. *European Psychiatry, 17*, 321–331.

Momoeda, M., Taketani, Y., Terakawa, N., Hoshiai, H., Tanaka, K., Tsutsumi, O., Osuga, Y., Maruyama, M., Harada, T., Obata, K., & Hayashi, K. (2002). Is endometriosis really associated with pain? *Gynecologic and Obstetric Investigation, 54*(Suppl 1), 18–23.

Monsen, K., & Havik, O. E. (2001). Psychological functioning and bodily conditions in patients with pain disorder associated with psychological factors. *British Journal of Medical Psychology, 74*, 183–195.

Muris, P., & Meesters, C. (2004). Children's somatization symptoms: Correlations with trait anxiety, anxiety sensitivity, and learning experiences. *Psychological Reports, 94*, 1269–1275.

Muris, P., Vlaeyen, J., & Meesters, C. (2001). The relationship between anxiety sensitivity and fear of pain in healthy adolescents. *Behaviour Research and Therapy, 39*, 1357–1368.

Ness, R. B., Soper, D. E., Holley, R. L., Peipert, J., Randall, H., Sweet, R. L., Sondheimer, S. J., Hendrix, S. L., Amortegui, A., Trucco, G., Songer, T., Lave, J. R., Hillier, S. L., Bass, D. C., & Kelsey, S. F. (2002). Effectiveness of inpatient and outpatient treatment strategies for women with pelvic inflammatory disease: Results from the Pelvic Inflammatory Disease Evaluation and Clinical Health (PEACH) randomized trial. *American Journal of Obstetrics and Gynecology, 186*, 929–937.

Newkirk, G. R. (1996). Pelvic inflammatory disease: A contemporary approach. *American Family Physician, 53*, 1127–1135.

Powell-Boone, T., Ness, T. J., Cannon, R., Lloyd, L. K., Weigent, D. A., & Fillingim, R. B. (2005). Menstrual cycle affects bladder pain sensation in subjects with interstitial cystitis. *The Journal of Urology, 174*, 1832–1836.

Propst, A. M., & Laufer, M. R. (1999). Endometriosis in adolescents: Incidence, diagnosis and treatment. *The Journal of Reproductive Medicine, 44*, 751–758.

Rasquin, A., Di Lorenzo, C., Forbes, D., Guiraldes, E., Hyams, J. S., Staiano, A., & Walker, L. S. (2006). Childhood functional gastrointestinal disorders: Child/adolescent. *Gastroenterology, 130*, 1527–1537.

Reed, B. D., Haefner, H. K., Punch, M. R., Roth, R. S., Gorenflo, D. W., & Gillespie, B. W. (2000). Psychosocial and sexual functioning in women with vulvodynia and chronic pelvic pain: A comparative evaluation. *The Journal of Reproductive Medicine, 45*, 624–632.

Rhee, H., Holditch-Davis, E., & Miles, M. S. (2005). Patterns of physical symptoms and relationships with psychosocial factors in adolescents. *Psychosomatic Medicine, 67*, 1006–1012.

Rickert, V. I., & Kozlowski, K. J. (2000). Pelvic pain: A SAFE approach. *Obstetrics and Gynecology Clinics of North America, 27*, 181–193.

Salmon, P., & Calderbank, S. (1996). The relationship of childhood physical and sexual abuse to adult illness behavior. *Journal of Psychosomatic Research, 40*, 329–336.

Samelius, L., Wijma, B., Wingren, G., & Wijma, K. (2007). Somatization in abused women. *Journal of Women's Health, 16*, 909–918.

Sanfilippo, J. S., & Black, A. (2003). Adolescent pelvic pain. *Best Practice & Research. Clinical Obstetrics & Gynaecology, 17*, 93–101.

Scialli, A. R., Barbieri, R. L., Glasser, M. H., Olive, D. L., & Winkel, C. A. (2000). *Chronic pelvic pain: An integrated approach. APGO educational series on women's health issues.* Washington DC: Association of Professors of Gynecology and Obstetrics.

Seng, J. S., Graham-Bermann, S. A., Clark, M. K., McCarthy, A. M., & Ronis, D. L. (2005). Posttraumatic stress disorder and physical comorbidity among female children and adolescents: Results from service-use data. *Pediatrics, 116*, e767–e776.

Silber, T. J., & Pao, M. (2003). Somatization disorders in children and adolescents. *Pediatrics in Review, 24*, 255–264.

Society for Pudendal Neuralgia (SPuN). (2008). www.spuninfo.org. Last updated 5 May 2008.

Solnik, M. J. (2006). Chronic pelvic pain and endometriosis in adolescents. *Current Opinion in Obstetrics & Gynecology, 18*, 511–518.

Song, A. H., & Advincula, A. P. (2005). Adolescent chronic pelvic pain. *Journal of Pediatric and Adolescent Gynecology, 18*, 371–377.

Startseva, N. V. (1980). Clinical immunological aspects of genital endometriosis [Russian]. *Akusherstvo i Ginekologiia, 3*, 23–26.

Stones, R. W., Selfe, S. A., Fransman, S., & Horn, S. A. (2000). Psychosocial and economic impact of chronic pelvic pain. *Bailliere's Best Practice & Research. Clinical Obstetrics & Gynaecology, 14*, 415–431.

Taylor, D. C., Szatmari, P., Boyle, M. H., & Offord, D. R. (1996). Somatization and the vocabulary of everyday bodily experiences and concerns: A community study of adolescents. *Journal of the American Academy of Child and Adolescent Psychiatry, 35*, 491–499.

Terre, L., & Ghiselli, W. (1997). A developmental perspective on family risk factors in somatization. *Journal of Psychosomatic Research, 42*, 197–208.

Thomson, J. C., & Redwine, D. B. (2005). Chronic pelvic pain associated with autoimmunity and systemic and peritoneal inflammation and treatment with immune modification. *The Journal of Reproductive Medicine, 50*, 745–758.

Tu, F. F., As-Sanie, S., & Steege, J. F. (2006). Prevalence of pelvic musculoskeletal disorders in a female chronic pelvic pain clinic. *The Journal of Reproductive Medicine, 51*, 185–189.

Tu, F., Bettendorf, B., & Shay, S. (2007). Dysmenorrhea: Contemporary perspectives. *Pain Clinical Updates, 15*, 1–4.

Venbrux, A. C., Chang, A. H., Kim, H. S., Montague, B. J., Hebert, J. B., Arepally, A., Rowe, P. C., Barron, D. F., Lambert, D., & Robinson, J. C. (2002). Pelvic congestion syndrome (pelvic venous incompetence): Impact of ovarian and internal iliac vein embolotherapy on menstrual cycle and chronic pelvic pain. *Journal of Vascular and Interventional Radiology, 13*, 171–178.

Wadhwa, L., Sharma, J. B., Arora, R., Malhotra, M., & Sharma, S. (2004). Severity, affect, family and environment (SAFE) approach to evaluate chronic pelvic pain in adolescent girls. *Indian Journal of Medical Sciences, 58*, 275–282.

Waldinger, R. J., Schulz, M. S., Barsky, A. J., & Ahern, D. K. (2006). Mapping the road from childhood trauma to adult somatization: The role of attachment. *Psychosomatic Medicine, 68*, 129–135.

Steve D. Wheeler and Elza Vasconcellos

Keywords

Primary headaches • Chronic daily headache diagnosis • Medication overuse headache • Migraine pathophysiology • Tension-type headache pathophysiology

Migraine Diagnosis

Migraine is a distinctively unique primary headache disorder with a neurobiology that is incompletely characterized. Migraine is not just about head pain; it is associated with environmental sensitivities to light, sound, taste, touch, smell, and movement, gastrointestinal symptoms, neurological dysfunction, disability, and comorbidity.

Headache diagnostic criteria were formalized successfully in 1988 by the Headache Classification Committee (HCC) of the International Headache Society (IHS) (1988) and updated in 2004 as the International Classification of Headache Disorders, 2nd Edition (ICHD-II) (Headache Classification Subcommittee (HCS) of the IHS 2004). Migraine can be divided into six major subtypes (Tables 10.1–10.4), however, these migraine subtypes were defined for adults, and illustrate how

S.D. Wheeler (✉)
Ryan Wheeler Headache Treatment Center, 5975 Sunset Drive, Suite 501, Miami 33143, FL, USA
and
University of Miami, Miller School of Medicine,
Miami, FL, USA
e-mail: DrHeadache@aol.com

little is known about childhood headache and pediatric-specific diagnostic criteria.

The 1988 IHS criteria excluded children and the 2004 ICHD-II criteria relegated children to discussion in the notes section. Childhood migraine was distinguished from adult migraine in that "attacks may last 1–72 h," "headache is commonly bilateral," and "photophobia and phonophobia may be inferred from their behavior" (Table 10.5).

Adult migraine is recognized as a benign, recurrent primary headache disorder lasting 4–72 h untreated or unsuccessfully treated, associated with unilateral, pulsatile pain of moderate to severe intensity, photophobia and phonophobia or nausea, and aggravated by movement (Table 10.5). Migraine can be associated with aura in 10% of unselected and 30% of office populations, (Table 10.6).

Although the current migraine diagnostic criteria are not sufficiently sensitive for children, recommendations have been suggested to adapt adult criteria to children. Hershey et al. (2005) recently reviewed headache characteristics in 260 children with migraine and noted that modified diagnostic criteria improved diagnostic sensitivity from 61.9% for ICHD-II criteria to 84.4%. Modified migraine diagnostic criteria for children include the following headache features: (1) attacks

B.C. McClain and S. Suresh (eds.), *Handbook of Pediatric Chronic Pain:*
Current Science and Integrative Practice, DOI 10.1007/978-1-4419-0350-1_10,
© Springer Science+Business Media, LLC 2011

Table 10.1 ICHD-II Migraine diagnoses (HCS IHS 2004)

1.1. Migraine without aura

1.2. Migraine with aura

    1.2.1. Typical aura with migraine headache

    1.2.2. Typical aura with non-migraine headache

    1.2.3. Typical aura without headache

    1.2.4. Familial hemiplegic migraine (FHM)

    1.2.5. Sporadic hemiplegic migraine

    1.2.6. Basilar-type migraine

1.3. Childhood periodic syndromes that are commonly precursors of migraine

    1.3.1. Cyclical vomiting

    1.3.2. Abdominal migraine

    1.3.3. Benign paroxysmal vertigo of childhood

1.4. Retinal migraine

1.5. Complications of migraine

    1.5.1. Chronic migraine

    1.5.2. Status migrainosus

    1.5.3. Persistent aura without infarction

    1.5.4. Migrainous infarction

    1.5.5. Migraine-triggered seizure

1.6. Probable migraine

    1.6.1. Probable migraine without aura

    1.6.2. Probable migraine with aura

    1.6.5. Probable chronic migraine

Table 10.2 Cyclical vomiting criteria (ICHD-II, HCS IHS 2004)

1.3.1. Cyclical vomiting

Diagnostic criteria:

A. At least five attacks fulfilling criteria B and C

B. Episodic attacks, stereotypical in the individual patient, of intense nausea and vomiting lasting from 1 h to 5 days

C. Vomiting during attacks occurs at least four times/h for at least 1 h

D. Symptom-free between attacks

E. Not attributed to another disorder

Table 10.3 Abdominal migraine criteria (ICHD-II, HCS IHS 2004)

1.3.2. Abdominal migraine

Diagnostic criteria:

A. At least five attacks fulfilling criteria B–D

B. Attacks of abdominal pain lasting 1–72 h (untreated or unsuccessfully treated)

C. Abdominal pain has all of the following characteristics:

    1. Midline location, periumbilical or poorly localized

    2. Dull or "just sore" quality

    3. Moderate or severe intensity

D. During abdominal pain at least two of the following:

    1. Anorexia

    2. Nausea

    3. Vomiting

    4. Pallor

E. Not attributed to another disorder

Table 10.4 Benign paroxysmal vertigo of childhood criteria (ICHD-II, HCS IHS 2004)

1.3.3. Benign paroxysmal vertigo of childhood

Diagnostic criteria:

A. At least five attacks fulfilling criterion B

B. Multiple episodes of severe vertigo, occurring without warning and resolving spontaneously after minutes to hours

C. Normal neurological examination and audiometric and vestibular functions between attacks

D. Normal electroencephalogram

Tension-Type Headache Diagnosis

Tension-type headache (TTH), like or similar to migraine, is a primary headache. It was previously known as muscle or scalp muscle contraction headache, tension headache, and psychogenic headache. Although a pathophysiologic connection between muscle tension, emotional state, and headache is suggested, any relationship is either spurious, coincidental, or of no etiological significance. Unfortunately, physicians often make the diagnosis of TTH based on the presence of neck pain, stress, or psychological issues which likely reflect exacerbating, associated, or secondary features,

last 1–72 h (untreated or unsuccessfully treated); (2) at least two of the four following characteristics: focal location (unilateral, bifrontal, bitemporal, or biparietal), pulsating quality, moderate or severe pain intensity, and pain worsening or limiting physical activity; (3) nausea and/or vomiting or two of the five following symptoms: photophobia, phonophobia, difficulty thinking, lightheadedness, or fatigue (Table 10.5).

Table 10.5 Diagnostic criteria for migraine without aura in adults (ICHD-II, HCS IHS 2004) and modified proposed criteria in children (Hershey et al. 2005)

Migraine without aura in adults	Migraine without aura in children
A. At least five attacks fulfilling criteria B–D	A. At least five attacks fulfilling criteria B–D
B. Headache attacks lasting 4–72 h (untreated or unsuccessfully treated)	B. Headache attacks lasting 1–72 h (untreated or unsuccessfully treated)
C. Headache has at least two of the following characteristics:	C. Headache has at least two of the following characteristics:
1. Unilateral location	1. Focal location (unilateral, bifrontal, bitemporal, or biparietal)
2. Pulsating quality	2. Pulsating quality
3. Moderate or severe pain intensity	3. Moderate or severe pain intensity
4. Aggravation by or causing avoidance of routine physical activity (e.g., walking or climbing stairs)	4. Worsening or limiting physical activity
D. During headache at least one of the following:	D. Nausea and/or vomiting or two of the five following symptoms:
1. Nausea and/or vomiting	1. Photophobia
2. Photophobia and phonophobia	2. Phonophobia
	3. Difficulty thinking
	4. Lightheadedness
	5. Fatigue
E. Not attributed to another disorder	E. Not attributed to another disorder

Table 10.6 Diagnostic criteria for typical aura with migraine headache (ICHD-II, HCS IHS 2004)

1.2.1. Typical aura with migraine headache
A. At least two attacks fulfilling criteria B–D
B. Aura consisting of at least one of the following, but no motor weakness:
1. Fully reversible visual symptoms including positive features (e.g., flickering lights, spots or lines) and/or negative features (i.e., loss of vision)
2. Fully reversible sensory symptoms including positive features (i.e., pins and needles) and/or negative features (i.e., numbness)
3. Fully reversible dysphasic speech disturbance
C. At least two of the following:
1. Homonymous visual symptoms and/or unilateral sensory symptoms
2. At least one aura symptom develops gradually over ≥5 min and/or different aura symptoms occur in succession over ≥5 min
3. Each symptom lasts ≥5 and ≤60 min
D. Headache fulfilling criteria B–D for 1.1 *Migraine without aura* begins during the aura or follows aura within 60 min
E. Not attributed to another disorder

not etiology. Moreover, since neck pain can occur in migraine, its presence cannot exclude the migraine diagnosis.

TTH can be divided into four major subtypes (Tables 10.7–10.10) that are defined by criteria that were developed for adults and generally classify TTH as the opposite of migraine (Table 10.9).

In an effort to classify headaches in children under the age of 6 years, Balottin et al. (2005) prospectively and longitudinally evaluated 25 patients with headache referred to a child neurology department in Italy. Balottin et al. (2005) found that only four patients met ICHD-II criteria for tension-type headache, yet 12 were

Table 10.7 Tension-type headaches (ICHD-II, HCS IHS 2004)

2.1. Infrequent episodic tension-type headache
    2.1.1. Infrequent episodic tension-type headache associated with pericranial tenderness
    2.1.2. Infrequent episodic tension-type headache not associated with pericranial tenderness
2.2. Frequent episodic tension-type headache
    2.2.1. Frequent episodic tension-type headache associated with pericranial tenderness
    2.2.2. Frequent episodic tension-type headache not associated with pericranial tenderness
2.3. Chronic tension-type headache
    2.3.1. Chronic tension-type headache associated with pericranial tenderness
    2.3.2. Chronic tension-type headache not associated with pericranial tenderness
2.4. Probable tension-type headache
    2.4.1. Probable infrequent episodic tension-type headache
    2.4.2. Probable frequent episodic tension-type headache
    2.4.3. Probable chronic tension-type headache

Table 10.8 Tension-type headache: ICHD-II criteria in adults versus alternative criteria of Balottin et al. (2005) in children

Attack criteria	Tension-type headache (ICHD-II)	Tension-type headache in children (Balottin alternative criteria)
A. Frequency	>10	>10
B. Duration	30 min to 7 days	<30 min to days
C.	At least 2 of 4	At least 2 of 4
1. Location	Bilateral	Bilateral
2. Pain	Pressing/tightening	Pressing or tightening
3. Intensity	Mild or moderate	Mild or moderate
4. Movement aggravation	Not aggravated by routine physical activity	Not aggravated by routine physical activity
D. 1. Nausea and/or vomiting	No	No
2. Photophobia or phonophobia	No	No more than one of photophobia or phonophobia

Table 10.9 Modified criteria (Hershey et al. 2005) for migraine without aura versus alternative criteria (Balottin et al. 2005) for tension-type headache in children

Attack criteria	Migraine without aura in children (Modified criteria)	Tension-type headache in children (Alternative criteria)
Frequency	>5	>10
Duration	1–72 h (untreated or unsatisfactorily treated)	<30 min to days
Nausea and/or vomiting	Yes	No
	At least 2 of 4	**At least 2 of 4**
Location	Bilateral > unilateral	Bilateral
Pain	Pulsatile	Pressing or tightening
Intensity	Moderate or severe	Mild or moderate
Movement aggravation	Worsening or limiting physical activity	Not aggravated by routine physical activity
	At least 2 of 5	
Photophobia	Yes	No more than one of photophobia or phonophobia
Phonophobia	Yes	
Difficulty thinking	Yes	No
Lightheadedness	Yes	No
Fatigue	Yes	No

Table 10.10 Chronic tension-type headache criteria (ICHD-II, HCS IHS 2004)

2.3. Chronic tension-type headache
A. Headache occurring on ≥15 days per month on average for >3 months (≥180 days per year) and fulfilling criteria B–D
B. Headache lasts hours or may be continuous
C. Headache has at least two of the following characteristics:
1. Bilateral location
2. Pressing/tightening (non-pulsating) quality
3. Mild or moderate intensity
4. Not aggravated by routine physical activity such as walking or climbing stairs
D. Both of the following:
1. No more than one of photophobia, phonophobia, or mild nausea
2. Neither moderate or severe nausea nor vomiting
E. Not attributed to another disorder

diagnosed with TTH utilizing alternative criteria (Tables 10.8–10.9). Laurell et al. (2004), in a Swedish prevalence study in 7–15–year-old school children, suggested that TTH diagnostic criteria ought to be modified by eliminating criteria A (attack frequency) and criteria B (attack duration). Interestingly, the major change, attack duration, is in keeping with the Balottin et al. (2005) alternative criteria. Eliminating criteria A is problematic since it relates to the recurrent and presumably benign nature of this primary headache and therefore the Balottin et al. (2005) criteria seem appropriate. Thus, using the Balottin et al. (2005) criteria, TTH in children can be differentiated from adult TTH (Table 10.9) by attack duration, less than 30 min to days, and allowing either photophobia or photophobia.

Selected Primary Headaches

Cluster Headache

Cluster headache is a primary headache characterized by severe unilateral orbital, supraorbital, or temporal pain of short duration (15–180 min untreated) that is associated with ipsilateral orbital-nasal autonomic dysfunction or restlessness (Table 10.11). Although, the diagnosis of cluster headache can be difficult, short duration and biological clock or behavioral disturbances are highly suggestive. The biological clock disturbances produce attack periodicity wherein headaches occur at certain times of the day, week, month, season, or year, and are predisposed to awaken sufferers from sleep early in the morning. Additionally, behavioral disturbances manifested by restlessness, agitation, pacing, rocking, or head banging support the cluster headache diagnosis. Maytal et al. (1992) reviewed 35 patients with cluster headache onset before age 18 and noted no difference between childhood and adult forms. Thus, there probably is no need to modify cluster headache diagnostic criteria for children.

Paroxysmal Hemicranias

The paroxysmal hemicranias (Table 10.12) are indomethacin-responsive primary headaches characterized by severe attacks of unilateral, orbital-region pain of short duration (2–30 min), associated with ipsilateral orbital-nasal autonomic dysfunction, and typically occur ≥8 times daily. Like primary stabbing headache, cluster and SUNCT (short-lasting unilateral neuralgiform headache with conjunctival injection and tearing), the paroxysmal hemicranias are short-duration headaches with fairly specific features that allow clinical differentiation (Table 10.13).

Primary Stabbing Headache

Primary stabbing headache (Table 10.14), another indomethacin-responsive primary headache, was

Table 10.11 Episodic and chronic cluster headache criteria (ICHD-II, HCS IHS 2004)

3.1. Cluster headache diagnostic criteria
A. At least five attacks fulfilling criteria B–D
B. Severe or very severe unilateral orbital, supraorbital and/or temporal pain lasting 15–180 min if untreated
C. Headache is accompanied by at least one of the following ipsilaterally:
1. Conjunctival injection and/or lacrimation
2. Nasal congestion and/or rhinorrhea
3. Eyelid edema
4. Forehead and facial sweating
5. Miosis and/or ptosis
6. A sense of restlessness or agitation
D. Not attributed to another disorder
E. Attacks have a frequency from one every other day to eight per day
3.1.1. Episodic cluster headache
Diagnostic criteria:
A. Attacks fulfilling criteria A–E for 3.1 *Cluster headache*
B. At least two cluster periods lasting 7–365 days and separated by pain-free remission periods of ≥1 month
3.1.2. Chronic cluster headache
Diagnostic criteria:
A. Attacks fulfilling criteria A–E for 3.1 *Cluster headache*
B. Attacks recur over >1 year without remission periods or with remission periods lasting <1 month

Table 10.12 Paroxysmal hemicrania diagnostic criteria, adapted (ICHD-II, HCS IHS 2004)

3.2. Paroxysmal hemicranias
A. At least 20 attacks fulfilling B–F
B. Attacks of severe unilateral orbital, supraorbital or temporal pain lasting 2–30 min
C. Headache is accompanied by at least one of the following:
1. Ipsilateral conjunctival injection and/or lacrimation
2. Ipsilateral nasal congestion and/or rhinorrhea
3. Ipsilateral eyelid edema
4. Ipsilateral forehead and facial sweating
5. Ipsilateral miosis and/or ptosis
D. Attacks have a frequency above five per day for more than half of the time, although periods with lower frequency may occur
E. Attacks are prevented completely by therapeutic doses of indomethacin (≥150 mg/day to rule out incomplete response)
F. Not attributed to another disorder
3.2.1. Episodic paroxysmal hemicranias
A. Attacks fulfilling criteria A–F for 3.2 *Paroxysmal hemicrania*
B. At least two attack periods lasting 7–365 days and separated by pain-free remission periods of ≥1 month
3.2.2. Chronic paroxysmal hemicranias
A. Attacks fulfilling criteria A–F for 3.2 *Paroxysmal hemicrania*
B. Attacks recur over >1 year without remission periods or with remission periods lasting <1 month

previously known as idiopathic stabbing headache, jabs-and-jolts syndrome, ice pick headache, ice cream headache, or brain freeze. In adults, it occurs most frequently in migraine sufferers. Severe pain occurs suddenly and patients often grab the painful head region. Although the severity

Table 10.13 Differential diagnosis of short-lasting headaches and trigeminal (cranial) autonomic cephalalgias, adapted from ICHD-II, HCS IHS 2004

Headache	Severe attack duration	Attack frequency	Ipsilateral orbital-nasal autonomic dysfunction	Indomethacin-responsive
Cluster headache	15–180 min	0.5–8/day (<5/day)	Yes	No
Hemicrania continua	1 s to 1–2 weeks	Continuous headache	Yes	Yes
Paroxysmal hemicranias	2–30 min	>5/day	Yes	Yes
Primary stabbing headache	1–3 s	Variable	No	Yes
SUNCT (short-lasting unilateral neuralgiform headache with conjunctival injection and tearing)	5–240 s	3–200/day	Yes	No

Table 10.14 Primary stabbing headache criteria (ICHD-II, HCS IHS 2004)

4.1. Primary stabbing headache
Diagnostic criteria:
A. Head pain occurring as a single stab or a series of stabs and fulfilling criteria B–D
B. Exclusively or predominantly felt in the distribution of the first division of the trigeminal nerve (orbital, temple and parietal area)
C. Stabs last for up to a few seconds and recur with irregular frequency ranging from one to many per day
D. No accompanying symptoms
E. Not attributed to another disorder

and abruptness are rather frightening and patients often are concerned about aneurysm rupture, this headache is rarely ever caused by serious disorders.

In children, primary stabbing headache differs from that seen in adults (Fusco et al. 2003; Soriani et al. 1996; Vieira et al. 2006; Vasconcellos and Luzondo 2007). Childhood stabbing headaches are not exclusively localized to a trigeminal distribution, most patients have no significant disability and indomethacin is seldom necessary. These headaches typically start early in life, often as early as 1.5 years, but only about one third of the patients have migraine, and others may have benign paroxysmal vertigo. However, there is a strong family history of migraine, and nearly half of the patient's mothers who suffer from migraine report stabbing headaches (Vasconcellos and Luzondo 2007). In children, extra-trigeminal short-lasting stabbing headaches are usually related to physical activity and changes in head position, but can be symptomatic of Chiari-I malformation or C1-C2 subluxation with spinal cord compression (Vieira et al. 2006) and appropriate neuroimaging should be obtained.

Chronic Daily Headache Diagnosis

Chronic daily headache (CHD) is a syndrome that is defined by headache frequency with attacks occurring daily or near daily, but definitely on 15 or more days per month, and each untreated attack lasts at least 4 h (Koenig et al. 2002). The differential diagnosis of the CDH syndrome includes: chronic migraine, hemicrania continua, new daily persistent headache, and chronic tension-type headache.

Chronic Migraine

Chronic migraine (Table 10.15) represents a migraine complication wherein there is a transformation to a daily or near daily headache process that usually takes place over months to years. It is the most frequent CDH seen in 13–17 year olds in headache clinics in the USA (Bigal et al. 2005). Recent ICHD-II diagnostic criteria (IHS HCC 2006) define chronic migraine to occur in a known migraine sufferer who

Table 10.15 Revised IHS criteria for chronic migraine (HCC IHS 2006)

A1.5.1 Revised IHS criteria for chronic migraine
A. Headache (tension-type and/or migraine) on ≥15 days per month for at least 3 months
B. Occurring in a patient who has had at least five attacks fulfilling criteria for 1.1 Migraine without aura
C. On ≥8 days per month for at least 3 months headache has fulfilled C1 and/or C2 below, that is, has fulfilled criteria for pain and associated symptoms of migraine without aura
1. Has at least two of a–d
(a) Unilateral location
(b) Pulsating quality
(c) Moderate or severe pain intensisy
(d) Aggravation by or causing avoidance of routine physical activity (e.g., walking or climbing stairs) and at least one of a or b
(a) Nausea and/or vomiting
(b) Photophobia and phonophobia
2. Treated and relieved by triptan(s) or ergot before the expected development of C1 above
D. No medication overuse and not attributed to another causative disorder

Table 10.16 Hemicrania continua diagnostic criteria, adapted from ICHD-II, HCS IHS 2004

4.7 Hemicrania continua
Diagnostic criteria:
A. Headache for >3 months, fulfilling criteria B–D
B. All of the following characteristics:
1. Unilateral pain without side-shift
2. Daily and continuous, without pain-free periods
3. Moderate intensity, but with exacerbations of severe pain
C. At least one of the following autonomic features occurs during exacerbations and ipsilateral to the side of the pain
1. Conjunctival injection and/or lacrimation
2. Nasal congestion and/or rhinorrhea
3. Ptosis and/or miosis
D. Complete response to therapeutic doses of indomethacin (≥150 mg/day to rule out incomplete response)
E. Not attributed to another disorder

experiences ≥15 all-type headache attacks per month for ≥3 months, continues to experience ≥8 migraine attacks/month, or successfully treats attacks with a migraine specific drug (triptan, e.g., almotriptan, eletriptan, frovatriptan, naratriptan, rizatriptan, sumatriptan, or zolmitriptan; or ergot, e.g., ergotamine or dihydroergotamine), and does not have medication overuse headache (MOH).

Hemicrania Continua

Hemicrania continua (Table 10.16) is an indomethacin-responsive primary headache disorder that is underappreciated (Peres et al. 2001). It is characterized by continuous mild to moderate unilateral pain with superimposed attacks of moderate to severe pain associated with ipsilateral orbital-nasal autonomic dysfunction. Many individuals will be diagnosed with chronic daily headache, chronic TTH, or chronic migraine; however, diagnostic errors can be limited by recognizing that chronic TTH is not unilateral, chronic migraine generally is not strictly unilateral, and neither is consistently associated with ipsilateral orbital-nasal autonomic dysfunction during pain exacerbations.

Hemicrania continua is important to consider since it is generally refractory to all therapeutic regimens except nonsteroidal anti-inflammatory drugs (NSAIDs), typically responding superiorly to the highly potent agent indomethacin.

New Daily Persistent Headache

New daily persistent headache (NDPH) most often occurs in non-headache-prone individuals, usually starts out of the blue, patients typically know the exact date of onset, and continues on a daily basis for ≥3 months (Table 10.17). NDPH is often symptomatic, e.g., produced by syndromes of low cerebral spinal fluid volume or high intracranial pressure, but can be primary. Most primary cases are associated with viral infections, typically EBV, and remit spontaneously. Unfortunately, cases presenting to specialists typically are refractory to most treatments. Recent studies suggest that NDPH is associated with allergies, asthma, alcohol, and hypothyroidism,

but treatment of the latter condition may prove therapeutic in the future (Bigal et al. 2002b).

Secondary Headaches

Secondary headaches represent a symptom of a pathologic process and may be attributed to a multitude of disorders, including serious or life-threatening causes. Fortunately, most headache complaints are due to primary headache disorders. A detailed history and physical examination help distinguish primary from secondary headaches, and ICHD-II (2004) criteria define eight major groups of secondary headaches (Table 10.18).

Secondary headaches in children often present as acute, sudden onset headache or as chronic progressive headache with gradually increasing frequency and severity. Acute recurrent headache

Table 10.17 New daily persistent headache (ICHD-II, HCS IHS 2004)

4.8. New daily persistent headache
A. Headache for >3 months, fulfilling criteria B–D
B. Headache is daily and unremitting from onset or from <3 days from onset
C. At least two of the following pain characteristics:
1. Bilateral location
2. Pressing/tightening (non-pulsating) quality
3. Mild or moderate intensity
4. Not aggravated by routine physical activity such as walking or climbing stairs
D. Both of the following:
1. No more than one of photophobia, phonophobia, or mild nausea
2. Neither moderate or severe nausea nor vomiting
E. Not attributed to another disorder

Table 10.18 Secondary headache diagnostic groups (ICHD-II, HCS IHS 2004)

Secondary headaches
5. Headache attributed to head and neck trauma
6. Headache attributed to cranial or cervical vascular disorder
7. Headache attributed to nonvascular intracranial disorder
8. Headache attributed to a substance or its withdrawal
9. Headache attributed to infection
10. Headache attributed to disturbance of homeostasis
11. Headache or facial pain attributed to disorder of cranium, neck, eyes, ears, nose, sinuses, teeth, mouth, or other facial or cranial structures
12. Headache attributed to psychiatric disorder

in a healthy child typically represents migraine or episodic TTH (Rothner 1995). However, an acute change of headache pattern should trigger an investigation for secondary headaches.

The majority of children (77%) presenting to an emergency department (ED) have secondary headaches as compared to 16–20% of adults. In a study of 150 consecutive children presenting to the ED with a chief complain of acute headache, 59% of patients had upper respiratory infections (39% viral upper respiratory infection, 9% sinusitis, 9% streptococcal pharyngitis), 18% had migraine, and 14% had more serious conditions, including meningitis (9%), posterior fossa tumor (2.6%), ventriculoperitoneal shunt malfunction (1.3%), intracranial hemorrhage (1.3%), concussion (1%), and post-seizure state (1%) (Lewis and Qureshi 2000; Schobitz et al. 2006). The evaluation of a child with headache in the ED should be directed toward ruling out organic causes, particularly life-threatening illness, and relieving pain (American College of Emergency Physicians 1996).

Causes of chronic progressive headaches in children include neoplasm, brain abscess, hydrocephalus, hematomas, Arnold-Chiari malformations, pseudotumor cerebri, hypertension, and MOH (Gladstein 2006). The first five entities can be diagnosed by neuroimaging. Clinically, warning signs or red flags suggest secondary headaches and are an indication for further investigation and neuroimaging (Table 10.19).

MRI of the brain is the test of choice in children with a high risk for secondary headache. However, in low-risk patients, close clinical observation with periodic reassessment is a reasonable strategy (Medina et al. 2003). Brain computed tomography (CT) is indicated for new-onset headache or acute headache, particularly if there is any suggestion of subarachnoid hemorrhage. The brain CT has advantages in the ED, but MRI or CT should always be performed before a lumbar puncture, except in cases where acute bacterial meningitis is suspected and time is critical. Lumbar puncture is diagnostic for meningitis, encephalitis, meningeal carcinomatosis, subarachnoid hemorrhage, and high or low intracranial pressure (Evans 2001). An electroencephalogram (EEG) is not useful in the routine evaluation of headache, except in cases where atypical migraine aura, or episodic loss of consciousness, is suggestive of a seizure disorder

Table 10.19 Red flags: Indications for investigation and neuroimaging in children with headaches

- Persistent headaches of less than 6 months duration that do not respond to medical treatment[a,b]
- Headaches associated with an abnormal neurologic finding, especially if accompanied by papilledema, nystagmus, or gait or motor abnormalities[a,b]
- Persistent headaches associated with a negative family history of migraine[a,b]
- Persistent headaches associated with substantial episodes of confusion, disorientation, or emesis[a,b]
- Headache that persistently awakens a child from sleep or occurs immediately on awakening[a,b]
- Family and medical history of disorders that predispose to CNS lesions and clinical laboratory findings that suggest CNS involvement[a,b]
- Headaches with fever that is otherwise unexplained[c,d,e]
- Headache in an immune-compromised, cancer, or ventriculo-peritoneal shunt patient[c,d]
- Headache with exclusive and persistent unilaterality[e]
- Headache triggered by increasing intracranial pressure maneuvers such as Valsalva, cough, squatting, exertion, etc[e,f,g]
- Sudden onset of first severe or worst headache (thunderclap headache)[g]

[a] Medina et al. (1997)
[b] Medina et al. (2001)
[c] Newman and Lipton (1998)
[d] Dodick (1997)
[e] Joubert (2005)
[f] Sobri et al. (2003)
[g] Evans (2001)

(Lewis et al. 2002). For primary headache, blood tests generally are not indicated, but may be useful when toxic, metabolic, nutritional, infectious, or inflammatory etiologies are suspected.

Idiopathic intracranial hypertension (IIH) (pseudotumor cerebri) is characterized by elevated intracranial pressure without evidence of infection, mass lesion, or hydrocephalus. Patients usually have headache and papilledema, although IIH without papilledema has been reported (Marcelis and Silberstein 1991). Associated symptoms can include sixth nerve palsy, diplopia, tinnitus, or blind spot enlargement. The incidence of IIH seems to be increasing among adolescent children, and among older children its clinical picture is similar to that of adult IIH showing a strong female and obese preponderance (Gordon 1997; Kesler and Fattal-Valevski 2002; Rangwala and Liu 2007). In prepubertal children, IIH does not occur predominantly in females and is not associated with obesity.

Brain CT or MRI may show small ventricles or an empty sella in IIH, but is usually normal. The diagnosis is established by a lumbar puncture that shows normal chemistry (with exception of a low protein) and cellularity, but pressures are elevated to >20 cm H_2O in nonobese and >25 cm H_2O in obese patients (HCS IHS 2004).

In children with IIH, associated conditions sometimes can be found, but is discussed elsewhere (Kesler and Fattal-Valevski 2002; Rangwala and Liu 2007; Scott et al. 1997; Friedman et al. 2008).

Treatment consists of removing the offending agent, treating associated conditions, utilizing diuretics, steroids, or repeated lumbar puncture with removal of sufficient CSF to return pressure to normal. Optic nerve fenestration or lumbar peritoneal shunt is reserved for those with visual field loss or intractable headache.

Medication Overuse Headache

Medication overuse headache (MOH) (analgesic rebound headache) is a secondary cause of chronic daily headache and has been recognized as the major cause of CDH in adults for decades (Kudrow 1982; Rapoport 1988; Mathew et al.

1990). In children, the frequent use of analgesics has been linked to the development of daily or near-daily headaches (Vasconcellos et al. 1998; Hering-Hanit et al. 2001). MOH is a frequent problem seen among new patients in pediatric headache clinics. Patients often have a history of migraine, then illness or injury precipitates headache deterioration, and patients progressively consume analgesics on a daily or near daily basis. These analgesics result in chronic, daily, or near daily, TTH, migraine or migraine-like attacks that persist for years. MOH only improves after the patient has ceased using all agents containing acetaminophen, aspirin, butalbital, ergotamine, NSAIDs, opiates, or triptans (Mathew 1993; Saper and Jones 1986). However, the benefit of discontinuing analgesics is not immediate, most require several weeks before any reduction in headaches, and some improve over many months. During this period of enhanced nociception, the effectiveness of preventive medications is reduced (Kudrow 1982; Mathew et al. 1990).

The exact amount of medication and time needed to cause MOH is not well known. What is important is that treatment overuse occurs both frequently and regularly, i.e., on several days per week for a sufficient period of time. The ICHD-II criteria state that for ergotamine, triptan, opioid, or combination medication overuse, the substance intake must be present on ≥10 days per month for at least 3 months, but for simple analgesics that number is ≥15 days per month. The importance of the role of regular overuse of analgesics in the perpetuation of chronic headache is largely not recognized by pediatricians (Cuvellier et al. 2007). This point is particularly significant, since commonly prescribed analgesics, e.g., acetaminophen and ibuprofen, are the most common substances associated with MOH in children (Vasconcellos et al. 1998). In adults, the analgesic agents most often implicated in rebound in decreasing order of significance, include butalbital–caffeine–aspirin–acetaminophen combinations, caffeine containing analgesic combinations, opioids, and ergotamine. Although less frequent, all of the triptans have been reported to induce MOH. Therefore, specific limits on the use of acute medications are necessary to prevent MOH; acute treatments generally should be limited to twice weekly. Patient education and close follow-up are extremely important to improve adherence and success.

The mechanism of MOH is poorly understood. MOH is an interaction between a therapeutic agent used excessively and a susceptible patient. Analgesics most likely reset pain control mechanisms probably by enhancing on-cell activity and central sensitization through N-methyl-D-aspartate receptors, or blocking adaptive anti-nociceptive changes (Silberstein and Young 1995; Srikiatkhachorn 2006; Silberstein et al. 2008). Platelets of patients with MOH have lower serotonin levels, but a greater density of serotonin receptors than controls (Srikiatkhachorn et al. 1994). The resulting serotonin receptor and transporter regulatory dysfunction is a possible mechanism for MOH (Srikiatkhachorn et al. 2000).

The treatment of MOH usually is easier in children than in adults, in part due to the fact that most children use simple analgesics. Successful withdrawal of the offending agent typically can be achieved without hospitalization or significant interference in daily life (Hering-Hanit et al. 2001). Preventive medications can be started concomitantly and likely enhance treatment success (Vasconcellos et al. 1998). Simple analgesics and triptans can be discontinued abruptly. Caffeine and low-dose opioids or butalbital can be gradually tapered. However, high-dose opioids or butalbital should be discontinued carefully due to serious withdrawal risks. Clonidine can be used to treat opioid withdrawal and a longer-acting barbiturate, e.g., phenobarbital, can treat butalbital withdrawal. In more severe cases, short-term transitional or "bridge" therapies can be used successfully during the abrupt cessation of painkillers. Although these therapies have not been studied fully in children, outpatient "bridge" therapies that can break the cycle of headache in adults include a short tapering oral course of prednisone 60 mg/day for 2 days, 40 mg/day for 2 days, then 20 mg/day for 2 days (Krymchantowski and Barbosa 2000), naproxen sodium 550 mg twice daily for 1 week, a 3-day course of nasal, subcutaneous (SQ) or intramuscular (IM) dihydroergotamine (Mathew 2005), or a short course of a triptan such as naratriptan or sumatriptan

(Krymchantowski and Moreira 2003; Drucker and Tepper 1998).

Triptans, naproxen sodium, or antiemetics such as promethazine can be used to treat breakthrough headaches during the withdrawal phase. Inpatient treatment is generally indicated for patients who fail outpatient treatment, consume large quantities of butalbital, opioids, or benzodiazepines, or if significant psychological or medical comorbidities exist.

Migraine Pathophysiology

Migraine is a multiform, multifactorial, polygenetic, neurobiological disease of unclear etiology, but cortical hyperexcitability, cortical spreading depression (CSD), brainstem dysfunction, and trigeminal activation are intimately involved in its pathogenesis.

Our current concepts of migraine pathophysiology are hypothetical and presume greater neurological than vascular involvement. Historically, migraine was thought to be a vascular disorder associated with constriction of intracranial arterials causing aura, followed by extracranial arterial dilation and pounding pain. It is now recognized that vascular events represent part of the final common pathway for migraine pain and are not etiologic. There is activation of the trigeminal vascular system, release of potent vasoactive substances, e.g., calcitonin gene-related polypeptide (CGRP), substance P, vasoactive intestinal peptide (VIP), and others, manifested as an inflammatory exudate, neurogenic edema or inflammation, and dilation of meningeal vessels. Activation of the trigeminal ganglion results in peripheral sensitization wherein trigeminal afferents from inflamed and dilated meningeal vessels are now able to "feel" the normal pulsations of blood and brain. Hence, pulsatile discomfort is the most common pain experienced by migraineurs.

Headache starts approximately 20 min after activation of the trigeminal ganglion and is followed within 60 min by activation of trigeminal nucleus caudalis (TNC) that is accompanied by central sensitization. Central sensitization is manifested clinically by cutaneous allodynia that generally starts ipsilateral to unilateral headache and is represented by the clinical phenomenon wherein normal sensations are uncomfortable or painful. Patients complain that their hair hurts and brushing or combing their hair is painful, as is wearing glasses, ties or snug collars, or touching or washing the face. As trigeminal activation continues, involvement of the thalamus occurs at approximately 120 min, and is followed by ascending central sensitization and greater cutaneous allodynia.

The presence of cutaneous allodynia appears to have some clinical importance since some studies show an association with poor triptan response (Burstein et al. 2004). Additionally, cutaneous allodynia may be associated with a poorer prognosis overall in some migraine populations (Kitaj and Klink 2005). Thus, chronic migraine risk may be related to abnormally prolonged cutaneous allodynia as a marker of active, self-perpetuating, or independent central sensitization that gives rise to dysfunctional brainstem pain modulation and exaggerated cortical hyperexcitability. Unfortunately, these alterations may transform episodic migraine to chronic migraine.

Migraine associated cortical hyperexcitability, brainstem dysfunction, and CSD seem to represent a disturbed pathophysiological substrate of neuronal modulation (Aurora et al. 1998; Palmer et al. 2000; Ayata et al. 2006). However, the causes of abnormal excitation and modulation are legend and characterized by alterations in serotonin (5HT), glutamate, gamma amino butyric acid (GABA), dopamine, nitric oxide, CGRP, magnesium, sodium and calcium channels, mitochondrial function, and probably other not appreciated neurotransmitters, receptors, ions, channels or factors.

Cortical hyperexcitability often is associated with photophobia, even when headache-free, and suggests that migraine attacks may be initiated by exaggeration of an excitable occipital cortex. Alternatively, dysfunction of brainstem modulation may produce cortical disinhibition and escalating cortical hyperexcitability. Experimental models of migraine aura produced by stimulating the cerebral cortex with topical potassium or a needle prick results in CSD which has been demonstrated to activate the trigeminal vascular system and produce dilation of meningeal vessels (Bolay et al. 2002).

Cortical spreading depression represents a long-lasting wave of cerebral hypoperfusion and hypoxia that is not generally severe enough to produce ischemia. CSD starts in the occipital cortex as neuronal and glial depolarization, has no respect for anatomical regions or vascular territories, and spreads forward along the cortex at the rate of 1–3 mm/minute. It is not associated with vascular constriction; instead maximal cerebral vasodilatation occurs in response to a hypoxia generated neuronal reflex. CSD is a misnomer since it is preceded by a short duration wave of excitability that is characterized by increased cortical hyperexcitability, hyperperfusion, and hyperoxia.

Migraine usually is not associated with clinically significant ischemia or vasoconstriction. However, CSD linked hypoperfusion may have vascular consequences under certain conditions, particularly when patients are dehydrated from vomiting or diarrhea, and especially if a prothrombotic state is present. Under these circumstances local small vessel involvement manifested by hypoperfusion, cellular and fibrin sludge, and concentrated clotting factors may produce subcortical ischemic alterations.

Functional brain imaging has demonstrated involvement of the cerebral cortex and pons in migraine (Weiller et al. 1995) and hypothalamus in cluster headache (May et al. 1999). Positron emission tomography (PET) in hemicrania continua interestingly reveals activation of ipsilateral rostral pons and contralateral inferior posterior hypothalamus (Matharu et al. 2004) which represents the exact opposite anatomical activations usually demonstrated in migraine, contralateral rostral pons, and ipsilateral inferior posterior hypothalamus in cluster. Additionally, PET in migraine has suggested iron deposition in the region of the midbrain dorsal raphe nucleus (Welch et al. 2001) and may represent the substrate for poor pain modulation resulting in increased cortical hyperexcitability. However, these midbrain pathological changes represent neuronal loss, and may possibly predispose to chronic migraine.

Neuronal loss may be the result of oxidative injury caused by hyperoxia and subsequent free radical liberation during the brief wave of cortical hyperexcitability preceding CSD.

Recent magnetic resonance imaging (MRI) and voxel-based morphometric studies have demonstrated significant reductions in cingulate cortex gray matter areas that are implicated in somatosensory cortex activation and pain transmission (Valfrè et al. 2008; Schmidt-Wilcke et al. 2008). Additionally, these studies show thickening of the caudal somatosensory cortex where the trigeminal region somatotopically represents the head and face (DaSilva et al. 2007). Although, distinct cortical regions are associated with migraine pathology, it is unknown whether these areas are primary or secondary.

The genetics of migraine are unclear. Even though it does not seem to be inherited in a dominant, recessive, sex linked, or mitochondrial fashion, it occurs with high penetrance in affected families. Familial hemiplegic migraine (FHM), a rare autosomal dominant disorder, has the best-understood genetics, but multiple mutations are present. FHM is associated with three known mutations: (1) *CACNA1A* gene encodes the pore-forming alpha 1-subunit of the neuronal P/Q type calcium channel (Mullner et al. 2004); (2) ATP1A2 gene encodes the Na,K-ATPase alpha 2-subunit (Segall et al. 2004); and (3) SCN1A gene encodes the neuronal voltage-gated sodium channel (Dichgans et al. 2005).

Most types of migraine (non-FHM) appear to be inherited through complex mechanisms that interact with environmental factors and susceptibility genes. Several mutations or single nucleotide polymorphisms (SNPs) have been associated with migraine and generally are believed to be migraine susceptibility genes. The best candidate susceptibility gene is the SNP that encodes the rate-limiting enzyme in the folic acid cycle, methylenetetrahydrofolate reductase (MTHFR), and the MTHFR C677T SNP is more highly associated with migraine, particularly migraine with aura, than the A1298C SNP (Scher et al. 2006; Kara et al. 2003). Furthermore, MTHFR SNPs are cardiovascular risk factors, and this cardiovascular risk is compounded by folic acid and

B12 deficiency, and to a lesser extent B2, and B6 deficiency (Kumar et al. 2005; Bottini et al. 2006). Additionally, SNPs of the estrogen receptor (ESR1 594A) and the progesterone receptor (PR) PROGINS (Colson et al. 2005) are recognized migraine susceptibility genes. Studies show that if subjects are at least heterozygous for both the ESR1 594A and PR PROGINS SNPs, then there is an unanticipated 3.2-fold increased risk for migraine. Altogether, migraine genetics may be dependent on the number, combination, characteristics, and environmental interplay of migraine susceptibility genes.

Tension-Type Headache Pathophysiology

Unlike migraine, the pathophysiology of TTH is poorly understood. Generally, evidence favors a peripheral origin mediated by pericranial muscle tenderness in episodic TTH. However, as headache frequency increases and transformation to chronic TTH occurs, a central mechanism with central sensitization becomes progressively operative even though initiated peripherally (Bendtsen 2000; Jensen 2001, 2003). Clearly, peripheral and central mechanisms are operative in tension-type headache; however, the interrelationships are unclear and too detailed to be discussed in this chapter.

Epidemiology of Pediatric Headache

Headache is a common disorder in children (Bille 1962). By the age of 3, headache occurs in 3–8% of children. At age 5, 20% of children have headache, by age 7, 37–51% have headache, and by the age of 15, the prevalence of headache ranges from 57% to 82% (Lewis et al. 2002).

The epidemiology of migraine has been closely examined and commonly begins in childhood. Migraine prevalence in children overall ranges between 6% and 10.5% (Bille 1962; Sillanpåå 1976, 1983; Mortimer et al. 1992; Abu-Arefeh, and Russell 1994; Rasmussen 1995; Barea et al. 1996; Lee and Olness 1997; Mavromichalis et al. 1999;

Wang et al. 2000; Al Jumah et al. 2002; Ayatollahi et al. 2002; Zwart et al. 2004; Kröner-Herwig et al. 2007; Akyol et al. 2007; Bigal et al. 2007). In adolescents, the migraine prevalence can reach 14–28% (Split and Neuman. 1999; Karli et al. 2006). Migraine begins earlier in males than in females, and migraine with aura begins earlier than migraine without aura (Stewart et al. 1991). In females, the incidence of migraine with aura peaks between 12 and 13 years and migraine without aura peaks between 14 and 17 years. In males, migraine with aura incidence peaks several years earlier, around 5 years, and migraine without aura between 10 and 11 years (Stewart et al. 1991). The prevalence of migraine headache steadily increases throughout childhood and the male-to-female ratio shifts during adolescence. In younger children, 3–7 years of age, migraine is more common in boys than girls. In children 7–11 years the prevalence becomes equal in boys and girls. However, girls become more affected later in puberty. In a large study, the 1-year prevalence of migraine in adolescents in the USA was 6.3% (5.0% in boys and 7.7% in girls). The prevalence was higher in girls older than 12 compared to boys, and in whites than African Americans (Bigal et al. 2007; Lipton et al. 2007; Lipton et al. 2001).

Recent population-based epidemiological studies employing ICHD-II criteria have improved our understanding of childhood headache. In Germany, where 8,800 households with children were surveyed, the 6-month prevalence of headache among children aged 7–14 years was 53% (Kröner-Herwig et al. 2007). Migraine was diagnosed in 7.5%, TTH in 18.5%, and a large proportion had unclassifiable headache. Recurrent headache (≥1/week) was experienced by 6.5% of the children. In 7,721 schoolchildren, aged 9–17 years, from the Menderes Region in Turkey, 79% of boys and 87% of girls suffered from headaches, and the migraine prevalence was 9.7% (Akyol et al. 2007).

The epidemiology of childhood TTH is less clear than migraine; however, recent IHS criteria–based studies are revealing. Zwart et al. (2004) in adolescents reported an 18% 1-year prevalence of TTH. Others have studied 7–15 year olds, and describe an overall prevalence of

10–18.5% (Laurell, et al. 2004; Kröner-Herwig et al. 2007; Wang et al. 2005). Although TTH is more prevalent than migraine in the general population (Lyngberg et al. 2005; Kröner-Herwig et al. 2007), migraine accounts for far more visits to physicians (Tepper et al. 2004).

In a large non-referred adolescent sample, the 1-year prevalence of CDH among 12–14 years old was 1.5% (Wang et al. 2006) and girls had a higher prevalence of CDH (2.4%) than boys (0.8%). About 72% of patients with CDH could be classified into either chronic TTH (65.6%) or chronic migraine (6.6%). However, the majority of adolescents (67%) with CDH had acute headache attacks that fulfilled criteria for migraine or probable migraine.

Headache Burden and Social Impact

Headache is the most common and one of the most disabling types of chronic pain in childhood. Given its high frequency, the impact of this disease on the lives of these children and their parents can be significant. A large study in elementary and high school students showed that nearly one third reported chronic pain. Headache was the most prevalent chronic pain affecting 60.5% of children, followed by abdominal pain in 43.3%, limb pain in 33.6%, and back pain in 30.2% (Roth-Isigkeit et al. 2005). Children with headache (43%) and abdominal pain (51%) were more likely to report school absences or inability to meet friends than children with other body pains. Headache patients reported taking pain medication significantly more often than those with all other types of pain. Peterson and Palermo (2004) reported that recurrent headaches produce more pain and had greater impact on functioning than other chronic diseases in children such as juvenile idiopathic arthritis or sickle cell disease.

Recurrent headaches impact children in many ways. Adolescents with recurrent headache experience increased school absences, reduction in performance, decreased home and family interactions, decreased peer socialization (Powers et al. 2003), inferior psychological functioning, more physical symptoms, poorer functioning status, and less satisfaction with life and health than healthy adolescents (Langeveld et al. 1996). A lower level of autonomy from their parents, and less healthy family functioning seems to be related to higher levels of functional impairment in adolescents with recurrent headache (Peterson and Palermo 2004). Adolescent migraineurs, who visited an ED in the previous year, are more likely to experience greater individual and family distress, more disability, and poorer quality of life (Tkachuk et al. 2003). Moreover, children with CDH have higher risk for medication overuse and emotional disorders including anxiety, depression, and somatization compared with controls (Pakalnis et al. 2007a).

Few validated scales in children offer ways to measure headache burden, impact, or quality of life. However, the Pediatric Migraine Disability Assessment Scale (PedMIDAS), a simple six question tool answered by the child, assesses headache disability at school, home, and play, is easily scored, and is used widely in routine evaluation, management and research (Hershey et al. 2004; Hershey et al. 2001). The Pediatric Quality of Life Inventory (PedsQL 4.0) is often used in patients with chronic illness, and has been validated in recurrent headache (Connelly and Rapoff 2006).

Acute Headache Treatement

Most migraine attacks start mild and progress to moderate or severe pain within several hours, but evidence from adult studies show that triptans used late in the attack are less effective. Early treatment with triptans ensures better pain-free responses since central sensitization sets the stage for headache recurrence and inconsistent response (Burstein et al. 2004). Additionally, relative gastroparesis occurs in migraineurs, resulting in poor passage of oral medication through the gastrointestinal tract and subsequently poor absorption (Aurora et al. 2007; Boyle et al. 1990; Volans 1978). Therefore, it becomes very important to ensure that children have early access to their acute symptomatic medications, particularly during school hours. To facilitate early intervention during school it is necessary to complete

appropriate forms authorizing administration of acute medications. Treating children at the beginning of the headache attack may prevent headache escalation, vomiting, and early school day release.

Most medications used to treat migraine attacks in children are available in oral form (Table 10.20). Rectal, nasal, SQ, or IM formulations can be utilized in cases associated with vomiting, particularly at onset, in rapidly escalating cases, or for severe attacks.

Despite the pharmacological options for the management of acute migraine, few randomized, controlled pediatric trials exist. To date, only ibuprofen and nasal sumatriptan are significantly more efficacious than placebo in obtaining headache relief in children and adolescents (Silver et al. 2008). Presently, there are no Food and Drug Administration (FDA)-approved medications for the acute treatment of migraine in children less than 18 years; thus, many recommendations in this section are observational.

Migraine Nonspecific Treatment

Acetaminophen and ibuprofen are considered first-line treatments for headaches in children. Ibuprofen (10 mg/kg) is significantly superior to acetaminophen (15 mg/kg) in eliminating the headache attack in 2 h (Hämäläinen et al. 1997b). Naproxen sodium (7–10 mg/kg) can be used effectively to treat migraine. A second dose can be repeated after 1 h if the headache persists, but no further dose should be used in the next 24 h. Ketorolac, another NSAID, can be used parenterally in the ED for severe headache attacks (Brousseau et al. 2004; Meredith et al. 2003). However, because of the Reye syndrome risk, aspirin should be avoided before age 15.

Combination analgesics containing caffeine, butalbital, or opioids should be used cautiously due to the high potential for MOH or abuse. These medications can be helpful at times, but should be reserved for children with infrequent headaches who need rescue agents if NSAIDs or triptans are contraindicated. Another combination analgesic containing

Table 10.20 Acute migraine-nonspecific medications

Acetaminophen[a]	10–15 mg/kg/dose Q 4–6 h
Ibuprofen	7–10 mg/kg/dose Q 6–8 h
Naproxen sodium	7–10 mg/kg/dose, may repeat dose in 1 h, maximum 15 mg/kg/day
Butalbital 50 mg + acetaminophen 325 mg + caffeine 40 mg[b]	12 years 1–2 tablets Q 4 h, maximum 6/day
	9–12 years 3/4 tablet Q 4 h
	6–9 years ½ tablet Q 4 h
	Weight >50 kg, maximum 5/day
	Weight <50 kg, maximum 3/day
Isometheptene mucate 65 mg + dichloralphenazone 100 mg + acetaminophen 325 mg[c]	>12 year 1–2 capsules at onset, repeat 1 capsule/h
	6–12 year 1 capsule at onset
	Weight >50 kg, maximum 5/day
	Weight <50 kg, maximum 3/day
Metoclopramide[d]	0.2 mg/kg to maximum 20 mg Q 6–8 h
Promethazine[a,d]	0.25–0.5 mg/kg Q 8 h, maximum 50 mg/dose
Prochlorperazine[a,d]	0.15 mg/kg Q 6–8 h, maximum 10 mg/dose

[a] Available in suppository
[b] Indicated only for children over 12 years and has high potential for MOH (limit number of tablets)
[c] Not FDA approved for children <18 years
[d] Extrapyramidal reactions may occur as side effects

isometheptene mucate, a sympathomimetic agent, acetaminophen and dichloralphenazone, a mild sedative, is useful for adolescents with migraine (Yuill et al. 1972).

Antiemetics with antidopaminergic effects not only treat the nausea and vomiting of migraine, but the pain also, and can be administered parenterally. In an ED randomized double-blind comparator study in children, intravenous prochlorperazine was shown to be superior to intravenous ketorolac in the acute treatment of migraine (Brousseau et al. 2004). Metoclopramide (0.2 mg/kg), promethazine (0.5 mg/kg), and prochlorperazine (0.15 mg/kg) are available in oral, IM, and intravenous (IV) formulations, and promethazine and prochlorperazine are available as rectal suppositories. These antiemetics can treat acute migraine attacks, particularly in the hospital or ED and although extrapyramidal side effects may occur, they can be reversed with diphenhydramine (1.25 mg/kg).

A miscellaneous group of agents can be used to treat more severe migraine attacks in adolescents and include IV valproate sodium rapidly infused over 10–20 min (10–15 mg/kg, to a maximum of 1,000 mg), IV magnesium sulfate (25 mg/kg to a maximum of 1 g per dose given over 15 min), and IM or IV steroids (dexamethasone, or

Table 10.21 Acute migraine-specific medications[a]

Nonselective 5HT agonists
Ergotamine (Cafergot®)[b]
Dihydroergotamine (DHE-45®, Migranal®)[b]
Selective 5HT$_{1B/1D}$ agonists (Triptans)
Almotriptan (Axert®)[b]
Eletriptan (Relpax®)[b]
Frovatriptan (Frova®)
Naratriptan (Amerge®)
Rizatriptan (Maxalt®)[b]
Sumatriptan (Imitrex®)[b]
Zolmitriptan (Zomig®)[b]

[a] None of these agents are FDA-approved for use in children
[b] Studies have been reported in pediatric populations

methylprednisolone). However, pediatric studies only exist for a small IV valproate series (Reiter et al. 2005).

Migraine-Specific Treatments

Migraine-specific drugs are used to treat acute attacks and have high affinity for serotonin (5HT) receptors, some selectively and others nonselectively (Tables 10.20–10.21). The triptans are selective agents and have high affinity for 5HT$_{1B/1D}$ receptors. In contrast, nonselective agents additionally have affinity for $5HT_2$, $5HT_3$, noradrenergic and dopaminergic receptors (Silberstein 1997).

Nonselective Serotonin Agonists

Ergotamine, a nonselective serotonin agonist, has not shown superiority to placebo in a double-blind, controlled study (Congdon and Forsythe 1979), but 60% of patients in the treatment group terminated early due to tolerability problems, e.g., nausea or vomiting. Hämäläinen et al. (1997a) showed oral dihydroergotamine (DHE) to be superior to placebo for therapy-resistant migraine attacks in children, but this is unavailable in the USA. Intravenous DHE is highly effective in adults for the treatment of acute, severe, or intractable migraine attacks (Raskin 1986; Callaham and Raskin 1986), and is available as a nasal spray (NS), or IM or SQ use.

IV DHE, preceded by oral or IV metoclopramide, can be used to treat prolonged, refractory, or acute migraine attacks in the ED in children 6 years and older; 80% of refractory headaches in children respond favorably to an inpatient protocol using these two drugs (Linder 1994). DHE seems to work even in the presence of central sensitization and is often used to break the cycle of MOH (Silberstein et al. 2007). Adverse effects of DHE include abdominal discomfort, nausea, vomiting, diarrhea, flushing, and vasoconstriction. Contraindications for the use of ergotamine tartrate or DHE include renal or hepatic failure, pregnancy, hypertension, sepsis, and coronary, cerebral, or peripheral vascular disease.

Selective Serotonin Agonists (Triptans)

The triptans are available in oral, nasal, and parenteral preparations. Two triptans, rizatriptan and zolmitriptan, are also available in an oral dissolving tablet that is not absorbed orally, instead it is absorbed via the gastrointestinal tract. Oral sumatriptan, rizatriptan, and eletriptan, have not shown efficacy in placebo-controlled trials in children, but a high placebo response likely contributes to their lack of efficacy (Visser et al. 2004; Winner et al. 2007). Oral zolmitriptan, 2.5 mg, showed efficacy compared to placebo in only one small (n = 32) crossover study in children (Evers et al.

2006). Almotriptan 6.25, 12.5, and 25 mg showed significantly higher 2 h pain relief compared to placebo in one multicenter trial (Winner et al. 2008). Since photophobia and phonophobia improved significantly with the 12.5 mg dose only, this is likely the most appropriate dose. Nasal and SQ sumatriptan have shown efficacy and tolerability in clinical trials in children over 6 years; however, placebo-controlled trials are only available for nasal sumatriptan in adolescents (Winner et al. 2008). Sumatriptan NS at 5 and 20 mg demonstrates significant headache relief in 2 h, and 20 mg showed efficacy as early as 30 min. The most frequent sumatriptan NS adverse events include taste disturbance, nausea, vomiting, and burning/stinging sensations, but pressure/tightness and chest symptoms were infrequent (1%) (Winner et al. 2006). Two open studies using sumatriptan (0.06 mg) SQ in children over 6 years, demonstrated good response rates (Linder 1996; MacDonald 1994). Adverse events occurred in up to 80% of patients, but were mild and transient and similar to those in adults. Zolmitriptan NS 5 mg in one controlled trial was well-tolerated and provided fast and effective relief of migraine symptoms (Lewis et al. 2007).

Triptan side effects include paresthesias, warm or cold sensations, and neck, throat, or jaw pain. Triptans are contraindicated in patients with coronary artery disease, peripheral vascular syndromes, or other underlying vascular syndromes or in patients with basilar or hemiplegic migraine (Physicians' Desk Reference 2007). Cases of life-threatening serotonin syndrome have been reported during combined use of triptans and selective serotonin reuptake inhibitors or serotonin-norepinephrine reuptake inhibitors (SSRI/SNRI); however, it is unclear whether this risk is truly increased (Shapiro and Tepper 2007).

Preventive Headache Treatement

Headache prevention represents a paradigm shift from acute treatment to long-term management. Headache prevention requires daily medication consumption with the major treatment goal being reduction in headache frequency. However, since disability represents the sum of frequency, duration, severity, and associated features, reduced headache frequency typically translates into reduced disability.

Three major issues with migraine prevention can impair successful treatment. First, the misconception that prevention works rapidly, just like acute treatment, must be corrected and clearly explained at the start of therapy, otherwise unreasonable expectations remain. Second, effective preventive therapy requires that medication be taken for an appropriate period of time, usually 2–3 months, at the appropriate, individualized dose. Third, early recognition of tolerability and safety issues is important. Timely management of dose and titration rate–dependent side effects can be accomplished by dose reduction and recognizing the admonition to start with a low dose and go slow, but if that is still too fast, then stop, wait, restart, and go slower.

Migraine prevention guidelines have been proposed by multiple organizations. The American Academy of Family Physicians/ American College of Physicians-American Society of Internal Medicine (AAFP/ACP-ASIM) Guidelines (Snow et al. 2002) are frequently quoted and taught, but for unclear reasons are not memorable. The AAFP/ACP-ASIM Guideline recommends that preventive treatment is indicated if (1) patients experience ≥ 2 attacks/month that produce disability lasting ≥ 3 days/month; (2) acute medication contraindications or failures; (3) use of acute medication > 2 times/week; or (4) presence of uncommon migraine conditions including hemiplegic migraine, migraine with prolonged aura, or migrainous infarction. However, the French Guidelines (Géraud et al. 2004) for migraine prevention are straightforward and suggest that treatment is indicated if (1) frequency or intensity of attacks impact activity of daily living or cause disability; or (2) when patients take 6–8 doses of acute migraine medication per month for ≥ 3 consecutive months, even if the medication is effective. Although the second French Guideline may engender premature preventive treatment, it encourages physicians to assess acute treatment goals, prevention needs, and MOH risk.

No migraine preventive medication is FDA-approved for pediatric populations aged less than 18 years. Evidence for migraine prevention in children obtained from randomized, controlled trials generally does not show active agents to be superior consistently to control or placebo. Topiramate was superior to placebo in a small trial (Lakshmi et al. 2007), it was not superior to placebo in a large intent-to-treat analysis, but it was superior to placebo in the per protocol or completers analysis (Winner et al. 2005), thus suggesting the importance of appropriate dose and treatment duration. Crossover, placebo-controlled trials with trazodone (Battistella et al. 1993) and nimodipine (Battistella et al. 1990) failed to differentiate active treatment from placebo. Additionally, there is little cyproheptadine data in children, but efficacy has been demonstrated in adults (Rao et al. 2000).

Observational studies consistently show effectiveness for all agents studied including vitamins and minerals (Tables 10.22–10.24). It is suspected that placebo response, carryover effect, inappropriate randomization (2:1), and publication bias may play a part in the negative controlled trials and placebo response and selection bias probably operates in the positive observational studies.

Existing clinical trials little assist migraine prevention treatment choice. Controlled trials do not demonstrate consistent efficacy and observational studies paradoxically demonstrate consistent effectiveness. There are few head-to-head trials that help decide whether one preventive agent is superior to another. Currently, treatment decisions often require assessment of comorbidity, then selecting a single agent that treats both migraine and the comorbid disorder, e.g., a tricyclic antidepressant for depression and migraine (Ashina et al. 2008). Likewise, tolerability and safety concerns may help decide the best or most appropriate migraine preventive (Table 10.25).

Vitamin, mineral, and supplement treatments, particularly when deficiencies are demonstrated, represent a reasonably safe choice for migraine prevention. Controlled trials with magnesium show improvement over baseline, but it is not superior to placebo (Wang et al. 2003). Observational studies

Table 10.22 Antiepilepsy drugs for pediatric migraine prevention

Antiepilepsy drug migraine preventives						
Migraine preventive	Age range or mean (years)	Active/ control (n)	50% Responder rate (%)	Headache frequency P value[a]	Open study	Maintenance dose (mg/kg/day)
Divalproex Na[b,c]	7–16	42/–	78.5	NA	Yes	15–45
Divalproex Na[b,d]	9–17	10/–	–	0.002	Yes	(500–1000 mg/ night)
Levetiracetam[b,e]	7–16	20/–	90	0.001	Yes	20–40
Levetiracetam[b,f]	3–17	19/–	NA	0.0001	Yes	(125–750 mg twice daily)
Topiramate[b,g]	6–15	112/50	54.6	0.061 ITT 0.033 PP	No	2
Topiramate[b,h,i]	8–14	21/21	95.2	0.002	No	(100 mg/day)
Topiramate[b,h,j]	14.9	75/–	NA	0.001	Yes	1.42–1.98
Zonisamide[b,h,k]	10–17	12/–	66.7	NA	Yes	5.8

NA Not applicable, *ITT* Intent-to-treat, *PP* Per protocol
[a] Active vs control or baseline
[b] Episodic migraine
[c] Caruso et al. (2000)
[d] Serdaroglu et al. (2002)
[e] Pakalnis et al. (2007b)
[f] Miller (2004)
[g] Winner et al. (2005)
[h] Chronic daily headache
[i] Lakshmi et al. (2007)
[j] Hershey et al. (2002)
[k] Pakalnis and Kring (2006)

Table 10.23 Antidepressant and antihypertensive drugs for pediatric migraine prevention

Antidepressant and antihypertensive migraine preventives						
Migraine preventive	Age range or Mean (years)	Active/ Control (n)	50% Responder rate (%)	Headache frequency P value[a]	Open study	Maintenance dose (mg/kg/day)
Amitriptyline[b,c,d]	12	146/–	NA	0.001	Yes	1
Nimodipine[b,e]	7–18	18/19 Crossover	NA	0.01	No	(30–60 mg/day)
Trazodone[b,f]	7–18	35/35 Crossover	NA	0.005	No	1
Propranolol[b,g,h]	3–15	57/58	69	<0.05	Yes	1–3

NA Not applicable
[a] Active vs control or baseline
[b] Episodic migraine
[c] Chronic daily headache
[d] Hershey et al. (2000)
[e] Battistella et al. (1990)
[f] Battistella et al. (1993)
[g] Ashrafi et al. (2005)
[h] Propranolol vs valproate

favor CoQ10 (Hershey et al. 2007), folic acid (DiRosa et al. 2007), and petasites hybridus (butterbur) (Pothmann and Danesch 2005) in children. Controlled trials in adults with riboflavin (Schoenen et al. 1998) and alpha lipoic acid (Delphine et al. 2007) demonstrate efficacy. However, feverfew, on the other hand, is not effective consistently in adult controlled trials (Pfaffenrath et al. 2002; Diener et al. 2005). It is likely that these effects in adults will be repeated in children.

Table 10.24 Vitamins, minerals, and supplements for pediatric migraine prevention

Vitamin, mineral and supplement migraine preventives						
Migraine preventive	Age range or mean (years)	Active/Control (n)	50% Responder rate (%)	Headache frequency P value[a]	Open study	Maintenance dose (mg/kg/day)
Butterbur[b,c,d]	6–17	108/–	77	NA	Yes	(50–150 mg/day)
CoQ10[b,c,e,f]	3–22	252/–	46.3	0.001	Yes	1–3
Folic acid[b,g,h]	8–18	16/–	100	–	Yes	(5 mg/day)
Magnesium oxide[b,i]	3–17	58/60	NA	0.0037 (baseline) and 0.88 (control)	No	9

NA Not applicable
[a] Active vs control or baseline
[b] Episodic migraine
[c] Chronic daily headache
[d] Pothmann and Danesch (2005)
[e] Migraine with CoQ10 deficiency
[f] Hershey et al. (2007)
[g] Migraine without aura associated with MTHFR SNP
[h] DiRosa et al. (2007)
[i] Wang et al. (2003)

Table 10.25 Serious adverse reactions for migraine preventives (Epocrates Rx 2008)

Serious adverse reactions for migraine preventives	
Preventive	Serious adverse reactions
Amitriptyline	Orthostatic hypotension, hypertension, syncope, ventricular arrhythmia, QT prolongation, torsades de pointes, AV block, myocardial infarction, stroke, seizures, extrapyramidal symptoms, ataxia, tardive dyskinesia, paralytic ileus, increased intraocular pressure, agranulocytosis, leukopenia, thrombocytopenia, hallucinations, psychosis exacerbation, hypomania/mania, depression worsening, suicidality, SIADH, hepatitis, angioedema, anticholinergic psychosis, hyperthermia
Divalproex Na	Hepatotoxicity, pancreatitis, hyponatremia, SIADH, pancytopenia, thrombocytopenia, myelosuppression, aplastic anemia, bleeding, hyperammonemia, erythema multiforme, Stevens-Johnson syndrome, toxic epidermal necrolysis, anaphylaxis, hallucinations, psychosis, suicidality, congenital neural tube effects, congenital anomalies, coma, polycystic ovary syndrome
Levetiracetam	Depression, hostility, aggressive behavior, psychosis, suicidality, leukopenia, neutropenia, pancytopenia, thrombocytopenia, withdrawal seizures
Nimodipine	EKG abnormalities, AV conduction abnormalities, congestive heart failure, thromboembolism, thrombocytopenia, anemia, gastrointestinal bleed, hepatitis, ileus, intestinal obstruction
Propranolol	CHF, heart block, severe bradycardia, Raynaud's phenomenon, bronchospasm, SLE, hypersensitivity reactions, Stevens-Johnson syndrome, toxic epidermal necrolysis, exfoliative dermatitis, erythema multiforme, anaphylactic/anaphylactoid reactions
Topiramate	Severe metabolic acidosis, nephrolithiasis, osteomalacia, osteoporosis, growth suppression, acute myopia, secondary angle closure glaucoma, oligohidrosis, hyperthermia, diabetes mellitus, leukopenia, anemia, psychosis, suicidality, severe skin reactions, hepatotoxicity, pancreatitis, deep vein thrombosis, pulmonary embolism
Trazodone	Priapism, orthostatic hypotension, arrhythmias, hypertension, syncope, bradycardia, tachycardia, stoke, myocardial infarction, extrapyramidal symptoms, tardive dyskinesis, hypomania/mania, psychosis exacerbation, depression worsening, suicidality, hallucinations, seizures, neutropenia, anemia, hepatitis, SIADH
Verapamil	CHF, severe hypotension, AV block, severe bradycardia, hepatotoxicity, paralytic ileus
Zonisamide	Stevens-Johnson syndrome, toxic epidermal necrolysis, aplastic anemia, agranulocytosis, oligohidrosis, hyperthermia, heat stroke, nephrolithiasis, pancreatitis, depression, psychosis, suicidality, withdrawal seizures, status epilepticus

Non-pharmacological and Behavioral Therapies

The addition of behavioral treatment components to a comprehensive pediatric headache care plan may lessen the need for medication, help maintain effects over the long term, and result in better clinical outcomes (Powers and Andrasik 2005). Non-pharmacological approaches that may reduce headache frequency include such lifestyle adjustments as good sleep hygiene, balanced diet, regular exercise, and identification and avoidance of migraine triggers (Van den Bergh et al. 1987; Stang et al. 1992). Skipping meals is one of the main migraine precipitants in adolescents; 7–44% of children and adults report migraine dietary triggers. In children, the principal dietary triggers are cheese, chocolate, and citrus fruits. Other dietary precipitants are processed meats, tyramine-containing food, yogurt, monosodium glutamate, aspartame, and alcoholic beverages. Every effort should be made to moderate caffeine intake since a link between caffeine and migraine has been established (Hering-Hanit and Gadoth 2003). Moreover, children who consume caffeine seem to be at increased risk for chronic daily headache (Vasconcellos and Muray 2005) and caffeine withdrawal headache is a well-recognized entity (HCS IHS 2004). Caffeine withdrawal can occur after only 2 weeks of regular caffeine consumption whenever there is an intake delay or interruption and the headache usually resolves within 7 days.

Interventions targeting good sleep habits may improve headache symptoms, and effective treatment of headaches in children may positively impact sleep. Children with migraine have a high prevalence of sleep disturbances compared to controls and include insufficient sleep (42%), bruxism (29%), co-sleeping with parents (25%), and snoring (23%) (Miller et al. 2003).

Regular exercise is recommended for children with migraine. Recent evidence shows that exercise has a significant and beneficial effect on all migraine aspects, especially in patients with low basal beta endorphin levels (Köseoglu et al. 2003).

Behavioral therapy available for the treatment of headache includes relaxation techniques, biofeedback training, and cognitive-behavioral therapy (stress management). A recent meta-analysis of these behavioral interventions in children and adolescents (Trautmann et al. 2006) showed a significant reduction in headache frequency, ≥50%, and long-term stability. In adults, a meta-analysis (Penzien et al. 2004) showed that biofeedback combined with relaxation training or cognitive-behavioral therapies are as effective as propranolol or flunarizine. Additionally, EMG biofeedback with or without relaxation was found superior to amitriptyline for the treatment of tension-type headache.

Future Considerations

Much remains to be understood about headache in children and adults. In the coming years, pediatric headache research will need to be directed to understanding these and related issues:

1. Headache diagnostic criteria. Further elaboration and validation are necessary since headache research requires that all involved speak the same diagnostic language.
2. Pathogenesis and pathophysiology. Do not be surprised if there are age-dependent differences between headache in pediatric and adult populations.
3. Acute and preventive treatment. Large, sufficiently powered, placebo-controlled trials with 1:1 randomization may be needed to demonstrate migraine efficacy in pediatric populations. Prospective observational studies may help define the most appropriate agents to be evaluated in these controlled trials.
4. Quality of life. All treatments will need to have a quantifiable and beneficial impact on quality of life.
5. Long-term complications. The risk of chronic daily headache, cardiovascular disease, and migraine comorbidities will need to be explored and defined longitudinally in pediatric populations.
6. Education. We must remember to educate future generations about the nature and impact of headache, particularly migraine, otherwise interest will fail and there will be little future to consider.

References

Abu-Arefeh, I., & Russell, G. (1994). Prevalence of headache and migraine in schoolchildren. *British Medical Journal, 309*, 765–769.

Akyol, A., Kiylioglu, N., Aydin, I., Erturk, A., Kaya, E., Telli, E., & Akyildiz, U. (2007). Epidemiology and clinical characteristics of migraine among school children in the Menderes region. *Cephalalgia, 27*, 781–787.

Al Jumah, M., Awada, A., & Al Azzam, S. (2002). Headache syndromes amongst school children in Riyadh, Saudi Arabia. *Headache, 42*, 281–286.

American College of Emergency Physicians. (1996). Clinical policy for the initial approach to adolescents and adults presenting to the emergency department with a children complain of headache. *Annals of Emergency Medicine, 27*, 821–844.

Ashina, S., Lipton, R. B., & Bigal, M. E. (2008). Treatment of comorbidities of chronic daily headache. *Current Treatment Options in Neurology, 10*, 36–43.

Ashrafi, M. R., Shabanian, R., Zamani, G. R., & Mahfelati, F. (2005). Sodium valproate versus propranolol in paediatric migraine prophylaxis. *European Journal of Paediatric Neurology, 9*, 333–338.

Aurora, S., Kori, S., Barrodale, P., Nelsen, A., & McDonald, S. (2007). Gastric stasis occurs in spontaneous, visually induced, and interictal migraine. *Headache, 47*, 1443–1446.

Aurora, S. K., Ahmad, B. K., Welch, K. M. A., Bhardhwaj, P., & Ramadan, N. M. (1998). Transcranial magnetic stimulation confirms hyperexcitability of occipital cortex in migraine. *Neurology, 50*, 1111–1114.

Ayata, C., Jin, H., Kudo, C., Dalkara, T., & Moskowitz, M. A. (2006). Suppression of cortical spreading depression in migraine prophylaxis. *Annals of Neurology, 59*, 652–661.

Ayatollahi, S. M., Moradi, F., & Ayatollahi, S. A. (2002). Prevalences of migraine and tension-type headache in adolescent girls of Shiraz (southern Iran). *Headache, 42*, 287–290.

Balottin, U., Termine, C., Nicoli, F., Quadrelli, M., Ferrari-Ginevra, O., & Lanzi, G. (2005). Idiopathic headache in children under six years of age: a follow-up study. *Headache, 45*, 705–715.

Barea, L. M., Tannhauser, M., & Rotta, N. T. (1996). An epidemiologic study of headache among children and adolescents of southern Brazil. *Cephalalgia, 16*, 545–549.

Battistella, P. A., Ruffilli, R., Cernetti, R., Pettenazzo, A., Baldwin, L., Bertoli, S., & Zacchello, F. (1993). A placebo-controlled crossover trial using trazadone in pediatric migraine. *Headache, 33*, 36–39.

Battistella, P. A., Ruffilli, R., Moro, R., Fabiani, M., Bertoli, S., Antolini, A., & Zacchello, F. (1990). A placebo-controlled crossover trial of nimodipine in pediatric migraine. *Headache, 30*, 264–268.

Bendtsen, L. (2000). Central sensitization in tension-type headache—possible pathophysiological mechanisms. *Cephalalgia, 20*, 486–508.

Bigal, M. E., Bordini, C. A., Tepper, S. J., & Speciali, J. G. (2002a). Intravenous magnesium sulphate in the acute treatment of migraine without aura and migraine with aura. A randomized, double-blind, placebo-controlled study. *Cephalalgia, 22*, 345–353.

Bigal, M. E., Lipton, R. B., Winner, P., Reed, M. L., Diamond, S., Stewart, W. F., & AMPP advisory group. (2007). Migraine in adolescents: association with socioeconomic status and family history. *Neurology, 69*, 12–13.

Bigal, M. E., Rapoport, A. M., Tepper, S. J., Sheftell, F. D., & Lipton, R. B. (2005). The classification of chronic daily headache in adolescents—a comparison between the second edition of the international classification of headache disorders and alternative diagnostic criteria. *Headache, 45*, 582–589.

Bigal, M. E., Sheftell, F. D., Rapoport, A. M., Tepper, S. J., & Lipton, R. B. (2002b). Chronic daily headache: identification of factors associated with induction and transformation. *Headache, 42*, 575–581.

Bille, B. S. (1962). Migraine in school children. A study of the incidence and short-term prognosis, and a clinical, psychological and electroencephalographic comparison between children with migraine and matched controls. *Acta Paediatrica, 51*(Suppl. 136), 1–151.

Bolay, H., Reuter, U., Dunn, A. K., Huang, Z., Boas, D. A., & Moskowitz, M. A. (2002). Intrinsic brain activity triggers trigeminal meningeal afferents in a migraine model. *Natural Medicines, 8*, 136–142.

Bottini, F., Celle, M. E., Calevo, M. G., Amato, S., Minniti, G., Montaldi, L., Di Pasquale, D., Cerone, R., Veneselli, E., & Molinari, A. C. (2006). Metabolic and genetic risk factors for migraine in children. *Cephalalgia, 26*, 731–737.

Boyle, R., Behan, P. O., & Sutton, J. A. (1990). Correlation between severity of migraine and delayed gastric emptying measured by an epigastric impedance method. *British Journal of Clinical Pharmacology, 30*, 405–409.

Brousseau, D. C., Duffy, S. J., Anderson, A. C., & Linakis, J. G. (2004). Treatment of pediatric migraine headaches: a randomized, double-blind trial of prochlorperazine versus ketorolac. *Annals of Emergency Medicine, 43*, 256–262.

Burstein, R., Collins, B., & Jakubowski, M. (2004). Defeating migraine pain with triptans: a race against the development of cutaneous allodynia. *Annals of Neurology, 55*, 19–26.

Callaham, M., & Raskin, N. H. (1986). A controlled study of dihydroergotamine as treatment of acute migraine headache. *Headache, 26*, 168–171.

Caruso, J. M., Brown, W. D., Exil, G., & Gascon, G. G. (2000). The efficacy of divalproex sodium in the prophylactic treatment of children with migraine. *Headache, 40*, 672–676.

Colson, N. J., Lea, R. A., Quinlan, S., MacMillan, J., & Griffiths, L. R. (2005). Investigation of hormone receptor genes in migraine. *Neurogenetics, 6*, 17–23.

Congdon, P. J., & Forsythe, W. I. (1979). Migraine in childhood. A review. *Clinical Pediatrics (Phila), 18*, 353–359.

Connelly, M., & Rapoff, M. A. (2006). Assessing health-related quality of life in children with recurrent headache: reliability and validity of the PedsQLTM 4.0 in a pediatric headache sample. *Journal of Pediatric Psychology, 31*, 698.

Cuvellier, J. C., Fily, A., Joriot, S., Cuisset, J. M., & Vallée, L. (2007). French general practitioners' management of children's migraine headaches. *Headache, 47*, 1282–1292.

DaSilva, A. F. M., Granziera, C., Snyder, J., & Hadjikhani, N. (2007). Thickening in the somatosensory cortex of patients with migraine. *Neurology, 69*, 1990–1995.

Delphine, M., Ambrosini, A., Sándor, P., Jacquy, J., Laloux, P., & Schoenen, J. (2007). A randomized double-blind placebo-controlled trial of thioctic acid in migraine prophylaxis. *Headache, 47*, 52–57.

Dichgans, M., Freilinger, T., Eckstein, G., Babini, E., Lorenz-Depiereux, B., Biskup, S., Ferrari, M. D., Herzog, J., van den Maagdenberg, A. M., Pusch, M., & Strom, T. M. (2005). Mutation in the neuronal voltage-gated sodium channel SCN1A in familial hemiplegic migraine. *Lancet, 366*, 371–377.

Diener, H. C., Pfaffenrath, V., Schnitker, J., Friede, M., & Henneicke-von Zepelin, H. H. (2005). Efficacy and safety of 6.25 mg t.i.d. feverfew CO2-extract (MIG-99) in migraine prevention—a randomized double-blind, multicentre, placebo-controlled study. *Cephalalgia, 25*, 1031–1041.

DiRosa, G., Attinà, S., Spanò, M., Ingegneri, G., Sgrò, D. L., Pustorina, G., Bonsignore, M., Trapani-Lombardo, V., & Tortorella, G. (2007). Efficacy of folic acid in children with migraine, hyperhomocysteinemia and MTHFR polymorphisms. *Headache, 47*, 1342–1351.

Dodick, D. (1997). Headache as a symptom of ominous disease. What are the warning signals? *Postgraduate Medicine, 101*, 46–50.

Drucker, P., & Tepper, S. (1998). Daily sumatriptan for detoxification from rebound. *Headache, 38*, 687–690.

Epocrates Rx [database for PDA]. Version 8.10. San Mateo (CA): Epocrates, Inc. c2008 [updated 15 Mar 2008; cited 15 Mar 2008]. Available from: http://www.epocrates.com.

Evans, R. W. (2001). Diagnostic testing for headache. *The Medical Clinics of North America, 85*, 865–885.

Evers, S., Rahmann, A., Kraemer, C., Kurlemann, G., Debus, O., Husstedt, I. W., & Frese, A. (2006). Treatment of childhood migraine attacks with oral zolmitriptan and ibuprofen. *Neurology, 67*, 497–499.

Friedman, D. I., Wall, M., & Silberstein, S. D. (2008). Headache associated with abnormalities in intracranial structure or function: high-cerebrospinal-fluid-pressure headache and brain tumor. In S. D. Silberstein, R. B. Lipton, & D. W. Dodick (Eds.), *Wolff's headache and other head pain* (pp. 489–511). New York: Oxford University Press.

Fusco, C., Pisani, F., & Faienza, C. (2003). Idiopathic stabbing headache: clinical characteristics of children and adolescents. *Brain & Development, 25*, 237–240.

Géraud, G., Lantéri-Minet, M., Lucas, C., Valade, D., & French Society for the Study of Migraine Headache (SFEMC). (2004). French guidelines for the diagnosis and management of migraine in adults and children. *Clinical Therapeutics, 26*, 1305–1318.

Gladstein, J. (2006). Secondary headaches. *Current Pain and Headache Reports, 10*, 382–386.

Gordon, K. (1997). Pediatric pseudotumor cerebri: descriptive epidemiology. *The Canadian Journal of Neurological Sciences, 24*, 219–221.

Hämäläinen, M. L., Hoppu, K., & Santavuori, P. R. (1997a). Oral dihydroergotamine for therapy-resistant migraine attacks in children. *Pediatric Neurology, 16*, 114–117.

Hämäläinen, M. L., Hoppu, K., Valkeila, E., & Santavuori, P. (1997b). Ibuprofen or acetaminophen for the acute treatment of migraine in children: a double-blind, randomized, placebo-controlled, crossover study. *Neurology, 48*, 103–107.

Headache Classification Committee of the International Headache Society. (1988). Classification and diagnostic criteria for headache disorders, cranial neuralgia, and facial pain. *Cephalalgia, 8*(Suppl 7), S1–S96.

Headache Classification Committee of the International Headache Society. (2006). New appendix criteria open for a broader concept of chronic migraine. *Cephalalgia, 26*, 742–746.

Headache Classification Subcommittee of the International Headache Society. (2004). The International Classification of Headache Disorders, 2nd Edition. *Cephalalgia, 24*(Suppl 1), S1–S160.

Hering-Hanit, R., & Gadoth, N. (2003). Caffeine-induced headache in children and adolescents. *Cephalalgia, 23*, 332–335.

Hering-Hanit, R., Gadoth, N., Cohen, A., & Horev, Z. (2001). Successful withdrawal from analgesic abuse in a group of youngsters with chronic daily headache. *Journal of Child Neurology, 16*, 448–449.

Hershey, A. D., Powers, S. W., Bentti, A. L., & deGrauw, T. J. (2000). Effectiveness of amitriptyline in the prophylactic management of childhood headaches. *Headache, 40*, 539–549.

Hershey, A. D., Powers, S. W., Vockell, A. L., LeCates, S. L., Ellinor, P. L., Segers, A., Burdine, D., Manning, P., & Kabbouche, M. A. (2007). Coenzyme Q10 deficiency and response to supplementation in pediatric and adolescent migraine. *Cephalalgia, 47*, 73–80.

Hershey, A. D., Powers, S. W., Vockell, A. L., LeCates, S. L., & Kabbouche, M. (2002). Effectiveness of topiramate in the prevention of childhood headaches. *Headache, 42*, 810–818.

Hershey, A. D., Powers, S. W., Vockell, A. L., LeCates, S., Kabbouche, M. A., & Maynard, M. K. (2001). PedMIDAS: development of a questionnaire to assess disability of migraines in children. *Neurology, 57*, 2034–2039.

Hershey, A. D., Powers, S. W., Vockell, A. L., LeCates, S. L., Segers, A., & Kabbouche, M. A. (2004). Development of a patient-based grading scale for PedMIDAS. *Cephalalgia, 24*, 844–849.

Hershey, A. D., Winner, P., Kabbouche, M. A., Gladstein, J., Yonker, M., Lewis, D., Pearlman, E., Linder, S. L., Rothner, D., & Powers, S. W. (2005). Use of the

ICHD-II criteria in the diagnosis of pediatric migraine. *Headache, 45*, 1288–1297.

Jensen, R. (2001). Mechanisms of tension-type headache. *Cephalalgia, 21*, 786–789.

Jensen, R. (2003). Peripheral and central mechanisms in tension-type headache: an update. *Cephalalgia, 23*(Suppl 1), S49–S52.

Joubert, J. (2005). Diagnosing headache. *Australian Family Physician, 34*, 621–625.

Kara, I., Sazci, A., Ergul, E., Kaya, G., & Kilic, G. (2003). Association of the C677T and A1298C polymorphisms in the 5, 10 methylenetetrahydrofolate reductase gene in patients with migraine risk. *Molecular Brain Research, 111*, 84–90.

Karli, N., Akiş, N., Zarifoğlu, M., Akgöz, S., Irgil, E., Ayvacioğlu, U., Calişir, N., Haran, N., & Akdoğan, O. (2006). Headache prevalence in adolescents aged 12 to 17: a student-based epidemiological study in Bursa. *Headache, 46*, 649–655.

Kesler, A., & Fattal-Valevski, A. (2002). Idiopathic intracranial hypertension in the pediatric population. *Journal of Child Neurology, 17*, 745–748.

Kitaj, M. B., & Klink, M. (2005). Pain thresholds in daily transformed migraine versus episodic migraine headache patients. *Headache, 45*, 992–998.

Koenig, M. A., Gladstein, J., McCarter, R. J., Hershey, A. D., & Wasiewski, W. (2002). Chronic daily headache in children and adolescents presenting to tertiary headache clinics. *Headache, 42*, 491–500.

Köseoglu, E., Akboyraz, A., Soyuer, A., & Ersoy, A. O. (2003). Aerobic exercise and plasma beta endorphin levels in patients with migrainous headache without aura. *Cephalalgia, 23*, 972–976.

Kröner-Herwig, B., Heinrich, M., & Morris, L. (2007). Headache in German children and adolescents: a population-based epidemiological study. *Cephalalgia, 27*, 519–527.

Krymchantowski, A. V., & Barbosa, J. S. (2000). Prednisone as initial treatment of analgesic-induced daily headache. *Cephalalgia, 20*, 107–113.

Krymchantowski, A. V., & Moreira, P. F. (2003). Outpatient detoxification in chronic migraine: comparison of strategies. *Cephalalgia, 23*, 982–993.

Kudrow, L. (1982). Paradoxical effects of frequent analgesic use. *Advances in Neurology, 33*, 335–341.

Kumar, J., Das, S. K., Sharma, P., Karthikeyan, G., Ramakrishnan, L., & Sengupta, S. (2005). Homocysteine levels are associated with MTHFR A1298C polymorphism in Indian population. *Journal of Human Genetics, 50*, 655–663.

Lakshmi, C. V. S., Singhi, P., Malhi, P., & Ray, M. (2007). Topiramate in the prophylaxis of pediatric migraine: a double-blind placebo-controlled trial. *Journal of Child Neurology, 22*, 829–835.

Langeveld, J. H., Koot, H. M., Loonen, M. C., Hazebroek-Kampschreur, A. A., & Passchier, J. (1996). A quality of life instrument for adolescents with chronic headache. *Cephalalgia, 16*, 183–196.

Laurell, K., Larsson, B., & Eeg-Olofsson, O. (2004). Prevalence of headache in Swedish schoolchildren, with a focus on tension-type headache. *Cephalalgia, 24*, 380–388.

Lee, L. H., & Olness, K. N. (1997). Clinical and demographic characteristics of migraine in urban children. *Headache, 37*, 269–276.

Lewis, D. W., Ashwal, S., Dahl, G., Dorbad, D., Hirtz, D., Prensky, A., Jarjour, I., & Quality Standards Subcommittee of the American Academy of Neurology; Practice Committee of the Child Neurology Society. (2002). Practice parameter: evaluation of children and adolescents with recurrent headaches: report of the Quality Standards Subcommittee of the American Academy of Neurology and the Practice Committee of the Child Neurology Society. *Neurology, 59*, 490–498.

Lewis, D. W., & Qureshi, F. (2000). Acute headache in children and adolescents presenting to the emergency department. *Headache, 40*, 200–203.

Lewis, D. W., Winner, P., Hershey, A. D., Wasiewski, W. W., & Pediatrics. Adolescent Migraine Steering Committee. (2007). Efficacy of zolmitriptan nasal spray in adolescent migraine. *Neurology, 120*, 390–396.

Linder, S. L. (1994). Treatment of childhood headache with dihydroergotamine mesylate. *Headache, 34*, 578–580.

Linder, S. L. (1996). Subcutaneous sumatriptan in the clinical setting: the first 50 consecutive patients with acute migraine in a pediatric neurology office practice. *Headache, 36*, 419–422.

Lipton, R. B., Bigal, M. E., Diamond, M., Freitag, F., Reed, M. L., Stewart, W. F., & on behalf of the AMPP Advisory Group. (2007). Migraine prevalence, disease burden, and the need for preventive therapy. *Neurology, 68*, 343–349.

Lipton, R. B., Stewart, W. F., Diamond, S., Diamond, M. L., & Reed, M. (2001). Prevalence and burden of migraine in the United States: data from the American Migraine Study II. *Headache, 41*, 646–657.

Lyngberg, A. C., Rasmussen, B. K., Jørgensen, T., & Jensen, R. (2005). Prognosis of migraine and tension-type headache: a population-based follow-up study. *Neurology, 65*, 580–585.

MacDonald, J. T. (1994). Treatment of juvenile migraine with subcutaneous sumatriptan. *Headache, 34*, 581–582.

Marcelis, J., & Silberstein, S. D. (1991). Idiopathic intracranial hypertension without papilledema. *Archives of Neurology, 48*, 392–399.

Matharu, M. S., Cohen, A. S., McGonigle, D. J., Ward, N., Frackowiak, R. S., & Goadsby, P. J. (2004). Posterior hypothalamic and brainstem activation in hemicrania continua. *Headache, 44*, 747–761.

Mathew, N. T. (1993). Chronic refractory headache. *Neurology, 43*(Suppl 3), S26–S33.

Mathew, N. T. (2005). Chronic daily headache. In R. W. Randolph & N. T. Mathew (Eds.), *Handbook of Headache* (pp. 113–138). Philadelphia: Lippincott Williams & Wilkins.

Mathew, N. T., Kurman, R., & Perez, F. (1990). Drug induced refractory headache–clinical features and management. *Headache, 30*, 634–638.

Mavromichalis, I., Anagnostopoulos, D., Metaxas, N., & Papanastassiou, E. (1999). Prevalence of migraine in school children and some clinical comparisons between migraine with and without aura. *Headache, 39*, 728–736.

May, A., Bahra, A., Büchel, C., Frackowiak, R. S., & Goadsby, P. J. (1999). Hypothalamic activation in cluster headache attacks. *Lancet, 352*, 275–278.

Maytal, J., Lipton, R. B., Solomon, S., & Shinnar, S. (1992). Childhood onset cluster headaches. *Headache, 32*, 275–279.

Medina, L. S., D'Souza, B., & Vasconcellos, E. (2003). Adults and children with headache: evidence-based diagnostic evaluation. *Neuroimaging Clinics of North America, 13*, 225–235.

Medina, L. S., Kuntz, K. M., & Pomeroy, S. (2001). Children with headache suspected of having a brain tumor: a cost-effectiveness analysis of diagnostic strategies. *Pediatrics, 108*, 255–263.

Medina, L. S., Pinter, J. D., Zurakowski, D., Davis, R. G., Kuban, K., & Barnes, P. D. (1997). Children with headache: clinical predictors of surgical space-occupying lesions and the role of neuroimaging. *Radiology, 202*, 819–824.

Meredith, J. T., Wait, S., & Brewer, K. L. (2003). A prospective double-blind study of nasal sumatriptan versus IV ketorolac in migraine. *The American Journal of Emergency Medicine, 21*, 173–175.

Miller, G. S. (2004). Efficacy and safety of levetiracetam in pediatric migraine. *Headache, 44*, 238–243.

Miller, V. A., Palermo, T. M., Powers, S. W., Scher, M. S., & Hershey, A. D. (2003). Migraine headaches and sleep disturbances in children. *Headache, 43*, 362–368.

Mortimer, M. J., Kay, J., & Jaron, A. (1992). Epidemiology of headache and childhood migraine in an urban general practice using Ad Hoc, Vahlquist and IHS criteria. *Developmental Medicine and Child Neurology, 34*, 1095–1101.

Mullner, C., Broos, L. A., van den Maagdenberg, A. M., & Striessnig, J. (2004). Familial hemiplegic migraine type 1 mutations K1336E, W1684R, and V1696I Alter Cav2.1 Ca2+ Channel gating: evidence for beta-subunit isoform-specific effects. *The Journal of Biological Chemistry, 279*, 51844–51850.

Newman, L. C., & Lipton, R. B. (1998). Emergency department evaluation of headache. *Neurologic Clinics, 16*, 285–303.

Pakalnis, A., Butz, C., Splaingard, D., Kring, D., & Fong, J. (2007a). Emotional problems and prevalence of medication overuse in pediatric chronic daily headache. *Journal of Child Neurology, 22*, 1356–1359.

Pakalnis, A., & Kring, D. (2006). Zonisamide prophylaxis in refractory pediatric headache. *Headache, 46*, 804–807.

Pakalnis, A., Kring, D., & Meier, L. (2007b). Levetiracetam prophylaxis in pediatric migraine—an open-label study. *Headache, 47*, 427–430.

Palmer, J. E., Chronicle, E. P., Rolan, P., & Muelleners, W. M. (2000). Cortical hyperexcitability is cortical underinhibition: evidence from a novel functional test of migraine patients. *Cephalalgia, 20*, 525–532.

Pfaffenrath, V., Diener, H. C., Fischer, M., Friede, M., & Henneicke-von Zepelin, H. H. (2002). The efficacy and safety of Tanacetum parthenium (feverfew) in migraine prophylaxis—a double-blind, multicentre, randomized placebo-controlled dose-response study. *Cephalalgia, 22*, 523–532.

Penzien, D. B., Rains, J. C., Lipchik, G. L., & Creer, T. L. (2004). Behavioral interventions for tension-type headache: overview of current therapies and reccomendations for a self-management model for chronic headache. *Current Pain and Headache Reports, 8*, 489–499.

Peres, M. F., Silberstein, S. D., Nahmias, S., Shechter, A. L., Youssef, I., Rozen, T. D., & Young, W. B. (2001). Hemicrania continua is not that rare. *Neurology, 57*, 948–951.

Peterson, C. C., & Palermo, D. M. (2004). Parental reinforcement of recurrent pain: the moderating impact of child depression and anxiety on functional disability. *Journal of Pediatric Psychology, 29*, 331–341.

Thompson PDR. (2007). *Physicians' Desk Reference* (61st ed.). Montvale: Thompson PDR.

Pothmann, R., & Danesch, U. (2005). Migraine prevention in children and adolescents: results of an open study with a special butterbur root extract. *Headache, 45*, 196–203.

Powers, S. W., & Andrasik, F. (2005). Biobehavioral treatment, disability, and psychological effects of pediatric headache. *Pediatric Annals, 34*, 461–465.

Powers, S. W., Patton, S. R., Hommel, K. A., & Hershey, A. D. (2003). Quality of life in childhood migraines: clinical impact and comparison to other chronic illnesses. *Pediatrics, 112*(1 Pt 1), e1–e5.

Rangwala, L. M., & Liu, G. T. (2007). Pediatric idiopathic intracranial hypertension. *Survey of Ophthalmology, 52*, 597–617.

Rao, B. S., Das, D. G., Taraknath, V. R., & Sarma, Y. (2000). A double blind controlled study of propranolol and cyproheptadine in migraine prophylaxis. *Neurology India, 48*, 223–226.

Rapoport, A. M. (1988). Analgesic rebound headache. *Headache, 28*, 662–665.

Raskin, N. H. (1986). Repetitive intravenous dihydroergotamine as treatment for intractable migraine. *Neurology, 36*, 995–997.

Rasmussen, B. K. (1995). Epidemiology of headache. *Cephalalgia, 15*, 45–68.

Reiter, P. D., Nickisch, J., & Merritt, G. (2005). Efficacy and tolerability of intravenous valproic acid in acute adolescent migraine. *Headache, 45*, 899–903.

Roth-Isigkeit, A., Thyen, U., Stöven, H., Schwarzenberger, J., & Schmucker, P. (2005). Pain among children and adolescents: restrictions in daily living and triggering factors. *Pediatrics, 115*, e152–e162.

Rothner, A. S. (1995). Miscellaneous headache syndromes in children and adolescents. *Seminars in Pediatric Neurology, 2*, 109–118.

Saper, J. R., & Jones, J. M. (1986). Ergotamine tartrate dependency: features and possible mechanisms. *Clinical Neuropharmacology, 9*, 244–256.

Scher, A. I., Terwindt, G. M., Verschuren, W. M., Kruit, M. C., Blom, H. J., Kowa, H., Frants, R. R., van den Maagdenberg, A. M., van Buchem, M., Ferrari, M. D., & Launer, L. J. (2006). Migraine and MTHFR C677T genotype in a population-based sample. *Annals of Neurology, 59*, 372–375.

Schmidt-Wilcke, T., Gänßbauer, S., Neuner, T., Bogdahn, U., & May, A. (2008). Subtle grey matter changes between migraine patients and healthy controls. *Cephalalgia, 28*, 1–4.

Schobitz, E., Qureshi, F., & Lewis, D. (2006). Pediatric headaches in the emergency department. *Current Pain and Headache Reports, 10*, 391–396.

Schoenen, J., Jacquy, J., & Lenaerts, M. (1998). Effectiveness of high-dose riboflavin in migraine prophylaxis: a randomized controlled trial. *Neurology, 50*, 466–470.

Scott, I. U., Siatkowski, R. M., Eneyni, M., Brodsky, M. C., & Lam, B. L. (1997). Idiopathic intracranial hypertension in children and adolescents. *American Journal of Ophthalmology, 124*, 253–255.

Segall, L., Scanzano, R., Kaunisto, M. A., Wessman, M., Palotie, A., Gargus, J. J., & Blostein, R. (2004). Kinetic alterations due to a missense mutation in the Na, K-ATPase alpha 2 subunit cause familial hemiplegic migraine type 2. *The Journal of Biological Chemistry, 279*, 43692–43696.

Serdaroglu, G., Erhan, E., Tekgul, H., Oksel, F., Erermis, S., Uyar, M., & Tutuncuoglu, S. (2002). Sodium valproate prophylaxis in childhood migraine. *Headache, 42*, 819–822.

Shapiro, R. E., & Tepper, S. J. (2007). The serotonin syndrome, triptans, and the potential for drug-drug interactions. *Headache, 47*, 266–269.

Silberstein, S. D. (1997). The pharmacology of ergotamine and dihydroergotamine. *Headache, 37*(Suppl 1), S15–S25.

Silberstein, S. D., Lipton, R. B., & Saper, J. R. (2008). Chronic daily headache including transformed migraine, chronic tension-type headache, and medication overuse headache. In S. D. Silberstein, R. B. Lipton, & D. W. Dodick (Eds.), *Wolff's Headache and Other Head Pain* (pp. 315–377). New York: Oxford University Press.

Silberstein, S. D., Young, W. B., Hopkins, M. M., Gebeline-Myers, C., & Bradley, K. C. (2007). Dihydroergotamine for early and late treatment of migraine with cutaneous allodynia: an open-label pilot trial. *Headache, 47*, 878–885.

Silberstein, S. D., & Young, W. B. (1995). Analgesic rebound headache. How great is the problem and what can be done? *Drug Safety, 13*, 133–144.

Sillanpää, M. (1976). Prevalence of migraine and other headache in Finnish children starting school. *Headache, 15*, 288–290.

Sillanpää, M. (1983). Changes in the prevalence of migraine and other headaches during the first seven school years. *Headache, 23*, 15–19.

Silver, S., Gano, D., & Gerretsen, P. J. (2008). Acute treatment of paediatric migraine: a meta-analysis of efficacy. *Paediatrics & Child Health, 44*, 3–9.

Snow, V., Weiss, K., Wall, E. M., & Mottur-Pilson, C. (2002). Pharmacologic management of acute attacks of migraine and prevention of migraine headache. *Annals of Internal Medicine, 137*, 840–849.

Sobri, M., Lamont, A. C., Alias, N. A., & Win, M. N. (2003). Red flags in patients presenting with headache: clinical indications for neuroimaging. *The British Journal of Radiology, 76*, 532–535.

Soriani, S., Battistella, P. A., Arnaldi, C., De Carlo, L., Cernetti, R., Corrà, S., & Tosato, G. (1996). Juvenile idiopathic stabbing headache. *Headache, 36*, 565–567.

Split, W., & Neuman, W. (1999). Epidemiology of migraine among students from randomly selected secondary schools in Lodz. *Headache, 39*, 494–501.

Srikiatkhachorn, A. (2006). Towards the better understanding about pathogenesis of chronic daily headache. *Journal of the Medical Association of Thailand, 89*(Suppl 3), S234–S243.

Srikiatkhachorn, A., Govitrapong, P., & Limthavon, C. (1994). Up-regulation of 5-HT2 serotonin receptor: a possible mechanism of transformed migraine. *Headache, 34*, 8–11.

Srikiatkhachorn, A., Tarasub, N., & Govitrapong, P. (2000). Effect of chronic analgesic exposure on the central serotonin system: a possible mechanism of analgesic abuse headache. *Headache, 40*, 343–350.

Stang, P. E., Yanagihara, P. A., Swanson, J. W., Beard, C. M., O'Fallon, W. M., Guess, H. A., & Melton, L. J., 3rd. (1992). Incidence of migraine headache: a population-based study in Olmsted County, Minnesota. *Neurology, 42*, 1657–1662.

Stewart, W. F., Linet, M. S., Celentano, D. D., Van Natta, M., & Ziegler, D. (1991). Age- and sex-specific incidence rates of migraine with and without visual aura. *American Journal of Epidemiology, 134*, 1111–1120.

Tepper, S. J., Dahlöf, C. G., Dowson, A., Newman, L., Mansbach, H., Jones, M., Pham, B., Webster, C., & Salonen, R. (2004). Prevalence and diagnosis of migraine in patients consulting their physician with a complaint of headache: data from the Landmark Study. *Headache, 44*, 856–864.

Tkachuk, G. A., Cottrell, C. K., Gibson, J. S., O'Donnell, F. J., & Holroyd, K. A. (2003). Factors associated with migraine-related quality of life and disability in adolescents: a preliminary investigation. *Headache, 43*, 950–955.

Trautmann, E., Lackschewitz, H., & Kröner-Herwig, B. (2006). Psychological treatment of recurrent headaches in children and adolescents–a meta-analysis. *Cephalalgia, 26*, 1411–1426.

Valfrè, W., Rainero, I., Bergui, M., & Pinessi, L. (2008). Voxel-based morphometry reveals gray matter abnormalities in migraine. *Headache, 48*, 109–117.

Van den Bergh, V., Amery, W. K., & Waelkens, J. (1987). Trigger factors in migraine: a study conducted by the Belgian Migraine Society. *Headache, 27*, 191–196.

Vasconcellos, E., & Luzondo, R. J. (2007). Primary Stabbing Headache in Children. *Headache, 47*, 807.

Vasconcellos, E., & Muray, M. J. (2005). Risk factors for chronic daily headache in children and adolescents. *Headache, 45*, 376.

Vasconcellos, E., Piña-Garza, J. E., Millan, E. J., & Warner, J. S. (1998). Analgesic rebound headache in children and adolescents. *Journal of Child Neurology, 13*, 443–447.

Vieira, J. P., Salgueiro, A. B., & Alfaro, M. (2006). Short-lasting headaches in children. *Cephalalgia, 26*, 1220–1224.

Visser, W. H., Winner, P., Strohmaier, K., Klipfel, M., Peng, Y., McCarroll, K., Cady, R., Lewis, D., Nett, R., & Rizatriptan Protocol 059 and 061 Study Groups. (2004). Rizatriptan 5 mg for the acute treatment of migraine in adolescents: results from a double-blind, single-attack study and two open-label, multiple-attack studies. *Headache, 44*, 891–899.

Volans, G. N. (1978). Migraine and drug absorption. *Clinical Pharmacokinetics, 3*, 313–318.

Wang, F., Van Den Eeden, S. K., Ackerson, L. M., Salk, S. E., Reince, R. H., & Elin, R. J. (2003). Oral magnesium oxide prophylaxis of frequent migrainous headache in children: a randomized, double-blind placebo-controlled trial. *Headache, 43*, 601–610.

Wang, S. J., Fuh, J. L., Juang, K. D., & Lu, S. R. (2005). Rising prevalence of migraine in Taiwanese adolescents aged 13–15 years. *Cephalalgia, 25*, 433–448.

Wang, S. J., Fuh, J. L., Lu, S. R., & Juang, K. D. (2006). Chronic daily headache in adolescents: prevalence, impact, and medication overuse. *Neurology, 66*, 193–197.

Wang, S. J., Fuh, J. L., Young, Y. H., Lu, S. R., & Shia, B. C. (2000). Prevalence of migraine in Taipei, Taiwan: a population-based survey. *Cephalalgia, 20*, 566–572.

Weiller, C., May, A., Limmroth, V., Juptner, M., Kaube, H., Schayck, R. V., Coenen, H. H., & Diener, H. C. (1995). Brainstem activation in spontaneous human migraine attacks. *Natural Medicines, 1*, 658–660.

Welch, K. M., Nagesh, V., Aurora, S. K., & Gelman, N. (2001). Periaqueductal gray matter dysfunction in migraine: cause or the burden of illness? *Headache, 41*, 629–637.

Winner, P., Linder, S. L., Lipton, R. B., Almas, M., Parsons, B., & Pitman, V. (2007). Eletriptan for the acute treatment of migraine in adolescents: results of a double-blind, placebo-controlled trial. *Headache, 47*, 511–518.

Winner, P., Pearlman, E. M., Linder, S. L., Jordan, D. M., Fisher, A. C., & Hulihan, J. (2005). Topiramate for migraine prevention in children: a randomized, double-blind, placebo-controlled trial. *Headache, 45*, 1304–1312.

Winner, P., Rothner, A. D., Wooten, J. D., Webster, C., & Ames, M. (2006). Sumatriptan nasal spray in adolescent migraineurs: a randomized, double-blind, placebo-controlled, acute study. *Headache, 46*, 212–222.

Winner, P. W., Hershey, A. D., & Zhicheng, L. (2008). Headaches in children. In S. D. Silberstein, R. B. Lipton, & D. W. Dodick (Eds.), *Wolff's Headache and Other Head Pain* (pp. 315–377). New York: Oxford University Press.

Yuill, G. M., Swinburn, W. R., & Liversedge, L. A. (1972). A double-blind crossover trial of isometheptene mucate compound and ergotamine in migraine. *The British Journal of Clinical Practice, 26*, 76–79.

Zwart, J. A., Dyb, G., Holmen, T. L., Stovner, L. J., & Sand, T. (2004). The prevalence of migraine and tension-type headaches among adolescents in Norway. The Nord-Trøndelag Health Study (Head-HUNT-Youth), a large population-based epidemiological study. *Cephalalgia, 24*, 373–379.

Sickle Cell Pain

Valerie E. Armstead
and Genevieve D'Souza

Keywords

Sickle cell pain • Sickle cell disease • Complications • Vaso-occlusive crises • Sickle cell trait • Therapy of sickle cell • Treatment of sickle cell pain

Introduction

"Pain and suffering are the hallmarks of sickle cell disease. For most patients who are afflicted with this illness, pain is their nemesis, their unpredictable master, and ruthless dictator. For many patients and their families, pain is a chore and a major component of routine activities of daily living. It has to be factored in to every plan, project, activity, dream, ambition, and relationship…Persistent, severe sickle cell pain is a poor prognostic sign and a predictor of death…I wish (Linus) Pauling had referred to sickle cell disease as the first painful molecular disease and not simply the first molecular disease. This descriptor might have emphasized the morbid clinical picture and stimulated more research on pain." (Ballas 1998)

– Samir K. Ballas, M.D., FACP, FASCP,
DABPM, FAAPM, 1938–

The preceding excerpt is from the preface to a tome that exemplifies integrative medicine, written by the preeminent hematologist and sickle cell researcher, Samir K. Ballas, M.D. Dr. Ballas was one of the first physicians to publish objective

information on the management problems for patients, healthcare providers, and loved ones dealing with sickle cell pain. By unabashedly using awkward, embarrassing terms such as prejudice, stereotyping, mistreatment and neglect to describe the problems encountered by the older sickle cell patient, Dr. Ballas helped shepherd in the much-needed, multi-disciplinary team approach in managing sickle cell pain and sickle cell disease (Epstein et al. 2006; Ballas 2005; Ballas 1995; Ballas 1990). This chapter is dedicated to Dr. Ballas who has devoted his professional life to sickle cell patients while sharing his time, generosity, and wisdom with any medical specialty interested in studying any aspect of sickle cell disease.

Background

Sickle cell disease is an inherited disorder of hemoglobin synthesis. The first description of sickle cell disease was published in 1910 (Herrick 1910). Sickle cell disease was named by West African tribes in a manner that universally described the pain excruciating, biting or gnawing pain that lasts for days. The painful episode is the most common malady affecting patients suffering from sickle cell disease and is the most

V.E. Armstead (✉)
St. Joseph's Regional Medical Center,
703 Main Street, Paterson, NJ 07503, USA
e-mail: vearmstead@gmail.com

B.C. McClain and S. Suresh (eds.), *Handbook of Pediatric Chronic Pain:
Current Science and Integrative Practice*, DOI 10.1007/978-1-4419-0350-1_11,
© Springer Science+Business Media, LLC 2011

frequent cause of emergency department visits and hospital admissions (Epstein et al. 2006). Sickle cell disease is a global health issue, with over 95% of affected individuals living outside of the United States (Ballas 2005).

Pathophysiology and Natural History

Sickle cell syndromes are caused by inheritance of homozygous hemoglobin S or compound heterozygosity for hemoglobin S, hemoglobin C, thalassemia or other structural variants (Weatherall 1985; Zago and Costa 1985). Sickle cell disease usually results from a single amino acid substitution (valine for glutamate) in position 6 of the beta chain of hemoglobin (Ballas 1995; Ballas 1990). This genetic alteration allows for polymerization of the hemoglobin during hypoxia yielding an unstable, sickle-shaped red blood cell with a shortened survival (Herrick 1910). The bizarre and somewhat whimsical variations in the deformities of red blood cells as a result of sickle cell disease are represented in the background of Fig. 11.1.

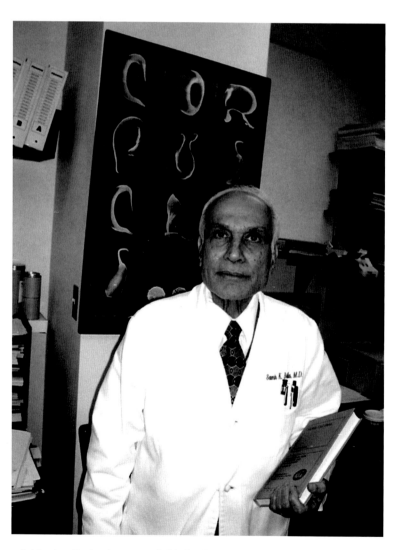

Fig. 11.1 The red blood cells in the poster behind Dr. Samir K. Ballas represent the variety of shapes sickled cells. The cells spell out the word, "CORPUSCLE". Dr. Ballas is holding a copy of his textbook entitled *Sickle Cell Pain* (Photograph by V. Armstead)

People who inherit two Hb S genes from their parents have sickle cell disease. However, there is significant phenotypic diversity among individuals with sickle cell disease such that the hemoglobin S mutation is necessary but insufficient to account for disease pathophysiology (Zago and Costa 1985; Marchant and Walker 2003; Amrolia et al. 2003a). Many other modifier genes determine disease phenotype; some of these act uniformly, influencing more than one sub-phenotype, while others are phenotype-specific. These genes and their variants determine disease severity by modulating the effects of the hemoglobin S mutation and interacting with each other and the environment (Amrolia et al. 2003a; Embury 1986).

The symptoms of sickle cell disease arise from the peculiar properties of the abnormal hemoglobin and from hemolytic anemia. Table 11.1 lists the variety of symptoms of sickle cell disease (Marchant and Walker 2003; Fosdal and Wojner Alexandrov 2007). Deoxygenated sickle hemoglobin forms rigid polymers that deform

red cells causing vaso-occlusion in the smaller vessels. Adherence of sickle cells to vascular endothelium results in intimal hyperplasia in larger vessels causing altered blood flow (Smith et al. 2002; Charache 1996).

Patients with sickle cell disease adapt to a lower hematocrit. However, with chronic severe anemia, children develop coexistent cardiomegaly as a result of increased cardiac output (Kerle and Nishimura 1996; Murray and Evans 1996; Dimashkieh et al. 2003; Setty et al. 2001).

In all infants, the spleen provides a line of defense against bacterial invasion; it is also a source of opsonins and fixed-tissue macrophages, as well as antibody production. From the age of a few months on, children with sickle disease have increasing splenic dysfunction as the organ is at first intermittently and then chronically occluded with sickled cells (Kerle and Nishimura 1996; Murray and Evans 1996; Dimashkieh et al. 2003; Setty et al. 2001).

The clinical course of for most patients with sickle cell disease is one of chronic illness precipitated by multiple acute exacerbations that can become life threatening at any time (Fig. 11.2). With current treatment advances approximately 50% of patients survive beyond the fifth decade. One third of deaths occur during an acute crisis in patients who are clinically free of organ failure. Infection is the leading cause of death in affected children aged 1–3 years (Amrolia et al. 2003a). The advent of early screening, penicillin prophylaxis and prompt treatment has now reduced the mortality rate from infection. Strokes and trauma are the leading causes of death in patients aged 10–20 years. Children in this age range also die from acute chest syndrome (Figs. 11.3 and 11.4), splenic sequestration crisis, and aplastic crisis (Embury 1986; Fosdal and Wojner-Alexandrov 2007).

Table 11.1 Systemic manifestations of sickle cell disease (With permission from Marchant and Walker 2003)

Hemolysis	Megaloblastic erythropoiesis
	Aplastic crisis
	Clinical jaundice and gallstones, liver dysfunction
Vaso-occlusion	Splenic manifestations
	Stroke
	Sickle retinopathy
	Impaired growth
	Complications in pregnancy
Skeletal	Painful crisis
	Dactylitis
	Bone marrow infarcts
	Osteomyelitis
	X-ray evidence of osteoporosis
Cardiopulmonary	Cardiomegaly
	Acute chest syndrome
	Pulmonary infarcts
Neurological	Stroke
	Cranial nerve neuropathies
Genitourinary	Poor urine concentrating ability
	Renal infarction
	Hematuria
	Renal failure
	Priapism

Sickle Cell Trait

People with only one gene for hemoglobin S (Hb S) are carriers of the recessive gene. These individuals have a mild phenotypical abnormalities and the condition is commonly known as sickle cell trait or sickle trait (Weatherall 1985).

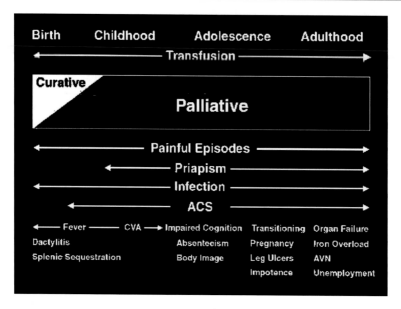

Fig. 11.2 Sequence of complications of sickle cell anemia from birth through adult life. Cure is possible in selected children. The mainstay of management in most patients is palliative, with pain management being most important. ACS, acute chest syndrome; AVN, avascular necrosis; CVA, cerebrovascular accident (Modified from Ballas 2005, with permission)

Sickle cell disease and certain types of malaria occur in the same geographic areas. It also has been shown that persons with sickle cell trait have an innate immunity to cerebral malaria and that the sickle-shaped stage of a malarial parasite (m. plasmodium falciparum) can not survive in sickle trait red cells (Smith et al. 2002). The incidence of the trait is 7–10% of Black African-Americans. The life span of people with this trait is normal, and serious complications are very rare. The complete blood cell count is within the normal range although the peripheral blood slide smear is abnormal.

Complications of sickle cell trait include sudden death during rigorous exercise, splenic infarcts at high altitude, hematuria, hyposthenuria, bacteriuria, and intraocular bleeding leading to blindness (Smith et al. 2002; Charache 1996; Kerle and Nishimura 1996; Murray and Evans 1996). A rare cancer, renal medullary carcinoma, is also associated with sickle cell trait (Dimashkieh et al. 2003)

Frequency

Sickle cell disease is the most common single gene disorder in black Americans in the U.S. occurring in 1 in 675 live births (Ballas 2005). Approximately 8–10% of black Americans in the population carry the HbS gene. Homozygous (SS) sickle disease occurs in about 0.15% of Black American newborns. Sickle cell disease also occurs in people who are Hispanic, Middle Eastern, Indians, individuals of Mediterranean descent and other Caucasians, with reported cases in every ethnic or racial group (Ballas 1998).

Age

Symptoms of sickle cell disease can be evident as early as the age of 10 weeks, though usually delayed until the age of 6–12 months because of high levels of circulating fetal hemoglobin (Hb F)

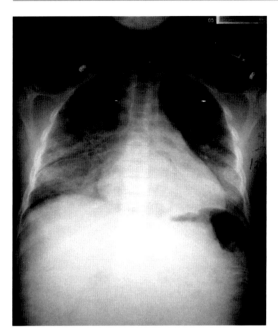

Fig. 11.3 Anterior-posterior x-ray showing diffuse bilateral alveolar and interstitial infiltrates in an 18 year-old male with sickle cell disease presenting with bilateral pleuritic chest pain, hypoxemia and other symptoms consistent with acute chest syndrome. Noticeable are other signs of sickle cell disease: Hepatomegaly, cardiomegaly, absent spleen from autoinfarction and osteonecrotic collapse of multiple thoracic vertebral end plates, giving the appearance of "fish vertebrae" (Image courtesy of Dr. Johnson Haynes, Jr.,Director, USA Sickle Center, Univ. of South Alabama College of Medicine)

(Setty et al. 2001; Steinberg 1996). After infancy, erythrocytes of patients with sickle cell anemia contain approximately 90% hemoglobin S (HbS), 2–10% hemoglobin F (HbF), a normal amount of minor fraction of adult hemoglobin (HbA2), and no hemoglobin A (HbA) (Lefevre-Witier 1985; Weatherall et al. 1985).

Clinical Manifestations

Painful vaso-occlusive crises is the most frequent clinical symptoms of sickle cell disease. In infants dactylitis or hand-foot syndrome caused by infarctions of the small bones may be the initial manifestation of sickle cell anemia. The findings include painful, usually symmetric, swelling of the hands and feet. The underlying abnormality is ischemic necrosis of the small bones, believed to be caused by occlusion of the blood supply as a result of the rapidly expanding bone marrow (Cordner and De 2003). Most bony vaso-occlusive events are multi-focal and occur primarily in the bone marrow cavity and are associated with exquisite tenderness and localized edema. As the child matures and hematopoiesis in the small bones of the hands and feet ceases, the painful episodes usually affect the joints, especially the hips and knees and those of the chest wall and back (Cordner and De 2003; Steiner et al. 1990; Terk et al. 1996). The acute bone pain crises are described as gnawing or biting and are associated with local swelling (Ballas 1998). Graphic descriptions of crises in patient diaries give lasting appreciation (Ballas 1998; Lane 1996) of the suffering. Later stages of osteonecrosis lead to chronic pain which is often associated with necrosis of the femoral head (Fig. 11.5) (Ballas 1995).

Children may experience frequent, maybe daily episodes of acute painful episodes. Some may require frequent hospitalizations for these acute painful episodes. Intercurrent illnesses accompanied by fever, hypoxia, and acidosis, which promote sickling, may precipitate sickle pain episodes, but acute pain also develops frequently without an apparent antecedent event. Other factors can also precipitate vaso-occlusion. Dehydration, hypothermia and infections are also known precipitating factors (Dickerhoff and von 1995; Hebbel 1985).

Painful splenic infarcts contributing to the process of autosplenectomy are common in children. Pulmonary infarction may occur in association with pneumonitis or microscopic fat emboli (from bone marrow infarction), producing the severe clinical picture of acute chest syndrome (Figs. 11.3 and 11.4). Acute chest syndrome is associated with increased phospholipase A2 levels and should be suspected with the constellation of chest pain, tachypnea, and hypoxia that can progress to global systemic vascular injury, cardiovascular collapse and death (Lane 1996).

Hemiplegia from stroke caused by cerebrovascular occlusion is among the most catastrophic acute events in children (Carvalho and Garg 2002; Nowak-Gottl et al. 2003). Similar ischemic

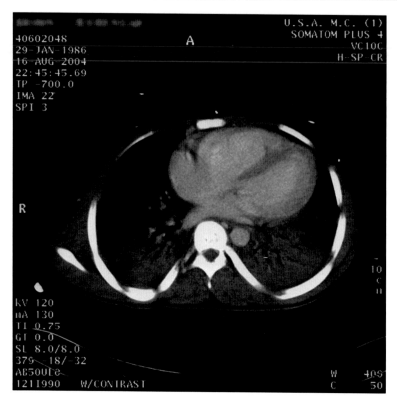

Fig. 11.4 MRI of chest from patient in Fig. 11.3. 18 year-old male with sickle cell disease presenting with bilateral pleuritic chest pain and hypoxemia. Cross-sectional image showing diffuse bilateral alveolar and interstitial infiltrates with decreased air entry consistent with acute chest syndrome (Image courtesy of Dr. Johnson Haynes, Jr.,Director, USA Sickle Center, Univ. of South Alabama College of Medicine)

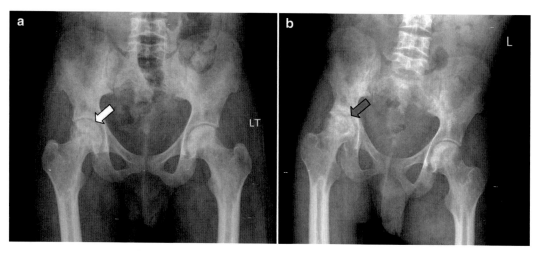

Fig. 11.5 (**a** and **b**) Plain radiograph indicating avascular necrosis of the right femoral head evidenced by joint narrowing (*white arrow*) compared to the left hip joint space. Figure (**b**) of the same patient shows progression to collapse of the femoral head and joint space (*shaded arrow*). Note that the patient's posture now favors the less-involved left leg. These radiographs are show evidence of central collapse of the vertebral joints with fish mouth deformity of the disc spaces

episodes occur in other organs like liver, heart and kidney.

Priapism is a frequent complication from venous obstruction causing pooling of blood in the corpora cavernosa of the penis. If not treated aggressively after 2 h of sustained priapism, this condition can lead to impotency from fibrosis (Molitierno 2003).

Anemia is a common lifelong problem, starting in the first year of life once the drop in fetal hemoglobin level begins. The average red cell survival is reduced from a normal of 120 days down to an average of 10–20 days in sickle cell anemia. This produces anemia, a high reticulocyte count, and a striking proliferation of red cell precursors in the bone marrow to compensate for the hemolysis. Other problems related to the anemia are jaundice (elevated bilirubin), changes in bone structure, and high lactic dehydrogenase levels (Ballas and Marcolina 2006). Many infectious complications can cause partial suppression of erythrocyte production increasing the anemia in patients with sickle syndromes. Acute anemia can be caused by an aplastic episode, sequestration, G6PD deficiency, acute chest syndrome, an allo-antibody, renal failure, or folate deficiency. Urinary tract infections are more common and can lead to bactericidal. Viral pneumonia and reactive airways disease can rapidly progress to acute chest syndrome. Children may present with increasing splenic enlargement leading to hypersplenism associated with worsening anemia and thrombocytopenia. Following an acute febrile illness, splenic sequestration may occur in young children. Large amounts of blood get acutely pooled in the spleen, which becomes massively enlarged, and signs of circulatory collapse rapidly develop (Lane 1996; Owusu-Ofori and Riddington 2002). Acute splenic sequestration has a peak incidence between 6 months to 3 years of age and can be rapid in onset and lead to death. Altered splenic function also leads to increased susceptibility to infections mainly caused by Pneumococci, H. Infleunzae and other virulent bacterial/viral infections (Moore et al. 1996).

In older children greater than 5 years, other complications of sickle cell disease are more common. Stroke, more frequent vaso-occlusive episodes with increased severity, avascular necrosis involving hip, shoulder joints, or vertebrae as well as cholelithiasis requiring cholecystectomy may occur. School-aged children get exposed to more severe infections including parvovirus (Pandit 1996; Wald 1985). Chronic anemia leads to more frequent blood transfusions which carry risk of blood borne infection with hepatitis and HIV viruses.

Patients with sickle cell anemia or sickle cell-b thalassemia are also at risk for iron overload if chronically given transfusions for the prevention of recurrent complications. The most important recent development in the management of patients with sickle cell disorders has been the demonstration that transfusion greatly reduces the risk of a first stroke in children with sickle cell anemia who have abnormal results on transcranial Doppler. The preventive use of red cell transfusions in patients with sickle cell disease will greatly increase the number of patients in the U.S. with transfusional iron overload (Fung et al. 2007).

Adolescents begin to develop chronic sequelae of sickle cell disease. These children may have increased urinary tract infections, severe episodes of priapism leading to impotence, frequent acute chest syndrome causing pulmonary hypertension, avascular necrosis of hip, chronic renal failure from sickle nephropathy, retinopathy and other sequelae including stroke. With severe infections like parvovirus B19, other viral and bacterial infections, children may have aplastic crisis (Pandit 1996). Older children usually have sickle cell related-cardiomyopathy causing cardiomegaly and parenchymal damage to major organs from increased iron absorption (Fung et al. 2007).

Leg ulcers cause chronic disability in 10–15% of older children and adults with sickle cell anemia (Blaylock 1996). They are likely related to vascular stasis explaining the chronicity and recurrence of sickle cell disease. Leg ulcers are more common in men and older patients and less common in patients with α-gene deletion, high total Hb level, or high levels of Hb F.

Avascular necrosis is the most commonly observed complication of sickle cell disease in 'adolescent patients and adults. The stages of progression have been characterized by different authors but the pattern is that of asymptomatic changes to painful joint deformities that necessitate surgical intervention (Hungerford and Lennox 1985). Although osteonecrosis, as it is also termed, tends to be most severe and disabling in the hip area, it is a generalized bone disorder in that the femoral and humeral heads and the vertebral bodies may be equally affected (Rao et al. 1991). Modern radiologic imaging techniques, such as high-resolution magnetic resonance imaging (MRI) provide excellent opportunities to correlate acute and chronic pathology because ischemic marrow changes are evident before x-ray bone changes are apparent (Fig. 11.6). The limited terminal arterial blood supply and the paucity of collateral circulation make these three areas especially vulnerable to sickling and subsequent bone damage. Patients with sickle cell anemia and α-gene deletion have a higher incidence of avascular necrosis, because their high hematocrit increases blood viscosity and thus enhances microvasculopathy in the aforementioned anatomic sites (Ballas et al. 1997).

As in most individuals affected by chronic medical illnesses children may suffer from depression (Walco and Dampier 1987). The day-to-day stresses associated with the illness may contribute to feelings of helplessness, a feeling of not being in control, and create a vulnerability to develop depressive symptoms (Eccleston et al. 2003; Jacob et al. 2006).

Sensorineural hearing loss (SNHL) has been associated with sickle cell disease (SCD) in older children and adults and may affect up to 40% of the population (Chiodo et al. 1997). Desferroxamine used for chelation therapy for transfusion related iron overload can also cause ototoxicity (Chiodo et al. 1997; Chen et al. 2005; Styles and Vichinsky 1996).

Laboratory Studies

Specific diagnosis of sickle cell is made using hemoglobin electrophoresis and is often picked up through newborn screening programs (Bardakdjian-Michau 2003; Labie and Elion 1996a; Labie and Elion 1996b; Laird et al. 1996). Peripheral blood smear shows evidence of target cells, elongated cells and sickle eyrthrocytes. Genetic laboratory analysis may be necessary to further characterize the defect or defects (Weatherall 1985; Labie and Elion 1996a; Brousseau et al. 2007; Sing et al. 1985). Clinical blood count for hemoglobin, hematocrit, white blood cell count, platelet count, reticulocyte count can be performed.

Treatment

Due to the increased hemolysis in the spleen, splenectomy can alleviate the increased hemolysis of the disease. Vaccines for encapsulated organisms such as pneumococcus, meningococcus, and Haemophilus influenza type b should be administered before splenectomy, and oral prophylactic penicillin V (age <5 year: 125 mg twice daily; age ≥5 year through adulthood: 250 mg twice daily) administered thereafter (Chulamokha et al. 2006; Serjeant 1996).

Hydration and analgesia is the cornerstone of therapy for vaso-occlusive crises (Ballas and Mohandas 1996; Kaul et al. 1996). Analgesic modalities for pain are discussed later in this chapter. More prolonged and constant pain can be seen with bone infarction, sickle arthritis, and aseptic necrosis of the femur or humerus (Fig. 11.6). With chronic pain, non-steroidal anti-inflammatory medications with renal sparing properties should be administered continuously to maintain analgesic blood levels during these episodes. Transcutaneous electrical nerve stimulation (TENS) units, relaxation techniques, occupational and physical therapy approaches may be useful in reducing pain and maintaining a functional lifestyle (Eccleston et al. 2003). Education and support are often required to prevent the inappropriate continuous use of opiate analgesics for these chronic pain states (Barakat et al. 2007; Dumaplin 2006; Mitchell et al. 2007).

Acute chest syndrome is an ominous complication of SCD resulting from vaso-occlusive episodes. Patients with acute chest syndrome require judicious hydration, analgesia, antibiotics, and oxygen supplementation with respiratory support. With severe respiratory distress, Inhalation

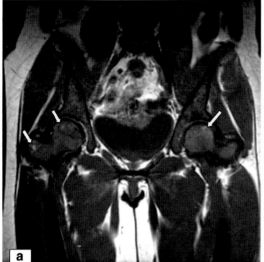 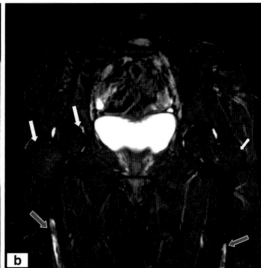

Fig. 11.6 (**a** and **b**) Bilateral avascular necrosis with collapse involving the femoral joints with areas of necrosis in femoral heads and trochanteric regions (*white arrows*) in the MRI (**a** & **b**). In the MRI image of the same patient there is evidence of persistent red marrow and iron overload (*dark marrow signals*) which can have similar appearances (**b**). There are also infarcts that appear as white streaks within the femoral shafts (Images courtesy of Dr. William D. Morrison, Director MSK imaging, Thomas Jefferson Univ. Hosp., Department of Radiology, Philadelphia)

of nitric oxide (NO) to replenish the endogenous gas consumed by free plasma Hb corrects the relative NO deficiency that occurs in sickle cell patients including the pulmonary vasculature, stimulates vasodilation, and reduces the pulmonary blood pressure. Other therapies include oral administration of arginine (the natural substrate for synthesis of NO) and l-carnitine, an analog of the naturally occurring fatty acid carnitine, which is thought to stabilize the red cell membrane, and thereby inhibits hemolysis (Ballas 1990).

Treatment of chronic leg ulcers includes daily saline wet-to-dry debridement, compressive dressings such as Unna's boots, hydroscopic dressings, hyperbaric oxygen therapy and antibiotics for cellulitis (Blaylock 1996). Transfusion and skin grafts may be of benefit in difficult cases.

Priapism is treated with hydration, analgesia, surgical intervention and exchange transfusion as appropriate (Molitierno 2003).

There is controversy over desired minimum hemoglobin for patients with sickle cell disease presenting for surgery. The type of surgery, anticipated blood loss, and sickle cell symptoms

must be considered. Circumstances may necessitate routine preoperative transfusions to raise the hemoglobin to the acceptable level. These simple transfusions are safe and as effective in preventing postoperative complications as is exchange or aggressive transfusions to decrease the hemoglobin S level below 30%. Postoperative complications from these frequent transfusions such as acute chest syndrome, fever, iron overload, and alloimmunization with delayed transfusion reactions are common.

Daily administration of oral hydroxyurea (Hydrea) is the first effective pharmacological intervention documented to provide clinically significantly prevention of complications in Sickle cell disease like vaso-occlusive pain crisis and acute chest syndrome (Herrick 1910). Treatment with hydroxyurea has recently been shown to reduce pain events, hospital admissions and the need for blood transfusions by 50% (Ballas et al. 2006). Hydroxyurea is a chemotherapeutic agent with potent effects on the bone marrow. Hydroxyurea was used for many years to treat people with certain malignancies before being used for sickle cell disease (Ballas et al. 2006; Halsey and Roberts 2003; Huang et al. 2003; Yang and Pace 2001). The primary side-effect of hydroxyurea is suppression of blood counts, particularly the white blood cells (neutropenia) and platelets (thrombocytopenia). Neutropenia and thrombocytopenia respectively place patients at risk for infection and bleeding.

In a placebo-controlled pilot trial, oral supplements of two omega-3 polyunsaturated fatty acids (PUFA)— docosahexanoic acid (DHA) and eicosapentanoic acid (EPA)—reduced the mean number of sickle cell crises requiring hospital attendance from 7.8 per year to 3.8 per year in 5 HbSS individuals (Weatherall 1985).

The Gardos channel is a calcium-dependent mechanism for potassium transport across cell membranes while regulating K^+ ion and water loss from erythrocytes. In humans and animal models who have Sickle cell disease, inhibition of this potassium flux system with the antifungal drug, clotrimazole, prevented intra-cellular dehydration of erythrocytes and reduced the polymerization of HbS and sickling of red blood cells (De Franceschi et al. 1994). An analog of clotrimazole that is less toxic to the liver and urinary tract because it has no imidazole moiety, ICA-17043 is a more potent Gardos channel inhibitor and specifically blocks potassium efflux from red blood cells mediated by this transport mechanism (Chulamokha et al. 2006; Kooy et al. 1996).

All female patients should receive accurate information about risks of pregnancy, genetic transmission of sickle syndromes, methods of contraception, prenatal diagnosis, prevention of sexually transmitted disease and the increased responsibility of raising children at puberty and periodically throughout their reproductive lives.

Acute and Chronic Pain in Sickle Cell Disease

The hallmark of pain in sickle cell disease is its extreme variability and unpredictability in timing, location and intensity (Marchant and Walker 2003). The normal baseline for pain is sickle cell disease ranges from no pain to daily discomfort which may be tolerable and intermittent acute exacerbations. Painful episodes may be precipitated by infection, stress, hypoxemia, dehydration, acidosis, fatigue, strenuous exercise, cold exposure, menses and pregnancy. Most episodes have no precipitant factors.

A tailored multidisciplinary approach to pain management is essential for treatment of painful episodes. An effective strategy to prevent delay in treatment is for patients or their care givers is to carry and provide plastic-laminated cards that provide photo identification and effective pain management regimen that work Opioids are considered the major therapy for these pain syndromes and are continued throughout adult life. The stepwise approach for management of cancer pain recommended by the World Health Organization is also A stepwise approach to pain management in sickle cell disease is represented in the algorithm in Fig. 11.7. Hydration and analgesia are the cornerstone of therapies for vaso-occlusive crises.

NSAIDS. Many patients use daily NSAIDs or acetaminophen at home to manage their baseline pain. NSAID use may lead to nephropathy and renal failure which are also the sequelae of vaso-occlusive disease (Scheinman 2003). Hence regular monitoring of renal function is necessary in sickle cell patients taking NSAIDs.

Opioids. Oral opioids are preferable for treatment of pain. Parenteral administration should be reserved for patients in severe pain, inability to take oral medications due to vomiting, severe dehydration etc. Opioids used range from codeine and oxycodone as first line therapy, followed by equianalgesic doses of morphine or hydromorphone. Oral methadone is also a modality of treatment for some patients. Tramadol has also been used with success to avoid more potent opiod in children in crisis however clinical trials for this indication have been completed (Erhan et al. 2007). Meperidine was widely used for therapy in management of sickle cell pain. Problems with its use are its long-acting metabolite normeperidine with its association with dysphoria, hallucinations and seizures (Ballas 1997; Ballas 2008). Meperidine is not recommended in patients with potential for renal disease.

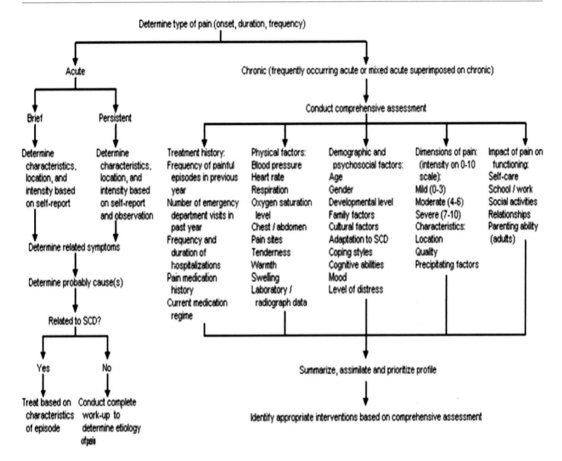

Fig. 11.7 A flow chart for sickle cell pain assessment. *SCD* sickle cell disease (Reprinted with permission from Benjamin LJ, Dampier CD, Jacox AK, Odesina V, Phoenix D, Shapiro B, et al., Guideline for the management of acute and chronic pain in sickle cell disease. APS Clinical Practice Guidelines Series, No. 1. Glenview: American Pain Society, 1999:12–13)

Parenteral opioids for hospital admissions can be administered PRN (not recommended), continuous infusions with PRN rescue doses, and Patient Controlled Analgesia (PCA). The opioid dose should be carefully titrated according to the extent of analgesia and sedation with pulse oximetry monitoring for in the hospital, emergency department, or other unit where patient monitoring is in place.

Other therapeutic modalities. Adjuvant drugs like tricylic antidepressants, stimulants and benzodiazepines are of some benefit in a few patients. The more commonly-used adjuvant drugs are compiled in Table 11.2 (Erhan et al. 2007; Mankad 2001; Stinson and Naser 2003). Epidural analgesia has been used for the treatment of pain (Zago and Costa 1985). Cognitive –behavioral and psychological interventions may be of added benefit in all patients. Patient and family education should be ongoing part of therapy. Physical therapy, transcutaneous electrical nerve stimulation, massage, heat therapy, hypnosis, may help in coping with pain.

Prognosis

The patient with sickle cell disease is faced with a myriad of potentially life-threatening and unpredictable complications. Most patients and families

Table 11.2 Adjuvant drugs commonly used to treat sickle cell pain (Erhan et al. 2007; Mankad 2001; Stinson and Naser 2003)

Antihistamines
- Hydroxyzine
- Diphenhydramine

Benzodiazepines
- Diazepam
- Alprazolam

Tricyclic Antidepressants
- Amitriptyline
- Nortriptyline
- Doxepin

Anticonvulsants
- Phenytoin
- Carbamazepine
- Gabapentin
- Topiramate
- Clonazepam

Phenothiazines
- Prochlorperazine
- Promethazine

with a good understanding of the disease process can have improved outcomes compared to the twentieth century due to compliance with medication regimes and multi-disciplinary support that promotes well-being. Still, the transition from pediatric to adulthood is difficult for those individuals who experience more sickle cell-related health problems that are translated into socioeconomic problems. Furthermore, the adolescent and adult sickle cell patient can suffer psychological setbacks due to historically dire health predictions associated with longevity, loss of friends with sickle cell as they advance in age such that birthdays are dreaded and the future appears bleak (Ballas 1995; Walco and Dampier 1987).

There are many promising ways to apply genomics tools and approaches to sickle cell disease. Given the phenotypic diversity of sickle cell disease, identification of genetic modifiers is a particularly promising approach. Methods to further study gene manipulation may include case/control studies and/or studies of twins, of sibling pairs and of individuals with unusually mild phenotypes. A search for genetic modifiers in applicable transgenic animal models might also prove beneficial (Yang and Pace 2001; Amrolia et al. 2003b; Beuzard 1996; Gaziev and Lucarelli 2003; Naffakh and Danos 1996).

Pharmacogenomics may also be a useful tool. Small molecule screens can be utilized to investigate possible new targets for therapeutics for sickle cell disease. Target-based compound screens to explore such possibilities as hemoglobin F induction, nitric oxide, antithrombotics/anticoagulants and other agents that might affect adhesion, inflammation, or oxidation would also be useful. Another genomic opportunity is performing proteomic and mRNA microarray-based analyses of bone marrow (if available), leukocytes, erythrocytes and their precursors, endothelial cells, etc. from a variety of patients with differing disease involvement. Promising results with selected pediatric and even adult sickle cell patients with bone marrow transplants from sibling donors using modified immunosuppression indicate that a more aggressive stance should be taken to implement this type of therapy more widely.

Summary

Sickle cell pain management requires an understanding of the complex sickle cell disease processes that vary with age, genomics, socioeconomics, environment, psychology, and therapy. Modern imaging techniques help elucidate the cause and location of pain as well as direct therapy. Treatments to prevent acute, life-threatening problems and pain can, ironically, create other serious chronic and acute challenges such as iron overload and complex pain syndromes. As the root cause is genetic, translational and integrative medical breakthroughs hold the most promise for optimal therapy and cure for sickle cell disease pain.

Acknowledgments The authors would like to thank Dr. Samir K. Ballas, Dr. Johnson Haynes, Jr., Director, USA Sickle Center, Univ. of South Alabama College of Medicine, Dr. William D. Morrison, Director of Musculoskeletal (MSK) Radiology, Jefferson Medical College, Philadelphia and Dr. Carlton Dampier, Director, Marian Anderson SCC Hematology/Oncology, St. Christopher's Hospital for Children, Philadelphia for sharing their expertise and materials in the preparation of this chapter.

References

Amrolia, P. J., Almeida, A., Davies, S. C., & Roberts, I. A. (2003a). Therapeutic challenges in childhood sickle cell disease. Part 2: a problem-orientated approach. *British Journal Haematology, 120,* 737–743.

Amrolia, P. J., Almeida, A., Halsey, C., Roberts, I. A., & Davies, S. C. (2003b). Therapeutic challenges in childhood sickle cell disease. Part 1: current and future treatment options. *British Journal Haematology, 120,* 725–736.

Ballas, S. K. (1990). Treatment of pain in adults with sickle cell disease. *American Journal of Hematology, 34,* 49–54.

Ballas, S. K. (1995). The sickle cell painful crisis in adults: phases and objective signs. *Hemoglobin, 19,* 323–333.

Ballas, S. K. (1997). Management of sickle pain. *Current Opinion in Hematology, 4,* 104–111.

Ballas, S. K. (1998). *Sickle cell pain* (p. ix). Seattle: International Association for the Study of Pain Press.

Ballas, S. K. (2005). Pain management of sickle cell disease. *Hematology/Oncology Clinics of North America, 19,* 785–802.

Ballas, S. K. (2008). Meperidine for acute sickle cell pain in the emergency department: revisited controversy. *Annals of Emergency Medicine, 51,* 217.

Ballas, S. K., & Marcolina, M. J. (2006). Hyperhemolysis during the evolution of uncomplicated acute painful episodes in patients with sickle cell anemia. *Transfusion, 46,* 105–110.

Ballas, S. K., & Mohandas, N. (1996). Pathophysiology of vaso-occlusion. *Hematology/Oncology Clinics of North America, 10,* 1221–1239.

Ballas, S. K., Cai, S. P., Gabuzda, T., & Chehab, F. F. (1997). Molecular basis of asymptomatic beta-thalassemia major in an African American individual. *American Journal of Medical Genetics, 69,* 196–199.

Ballas, S. K., Barton, F. B., Waclawiw, M. A., Swerdlow, P., Eckman, J. R., Pegelow, C. H., Koshy, M., Barton, B. A., & Bonds, D. R. (2006). Hydroxyurea and sickle cell anemia: effect on quality of life. *Health and Quality of Life Outcomes, 4,* 59.

Barakat, L. P., Patterson, C. A., Weinberger, B. S., Simon, K., Gonzalez, E. R., & Dampier, C. (2007). A prospective study of the role of coping and family functioning in health outcomes for adolescents with sickle cell disease. *Journal of Pediatric Hematology/Oncology, 29,* 752–760.

Bardakdjian-Michau, J. (2003). Neonatal detection of sickle cell disease. *Journal de Gynecologie, Obstetrique et Biologie de la Reproduction (Paris), 32*(1), S61–S64.

Beuzard, Y. (1996). Towards gene therapy of hemoglobinopathies. *Seminars in Hematology, 33,* 43–52.

Blaylock, B. (1996). Sickle cell leg ulcers. *Medsurg Nursing, 5,* 41–43.

Brousseau, D. C., McCarver, D. G., Drendel, A. L., Divakaran, K., & Panepinto, J. A. (2007). The effect of CYP2D6 polymorphisms on the response to pain treatment for pediatric sickle cell pain crisis. *Jornal de Pediatria, 150,* 623–626.

Carvalho, K. S., & Garg, B. P. (2002). Arterial strokes in children. *Neurologic Clinics, 20,* 1079–1100. vii.

Charache, S. (1996). Treatment of sickling disorders. *Current Opinion in Hematology, 3,* 139–144.

Chen, S. H., Liang, D. C., Lin, H. C., Cheng, S. Y., Chen, L. J., & Liu, H. C. (2005). Auditory and visual toxicity during deferoxamine therapy in transfusion-dependent patients. *Journal of Pediatric Hematology/Oncology, 27,* 651–653.

Chiodo, A. A., Alberti, P. W., Sher, G. D., Francombe, W. H., & Tyler, B. (1997). Desferrioxamine ototoxicity in an adult transfusion-dependent population. *The Journal of Otolaryngology, 26,* 116–122.

Chulamokha, L., Scholand, S. J., Riggio, J. M., Ballas, S. K., Horn, D., & DeSimone, J. A. (2006). Bloodstream infections in hospitalized adults with sickle cell disease: a retrospective analysis. *American Journal of Hematology, 81,* 723–728.

Cordner, S., & De, C. K. (2003). Musculoskeletal manifestations of hemoglobinopathies. *Current Opinion in Rheumatology, 15,* 44–47.

De Franceschi, L., Saadane, N., Trudel, M., et al. (1994). Treatment with oral clotrimazole blocks Ca^{2+}-mediated K^+ transport and reverses erythrocyte dehydration in transgenic SAD mice: a model for therapy of sickle cell disease. *The Journal of Clinical Investigation, 93,* 1670–1676.

Dickerhoff, R., & von, R. A. (1995). Pain crises in patients with sickle cell diseases. Pathogenesis, clinical aspects, therapy. *Klinische Pädiatrie, 207,* 321–325.

Dimashkieh, H., Choe, J., & Mutema, G. (2003). Renal medullary carcinoma: a report of 2 cases and review of the literature. *Archives of Pathology & Laboratory Medicine, 127,* e135–e138.

Dumaplin, C. A. (2006). Avoiding admission for afebrile pediatric sickle cell pain: pain management methods. *Journal of Pediatric Health Care, 20,* 115–122.

Eccleston, C., Yorke, L., Morley, S., Williams, A. C., & Mastroyannopoulou, K. (2003). Psychological therapies for the management of chronic and recurrent pain in children and adolescents. *Cochrane Database System Reviews, 99,* 157–65. CD003968.

Embury, S. H. (1986). The clinical pathophysiology of sickle cell disease. *Annual Review of Medicine, 37,* 361–376.

Epstein, K., Yuen, E., Riggio, J. M., Ballas, S. K., & Moleski, S. M. (2006). Utilization of the office, hospital and emergency department for adult sickle cell patients: a five-year study. *Journal of the National Medical Association, 98,* 1109–1113.

Erhan, E., Inal, M. T., Aydinok, Y., Balkan, C., & Yegul, I. (2007). Tramadol infusion for the pain management in sickle cell disease: a case report. *Paediatric Anaesthesia, 17,* 84–86.

Fosdal, M. B., & Wojner-Alexandrov, A. W. (2007). Events of hospitalization among children with sickle cell disease. *Journal of Pediatric Nursing, 22,* 342–346.

Fung, E. B., Harmatz, P., Milet, M., Ballas, S. K., De, C. L., Hagar, W., Owen, W., Olivieri, N., Smith-Whitley, K., Darbari, D., Wang, W., & Vichinsky, E. (2007). Morbidity and mortality in chronically transfused subjects with thalassemia and sickle cell disease: a report from the multi-center study of iron overload. *American Journal of Hematology, 82*, 255–265.

Gaziev, J., & Lucarelli, G. (2003). Stem cell transplantation for hemoglobinopathies. *Current Opinion in Pediatrics, 15*, 24–31.

Halsey, C., & Roberts, I. A. (2003). The role of hydroxyurea in sickle cell disease. *British Journal Haematology, 120*, 177–186.

Hebbel, R. P. (1985). Auto-oxidation and a membrane-associated 'Fenton reagent': a possible explanation for development of membrane lesions in sickle erythrocytes. *Clinics in Haematology, 14*, 129–140.

Herrick, J. B. (1910). Peculiar elongated and sickle-shaped red blood corpuscles in a case of severe anemia. *Archives of Internal Medicine, 6*, 517–521.

Huang, J., Zou, Z., Kim-Shapiro, D. B., Ballas, S. K., & King, S. B. (2003). Hydroxyurea analogues as kinetic and mechanistic probes of the nitric oxide producing reactions of hydroxyurea and oxyhemoglobin. *Journal of Medicinal Chemistry, 46*, 3748–3753.

Hungerford, D. S., & Lennox, D. W. (1985). The importance of increased intraosseous pressure in the development of osteonecrosis of the femoral head: implications for treatment. *The Orthopedic Clinics of North America, 16*, 635–654.

Jacob, E., Miaskowski, C., Savedra, M., Beyer, J. E., Treadwell, M., & Styles, L. (2006). Changes in sleep, food intake, and activity levels during acute painful episodes in children with sickle cell disease. *Journal of Pediatric Nursing, 21*, 23–34.

Kaul, D. K., Fabry, M. E., & Nagel, R. L. (1996). The pathophysiology of vascular obstruction in the sickle syndromes. *Blood Reviews, 10*, 29–44.

Kerle, K. K., & Nishimura, K. D. (1996). Exertional collapse and sudden death associated with sickle cell trait. *American Family Physician, 54*, 237–240.

Kooy, A., de Heide, L. J., ten Tije, A. J., Mulder, A. H., Tanghe, H. L., Kluytmans, J. A., & Michiels, J. J. (1996). Vertebral bone destruction in sickle cell disease: infection, infarction or both. *The Netherlands Journal of Medicine, 48*, 227–231.

Labie, D., & Elion, J. (1996a). Sickle cell anemia: model of variability in expression of monogenic disease. *Archives of Pediatrics, 3*, 101–103.

Labie, D., & Elion, J. (1996b). Sequence polymorphisms of potential functional relevance in the beta-globin gene locus. *Hemoglobin, 20*, 85–101.

Laird, L., Dezateux, C., & Anionwu, E. N. (1996). Neonatal screening for sickle cell disorders: what about the carrier infants? *British Medical Journal, 313*, 407–411.

Lane, P. A. (1996). Sickle cell disease. *Pediatric Clinics of North America, 43*, 639–664.

Lefevre-Witier, P. (1985). An anthropological perspective on the epidemiology of hemoglobin defects and glucose-6-phosphate dehydrogenase deficiencies in the northern half of the African continent. *Progress in Clinical and Biological Research, 194*, 367–397.

Mankad, V. N. (2001). Exciting new treatment approaches for pathphysiologic mechanisms of sickle cell disease. *Pediatric Pathology & Molecular Medicine, 20*, 1–13.

Marchant, W. A., & Walker, I. (2003). Anaesthetic management of the child with sickle cell disease. *Paediatric Anaesthesia, 13*, 473–489.

Mitchell, M. J., Lemanek, K., Palermo, T. M., Crosby, L. E., Nichols, A., & Powers, S. W. (2007). Parent perspectives on pain management, coping, and family functioning in pediatric sickle cell disease. *Clinical Pediatrics (Philadelphia), 46*, 311–319.

Molitierno, J. A., Jr. (2003). Carson CC, III: urologic manifestations of hematologic disease sickle cell, leukemia, and thromboembolic disease. *The Urologic Clinics of North America, 30*, 49–61.

Moore, C. M., Ehlayel, M., Leiva, L. E., & Sorensen, R. U. (1996). New concepts in the immunology of sickle cell disease. *Annals of Allergy, Asthma & Immunology, 76*, 385–400.

Murray, M. J., & Evans, P. (1996). Sudden exertional death in a soldier with sickle cell trait. *Military Medicine, 161*, 303–305.

Naffakh, N., & Danos, O. (1996). Gene transfer for erythropoiesis enhancement. *Molecular Medicine Today, 2*, 343–348.

Nowak-Gottl, U., Straeter, R., Sebire, G., & Kirkham, F. (2003). Antithrombotic drug treatment of pediatric patients with ischemic stroke. *Paediatric Drugs, 5*, 167–175.

Owusu-Ofori, S., & Riddington, C. (2002). Splenectomy versus conservative management for acute sequestration crises in people with sickle cell disease. *Cochrane Database System Reviews*, PubMed, CD003425.

Pandit, H. M. (1996). Viruses–a conundrum. *Physiological Chemistry and Physics and Medical NMR, 28*, 29–33.

Rao, V. M., Sebes, J. I., Steiner, R. M., & Ballas, S. K. (1991). Noninvasive diagnostic imaging in hemoglobinopathies. *Hematology/Oncology Clinics of North America, 5*, 517–533.

Scheinman, J. I. (2003). Sickle cell disease and the kidney. *Seminars in Nephrology, 23*, 66–76.

Serjeant, G. R. (1996). The role of preventive medicine in sickle cell disease. The Watson Smith lecture. *Journal of the Royal College of Physicians of London, 30*, 37–41.

Setty, B. N., Kulkarni, S., Dampier, C. D., & Stuart, M. J. (2001). Fetal hemoglobin in sickle cell anemia: relationship to erythrocyte adhesion markers and adhesion. *Blood, 97*, 2568–2573.

Sing, C. F., Boerwinkle, E., & Moll, P. P. (1985). Strategies for elucidating the phenotypic and genetic heterogeneity of a chronic disease with a complex etiology. *Progress in Clinical and Biological Research, 194*, 39–66.

Smith, T. G., Ayi, K., Serghides, L., Mcallister, C. D., & Kain, K. C. (2002). Innate immunity to malaria caused by Plasmodium falciparum. *Clinical and Investigative Medicine, 25*, 262–272.

Steinberg, M. H. (1996). Modulation of the phenotypic diversity of sickle cell anemia. *Hemoglobin, 20*, 1–19.

Steiner, R. M., Mitchell, D. G., Rao, V. M., Murphy, S., Rifkin, M. D., Burk, D. L., Jr., Ballas, S. K., & Vinitski, S. (1990). Magnetic resonance imaging of bone marrow: diagnostic value in diffuse hematologic disorders. *Magnetic Resonance Quarterly, 6*, 17–34.

Stinson, J., & Naser, B. (2003). Pain management in children with sickle cell disease. *Paediatric Drugs, 5*, 229–241.

Styles, L. A., & Vichinsky, E. P. (1996). Ototoxicity in hemoglobinopathy patients chelated with desferrioxamine. *Journal of Pediatric Hematology/Oncology, 18*, 42–45.

Terk, M. R., Zee, C. S., Colletti, P. M., & Haywood, L. J. (1996). The application of magnetic resonance techniques to the evaluation of the patient with sickle-cell disease. *Biomedical Instrumentation & Technology, 30*, 349–353.

Walco, G. A., & Dampier, C. D. (1987). Chronic pain in adolescent patients. *Journal of Pediatric Psychology, 12*, 215–225.

Wald, E. R. (1985). Risk factors for osteomyelitis. *The American Journal of Medicine, 78*, 206–212.

Weatherall, D. J. (1985). WWJRCJB: The developmental genetics of human hemoglobin. *Progress in Clinical and Biological Research, 191*, 3–25.

Weatherall, D. J., Old, J. M., Thein, S. L., Wainscoat, J. S., & Clegg, J. B. (1985). Prenatal diagnosis of the common haemoglobin disorders. *Journal of Medical Genetics, 22*, 422–430.

Yang, Y. M., & Pace, B. (2001). Pharmacologic induction of fetal hemoglobin synthesis: cellular and molecular mechanisms. *Pediatric Pathology & Molecular Medicine, 20*, 87–106.

Zago, M. A., & Costa, F. F. (1985). Hereditary haemoglobin disorders in Brazil. *Transactions of the Royal Society of Tropical Medicine and Hygiene, 79*, 385–388.

Pain Management in Pediatric Palliative Care

12

Tamara Vesel, Patricia O'Malley,
and Benjamin Howard Lee

Keywords

Family-centered in approach • Palliative care, goals • Conflicts in ethical practice • WHO principles by the ladder • "Double effect" • Comfort sedation

Introduction

Pediatric palliative care is an approach to delivering comprehensive, symptom-based, compassionate care to children with chronic complex conditions (CCC) and/or life-threatening conditions which treats the patient and his/her family as the unit of care (family-centered in approach). Palliative care is focused on providing a systematic approach to enhancing quality of life, minimizing suffering, optimizing function, and providing opportunities for personal and spiritual growth (Friebert 2009). Palliative care is concerned with the physical, psychosocial, and spiritual care of children with a life-limiting or life-threatening illness. The goal of palliative medicine is to provide the best possible quality of life by providing holistic care at every stage of the illness and, as such, this care is not reserved only for the imminently dying patient.

Each year in the USA, approximately 50,000 children die and 500,000 children live with life-threatening illness. Palliative care medicine developed initially in response to the physical, emotional, psychological, and spiritual needs of adults dying from cancer. Of necessity, pediatric palliative care must have a broader scope because of the heterogeneity of life span–limiting conditions that affect children and the varying trajectories of health and illness these conditions follow (Himelstein et al. 2004). In 1993, the World Health Organization defined pediatric palliative care as compassionate and all-inclusive care when curative treatments are no longer possible. Since then, pediatric palliative care has broadened into family-centered care aimed at enhancing quality of life and minimizing suffering of all children with life-threatening conditions, no matter what the outcome of the illness is (American Academy of Pediatrics 2000).

Pain control and symptom management are integral aspects of quality palliative care. Assessment and management of pain and suffering should always consider the larger context of social, emotional, physical, and spiritual meaning, especially in the context of treating a child's pain at end-of-life. Many physical and psychological symptoms are common at the end-of-life. Optimum treatment will entail comprehensive and timely assessment, use of pharmacological

T. Vesel (✉)

Dana–Farber Cancer Institute, 450 Brookline Avenue, Boston, MA 02215, USA

e-mail: Tamara_vesel@dfci.harvard.edu

B.C. McClain and S. Suresh (eds.), *Handbook of Pediatric Chronic Pain: Current Science and Integrative Practice*, DOI 10.1007/978-1-4419-0350-1_12, © Springer Science+Business Media, LLC 2011

and non-pharmacological interventions, and an expert multidisciplinary team of health-care providers. Parents and patients will often tolerate significant pain and suffering in the context of potential curative therapy if there is hope for recovery; however, tolerance for pain and suffering can change when the outcome of illness is more clearly pointing to failure of therapy and likely death.

The frequent struggle to balance the desire for a child's comfort with the goal for an awake and interactive child is always difficult, but can become particularly poignant at end-of-life if the family and the patient recognize that life span is significantly limited. The measurement of the benefits and burdens of life-extending technologies such as medically supplied nutrition and hydration or ventilatory support may also shift with end-of-life care, particularly if they are seen as contributing to a child's discomfort or distress. Suffering resulting from a child's pain and illness will often extend beyond the patient to involve his or her family, friends, and providers. A central tenet of palliative care is that the family is the unit of care, and this is truly the case when managing a child's pain at end-of-life.

Pain and Suffering in Children with Life-Threatening Illness

Despite increasing awareness about pain assessment and treatment over the most recent few decades, most children with advanced illness still experience pain. The high prevalence of pain in children with cancer has been recognized for many years. In a study by Miser et al. (1987a), the prevalence of pain in children with cancer in the outpatient clinic was 25%, and 50% of inpatients with cancer had pain. Most of the pain was associated with treatment for the disease. In a further study by Miser et al. (1987b), pain was the presenting symptom in 62% of children with newly diagnosed cancer, and this pain was present for a long time prior to diagnosis (median 74 days before cancer treatment). Many patients with moderate to severe pain were not receiving any analgesic therapy. Pain is also common with chronic conditions

such as cystic fibrosis (dyspnea, chest wall and abdominal pain, sinusitis, and headaches), neuromuscular and neurodegenerative diseases (contractures, back pain from scoliosis and facet joint arthritis, gastroesophageal reflux, osteoarthritis, nerve entrapment, or nerve injury), and HIV/AIDS (neuropathic pain).

Frequent Symptoms of Dying Children

Recently, we have gained more information about the symptoms of dying children through research focused on end-of-life care of children. However, there are few reports of the symptoms experienced by dying children, likely due to the difficulties inherit in conducting research involving fragile children, and most of these reports are retrospective. Pain is a common symptom in children at the end-of-life. Robinson et al. (1997) describe frequent use of opioids in the end-of-life care of 44 children with cystic fibrosis, noting that 86% received an opioid medication at the time of death. The indication for opioid use in these children was for treatment of chest pain and/or dyspnea. Unfortunately, the authors do not describe the effectiveness of opioid therapy in this report. Sirkia et al. (1998) reported their evaluation of the need for pain management and the adequacy of analgesia for children who died receiving palliative care. This retrospective study of medical records and a structured interview of both parents indicated that most children (89%) received treatment for pain, and adequate analgesia was achieved in the majority (81%) of children with cancer. In stark contrast are the findings of Wolfe at al. (2000) in a retrospective study of 103 parents of children who died of cancer between 1990 and 1997 at Children's Hospital, Boston and the Dana–Farber Cancer Institute. Wolfe reports that 89% of parents felt their child suffered "a lot" or "a great deal" from at least one symptom in the last month of life. The most common symptoms were pain, fatigue, and dyspnea.

Drake at al. (2003) examined the symptom prevalence, characteristics and distress of 30 children dying in the hospital. Symptoms during the last week of life were obtained from medical records, and symptoms and their characteristics during the last day of life were determined by nurse interview. The mean number of symptoms per patient in the last week of life was 11.1 ± 5.6 with six symptoms occurring with a prevalence of $\geq 50\%$. The location of death had a significant impact on the mean number of symptoms: ward (14.3 ± 6.1) versus intensive care (9.5 ± 4.7). In general, symptoms in the last day of life were not associated with a high level of distress. Jalmsell at al. (2006) aimed to study symptoms in children with cancer the last month of their lives. This study was a population-based national survey in Sweden of 449 of 561 eligible parents who lost children during a 6-year period. The symptoms most frequently reported by parents with a high or moderate impact on the child's well-being were physical fatigue (86%), reduced mobility (76%), pain (73%), and decreased appetite (71%). The prevalence of pain in dying children is quite significant, and inadequately treated pain is a common finding in the literature.

Palliative Care

What Children Want

Although many inferences have been drawn from communication via play, art, and storytelling (Pazola and Gerberg 1990) regarding the likelihood that dying children have very similar desires to those of dying adults, there are few direct interviews of children to ascertain their feelings and wishes at the end-of-life. In an interview with 14-year-old Mattie Stepanek, a poet who died of muscular dystrophy, Mattie speaks compellingly of the wish to have choices in aspects of his treatment, and to have a sense that people are listening to his wishes and worries (Education Development Center 2003). Similar to dying adults, dying children may likely wish for autonomy, dignity, comfort, and the opportunity to make meaning of their lives and leave a legacy to those they love, as well as an opportunity to resolve conflicts prior to their death. Despite our understanding of the developmental evolution of the child's concept of death and dying (Himelstein et al. 2004), it may be presumptuous to assume that children do not struggle with the same end-of-life issues as adults. Children often are constrained from sharing their concerns for fear that they will add to their parents' and family's distress; they may decline the opportunity for better pain management because they may feel it is a sign of giving up or disappointing their family. For some children, pain (as well as the underlying condition) may be perceived as deserved punishment.

What Parents/Families Want

Pain management at end-of-life cannot happen in isolation from other central aspects of end-of-life care. In the hospital setting, parents identify pain management as one of the most important aspects of end-of-life care for their child, but they also place high value on the following: complete and honest information, ready access to staff, coordination of the communication from multiple providers, emotional expression and empathetic support from staff, preservation of the integrity of the parent–child relationship, and acknowledgment of the role of faith and meaning-making (Meyer et al. 2002). Contrary to many providers' beliefs, parents may derive greater hope from full disclosure of a child's prognosis than from communication which attempts to shield the parents from the provider's full understanding of a child's likelihood of recovery (Mack et al. 2006). Perception of their child's suffering and pain is a touchstone for parents' decision making, along with their broader assessment of quality of life and expected neurological recovery (Wolfe et al. 2000; Meyer et al. 2006). In end-of-life care in the home setting, parents report that having a medical provider present at time of death is very comforting. Family-centered care is also concerned with the care and emotional well-being of the patient's siblings. Siblings often fear that they are responsible for, or vulnerable to, the same suffering as the affected child, and often have difficulty finding a safe place in which to reveal those fears.

What Clinicians Want

A recently published survey of pediatric residents in a single program identified better skills in pain management as the primary education need expressed by residents caring for children at end-of-life. Their comments implicitly recognize that pain management does not happen in isolation, and communication skills were listed as the next four most important education needs, namely to be able to communicate regarding prognosis, bad news, code status, and to be able to talk with a child about dying (Kolarik et al. 2006).

Nurses often report conflicts in ethical practice, in providing adequate pain management versus hastening death, and in truth telling to children whose parents are not willing or able to disclose the likelihood of their child's impending death (Solomon et al. 2005).

A disparity between family and provider' perceptions regarding adequacy of pain management at end-of-life was noted by Contro et al. (2004). A majority of families reported feeling that all that could be done to manage their child's pain had been done, whereas the majority of staff revealed concerns that their pain management skills were inadequate to the task of caring for a dying child. Clinicians from different disciplines report the need for more personal support during the difficult task of providing compassionate end-of-life care to children.

Quality Pediatric Palliative Care

Recently, health-care providers are involved in the attempt to provide care that is both clinically effective and results in an improvement in patient-reported outcomes. There has been a renewed emphasis on the quality of care rendered to patients as identified by measuring process and outcomes for patient care. Quality pediatric palliative care is timely (occurring at the point of need and not just at end-of-life), beneficial (safe care with positive influence on process and outcomes), effective (evidence-based when possible), efficient (process of care meets the needs of the patient), accessible (available to all who need it), and is patient centered.

Principles of Pain Control in Pediatric Palliative Care

Pain assessment and management is an integral component of high-quality, clinically effective palliative care. There may be many sources of pain for the patient including progressive disease, symptoms/side effects of the therapy, and pain associated with invasive procedures. The pain may be nociceptive or neuropathic in character. The perception of pain by children is affected by their age and cognitive level, previous pain experiences, ability to control the environment, their expectations regarding potential recovery, and the relevance of pain or the disease causing pain. Pain assessment should occur with regular frequency to gauge the severity of the pain and its response to intervention. Appropriate analgesics should be available and should be given on a fixed, regular dosing interval. Adjunctive therapy is needed for the treatment of analgesic side effects/adverse events as well as for neuropathic pain syndromes. The use of non-pharmacological adjunctive therapy to modify situational factors may also be useful. The focus of treatment is child-centered and family centered.

There are many potential barriers to effective pain management for children. The providers may withhold treatment for fear of potential harm to the patient. Providers often worry about the likelihood of respiratory depression and serious adverse effects. There remains a significant lack of education to providers in the principles of pain assessment and treatment. There remains a fear of patient addiction and abuse as well as the concern over possible drug diversion. Initiating opioid dosing for pain control may be perceived by the patient or the family as a sign of "giving up." There may be a lack of clear goals elicited from the patient and/or family resulting in confusion over methods to achieve adequate pain control. Issues such as preservation of normal routines, location of treatment (home vs. hospital), and level of alertness desired at the time of imminent death may impact the use of medications for pain control.

In order to achieve effective pain management, the provider needs a comprehensive, age-appropriate pain assessment strategy, an individualized treatment plan, and a regular review and adjustment of the plan as needed. A thorough pain assessment will include a description of the sensory characteristics of the pain (onset, duration, intensity, character, location, precipitating factors) as well as potential behavioral factors (coping style, learned pain behaviors, distress level, social dimensions). Age-appropriate tools for measurement of pain in children may be classified as self-report, behavioral, or physiologic measures. Self-report scales (visual analog scale, numerical rating scale, Bieri faces scale, Wong-Baker faces scale) are the "gold standard" for measurement of pain. In infants, tools that use behavioral and physiological measures are commonly used for pain in the very young. For cognitively impaired children, there are validated tools to elicit pain measurement such as the Gauvain-Piquard Scale (Gauvain-Piquard et al. 1999) or the Non-Communicating Children's Pain Checklist (Breau et al. 2002).

Although there are several guidelines for providing pain management for children in the palliative care setting, many practitioners will use the "analgesic ladder" endorsed by the World Health Organization (WHO) and the International Association for the Study of Pain (IASP) in 1998 (World Health Organization 1998). This graded or stepwise approach to pain management recommends a strategy for using nonopioid analgesics for mild pain, and progressing to stronger opioids and invasive therapy for severe and refractive pain (Fig. 12.1). Mild pain is treated with non-pharmacologic methods (cognitive therapies) and nonsteroidal anti-inflammatory agents (NSAIDs) or acetaminophen (APAP). Moderate pain is treated with NSAIDs/APAP with an oral opioid (oxycodone/hydrocodone/codeine), and severe pain is treated with potent oral or parenteral opioids (morphine/hydromorphone/methadone). In appropriate patients with refractory pain, the provider may consider invasive methods for pain control such as regional neurolytic blockade, neuraxial analgesics (local analgesics with opioids and/or clonidine), or neurosurgical techniques for pain management. Adjuvant medications, a diverse group of medications that may enhance the effects of nonopioid or opioid analgesics, have independent analgesic activity in

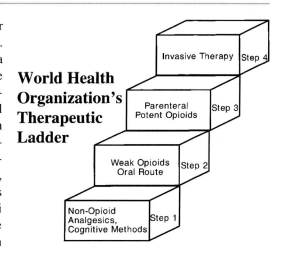

World Health Organization's Therapeutic Ladder

Fig. 12.1   WHO analgesic ladder for cancer pain relief and palliative care

certain pain syndromes or conditions, or counteract the side effects of analgesics, may be introduced at any point along the analgesic ladder if the patient's pain is likely to be responsive to these medications. They represent multiple drug classes including the following: antidepressants, anticonvulsants, local anesthetics, corticosteroids, antispasmodic agents, benzodiazepines, alpha-2 adrenergic agents, NMDA-receptor antagonists, stimulants, skeletal muscle relaxants, bisphosphonates, calcitonin, radionucleotides, and cannabinioids. For many of these agents, their primary indication is for conditions other than pain.

The WHO recommends four principles to guide analgesic administration for children in the palliative care setting: "by the ladder," using the WHO analgesic ladder with adjuvant drugs as needed; "by the clock," with analgesics being given on a regular schedule (not *pro re nata* [*prn*]); "by the child," with individualized therapy and regular assessment and updates as needed; and "by the mouth," with administration by the simplest and most effective route (orally for most patients).

Acetaminophen (APAP) and NSAIDs are often used for the treatment of mild pain. The mechanism of action of acetaminophen is largely by the central inhibition of the cyclo-oxygenase pathway in the central nervous system resulting in analgesia with minimal peripheral anti-inflammatory effects.

APAP is generally well-tolerated in children and is inexpensive. Disadvantages of use include the potential to mask a fever as sign of infection with potential risks in immunocompromised individuals as well as potential hepatic toxicity with prolonged use, especially in large doses. NSAIDs have moderately good analgesic properties with no physical dependency or sedation associated with use. NSAIDs principally inhibit the cyclooxygenase and lipoygenase pathways in peripheral nociceptors leading to analgesia. There are also minor centrally mediated effects via endogenous opioid peptides, cyclo-oxygenase inhibition, and serotonergic-mediated effects. NSAIDs are useful for bone pain and inflammation; however, they may inhibit platelet function, mask fever, and have potential GI and renal toxicity associated with prolonged use.

Opioid analgesics are very commonly used in the palliative care of children, especially at the end-of-life. Opioid analgesics will decrease or modify the perception of pain in the central nervous system, and these medications are titrated to effect as they have no ceiling effect for dose. Opioids provide analgesia principally via the mu, kappa, and delta opioid receptors by mimicking the actions of the endogenous opioid peptides resulting in membrane hyperpolarization and analgesia. Side effects are often dose-dependent and may involve sedation and respiratory depression in some patients. Thus, patients who are taking opioid medications for pain need to be monitored regularly for efficacy and adverse effects. There is no evidence that one opioid is more effective clinically than another, and the choice of opioid is individualized with respect to the patient's clinical state, previous responses to the agent, and potential for side effects. Providers should administer the agent at regular intervals with "rescue" dosing for breakthrough pain. The typical "rescue" dose is 5–10% of the daily requirement of the opioid which can be given as frequently as every 1 h for unrelieved pain. Escalation of dosing with incorporation of the breakthrough doses is encouraged to titrate to effect or side effects. Key concepts for the use of opioids for pain management include titration to effect, a goal for steady-state analgesia, anticipation and treatment of side effects, and use

of equianalgesic doses when switching opioids in patients who are opioid-naïve.

Codeine and tramadol are used often for mild to moderate pain and are so-called weak opioids due to their ceiling effect (an increase in dose will cause side effects at some point but not increased analgesia). Codeine has a variable bioavailability (15–80%) but also is an inactive prodrug that has analgesic efficacy only via metabolism to morphine. This metabolism is dependent on the mixed function oxidases with the cytochrome P450 2D6 enzyme isomer. There are slow metabolizers of codeine (Caucasian 10%, Chinese 30%), and the drug is ineffective for these patients while 5% of the population will be ultra-rapid metabolizers with increased concentrations of morphine (Williams et al. 2001). Tramadol is a weak mu-receptor opioid agonist and norepinephrine/serotonin reuptake inhibitor used for mild to moderate pain. It has been used in Europe for many decades and is becoming more popular in the USA. Tramadol is largely eliminated by the kidney and has nausea/vomiting, dizziness, constipation, and sedation as common side effects. It should be used cautiously in patients with a history of seizure disorder or with medications that potentially lower the seizure threshold. It has also been associated with serotonergic syndrome in some patients with concomitant risk factors.

Potent opioids are used for the treatment of moderate to severe pain. Oral dosing is the most common route of administration; however, intravenous, subcutaneous injection/infusion, rectal dosing, and transdermal dosing options are used as needed. Morphine is the "gold standard" for palliative care pain management due to the long track record of safe use, the availability of the agent in various formulations, and its hydrophilicity. Morphine has active metabolites so should be used cautiously in the presence of renal disease/failure. Morphine has poor oral bioavailability, has histamine release associated with its use, and may cause vasodilatation with hypotension in hypovolemic patients. Hydromorphone is more potent than morphine with minimal active metabolites so it may be useful in patients with renal disease. Fentanyl is highly lipid soluble with a rapid onset of action. It is 50–100 times more potent than morphine and has no active metabolites. Tolerance and dependence may occur rapidly, and fentanyl is available as a transdermal patch for patients with chronic pain. It is also available as a buccal transmucosal oralet for use for procedural pain or as a breakthrough agent (Table 12.1).

Methadone is a unique long-acting opioid that is a racemic mixture of two isomers. The drug is a μ-receptor opioid agonist with some activity also at the δ and κ receptors; it is also an N-methyl-D-aspartate (NMDA) receptor antagonist. The L-isomer of methadone inhibits serotonin and norepinephrine reuptake as well. The drug is lipophilic with high oral bioavailability (80–90%)

Table 12.1 Commonly used mu agonist drugs

Agonist	Equipotent IV dose (mg/kg)	Duration (hr)	Bioavailability (%)	Comments
Morphine	0.1	3–4	20–40	• "Gold Standard," very inexpensive • Can cause seizures in newborns • Histamine release, vasodilation (avoid in asthmatics and in circulatory compromise) • MS-Contin® 8–12 h duration (pill), cannot be crushed or given via a gastric tube • Liquid morphine 2–20 mg/mL
Meperidine	1	3–4	40–60	• Catastrophic interactions with MAO Inhibitors • Tachycardia; negative inotrope • Metabolite produces seizures • 0.25 mg/kg effectively treats shivering • **Not recommended for routine use**
Hydromor-phone (Dilaudid)	0.015	3–4	50–70	• Less itching and nausea than morphine, commonly used when morphine produces too many of these systemic side effects
Fentanyl	0.001	0.5–1		• Very effective for short painful procedures • Bradycardia; minimal hemodynamic alterations • Chest wall rigidity (>5 mcg/kg rapid IV bolus). R_x naloxone or succinylcholine or pancuronium • Oral transmucosal dose 10–15 mcg/kg
Methadone	0.1	4–24	70–100	• Liquid preparation available • Long duration of action makes it ideal for cancer pain, weaning dependent patients, etc. weaning
Codeine	1.2	3–4	40–70	• PO only • Prescribe with acetaminophen
Hydrocodone	0.1	3–4	60–80	• PO only • Usually prescribed with acetaminophen • Less nausea than codeine
Oxycodone	0.1	3–4	60–80	• PO only • Sustained-release tablet available • Usually prescribed with acetaminophen • Less nausea than codeine

and is slowly metabolized in the liver. The metabolites of methadone are not pharmacologically active. This agent has a long and unpredictable elimination half-life ranging from 12 to 200 h. The analgesic efficacy is much shorter than the elimination half-life. The potency of methadone is roughly equal for opioid-naïve patients; however, the potency of methadone is 4–20 times that of oral morphine with opioid-tolerant patients. The conversion of oral morphine to methadone is dose-dependent and is as follows (Houlahan et al. 2006):

Oral morphine (mg/24 h)	Oral morphine/ oral methadone ratio
<100 mg	4:1
101–300 mg	8:1
301–600	10:1
601–1,000	15:1
>1,000	20:1

The practitioner must use caution when switching from another opioid to methadone. After using the table to calculate equianalgesic dose of methadone, the calculated dose should be decreased by 50%, because of methadone inhibition of NMDA receptor. The agent is usually given as BID or TID dosing.

Adverse effects due to opioids are not uncommon, and constipation is a predictable side effect with prolonged use. It occurs in virtually all cases, so a prescription to treat constipation should be administered as soon as an opioid is started. Sedation with opioid use is common and can significantly impact the child and the family's quality of life. If sedation does not dissipate after a few days, add an adjuvant drug and decrease the opioid dose, give the patient a stimulant such as methylphenidate or dextroamphetamine, or consider switching to a different opioid. Nausea and/or vomiting may occur with opioid use and can be treated by opioid rotation, the use of selective 5-HT$_3$ receptor antagonists such as ondansetron, the addition of a bowel stimulant such as metoclopramide, or the use of an ultra-low dose naloxone infusion (0.25–1 mcg/kg/h) in patients with IV access. Pruritis is treated by opioid rotation, use of adjuvants to decrease opioid dose, or antipruretics such as naloxone, nalbuphene, or diphenhydramine. Respiratory depression is another

Table 12.2 Equianalgesic conversion of opioid analgesics

Oral/rectal dose (mg)	Analgesic	Parenteral dose (mg)
150	Codeine	50
150	Meperidine	50
150	Tramadol	–
15	Hydrocodone	–
15	Morphine	5
10	Oxycodone	–
3	Hydromorphone	1
2	Levorphanol	1
–	Fentanyl	0.05

potential side effect of opioids and is often cited by practitioners as a reason for not prescribing opioid analgesics for pain. However, an opioid-induced respiratory depression is less common than many practitioners believe and can largely be avoided with standard dosage titration and frequent monitoring in at-risk patients. Respiratory depression, if it does occur, is treatable with an opioid antagonist, stimulation, and bag/mask ventilation if necessary. Unless the patient is experiencing severe respiratory depression with hypoxia, small doses of naloxone (1–2 mcg/kg/dose) given every few minutes will often improve sedation without reversing the analgesic effects of the opioid. The patient will usually develop tolerance to the analgesic efficacy and the adverse effects of opioids with prolonged use with the exception of constipation. Frequent monitoring for efficacy and the development of adverse effects is needed, and, if the patient is developing tolerance to the medication, then the provider should consider opioid rotation. Switching to another agent will take advantage of the phenomenon of incomplete cross-tolerance in which lower doses vis-à-vis the recommended equianalgesic dose can be used with analgesic efficacy (Table 12.2).

Neuropathic Pain in Children with Cancer and Life-Limiting Illnesses

Neuropathic pain is associated with injury, dysfunction, or altered excitability of portions of the peripheral, central, or autonomic nervous system, and it is not associated with ongoing tissue inflammation or injury. Patients will present with sensory disturbances (allodynia, hyperpathia, hyperalgesia, cold hypersensitivity, and focal sensory deficits), motor disturbances (spasms, tremors, fasciculations, weakness, and atrophy), and autonomic disturbances (cyanosis, erythema, mottling, hyperhidrosis, and edema). Patients with neuropathic pain will often describe the pain as lancinating, burning, tingling, shooting, and/or electric-shock like in nature. The most common cause of neuropathic pain in patients with cancer is painful peripheral neuropathy caused by chemotherapeutic agents such as vincristine and cisplatin. Painful dysesthesias in the hands and feet are commonly seen associated with decreased deep tendon reflexes. This pain usually resolves within a few weeks after the removal of the chemotherapy; however, the pain may persist for months (Jacob 2004). In a review of children in hospice with neuropathic pain, Dougherty and Braun reported that dying children with neuropathic pain syndromes had higher baseline requirements for morphine and needed more aggressive dose escalation prior to their death (Dougherty and DeBaun 2003). Collins et al. described a greater likelihood of neuropathic pain in children with solid tumors that had involvement of nerve tissue or the central nervous system. In many cases, these patients had pain that was resistant to large doses of opioids (Collins et al. 1995, 1996; Collins 1996). Patients with HIV infection may also exhibit peripheral neuropathies with paresthesias and lancinating or burning pain, and patients may develop neuropathic pain from antiretroviral therapy for the HIV infection (Hirschfeld 1998). Other causes of neuropathic pain in patients with life-threatening illnesses include radiation therapy, surgical trauma, mechanical entrapment of nerves, and tumor encroachment (Galloway and Yaster 2000).

In a review of analgesics for the treatment of neuropathic pain in adults, Finnerup reported on the number needed to treat (NNT) to obtain one patient with 50% pain relief, and the most effective medications in descending order of efficacy were as follows: carbamezepine (2.0), "strong" opioids (2.5), valproate (2.8), tricyclic antidepressants [TCAs] (3.1), tramadol (3.9), lidocaine patch (4.4), gabapentin (4.7), SSRIs (6.8), and

topiramate (7.4) (Finnerup et al. 2005). There are randomized controlled trials indicating the efficacy of potent opioids and tramadol for the treatment of neuropathic pain in adults. There is evidence of the efficacy of TCAs for the treatment of painful diabetic neuropathy and postherpetic neuralgia. Calcium-channel alpha-2-delta ligands such as gabapentin and pregabalin have been shown to be useful for the treatment of phantom limb pain, neuropathic cancer pain, and peripheral neuropathies. There are a few case reports describing the utility of gabapentin and pregabalin for the treatment of neuropathic pain in children (Dayioglu et al. 2008; Butkovic et al. 2006; Lauder and White 2005; Carrazana and Mikoshiba 2003; Vondracek et al. 2009). NMDA-receptor blocking agents such as ketamine have been shown to decrease opioid requirements and improve pain control in a few case reports (Finkel et al. 2007). Evidence-based recommendations for the pharmacological management of neuropathic pain are the use of tricyclic antidepressants and serotonin/norepinephrine reuptake inhibitors (e.g, duloxetine), calcium-channel α2-δ ligands (gabapentin/pregabalin), and opioids for select clinical circumstances. Second- and third-line therapies involve treatment with opioids, antiepileptics and antidepressants for specific clinical issues, mexilitene, NMDA-receptor antagonists, and/or topical capsaicin (Dworkin et al. 2007). A potential stepwise approach to the treatment of neuropathic pain suggested by Friedrichsdorf is as follows (Zernikow et al. 2009; Friedrichsdorf and Kang 2007):

1. Identify and treat underlying disease process
2. Integrative therapies; manage comorbidities (anxiety/sleep disturbances)
3. Opioid (+ nonopioid) analgesics (consider tramadol vs. methadone)
4. Tricyclic antidepressants (or calcium-channel α2-δ ligands ± ketamine)
5. Tricyclic antidepressants and calcium-channel α2-δ ligands
6. Lidocaine patch
7. NMDA-receptor channel blocker, (benzodiazepines?)
8. Regional anesthesia

When possible, the initial management of neuropathic pain is to treat the underlying cause.

Table 12.3 Adjuvant medications to treat neuropathic pain (From Krane et al. (2003) used with permission)

Drug	Indications and uses	Pediatric dosing	Toxicity and notes
Lidocaine	Neuropathic pain, refractory, visceral pain	150 mcg/kg/h	Measure plasma level every 8–12 h and maintain 2–5 μg/mL
Mexiletine	See lidocaine	10–15 mg/kg	Sedation, fatigue, confusion, nausea, hypotension
Carbamazepine	Trigeminal neuralgia, neuropathic pain, migraine prophylaxis	15–30 mg/kg	Blood dyscrasias, monitor plasma level and periodic CBC
Valproate	Neuropathic pain, migraine prophylaxis, mood lability	10–60 mg/kg	Blood dyscrasias, hepatotoxicity, dose divided t.i.d., monitor plasma level periodic CBC and LFTs
Gabapentin	Neuropathic pain, migraine prophylaxis	5–30 mg/kg	Dose divided t.i.d. or q.i.d., escalate dose over several weeks to target dose
Amitriptyline, Nortriptyline	Neuropathic pain, migraine prophylaxis	0.05–2 mg/kg	Escalate dose over several weeks to target dose, does given h.s., obtain screening ECG before use, contraindicated in prolonged QTc
Venlafaxine	Chronic pain with depression, neuropathic pain	1–2 mg/kg	Dose divided b.i.d. or t.i.d., caution when used with TCAs or other SSRIs because of reported arrhythmias
Clonidine	Neuropathic pain, visceral pain, postoperative pain	0.05–0.2 mcg/kg/hr	By oral, transdermal, or continuous epidural infusion; may produce hypotension, bradycardia, somnolence

CBC complete blood count, *t.i.d.* three times a day, *LFTs* liver function tests, *q.i.d.* four times daily, *h.s.* at bedtime, *ECG* electrocardiogram, *b.i.d.* twice a day, *TCAs* tricyclic antidepressants, *SSRIs* selective serotonin reuptake inhibitors

Potential etiologies for neuropathic pain include neurodegenerative conditions, postsurgical pain, phantom limb pain, chemotherapy-induced pain, and tumor progression; potential therapies to treat the cause of neuropathic pain may include palliative radiation therapy, bisphosphonates for bone pain, corticosteroids, or surgery. Non-pharmacologic therapies include cognitive-behavioral interventions, acupuncture, transcutaneous nerve stimulation (TENS), massage, and physical therapy.

There are no randomized controlled trials for the use of pharmacologic agents for the treatment of neuropathic pain in children. Recommendations for therapy have evolved from a combination of studies of adult patients and case reports of efficacy in children. Opioids are commonly used for the management of neuropathic pain in the palliative care setting. Methadone is a useful agent due to its opioid receptor agonist activity and NMDA-receptor antagonist activity. Tramadol, a weak μ-receptor agonist and serotonin/norepinephrine reuptake inhibitor, is also a potentially useful agent for the treatment of neuropathic pain.

Adjuvant agents are often used for the management of neuropathic pain (Table 12.3). The effectiveness of tricyclic antidepressants (TCA) for the management of neuropathic pain is well established in adults. The mechanism of action of these agents is to inhibit the reuptake of serotonin and norepinephrine; common adverse effects of these agents include sedation, dry mouth, orthostatic hypotension, constipation, urinary retention, and tachycardia. Patients should receive an ECG prior to the initiation of TCA therapy to determine if there are any preexisting rhythm disturbances that may be exacerbated by TCA therapy (Table 12.4).

The calcium-channel α-2-δ ligands (gabapentin/pregabalin) are common first-line agents in adults, and gabapentin is commonly used in pediatric pain management (Dayioglu et al. 2008; Butkovic et al. 2006). There are few studies of pregabalin in pediatric patients for pain management (Vondracek et al. 2009). These agents affect the voltage-gated calcium channel resulting in decreased release of glutamine, norepinephrine,

Table 12.4 Sample dose titration regimen for nortriptyline and gabapentin for neuropathic pain (From Berde et al. (2003) used with permission)

1. Slow titration (e.g., ambulatory outpatients who are not debilitated)		
	<50 kg	
a. Nortriptyline or amitriptyline	Obtain baseline ECG	
Days 1–4	0.2 mg/kg q.h.s.	
Days 5–8	0.4 mg/kg q.h.s.	
Increase as tolerated every 4–6 days until		
i. Good analgesia		
ii. Limiting side effects or		
iii. Dosing reaches 1 mg/kg/d (<50 kg) or 50 mg (>50 mg)		
iv. If condition iii, consider measuring plasma concentration and ECG before further does escalation.		
Consider twice-daily dosing (25% in morning, 75% in evening).		
b. Gabapentin	<50 kg	>50 mg
Days 1–2	2 mg/kg q.h.s.	100 mg q.h.s.
Days 3–4	2 mg/kg b.i.d.	100 mg b.i.d.
Days 4–6	2 mg/kg t.i.d.	100 mg t.i.d.
Days 7–9	2, 2, 4 mg/kg (t.i.d. schedule)	100, 100, 200 mg
Increase as tolerated every 3 days (with 50% of daily dose in the evening) until		
i. Good analgesia		
ii. Limiting side effects or		
iii. Dosing reaches 60 mg/kg daily (<50 kg) or 3 g daily (>50 kg)		
2. Rapid titration (e.g., nonambulatory patients with widely metastatic cancer)		
a. Tricyclics: begin at 0.2 mg/kg (10 mg for >50 kg) and titrate up every 1–2 days in steps according to the slow titration regimen		
b. Gabapentin: begin at 6 mg/kg b.i.d. (300 mg b.i.d. for >50 kg) for 1–2 days, 6 mg/kg t.i.d. (300 mg t.i.d. for >50 kg) for 1 to days, 6 mg/kg morning and midday, 12 mg/kg q.h.s (300, 300, 600 mg for >50 kg) for 1–2 days, and increase as tolerated to 60 mg/kg daily (3 g/d for >50 kg) over 5–10 days		

ECG electrocardiogram, *q.h.s.* once daily at bedtime, *b.i.d.* twice daily, *t.i.d.* three times daily

and substance P. Dosing frequency is greater for these medications compared to the tricyclic antidepressants, and common adverse effects include sedation and ataxia (Table 12.4).

Ketamine is an NMDA-receptor antagonist that is used as an analgesic adjuvant in poorly controlled pain (Finkel et al. 2007). Ketamine is also an opioid-receptor agonist and a serotonin/norepinephrine reuptake inhibitor. Subtherapeutic dosing (0.25–0.5 mg/kg loading dose over 30 min is followed by a continuous infusion between 0.14 and 0.5 mg/kg/h) may be useful for neuropathic pain as well as attenuation of opioid-induced hyperalgesia (Tsui et al. 2004). Ketamine likely provides an additive analgesic effect as well as reversing opioid tolerance. Other NMDA-antagonists such as dextromethorphan and memantine have not been commonly used for children with neuropathic pain.

Membrane-stabilizing agents (lidocaine, mexiletene) are potentially useful in the treatment of neuropathic pain (Tremont-Lukats et al. 2006; Ferrini 2000; Nathan et al. 2005; Kastrup et al. 1987). There are sporadic case reports of the use of a lidocaine infusion for refractory pain in pediatric cancer patients (Massey et al. 2002). More commonly, the 5% transdermal lidocaine patch is applied for 12 h/day with a maximum use of three patches at one time in the adult-sized patient. The patch may be cut to size without loss of agent, and used over multiple areas topically. There are minimal systemic effects and plasma concentrations (1/10 for cardiac effects and 1/32 for toxicity). Alpha-2 agonists have demonstrated efficacy with epidural use for neuropathic pain associated with cancer. The mechanism of action is to act on the dorsal horn to facilitate the descending inhibitory pathway and the typical dose is 2–4 μg/kg every

4–6 hrs. This agent can also be given orally or via a transcutaneous patch.

Pain at the End-of-Life in the ICU

When parents were asked by researchers (Meyer et al. 2002) about the end-of-life care received by their children in a study of three major intensive care units in Boston between 1994 and 1996, they were able to place the highest priority on quality of life, likelihood of improvement, and perception of their child's pain when considering withdrawal of life support. In 2001, the Ethics Committee of the Society of Critical Care Medicine published recommendations for end-of-life care in the intensive care unit (Truog et al. 2001). They concluded that "palliative care and intensive care are not mutually exclusive options but rather should be coexistent." In the committee's recommendations, it became evident that both principles of intensive and palliative care are always present to some degree in the care of the critically ill patient. It became clear that there is a significant need for preparation of the patient, the family, and the clinical team for end-of-life events. The adult critical care literature identified important needs of the patients and these are summarized in Table 12.5.

Despite all the progress, many patients still die with treatable pain in the intensive care unit (1995). We think that one of the reasons is a strong bias in medicine toward curative therapy and less concentration on the symptom management. Palliative care medicine stresses the priority of symptom management at the end-of-life. The other reason for the undertreatment is that pain is a subjective phenomenon and, despite all

Table 12.5 Domains of good end-of life care

- Receiving adequate pain and symptom management
- Avoiding inappropriate prolongation of dying
- Achieving a sense of control
- Relieving burden
- Strengthening relationship with loved one

the efforts with pain assessment, in the process of dying in the intensive care unit we often rely on evaluation of consciousness and awareness, breathing patterns and hemodynamic parameters. In some circumstances a use of bispectral analysis (BIS monitoring), which uses an electroencephalographic signal to assess patient's level of consciousness is appropriate at the end-of-life, including the special circumstance of a patient having a neuromuscular blocking agent administered at the end-of-life. The assessment of the breathing pattern/dyspnea and related pain/discomfort is very complicated and not uniformly treated in the intensive care unit for the dying patient. Irregular breathing called "agonal breathing" in an unconscious patient and "death rattle" may be very distressing to the family members and child's parents. The controversy still persists around whether the clinician should treat the patient primarily to relieve the distress of the family.

The assessment of pain in dying neonates and small infants in the Neonatal Intensive Care Unit deserves special attention. Recognition of the clinical importance of neonatal pain and stress has been delayed by outdated professional attitudes (Anand 1998) (that newborns are less sensitive to pain), lack of education, need for accurate assessment methods, and lack of evidence for the safety and efficacy of management approaches that can be applied to the dying neonate. The literature (Schechter 1989) extends the same emphasis on relief of pain and suffering that has become mandatory for adults to the clinical management of dying newborns and children. Opioids have been the mainstay of therapy for pain at the end-of-life; thus, morphine, hydromorphone, and fentanyl are preferred agents to be used at the end-of-life according to the recommendations of the Society of Critical Care Medicine (SCCM).

Hampe and al. (Hampe 1975) conducted interviews with families in adult intensive care units and identified eight needs of spouses of dying patients in the hospital settings. Meta-analysis of several studies that used the Critical Care Family Inventory (Leske 1986) led to the summary listed

Table 12.6 Important needs of families of critically ill patients

To be with the person
To be helpful to the dying person
To be informed of the dying person's condition
To understand what is being done and why
To be assured of the patient's comfort
To be comforted
To ventilate emotions
To be assured that their decisions were right
To find meaning in the dying of their loved one
To be fed, hydrated, and rested

in Table 12.6. Based on clinical practice and literature we are aware that there are difficulties in this area. A summary of the existing literature related to moral distress and the pediatric intensive care unit (PICU) reveals a high-tech, high-pressure environment in which effective teamwork can be compromised by moral distress arising from different situations related to consent for treatment, futile care, end-of-life decision making, formal decision-making structures, training and experience by discipline, individual values and attitudes, and power and authority issues. Attempts to resolve moral distress around the end-of-life care in pediatric ICUs have included the use of administrative tools such as shift worksheets, the implementation of continuing education, and encouragement to report and debrief (Austin et al. 2009).

Pain at the End-of-Life for the Pediatric Cancer Patient

Pain in children with cancer may be due to disease progression, as a side effect of treatment, or be associated with procedures to provide therapy. Most dying children with cancer can be made comfortable with titrated oral doses of opioids and non-steroidal medications (Berde and Sethna 2002). If oral administration is not tolerated or is not desired by the patient and/or family, intravenous, rectal, subcutaneous, and transdermal routes can also be used. In addition, the use of non-pharmacologic interventions (cognitive therapy, relaxation,

imagery) is strongly encouraged. An initial pain assessment should be made with consideration of the following six principles:

- The patient and parents are the experts.
- A comprehensive pain assessment should be performed.
- Obtaining a history of previous pain management is critical.
- Pain assessment should identify all factors (physiological and non-physiological) contributing to a child's pain and suffering.
- A pain measurement tool should be used consistently and must be appropriate for the child's developmental stage.
- Pain must be reassessed following any intervention until desired clinical effect, and must continue on a regular basis thereafter.

The provider should discuss with the patient goals for pain therapy and ensure that the patient understands how to measure his/her pain and treat it, if the patient is cognitively and developmentally capable. Asking the child's parents what their goals and expectations regarding the child's pain and symptom management is important in order to have realistic goals and targets for appropriate patient/family-directed outcomes. The provider should provide information and council in order to teach the child and family about the significance of pain control in childhood cancer. Pain may frequently be associated with sleep disturbances, mood disturbances, and other significant symptoms.

The child or his/her parents may be hesitant or afraid to use opioid pain medications because of fears of addiction, overdose, side effects, or the symbolism of using a opioid which may be interpreted as "giving up" on curative therapy. The provider should encourage an open conversation about physical, psychological, and other aspects of pain and its management. The palliative care provider should recognize that there are often common fears and concerns of parents regarding opioid use, and should provide accurate information regarding misconceptions surrounding the use of opioids. The physician or provider should anticipate and respond to parents' concerns about addiction with opioids, common adverse side effects of opioids, risk of accidental overdose, and methods to ensure safety of use, the common myth of morphine's association with hastening death and dying, and the potential for drug theft and diversion. The health-care professional should consider addressing issues of tolerance, physical dependency, and addiction, explaining the difference between physical dependency and addiction while emphasizing that children would normally experience withdrawal symptoms if they are not tapered off opioid medication but that this is not the same thing as addiction (psychological craving for the medication).

If the patient presents with a new onset of pain or escalating pain, the provider should conduct a thorough pain assessment and initiate a STAT dose of an analgesic; reassessment of pain and pain relief should occur 15 min after IV/SC dosing or 30 min after oral dosing. If there is no relief, then give another dose and repeat until the pain is relieved or under control. The effective dose should be given as a scheduled dose (given around the clock, not prn), and a dose for breakthrough pain that would be approximately 1/10–1/6 of the daily dose given every hour prn. The scheduled doses and the breakthrough doses given over a 24 h period can be incorporated into larger scheduled doses of the immediate-release analgesic or can be replaced by dosing with a sustained release preparation of the medication (e.g., MSContin® or OxyContin®). If IV dosing is needed or desired, a PCA can be used with a continuous infusion of opioid which may be supplemented with PCA-bolus dosing as needed. If poor IV access and oral route is problematic, the practitioner may institute a subcutaneous (SC) infusion of opioid by using a small (25–27 gauge) needle placed SC in the thorax, abdomen, or thigh. Infusion rates should not exceed 1–3 cc/h, and the site should be rotated every 3 days. The SC dosing is the same as the IV dosing.

If the patient is experiencing poor analgesic relief from possible tolerance phenomenon or is having problematic adverse effects, consider opioid switching to another agent. The provider may consult a table for equianalgesic dosing to determine the dose of the new agent; however, incomplete cross-tolerance will guide the provider to reduce the dose of the new agent by 30–50%. If the provider would like to change his pain management regimen to a sustained-release opioid with a combination of immediate-release opioid, consult an equianalgesic table for opioid conversion (Abrahm 2005).

Anxiety is often associated with pain, suffering, and a life-threatening illness, and may be secondary to fear and uncertainty. An anxious patient will present with agitation, insomnia, restlessness, sweating, tachycardia, hyperventilation, panic disorder, tension, and worry. Benzodiazepines such as lorazepam (0.05 mg/kg PO,IV,or SL), midazolam (0.05 mg/kg IV, 0.5 mg/kg PO), clonazepam, and diazepam (0.1 mg/kg IV/PO) should be added to the regimen for anxiety that is associated with pain and suffering.

Pain and Symptom Management for the Imminently Dying Child/Palliative Sedation

As death approaches, pain may sometimes increase and become more refractory to treatment requiring rapid dose escalation of analgesics. The need for rapid escalation protocols has been examined by a few centers around the country. The Dana–Farber Cancer Institute/Children's Hospital, Boston Cancer Care Program has made it a priority to create a process of care that includes identifying barriers to care and the development of an end-of-life (EOL) rapid response model (Houlahan et al. 2006) that includes guidelines and standardized orders for the rapid escalation of opioids. The goal of this quality-improvement initiative was to develop a model of care that would enable the caregivers to provide effective comfort care to any patient experiencing symptoms of rapid escalation of pain, dyspnea, and agitation. A model of care was created to overcome barriers to care. Staff feedback was solicited relative to the content, format, and usability of the guidelines and standardized orders. The physician and nursing staff reported that they found the standardized orders and guidelines very helpful and effective. Our experience over the years suggests that templates are helpful but do not replace a highly educated clinician at the bedside of a dying child.

When physical suffering and pain are refractory to treatment with analgesics, the provider may want to consider the use of palliative sedation (terminal sedation) to relieve distress by inducing sedation and unconsciousness. The use of barbiturates for palliative sedation has been justified by ethicists and practitioners on the basis of reliable production of sedation and the principle of double effect. The American Academy of Pediatrics (AAP), in the policy on palliative care for children, recognizes that deep sedation may be needed to treat severe, progressive symptoms; however, the AAP guidelines are concerned to explicitly state that involuntary euthanasia or physician-assisted suicide is not supported (American Academy of Pediatrics 2000). Studies have shown that palliative sedation does not hasten death and is thus not euthanasia (Muller-Busch et al. 2003).

The principle of double effect states that the nature of the act must be good or at least morally neutral (providing sedation for comfort) and the intention of the agent is the good effect. The bad effect may be foreseen and tolerated, but not intended (providing sedation for comfort (good effect) and the patient dies from respiratory failure (bad effect) (Hawryluck et al. 2002). Requirements for palliative sedation include the following: use of all available effective treatments with documentation of patient suffering, use of the principle of double effect, understand and adhere to patient/family's wishes, document the plan, document the patient/family's consent, and seek an interdisciplinary team meeting with a hospital ethics consult. No consensus exists on the most appropriate medications for palliative sedation, and a variety of drugs have been used including barbiturates, benzodiazepines, and phenothiazines. Pentobarbital is commonly used with a typical loading dose of 1–4 mg/kg slow IV push followed by a continuous infusion of 1 mg/kg/h with titration to desired effect. The onset of action with IV dosing is within

1–5 min, and the duration of each IV injection is 15–45 min. Some practitioners will use the BIS monitor to guide level of sedation.

Pain at End of Life for the Neurologically Devastated Patient/Patient with Neurological Illness

Pediatric palliative care practitioners are often called upon to deal with rare or heterogeneous conditions for which there is little published experience in providing good symptom management at end-of-life (Labauge et al. 2007). Many children with neurological conditions will experience apparent pain which falls outside of the traditional categories of visceral, somatic, or neuropathic. The source of pain may be difficult to localize or manage, particularly if the child is unable to communicate easily; intestinal dysfunction exacerbated by feeding goals that are no longer applicable can often contribute considerable distress (Hauer et al. 2007). It will often be difficult to interpret what are causal and what are merely temporal effects without careful trial and experiment (Wusthoff et al. 2007). Often these are patients who are on a large number of medications for associated comorbidities, such as seizures, spasticity, respiratory secretions, bladder dysfunction, or intestinal dysfunction, and therefore untoward drug interactions will limit options for treatment and be difficult to predict.

In the setting of a progressive neurological disorder, pain takes on new meaning as a sign of potential progression of the underlying disease, and families will struggle with adhering to proposed medication plans because of the wish to keep a child awake and present, just as they may struggle with acceptance of hospice services as a sign of diminishing time left. For families who have managed complex medical care at home, uncontrolled pain undermines the sense of control and competence that they have acquired. Siblings easily read the signs of parental distress in the face of unmanaged pain and may become frightened at what they are not able to control. Providing relief from the distress while optimizing the patient's time while awake can help restore a sense of control even when it cannot alter the fact of impending death.

Summary

Many patients with complex chronic conditions have pain and suffering associated with their condition, especially towards the end-of-life. Managing the pain of a child at end-of-life requires considerable skill for palliative care practitioners, in order to treat our patients, their families, and the team of providers involved in this difficult work. Frequent pain assessment and flexibility in treatment are essential aspects of quality pain management. Excellent pain and symptom management at end-of-life leaves a lasting legacy of comfort to those who have cared for a dying child. We hope that research in pediatric palliative care (Steele et al. 2008) will start to answer some of the questions at the bedside and improve the quality of pain management of end-of-life care.

Reference List

The SUPPORT Principal Investigators. (1995). A controlled trial to improve care for seriously ill hospitalized patients. The study to understand prognoses and preferences for outcomes and risks of treatments (SUPPORT). The SUPPORT Principal Investigators. *Journal of the American Medical Association, 274*(20), 1591–1598.

Abrahm, J. (2005). *A physician's guide to pain and symptom management in cancer patients* (2nd ed.). Baltimore: Johns Hopkins University Press.

American Academy of Pediatrics. (2000). Committee on bioethics and committee on hospital care. Palliative care for children. *Pediatrics, 106*(2 Pt 1), 351–357.

Anand, K. J. S. (1998). Clinical importance of pain and stress in preterm newborn infants. *Biology of the Neonate, 73*, 1–9.

Austin, W., Kelecevic, J., Goble, E., & Mekechuk, J. (2009). An overview of moral distress and the paediatric intensive care team. *Nursing Ethics, 16*(1), 57–68.

Berde, C. B., & Sethna, N. F. (2002). Analgesics for the treatment of pain in children. *The New England Journal of Medicine, 347*(14), 1094–1103.

Berde, C. B., Lebel, A. A., & Olsson, G. (2003). Neuropathic pain in children. In N. L. Schechter, C. B. Berde, & M. Yaster (Eds.), *Pain in infants, children, and adolescents* (2nd ed.). Philadelphia: Lippincott Williams, and Wilkins.

Breau, L. M., Finley, G. A., McGrath, P. J., & Camfield, C. S. (2002). Validation of the non-communicating children's pain checklist-postoperative version. *Anesthesiology, 96*(3), 528–535.

Butkovic, D., Toljan, S., & Mihovilovic-Novak, B. (2006). Experience with gabapentin for neuropathic pain in adolescents: Report of five cases. *Paediatric Anaesthesia, 16*(3), 325–329.

Carrazana, E., & Mikoshiba, I. (2003). Rationale and evidence for the use of oxcarbazepine in neuropathic pain. *Journal of Pain and Symptom Management, 25*(5 Suppl), S31–S35.

Collins, J. J. (1996). Intractable pain in children with terminal cancer. *Journal of Palliative Care, 12*(3), 29–34.

Collins, J. J., Grier, H. E., Kinney, H. C., & Berde, C. B. (1995). Control of severe pain in children with terminal malignancy. *Jornal de Pediatria, 126*(4), 653–657.

Collins, J. J., Grier, H. E., Sethna, N. F., Wilder, R. T., & Berde, C. B. (1996). Regional anesthesia for pain associated with terminal pediatric malignancy. *Pain, 65*(1), 63–69.

Contro, N. A., Larson, J., Scofield, S., Sourkes, B., & Cohen, H. J. (2004). Hospital staff and family perspectives regarding quality of pediatric palliative care. *Pediatrics, 114*(5), 1248–1252.

Dayioglu, M., Tuncer, S., & Reisli, R. (2008). Gabapentin for neurophatic pain in children: A case report. *Agri, 20*(2), 37–40.

Dougherty, M., & DeBaun, M. R. (2003). Rapid increase of morphine and benzodiazepine usage in the last three days of life in children with cancer is related to neuropathic pain. *Jornal de Pediatria, 142*(4), 373–376.

Drake, R., Frost, J., & Collins, J. J. (2003). The symptoms of dying children. *Journal of Pain and Symptom Management, 26*(1), 594–603.

Dworkin, R. H., O'Connor, A. B., Backonja, M., et al. (2007). Pharmacologic management of neuropathic pain: Evidence-based recommendations. *Pain, 132*(3), 237–251.

Education Development Center. (2003). What matters to families: Part 3: Big choices, little choices IPPC videos. [Video] Education Development Center, Inc.

Ferrini, R. (2000). Parenteral lidocaine for severe intractable pain in six hospice patients continued at home. *Journal of Palliative Medicine, 3*(2), 193–200.

Finkel, J. C., Pestieau, S. R., & Quezado, Z. M. (2007). Ketamine as an adjuvant for treatment of cancer pain in children and adolescents. *The Journal of Pain, 8*(6), 515–521.

Finnerup, N. B., Otto, M., McQuay, H. J., Jensen, T. S., & Sindrup, S. H. (2005). Algorithm for neuropathic pain treatment: An evidence based proposal. *Pain, 118*(3), 289–305.

Friebert, S. (2009). *NHPCO facts and figures: Pediatric palliative and hospice care in America*. National Hospice and Palliative Care Organization.

Friedrichsdorf, S. J., & Kang, T. I. (2007). The management of pain in children with life-limiting illnesses. *Pediatric Clinics of North America, 54*(5), 645–672. x.

Galloway, K. S., & Yaster, M. (2000). Pain and symptom control in terminally ill children. *Pediatric Clinics of North America, 47*(3), 711–746.

Gauvain-Piquard, A., Rodary, C., Rezvani, A., & Serbouti, S. (1999). The development of the DEGR(R): A scale to assess pain in young children with cancer. *European Journal of Pain, 3*(2), 165–176.

Hampe, S. O. (1975). Needs of the grieving spouses in a hospital setting. *Nursing Research, 24*, 113–120.

Hauer, J. M., Wical, B. S., & Charnas, L. (2007). Gabapentin successfully manages chronic unexplained irritability in children with severe neurologic impairment. *Pediatrics, 119*(2), e519–e522.

Hawryluck, L. A., Harvey, W. R., Lemieux-Charles, L., & Singer, P. A. (2002). Consensus guidelines on analgesia and sedation in dying intensive care unit patients. *BMC Medical Ethics, 3*, E3.

Himelstein, B. P., Hilden, J. M., Boldt, A. M., & Weissman, D. (2004). Pediatric palliative care. *The New England Journal of Medicine, 350*(17), 1752–1762.

Hirschfeld, S. (1998). Pain as a complication of HIV disease. *AIDS Patient Care and STDs, 12*(2), 91–108.

Houlahan, K. E., Branowicki, P. A., Mack, J. W., Dinning, C., & McCabe, M. (2006). Can end of life care for the pediatric patient suffering with escalating and intractable symptoms be improved? *Journal of Pediatric Oncology Nursing, 23*(1), 45–51.

Jacob, E. (2004). Neuropathic pain in children with cancer. *Journal of Pediatric Oncology Nursing, 21*(6), 350–357.

Jalmsell, L., Kreicbergs, U., Onelov, E., Steineck, G., & Henter, J. I. (2006). Symptoms affecting children with malignancies during the last month of life: A nationwide follow-up. *Pediatrics, 117*(4), 1314–1320.

Kastrup, J., Petersen, P., Dejgard, A., Angelo, H. R., & Hilsted, J. (1987). Intravenous lidocaine infusion–a new treatment of chronic painful diabetic neuropathy? *Pain, 28*(1), 69–75.

Kolarik, R. C., Walker, G., & Arnold, R. M. (2006). Pediatric resident education in palliative care: A needs assessment. *Pediatrics, 117*(6), 1949–1954.

Krane, E. J., Leong, M. S., Golianu, B., & Leong, Y. Y. (2003). Treatment of pediatric pain with nonconventional analgesics. In N. L. Schechter, C. B. Berde, & M. Yaster (Eds.), *Pain in infants, children, and adolescents* (2nd ed.). Philadelphia: Lippincott Williams, & Wilkins.

Labauge, P., Fogli, A., Niel, F., Rodriguez, D., & Boespflug-Tanguy, O. (2007). CACH/VWM syndrome and leucodystrophies related to EIF2B mutations. *Revue neurologique, 163*(8–9), 793–799.

Lauder, G. R., & White, M. C. (2005). Neuropathic pain following multilevel surgery in children with cerebral palsy: A case series and review. *Paediatric Anaesthesia, 15*(5), 412–420.

Leske, J. S. (1986). Needs of relatives of critically ill patients: A follow-up. *Heart & Lung, 15*(2), 189–193.

Mack, J. W., Wolfe, J., Grier, H. E., Cleary, P. D., & Weeks, J. C. (2006). Communication about prognosis between parents and physicians of children with cancer: Parent preferences and the impact of prognostic information. *Journal of Clinical Oncology, 24*(33), 5265–5270.

Massey, G. V., Pedigo, S., Dunn, N. L., Grossman, N. J., & Russell, E. C. (2002). Continuous lidocaine infusion for the relief of refractory malignant pain in a terminally ill pediatric cancer patient. *Journal of Pediatric Hematology/Oncology, 24*(7), 566–568.

Meyer, E. C., Burns, J. P., Griffith, J. L., & Truog, R. D. (2002). Parental perspectives on end-of-life care in the pediatric intensive care unit. *Critical Care Medicine, 30*(1), 226–231.

Meyer, E. C., Ritholz, M. D., Burns, J. P., & Truog, R. D. (2006). Improving the quality of end-of-life care in the pediatric intensive care unit: Parents' priorities and recommendations. *Pediatrics, 117*(3), 649–657.

Miser, A. W., McCalla, J., Dothage, J. A., Wesley, M., & Miser, J. S. (1987a). Pain as a presenting symptom in children and young adults with newly diagnosed malignancy. *Pain, 29*(1), 85–90.

Miser, A. W., Dothage, J. A., Wesley, R. A., & Miser, J. S. (1987b). The prevalence of pain in a pediatric and young adult cancer population. *Pain, 29*(1), 73–83.

Muller-Busch, H. C., Andres, I., & Jehser, T. (2003). Sedation in palliative care - a critical analysis of 7 years experience. *BMC Palliat Care, 2*(1), 2.

Nathan, A., Rose, J. B., Guite, J. W., Hehir, D., & Milovcich, K. (2005). Primary erythromelalgia in a child responding to intravenous lidocaine and oral mexiletine treatment. *Pediatrics, 115*(4), e504–e507.

Pazola, K. J., & Gerberg, A. K. (1990). Privileged communication–talking with a dying adolescent. *MCN. The American journal of maternal child nursing, 15*(1), 16–21.

Robinson, W. M., Ravilly, S., Berde, C., & Wohl, M. E. (1997). End-of-life care in cystic fibrosis. *Pediatrics, 100*(2 Pt 1), 205–209.

Schechter, N. L. (1989). The undertreatment of pain in children: An overview. *Pediatric Clinics of North America, 36*(4), 781–794.

Sirkia, K., Hovi, L., Pouttu, J., & Saarinen-Pihkala, U. M. (1998). Pain medication during terminal care of children with cancer. *Journal of Pain and Symptom Management, 15*(4), 220–226.

Solomon, M. Z., Sellers, D. E., Heller, K. S., et al. (2005). New and lingering controversies in pediatric end-of-life care. *Pediatrics, 116*(4), 872–883.

Steele, R., Bosma, H., Johnston, M. F., et al. (2008). Research priorities in pediatric palliative care: A Delphi study. *Journal of Palliative Care, 24*(4), 229–239.

Tremont-Lukats, I. W., Hutson, P. R., & Backonja, M. M. (2006). A randomized, double-masked, placebo-controlled pilot trial of extended IV lidocaine infusion for relief of ongoing neuropathic pain. *The Clinical Journal of Pain, 22*(3), 266–271.

Truog, R. D., Cist, A. F., Brackett, S. E., et al. (2001). Recommendations for end-of-life care in the intensive care unit: The Ethics Committee of the Society of Critical Care Medicine. *Critical Care Medicine, 29*(12), 2332–2348.

Tsui, B. C., Davies, D., Desai, S., & Malherbe, S. (2004). Intravenous ketamine infusion as an adjuvant to morphine in a 2-year-old with severe cancer pain from metastatic neuroblastoma. *Journal of Pediatric Hematology/Oncology, 26*(10), 678–680.

Vondracek, P., Oslejskova, H., Kepak, T., et al. (2009). Efficacy of pregabalin in neuropathic pain in paediatric oncological patients. *European Journal of Paediatric Neurology, 13*(4), 332–336.

Williams, D. G., Hatch, D. J., & Howard, R. F. (2001). Codeine phosphate in paediatric medicine. *British Journal of Anaesthesia, 86*(3), 413–421.

Wolfe, J., Grier, H. E., Klar, N., et al. (2000). Symptoms and suffering at the end of life in children with cancer. *The New England Journal of Medicine, 342*(5), 326–333.

World Health Organization. (1998). *Cancer pain relief and palliative care in children*. Geneva: World Health Organization.

Wusthoff, C. J., Shellhaas, R. A., & Licht, D. J. (2007). Management of common neurologic symptoms in pediatric palliative care: Seizures, agitation, and spasticity. *Pediatric Clinics of North America, 54*(5), 709–733. xi.

Zernikow, B., Michel, E., Craig, F., & Anderson, B. J. (2009). Pediatric palliative care: Use of opioids for the management of pain. *Paediatric Drugs, 11*(2), 129–151.

Cancer-Related Pain in Childhood

13

Brenda C. McClain

Keywords

Limb sparing procedures • Postthoracotomy pain syndrome • Postamputation syndrome • Chemotherapy–induced neuropathies (CIN) • Mucositis • Radiation therapy

Introduction

More than one million Americans are diagnosed annually with cancer. In adults and in children ages 1–4 years, cancer is the second and third most common cause of death, respectively. Cancer accounts for more than 1/2 million deaths each year. It has been reported that procedural pain due to cancer-related diagnostic and treatment measures is a greater problem for children than pain due to disease. However, studies show 50–78% of children experience pain as a presenting symptom at the time of oncological diagnosis (Miser et al. 1987). With disease progression, greater than 89% of children experience pain in advanced stages (Sirkia et al. 1998). Pain is one of the most feared aspects of cancer and has led to fierce debates regarding euthanasia in adults. Recent rulings in the Netherlands allows euthanasia in children aged 12 years or less, with newborns inclusive, if they are deemed to have incurable disease and unbearable suffering

(ZENIT 2004). A debate of medical ethics on pediatric euthanasia is beyond the scope of this chapter. However, with concerted efforts, up to 90% of cancer patients with pain can have adequate analgesia by non-invasive measures. With the institution of the World Health Organization Guidelines on Cancer Pain Relief and Palliative Care in Children most patients can experience respite from pain (McGrath 1996).

Reasons to Treat Pain

Uncontrolled pain can be devastating and limiting to one's activities and abilities (Hanks 1995). Sleep deprivation, fatigue, emotional despair, and/or a sense of helplessness may result from unrelieved pain (Mercadante 2004; Mercadante et al. 2004). Thus, the quality of life and sense of well-being are markedly affected and can result in distress and undue suffering for the child and family. Pain is an overriding concern and may affect parental decisions regarding therapy or acceptance of pain producing procedures and can lead to drop out from care or use of suboptimal cancer-treatment regimens (Yeh et al. 1999). Parental anxiety and disruption of family function may result from the ravages of cancer and cancer-related pain. It is not only humane to treat a child in pain, but it is also

B.C. McClain (✉)
Department of Anesthesiology, Yale University School of Medicine, 333 Cedar Street, TMP-3, 208051, New Haven, CT, USA 06520-8051
e-mail: brenda.mcclain@yale.edu

B.C. McClain and S. Suresh (eds.), *Handbook of Pediatric Chronic Pain: Current Science and Integrative Practice*, DOI 10.1007/978-1-4419-0350-1_13,
© Springer Science+Business Media, LLC 2011

sound medical practice because pain can result in nausea, vomiting, restless sleep, and hyperalgesia (Baghdoyan 2006; May et al. 2005).

It is an accepted fact that pain in cancer patients is under-treated and pediatric patients are at particular risk (Susman 2005; Ljungman et al. 1999). Reasons for inadequate care are multiple. Many physicians are not comfortable with the pharmacology and dosing of strong opioids. An appreciation of the implications of cross-tolerance, the effects of long-term opioid administration, and indications for opioid rotation is needed. Lack of thorough and/or infrequent pain assessment can result in false assumptions of adequate pain management. Fear of addiction and misinformation about side effects of analgesics and adjuvants lead to limited or less than appropriate use of the pain relief armamentarium (Susman 2005). Patients may also under-report pain, possibly due to the assumption that discomfort is an inseparable component of the oncology experience (Pfefferbaum et al. 1990).

The History and Physical

A thorough examination and physical is mandatory in patients with cancer. The initial encounter should be broadly based. Focus cannot be on the neoplasm alone. The history should include a review of the psychosocial, medical, and oncological records. A complete review of systems and physical exam may reveal co-morbidities that can impact the patient's well-being and pain experience. Hereditary neuropathies present at a frequency of 1 in 2,500 people (Chauvenet et al. 2003). Therefore, it is plausible that an unforeseen co-morbidity can go undetected if intake information is incomplete. For example, a child with undiagnosed Charcot-Marie-Tooth manifested at the induction of chemotherapy and resulted in profound peripheral neurotoxicity (Chauvenet et al. 2003). A history of subtle motor or neuropathic symptoms should be sought since an alteration of the treatment protocol may be needed to provide preventive care.

A battery of tests may seem daunting, but is required. Diagnostic tests rely on changes in normal structure. Imaging studies should start with the basic radiograph. Tomography may delineate tumor margins. Radionuclide studies are better for detecting metastatic disease. Magnetic resonance imaging is indicated for brain and spinal cord lesions. Laboratory data are essential to the diagnostic evaluation. Acid phosphatase is found in many tissues but is higher in prostate. Alkaline phosphatase is a useful tumor marker and is elevated in osteogenic sarcoma and Paget's disease (Shankar and Hosking 2006).

Pain Assessment

Pain assessment must be global and standardized for consistent comparisons throughout the care of the patient. The Memorial Symptom Assessment Scale (MSAS) has been validated in children ages 7-12 years (Collins et al. 2002). The Brief Pain Inventory (BPI) and the Memorial Pain Assessment Card (MPAC) are validated for cancer pain. The BPI is available in short and long forms for clinical- and research-use, respectively. The short form includes four pain items and seven items on pain interference with daily living and body diagrams are also included (Cleeland 2009). The MPAC can distinguish pain intensity from pain relief (Fishman et al. 1987). The short form of the McGill Pain Questionnaire (MPQ) evaluates the three main components of the gate control theory of pain which are the sensory, affective, and evaluative dimensions. The MPQ is best used for assessing current pain intensity (Melzack 1975). These three multidimensional assessments were originally designed for adults but can be applied to older children and young adults. Nine domains are rated in the Procedure Behavior Checklist which assesses distress at distinct times during procedures performed in children (LeBaron and Zeltzer 1984; Walco et al. 2005).

A diverse group of pain experts convened under the Initiative on Methods, Measurement, and Pain Assessment in Clinical Trials (IMMPACT). Key outcome domains and measures were identified for consideration in clinical trials of treatments for acute and chronic pain in children and adolescents. The recommendations for assessing outcomes in children with chronic pain included the following measures: pain intensity, physical functioning, emotional functioning, role functioning, symptoms and adverse events, satisfaction with treatment, sleep, and economic factors. While the IMMPACT recommendations are predominately for research trials, the cited domains are notable in cancer-related pain management (McGrath et al. 2008). The Pediatric Quality of Life Inventory™ (PedsQL™) 1.0 Generic Core Scales and Cancer Module by the Pediatric Quality of Life Inventory™ (PedsQL™), is a health-related quality of life measure that longitudinally assesses pain intensity and emotional distress in children with cancer. Varni has shown that pain management will not allay emotional distress and the latter should be dealt with in a direct manner (Varni et al. 2004).

Assessment of procedural pain can utilize acute pain measurement tools which are familiar to most pediatric sub-specialists. Subjective measures of self-report are preferred and remain the gold standard. Self-report can be obtained from children as young as 3 years of age. Age-appropriate tools with acceptable validity are available for the measurement of pain intensity and affect. The Faces Pain Scale-revised is widely used and addresses intensity and affect as it correlates the faces with metric values (Hicks et al. 2001) (see Fig. 13.1). Objective scales are indicated for infants, toddlers, and non-verbal children. One objective scale that has been utilized in pre-verbal and non-verbal children as well as in adults with dementia is the Faces Legs Arms, Cry, and Consolability (FLACC) scale (Nilsson et al. 2008). Other behavioral scales used in procedural

pain which measure distress associated with invasive procedures include the Procedural Behavior Rating Scale revised (PBRS-R) and the Observational Scale of Behavioral Distress (OSBD); both assess 11 behaviors of distress and pain as they occur throughout the procedure. The Behavioral Approach-Avoidance and Distress Scale (BAADS) is an observational scale for assessing a child's coping style as well as the degree of distress prior to, during and after a medical procedure (Bachanas and Blount 1996). The Child-Adult Medical Procedure Interaction Scale-Short Form (CAMPIS-SF) was validated in 60 children ages 3–7 years and revealed not only the child's distress and coping style but revealed the impact of the accompanying adult's behavior on the child's distress (Blount et al. 2001).

Causes of Pain

There are three causes for pain: as a presenting symptom in association with cancer, from therapy, or as an unrelated co-morbid finding (Coyle and Foley 1985). Solid tumors can cause pain as a result of tumor growth, expansion, and encroachment of neighboring tissues, including nerve impingement and ischemia. Additionally, up regulation of genes result in production and release of pro-inflammatory cytokines such as tumor necrosis factor-alpha or TNF-α, interleukin (IL) – 1B and IL-6 which directly or indirectly affect nociceptors (Fall-Dickson et al. 2007). Unfortunately,

Faces Pain Scale- Revised

Sources. Hicks CL, von Baeyer CL, Spafford P, van Korlaar I, Goodenough B. The Faces Pain Scale – Revised: Toward a common metric in pediatric pain measurement. Pain 2001;93:173-183. Bieri D, Reeve R, Champion GD, Addicoat L, Ziegler J. The Faces Pain Scale for the self-assessment of the severity of pain experienced by children: Development, initial validation and preliminary investigation for ratio scale properties. Pain 1990;41:139-150.

```
0          2          4       Pier    6          8          10
```

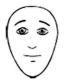 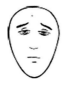

Fig. 13.1 Faces pain scale-revised (Sources: Hicks et al. 2001; Bieri et al. 1990)

treatment of the neoplasm can result in acute and even persistent pain.

Despite recent advances, the molecular mechanisms underlying the development and maintenance of cancer-evoked pain are not well understood. Tumors that secrete hematopoietic colony-stimulating factors act on myeloid cells as well as tumor cells. Receptors and signaling mediators of granulocyte- and granulocyte-macrophage colony-stimulating factors (G-CSF and GM-CSF) are found on sensory nerves. GM-CSF sensitized nerves to mechanical stimuli in vitro and in vivo, potentiated CGRP release, and caused sprouting of sensory nerve endings in the skin (Schweizerhof et al. 2009).

The mechanisms by which tumors produce pain include impingement and invasion of lymphatic and vascular channels, distension of a hollow viscous, edema, tissue inflammation, and necrosis. Injury to tissues results in the local release of numerous chemicals that mediate transmission of the pain stimulus. Cancer pain syndromes are classified by type (nociceptive or neuropathic) or duration (acute or chronic). Cancer pain characteristics provide some of the data essential for syndrome identification. These characteristics include intensity, quality, distribution, and temporal relationships (Portenoy and Waldman 1991). The principles of tumor-directed pain control include modifying the source of pain by treating the cancer and the inflammatory response to cancer, modulation at the neuraxis, altering the central perception of pain, and interfering with transmission of nociception within the central nervous system (Kocoglu et al. 2002).

Procedural Pain

The management of pediatric cancer requires the patient to undergo repeated procedures in the diagnosis, treatment, and follow-up of the disease. Repeated procedures become seemingly innumerable and are among the most memorable occurrences for many survivors of childhood cancer (Van Cleve et al. 1996). Children undergo multiple procedures such as venipunctures for administration of nutrition, antibiotics and blood products; lumbar punctures for obtaining cerebrospinal fluid or injection of intrathecal chemotherapy; bone marrow aspirates and biopsies for diagnosis and assessment of disease status. It is imperative that swift and effective pain treatment be given to avoid long-term psychological and physical consequences (Nayak et al 2008).

Current literature suggests that health care providers under-utilize pain management methods when performing painful procedures. Cancer-related procedural pain is probably as common in pediatric patients as intensive care procedures in neonates. Studies have documented more than ten noxious procedures per day being performed within the first few days of life (Stevens et al. 2003; Simons et al. 2003). In a study of 137 pediatric inpatients, 46 attributed their worst pain experienced to a procedure, with intravenous line placement being the most common procedure cited (Cummings et al. 1996). Another study of inpatients showed that 220 of 237 children experienced some type of procedural pain of at least moderate intensity (Ellis et al. 2002).

A study of 36 children undergoing dental procedures provides evidence which suggests that what a child recollects about a painful experience is more important in predicting future clinical behavior than the actual pain experienced (Rocha et al. 2009). Most children (85%) accurately recalled their pain. Temperament had no significant effect, but trait-anxious children showed a greater likelihood of recalling more pain than they initially reported (Rocha et al. 2009). State or situational anxiety was not mentioned. Children are generally capable of providing accurate reports of painful procedures that they have experienced. Fortunately, distress management interventions may have delayed benefits and positive influences on coping with future pain (Rocha et al. 2009). The use of pre-medication with benzodiazepines renders most patients into a cooperative, calm state. However, there is evidence that patients who pre-emptively received this drug class experienced more pain than those patients who did not receive premedicant or placebo prior to the procedures (Conte et al. 1999; Park et al. 2008). Ergo, a quiet patient is not necessarily a pain-free patient. Thus, a goal of administering only amnesia or sedation is inappropriate and inadequate for painful procedures.

A multimodal approach of psychological techniques, pharmacological agents, and family/patient education is preferred for painful and repeated procedures. Preparation for painful procedures requires adequate time allowance for effective use of psychological methods such as cognitive behavioral therapy (CBT). CBT distraction techniques such as non-procedural talking are coping-promoting while reassurance has been found to be distress-promoting (Blount et al. 1989). Hypnosis or distraction is most effective when performed by a therapist (Uman et al. 2008; Wild and Espie 2004). Topical anesthetics or oral analgesics should be given based on times to peak effects. Intravenous agents should be given in adequate amounts just prior to the noxious stimulus in a monitored setting.

Sedation guidelines have been developed by the American Academy of Pediatrics and the American Society of Anesthesiology in an effort to foster quality control for moderate and deep sedation. JCAHO Standards do not require certification in sedation, however, the ASA guidelines advise that individuals who are permitted to administer sedation should be able to rescue patients at whatever level of sedation or anesthesia is achieved whether the state was entered intentionally or unintentionally (www.JCAHO.org 2009). Certification in conscious or moderate sedation techniques by non-anesthesiologists may be an institutional requirement before such privileges are granted. Standardized competency-based training programs establish baseline educational requirements and ensure comparable training throughout a facility. Some state governments have outlined monitoring requirements for intravenous agents (Getter and Trieger 1996). Patient safety is the ultimate goal (Cote 2001). Separate personnel who are solely dedicated to monitoring the patient are needed during procedures. Post-sedation recovery also requires monitoring until the patient returns to baseline biophysical function.

Therapy-Related Pain

Surgical Interventions

New pain sites may occur as a result of surgical interventions. Procedures for implantation of central venous access and removal of such ports can be associated with pain well past the perioperative period. Hypertrophic scar formation, keloids, and mechanical problems can be painful. Pruritus, pain, and mechanical allodynia are common presentations in keloids and are associated with abnormalities in small nerve fiber function and suggest a small nerve fiber neuropathy as the cause of allokinesis and pain (Lee et al. 2004). Surgeons should consider the need for pre-emptive or postoperative scar management in patients with a history of hypertrophic scar or keloid formation.

Central venous access is often required for delivery of nutrition and/or chemotherapy. Catheter-related infections and malfunction of access ports and indwelling catheters may require multiple surgeries that compound the oncological experience (Ingram et al. 1991; Darbyshire et al. 1985). Surgery is used as a therapeutic modality primarily when there is a likelihood of achieving cure. However, surgical intervention may be limited to only biopsy for tissue diagnosis, especially when the tumor location or size presents extreme risk if complete excision was attempted. In advanced disease, partial excision and biopsy are indicated for palliative relief of tumor burden or for staging. Pain may persist due to tumor or surgical trauma to adjacent structures. Common surgically-related pain disorders seen in adults and children include postthoracotomy and postamputation syndromes.

Surgically – Induced Syndromes

Thoracotomy is well known to cause severe pain in the immediate postoperative period but in a significant number of patients it also produces long-term postthoracotomy pain syndrome. This syndrome often lasts for months or even years after surgery (Karmakar et al. 2004). Postthoracotomy syndrome is defined as pain that persists along the surgical scar for more than 2 months (Merskey et al. 1994) and occurs in 50–80% of adult patients. Characteristics of myofascial and neuropathic pain are often present (Wallace et al. 1996). Studies on pre-emptive analgesia show superior control of postoperative pain with administration of combined local anesthetic and opioid via thoracic epidural techniques when compared to intravenous opioids, however, the incidence or intensity of postthoracotomy syndrome was not affected in similar fashion in adults and children (Senturk et al. 2002; Doyle and Bowler 1998).

Postamputation syndrome can occur with amputation of any body part, not just of limbs. Postamputation syndrome has been described for teeth, tongue, breast, and even viscera (Dijkstra et al. 2007; Marbach 1996; Hanowell and Kennedy 1979). Current concepts on the pathophysiology on deafferentation and phantom limb pain as proposed by Flor (2008) suggest that phantom limb pain is due to neuroplastic changes along the neuraxis. There is a close correlation between changes in the homoncular mapping at the somatosensory cortex of the affected limb and somatosensory memories which manifest as phantom limb pain. Mechanisms underlying these maladaptive plastic changes are related to a loss of GABAergic inhibition, glutamate-mediated long-term potentiation and, axonal sprouting. The effects of neuroplastic changes in phantom limb pain seem worse than in those with chronic pain prior to amputation (Flor 2008).

The incidence of phantom limb pain in children is reported to be 12% in trauma-related cases, 28% in congenital limb loss cases, and up to 48% in cancer-related amputations (Lambert et al. 2001; Thompson 1995). Within 72 h of amputation, 76% of 67 children who received chemotherapy prior to or at the time of amputation, experienced phantom limb pain (Smith and Thompson 1995). This is not to be confused with stump pain or phantom sensation.

In the retrospective study of Wilkins et al., stump pain occurred in 88% of children experiencing amputation. This pain occurs as a result of surgically-induced nociception, neuroma formation, infection, and stretch at the stump site. Phantom sensation is the non-painful perception of the ongoing presence of the amputated limb and may be triggered by weather changes, emotions, and fear of touching the stump (Wilkins et al. 1998).

Limb Sparing Procedures

Limb sparing procedures (also known as limb salvaging) are indicated for sarcomas of the upper and lower extremities and are preferred when there is a chance for complete tumor excision, preservation of function, and reasonable cosmesis. Different types of limb-sparing procedures are available. These procedures include intercalary, intra-articular and extra-articular excisions for bony lesions (Marchese et al. 2006). Generally, wide excision of the tumor and its margins is followed by placement of a prosthesis and muscle flap with soft tissue reconstruction. The prosthesis may be one of several types depending on the location and functional concerns. For example, an extendable device could be placed if future limb length inequality is a concern (Marulanda et al. 2008).

The quality of life in patients with limb sarcomas has improved with the advent of improved neoadjuvant chemotherapy and improved limb-sparing procedures for children (Aksnes et al. 2008). The functionality of the operated limb is key to the child's sense of well being. Range of motion correlates with quality of life for pediatric patients who have undergone lower extremity sarcomas limb-sparing procedures. Musculoskeletal pain, decreased range of motion, and neuropathic pain may affect daily activities and well being (Marchese et al. 2006). Hence, the critical nature of insuring incorporation of range of motion exercises in the physical therapy regimen is essential for increased function and reduction of pain.

In other studies, patients reported limitations in physical activities, participation in sports, and cosmetic aspects as the most detrimental consequences of their disease and its treatment, especially where lower extremity weight bearing and gait are concerns (Bekkering et al. 2010). Current treatment for bone malignancies is complicated by an unexpectedly high incidence of infection. Orthopedic device infections were the most common reason for subsequent amputation and poor functional outcomes in a study of 104 cases (Gaur et al. 2005). African-American patients had the highest rate of infection and failure of limb salvage.

Shoulder subluxation and dislocation are concerns in children who have undergone upper extremity limb-sparing procedures of the proximal humerus (Hosalkar and Dormans 2004; Kim et al. 2010). Wittig et al. (2002) performed a 10-year follow-up of upper limb sparing procedure patients and found that hand positioning, dexterity, and lifting ability in the upper extremity are key in function and well being. No patient could lift an object above shoulder level; however, patients could carry objects with the humerus close to the body, and feed and groom themselves without assistance. Several patients participated in sports and one lifted weights, within limits (Wittig et al. 2002). Eight of twenty three patients experienced transient nerve palsies but no neuropraxia occurred in this longitudinal study.

Chemotherapy

Chemotherapy-induced neuropathies (CIN) affect peripheral nerves in the forms of myelinopathies and axonopathies, or more centrally, at the neuronal cell body as neuronopathies and can involve apoptosis of the dorsal root ganglion. The onset of CIN usually appears after undergoing several cycles of chemotherapy over weeks to months (Ocean and Vahdat 2004). Yet, some agents, such as granulocyte colony stimulating factor (GCSF), may cause acute pain. The use of combination chemotherapy has resulted in greater survival rates for many childhood cancers. However, the use of these strategies is not without adverse effects and the risk: benefit ratio varies with the type of drug combination and dosing schedules. The type and degree of neuropathy depends on the chemotherapeutic agent, dose intensity, and cumulative dose (Ocean and Vahdat 2004). If neuronal damage is severe, then pain may continue despite cessation of drug administration (Peltier and Russel 2002).

Cisplatin and oxaliplatin are platinum compounds that result in inhibition of DNA synthesis and induction of apoptosis of dorsal root ganglion cells. The clinical manifestation is a sensory neuropathy; however, doses higher than 400 mg/m^2 can result in sensory ataxia and impaired deep tendon reflexes. The neuropathy may persist for years after the termination of the drug (Chaudhry et al. 2003). Children receiving >500 mg/m^2 and at a higher dose rate can develop hypomagnesemia, hypocalcemia, and proximal nephron impairment (Elisaf et al. 1997). Paresthesias and seizures of metabolic origin can result from cisplatin-induced hypomagnesemia (Bellin and Selim 1988).

Ifosfamide is an alkylating agent used to treat solid tumors. Its neurotoxicity, manifesting as seizures and encephalopathy, can be precipitated by cisplatin administration in a dose-dependent manner. The occurrence of neurotoxicity can be related to previous cumulative dosages of cisplatin. Ninety seven children and adolescents with malignant solid tumors were treated with ifosfamide within a phase II protocol. One third of the patients who received more than 600 mg/m^2 of cisplatin developed some degree of encephalopathy. The increased risk of neurotoxicity in patients who received more than 600 mg/m^2 of cisplatin may be related to either a decreased clearance of ifosfamide itself or of the drug's active metabolites (Pratt et al. 1990). Ifosfamide is often given with mesna to protect against bladder complications.

The vinca alkaloids are extracts from the periwinkle plant and include vinorelbine, vindesine, vincristine, and vinblastine. The vinca alkaloids vincristine and vinblastine have similar structures but are effective in different types of cancers. Vincristine has been remarkable in its ability to cause complete remission of both lymphocytic and myelogenous acute leukemias of childhood (Duflos et al. 2002). Chemo-cytotoxic effects of these alkaloids lead to inhibition of mitosis and clinically result in distal axonopathies which present as chronic polyneuropathies with delayed recovery after cessation of the drug. Nerve conduction study abnormalities were seen in 29.7% of 37 surviving children who were longer than 2 years off from vincristine therapy for ALL.

Most children with an abnormal examination or nerve conduction study did not have subjective symptoms or a significantly impaired quality of life (Ramchandren et al. 2009). Peripheral neurological side effects include paresthesias, of the fingers or toes, abdominal pain, constipation, and muscle weakness. Animal studies reveal that vincristine causes disorganization of the axonal microtubule cytoskeleton, as well as an increase in the caliber of unmyelinated sensory axons in association with hyperalgesia and allodynia (Tanner et al. 1998) Ultimately, vincristine-induced apoptosis in ALL cells proceeds by a mitochondrial controlled pathway. Other cytotoxic effects include bone marrow suppression, hair loss, and clinical neuropathy. The scavenger ascorbic acid inhibits reactive oxygen species generation and cell death induced by vincristine (Groninger et al. 2002). Thus, vitamin C may play a future role in the treatment of CIN.

Bone pain is the most common toxicity from G-CSF administration (Froberg et al. 1999). Splenic rupture has occurred in healthy volunteers (Tigue et al. 2007; Nuamah et al. 2006). Hyperalgesia and muscle pain are generally short lived with G-CSF, from hours to a few days (see Table 13.1).

Mucositis is the ulceration of the mucosa of the alimentary system and affects the oral cavity and gastrointestinal tract. Although the signs in the mouth are most apparent, any part of the gastrointestinal tract may be involved. The clinical

signs and symptoms begin around Day 3 of chemotherapy with abdominal pain, bloating, and diarrhea with oral symptoms starting at Day 7 with burning and erythema of the mouth followed by intensely painful erosions of the mucosa (Keefe et al. 2000). Oral candidiasis, bacterial, and viral infections often complicate the experience (see Fig. 13.2). The World Health Organization's Oral Toxicity Assessment Scale is a grading system for oral mucositis and provides a common language for clinicians to assess the severity of disease (see Table 13.2). Another enteric complication seen in cancer patients is typhlitis, also known as inflammatory colitis or cecitis and may represent an entity in the spectrum of alimentary mucositis. Typhlitis is a painful condition that can require surgical intervention if supportive therapy fails. In a retrospective study of 843 cancer patients, the incidence of typhlitis was highest in patients with AML or Burkitt's lymphoma. The etiology of typhilitis is uncertain but may stem from chemotherapy-induced ulcerations or from inflammation related to the malignancy (Moran et al. 2009). While most chemotherapy agents have the potential to cause mucositis, those with a propensity for mucositis include cyclophosphamide, methotrexate, and the anthracycline antibiotics (e.g., aclarubicin, daunorubicin, doxorubicin, epirubicin, and pirarubicin) (Lothstein et al. 2001). Mucositis may result from radiotherapy or chemotherapy but is worse when the two treatments are combined (Yeoh et al. 2006).

Treatment of mucositis is supportive and aimed at symptom control. Preventive oral regimens which include pre-emptive dental rehabilitation, daily cleaning, and chlorhexidine mouthwash, nystatin and iodopovidine cause a reduction in the severity and incidence of mucositis by 38% (Cheng et al. 2001). Oral rinses with antiseptic and antifungal mouthwashes should be included in the routine, pre-emptive care but have little effect in established mucositis (Dodd et al. 2000). Mucosal coating agents such as oral sucralfate may increase the incidence of diarrhea (Barasch et al. 2006; Rubenstein et al. 2004). Capsaicin lollipops deplete substance P and can be effective if the child can tolerate the initial

Table 13.1 Chemotherapy-induced neuropathy and/or nociceptive pain

Agent	Type(s) of pain
Steroids	Muscle pain
	Gastric upset
Vinca alkaloids vincristine, vinblastine	Neuropathy predominately of the lower extremities
GCSF	Acute chest syndrome
	Bone pain
	Splenic rupture
Platinum compounds	Mono and polyneuropathies
	Sensory ataxia, loss of deep tendon reflexes

Chemotherapeutic agents that are commonly associated with pain which occurs as a dose-dependent dysfunction

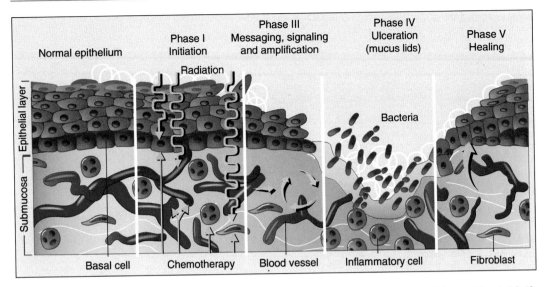

Fig. 13.2 Phases in the development of oral mucositis. (Adapted from Peterson DE: New strategies for management of oral mucositis in cancer patients, J Support Oncol; 4:9-13. Copyright the Mayo Foundation.)

Table 13.2 World Health Organization Oral Mucositis Assessment Scale

Grade	0	1	2	3	4
Signs and symptoms	None	Soreness ± erythema	Erythema, ulcers, and patient can swallow solid food	Ulcers with extensive erythema and patient cannot swallow solid food	Mucositis to the extent that alimentation is not possible

The WHO Oral Toxicity Scale takes into consideration appearance and function

burning sensation (Berger et al. 1995). Topical 2% lidocaine, viscous lidocaine "swish and expectorate" and nebulized lidocaine 4% can temporarily anesthetize the mouth and esophagus without evidence of toxic plasma levels, provided that the total daily dose is less than 240 mg of lidocaine per day (Elad et al. 1999; Yamashita et al. 2002).

Intravenous opioids are indicated for moderate to severe pain where the patient has limited or no ability to swallow secondary to the painful ulcerations (Rubenstein et al. 2004). The 2006 Cochrane Review on treatment of oral mucositis performed a meta-analysis and found 71 randomized studies of 29 interventions. Treatments that showed some benefit in established, moderately severe mucositis included amifostine, antibiotic paste, hydrolytic enzyme, and ice chips (Worthington et al. 2006).

Radiotherapy

The position of radiation therapy in pediatric oncology is usually after chemotherapy and surgery when the tumor volume has shrunk (Plowman et al. 2008). However, the concurrent use of chemotherapy and radiation therapy is increasing for some tumors.

Radiation therapy works by injury of the DNA in cells by two mechanisms: DNA strand breaks with subsequent mitotic interference and free radical formation with ensuing cell death. The damage is caused by elementary particles such as a photon, electron, proton, neutron, or ion beam directly or indirectly ionizing the DNA atoms. Free radicals are formed which then damage DNA targets leading to cell death (Shih et al. 2003). Oxygen heightens radiosensitivity, thus increasing the effectiveness of a given dose of radiation

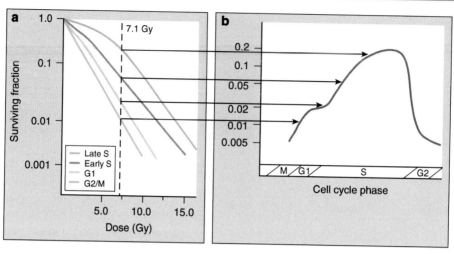

Fig. 13.3 (**a**) Cell survival curves for populations of Chinese hamster cells irradiated in different phases of the cycle cycle. (**b**) Graphic illustration of how these radiosensitive differences translate into age response patterns. (Adapted from Abeloff MD et. al., Basics of Radiation Therapy: *In* Abeloff's Clinical Oncology p. 428.)

by forming DNA-damaging free radicals. Solid tumors can outgrow their blood supply, causing a low-oxygen state. Tumor cells in a hypoxic environment may be more resistant to radiation damage than those in a normal oxygen environment (Harrison et al. 2002). Irradiated cancer cells generally are poorly differentiated and reproduce more, but with a diminished capacity to repair themselves when compared to most normally differentiated cells. The DNA damage caused by radiation therapy becomes inborn and causes the cancer cells to die or reproduce more slowly than healthy cells (see Fig. 13.3).

The dosimetry of radiation is measured in gray (Gy) and varies depending on the type and stage of cancer and whether the aim of treatment is cure or palliation. The total dose is fractionated usually as a 5-day course over several weeks in curative therapy. The purpose of dose fractionation is to allow time for recovery of normal cells while tumor cells remain damaged and radiosensitive (Whitelaw et al. 2008). Also, the time course of fractionation allows hypoxic, radioresistant tumor cells time to re-oxygenate and become vulnerable to radiation by the next cycle. The four Rs of radiotherapy are repair, re-assortment, repopulation, and re-oxygenation. Repair is the prompt cellular response to sublethal damage from radiation. The second R, re-assortment, occurs next with cell progression through the cell

cycle. The third R, repopulation, represents an increase in the fraction of surviving cells as a result of cell division, and the fourth R, re-oxygenation, occurs when recovery of hypoxic cells regain access to oxygen due to tumor shrinkage and improved blood supply (Yeoh et al. 2006). The lag time between repopulation and re-oxygenation will determine the tissues' tolerance of radiotherapy and this relationship is inversely proportional such that the longer the lag time, the lower the tolerance of the given tissue.

External beam radiation therapy is delivered by means of a linear accelerator. Linear accelerators are generators that create high energy X-rays for external beam radiation therapy. The linear accelerator contains lead shutters, called collimators, which focus and direct the X-ray vectors onto the tumor. The L-shaped design of the linear accelerator allows it to rotate, delivering radiation from all angles. This is the conventional mode of delivery for pediatric radiation therapy (Loeffler et al. 1990).

Conformational radiation therapy, also known as intensity modulated radiation therapy tomography, is a procedure that uses computerized three-dimensional pictures of the tumor in order to target the tumor as accurately as possible. Theoretically, this technique gives the highest possible dose of radiation at the target while sparing normal tissue the most. Disadvantages of IMRT include, "the low-dose bath" effect where the multiple entry/exit paths of radiation result in a larger proportion of the body receiving low doses, possibly resulting in late oncogenic risks and growth delay (Plowman et al. 2008). Longitudinal follow-up of children who received external or intra-abdominal radiotherapy for neuroblastoma later displayed delayed vascular development of the abdominal aorta. Vascular complications in seven children who received internal and external radiotherapy included hypertension (five), middle aortic syndrome (two), death due to mesenteric ischemia (one), and critical aortic stenosis (Sutton et al. 2009).

The gamma knife uses a concentrated radiation dose from Cobalt-60 sources. Over 200 beams of radiation intersect to form a powerful tool focused on a targeted area of abnormal or cancerous tissue within the brain. The gamma knife is considered radiosurgery due to its very precise nature as it damages and destroys unhealthy tissue while sparing adjacent normal, healthy brain tissues. This technique entails the use of cranial pinning in a vise and therefore, requires the administration of sedation and local anesthesia for adults. General anesthesia is often used in children to insure tolerance of restraint (Hirth et al. 2003).

There is a host of factors to consider in an attempt to limit radiation of normal tissue in growing children while insuring the delivery of the radiotherapy dose inclusive of tumor margins. The size of the child and location of the tumor are major concerns. For example, the exit corridor of normal tissue exposed when using a linear accelerator to treat a low thoracic neuroblastoma will expose a larger volume of normal tissue in an infant than in an adolescent with a tumor of the same location and relative volume. Vulnerability to radiation therapy increases during periods of rapid proliferation, therefore, sensitivity of surrounding structures also relates to individual tissue metabolic activity (Sutton et al. 2009). Thus, vulnerability to toxicity varies with the tissue type and the dose/volume of radiation. The cumulative dose of Gy each tissue type can tolerate is variable. A dose volume histogram (DVH) plots the delivery of high dose ionized radiation to the target tissue volume as well as estimates the risk of exposure of adjacent normal tissue.

Radiation therapy can be used in acute situations to palliate pain and related symptoms such as ulceration or obstruction and can provide rapid relief. However, chronic effects of radiation include tissue necrosis, burn pain, strictures, contractures, and neuropathy.

Regardless of the type of radiation therapy used, most infants and children will require sedation or general anesthesia (intravenous or inhalational) on a daily basis to insure cooperation and safety during treatment.

Pain Management Interventions

The Cancer Pain Relief Program of the World Health Organization (WHO) developed an analgesic ladder for the management of persistent cancer pain of increasing intensity (see Fig. 13.4). Zernikow et al. (2006) prospectively applied the WHO ladder to 224 pediatric cases of cancer (median age 9 years) and found that the guidelines provide effective relief for children with cancer. However, the combination of opioid plus non-opioid was not more effective than opioid alone (Zernikow et al. 2006).

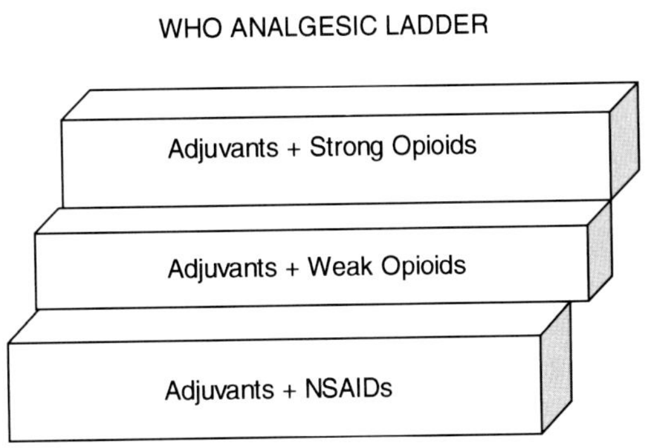

WHO ANALGESIC LADDER

Fig. 13.4 WHO analgesic ladder. Adjuvants can be added at any step. Adequate analgesia can be obtained for most patients; however, a fourth step for interventional procedures might address intractable pain

Mild Pain

The WHO pain relief guide recommends that care start with a non-opioid such as the para-aminophenols (e.g., paracetamol, acetaminophen) or non-steroidal anti-inflammatory drugs (NSAIDs) for mild pain. In general, NSAIDs are well tolerated in children; however, NSAIDs are contraindicated for patients who have renal insufficiency, intravascular volume depletion, congestive heart failure, or peptic ulcer disease. Those patients receiving steroids as part of their oncologic management are at increased risk of GI upset and hemorrhage when NSAIDs are concomitantly used. (Hernandez-Diaz and Rodriguez 2001).

The co-administration of serotonin selective reuptake inhibitor (SSRIs) antidepressants and NSAIDs show marked increased GI risks when compared to SSRI use alone and should be avoided. However, non-selective tricyclic antidepressants (TCAs) in combination with NSAIDs do not show similar increased GI risks (de Jong et al. 2003). The pediatric rheumatologic population is best studied for the safety and efficacy of NSAIDs. For bone and joint pain, diclofenac, ibuprofen, tolmetin, and naproxen are equal in their efficacy and tolerance. Salicylates and indomethacin are no more effective but are more toxic (Hollingworth 1993). NSAIDs have a ceiling effect and increasing doses will lead to side effects without additional benefits. Mu agonist opioids have no ceiling effect.

Mild to Moderate Pain

In the WHO ladder, moderate pain is treated with the addition of "weak" or mild opioids. Agents such as codeine and tramadol are used. In the US, codeine is the most frequently used opioid in children. Codeine and tramadol have similar potencies. Tramadol is metabolized in the liver yielding several metabolites among which is O-demethyltramadol, an active metabolite via the enzyme CYPD26 for which polymorphism affects about 10% of the Caucasian population (Garrido et al. 2006). Studies of compound medicines compared tramadol 37.5 mg/325 mg acetaminophen with codeine 30 mg/300 mg acetaminophen in

adults with chronic pain and found comparable efficacy (Mullican and Lacy 2001). In pediatric studies, tramadol at a starting dose of 1 mg/kg Q 4–6 hourly was tolerated in a 30-day duration of use study for surgical and medically-related pain. The maximum daily dose was not to exceed 8 mg/kg/day or 400 mg/day. Nausea, vomiting, and dizziness were among the main complaints but did not improve with the length of exposure to tramadol (Rose et al. 2003). Pharmacokinetic/pharmacodynamic modeling studies of tramadol's analgesic efficacy in children suggest that the analgesic effects seen in children are due to not only the mu receptor activity but to the serotonin and norepinephrine reuptake inhibition (Garrido et al. 2006). Tramadol should not be given to patients with a history of seizures. Co-administration with SSRIs can lead to seizure, hypertension, or serotonin syndrome. Respiratory depression appears to be less with tramadol when compared to other opioids (Silvasti et al. 1999). In a randomized, prospective study, children receiving tramadol for postoperative pain had less nausea than those who received morphine (Ozalevli et al. 2005). Tramadol is available in the US only in oral form but it is available in other countries for intravenous PCA and regional analgesia. The oral tramadol to morphine potency ratio is 10:1 and the tramadol to oxycodone potency ratio is approximately 8:1 in children.

Mixed agonists–antagonists are incorrectly considered as protective against respiratory depression but may have greater side effects. These mixed agonists also have a ceiling effect and are not first choice agents for cancer pain management. Partial agonists may have a place in the treatment paradigm regardless of the risk of ceiling effects for analgesia. Additionally, greater sedation is observed with partial agonists than with mixed agonists (Megabane et al. 2010).

Moderate to Severe Pain

For severe pain, strong opioids are used and morphine is generally considered the agent of choice. Around the clock administration is needed and compliance may be difficult for a host of reasons. Controlled release preparations for 12-hourly administration are available. Sustained release tablets should never be crushed or divided because this could lead to acute overdose. The exception to this rule is once daily capsule preparations of long acting morphine. These 24-hourly capsules can be opened and made into a solution if the child cannot swallow pills or capsules. Other strong opioids include oxycodone, hydrocodone, methadone, hydromorphone, and fentanyl. Oxycodone and hydrocodone are equipotent and well tolerated in children. Of these two agents, more literature exists regarding the use of oxycodone in children. Oxycodone is 1.5 times stronger than morphine for oral dosing; however, intravenous studies show equipotency for parenteral formulations of morphine and oxycodone (Silvasti et al. 1999). The initial dose for oxycodone is not standardized. Population pharmacokinetic studies in children 6 months to 7 years of age suggest 0.1 mg/kg as the initial oral dose for moderate to severe pain. Weight is a more important factor than age since clearance of oxycodone does not increase with age as expected (El-Tahtawy et al. 2006).

While most children with advanced disease can obtain adequate analgesia with oral opioids (Berde and Sethna 2002), many have an intolerance of oral analgesics due to adverse side effects that are unresponsive to intervention. Other feasible routes of delivery include transdermal systems and buccal mucosal delivery. Fentanyl is available in the US for intravenous, transdermal, and buccal routes. Long-term use of intravenous fentanyl is impractical, in part, due to the propensity for rapid tolerance. Transdermal therapeutic systems of fentanyl (i.e., TTS or fentanyl patch) are effective in patients with established, stable opioid requirements. A fentanyl depot concentrates in the upper dermis. Onset of analgesia is within 1–12 h (Grond et al. 2000). Steady state is not reached for 72 h, thus it is not a route for titration of analgesia, especially in the face of poorly determined opioid requirements. An intake of at least 45 mg of oral morphine equivalents per day is required for use of the 25 mcg/h transdermal system. Pediatric trials on fentanyl TTS have led to the approval of a 12.5 mcg system. A TTS should never be cut in an attempt to tailor dosage. Other opioids suitable for transdermal therapeutic systems include buprenorphine and sufentanil; however, more clinical data in children are needed.

Additional routes of delivery include intranasal, sublingual, subcutaneous infusion, and rectal administration. Intravenous administration is indicated for severe pain when oral analgesics cannot be tolerated due to emesis or if pain is inadequately controlled by other routes of administration. Adjuvants such as tricyclic antidepressants are added to improve sleep and enhance analgesia. Adjuvants may be added at any rung in the ladder (see Fig. 13.4).

A fourth step to the ladder has been suggested. It includes invasive therapies such as intraspinal narcotics, neuroablation, and neuromodulation. These techniques may be applicable when extraordinary dosage escalation is no longer effective or side effects are intolerable in spite of efforts. In these incidences, techniques such as chronic epidural and intrathecal catheters as tunneled or closed systems and neurolytic nerve blockade can be invaluable (Galloway and Yaster 2000). Neuraxial analgesia has been performed in supported fashion for several weeks outside the hospital setting, thus, allowing children to have comfort at home at the end of life (Collins et al. 1996).

Breakthrough pain is defined as a transitory flare of moderate to severe pain that interrupts otherwise controlled persistent pain. Breakthrough pain may last from seconds to hours and may be somatic, visceral, or neuropathic in origin. The early descriptions of this phenomenon observed that nearly 30% of the cases occurred just prior to the next scheduled dose of opioid (Portenoy et al. 1990). Breakthrough and precipitated, incident pain must be treated with "as needed" doses of immediate release analgesics in addition to the usual schedule of opioid administration. Transmucosal fentanyl has been investigated and found effective for breakthrough pain but can be associated with nausea and vomiting (Portenoy et al. 1999). Fears of addiction must be addressed for the patient and family. A clear differentiation of addiction, physical dependence, and tolerance must be offered.

An alternative to the WHO ladder is the Guideline for the Management of Cancer Pain in Adults and Children, an evidence-based clinical practice guideline. This algorithmic approach stresses individualization of care and timely implementation and pain control and therefore, is more adaptable to the dynamic nature of cancer and breakthrough pain (Miaskowski 2004) (see Chap. 19 for analgesic tables.)

Extraordinary Dosing

Children with advanced disease may experience marked increases in pain especially in the terminal stages. Predictors of increased pain include ongoing breakthrough pain, poor performance status, increasing disability, neuropathic pain symptoms, and frank nerve involvement (Caraceni and Portenoy 1999; Collins et al. 1995). While opioids are the mainstay, they can display pronociceptive properties (Bannister and Dickenson 2010). Opioid-induced hyperalgesia (OIH) may result from acutely increasing opioid doses or from chronic administration and is often seen in association with, but is separate from, opioid tolerance. The mechanism of OIH involves excitatory opioid receptors, NMDA receptors, and Cholecystokinin (CCK) activity (Xu et al. 2003).

Collins (1995) did a retrospective review of children with peripheral nerve or neuraxial involvement and found maximal intravenous opioid dosing ranged from 3.8–518 mg/kg/h of morphine equivalents with the highest dose required by a child who had periaqueductal gray involvement. Dougherty and DeBaun (2003) reported on 18 children during their final 72 h of life and found that children with neuropathic pain at end of life required up to 100-fold increase in opioid when compared to children whose pain was nonneuropathic at end of life.

Management of Opioid Side Effects

Opioids form the cornerstone of care and adequate knowledge of the pharmacology of the individual agents in this drug class is needed. Side effects are common and should be anticipated and addressed throughout the care plan. Stool stimulants, not stool softeners, are needed in many cases and should be prescribed hand in hand with opioids. Respiratory depression can

be addressed by rearrangement of schedules or fractionation of the dose, while sedation can be treated by the addition of psychostimulants. Low doses of amphetamines such as dextroamphetamine or methylphenidate given in the morning and mid-day can improve alertness and increase play activity (Westberg and Gobel 2004). The inherent analgesic properties can decrease opioid requirements. Amphetamine psychostimulants should not be given in the late afternoon because the arousal can interfere with sleep. Modafinil, a non-amphetamine stimulant, is considered a wakefulness-promoting agent and is approved for narcolepsy and obstructive sleep apnea. It does not have the same abuse potential of amphetamines; however, it causes euphoria and reinforcing behavior such as amphetamines. Modafinil is administered once daily and is not approved in children less than 16 years of age. Pediatric trials are notable for dysmenorrhea in girls age 12 and older (Rx List 2010) (see Table 13.3).

Opioids affect both the sleep and awakening systems and can result in sleep disturbances (Moore and Kelz 2009). Non-restorative sleep and inadequate sleep are implicated as causes of hyperalgesia. Kappa agonists do not affect the nucleus of the tractus solitarius in the medullary brain and have a positive impact on sleep (Reinoso-Barbero and de Andres 1995). Non-REM sleep is increased when kappa agonists are injected into the ventrolateral preoptic nucleus while mu agonists injected into the same area promote wakefulness (Greco et al. 2008). The effects of commercially available opioids may be variable in patients due to drug chemistry or genetics and enzyme polymorphism. Thus, an individuals' response to a given opioid may differ from one another with regards to analgesia, side effects, sleep interruption, or sleep restoration. Current research displays the importance of the arousal state in the management of pain.

Complementary and Alternative Medicine (CAM)

Complementary and alternative medicine (CAM), as defined by the National Center for Complementary and Alternative Medicine (NCCAM),

Table 13.3 Symptom management (Adapted from 2009 Yale University- pediatric pain management services guide)

Agent	Dose	Route	Regimen	Indication	Caution
Dextroamphetamine	0.1–0.15 mg/kg up to 10 mg/dose	PO	Q AM and Mid-day	Enhanced opioid analgesia; Inherent analgesia Therapy for opioid sedation	Addictive Prolonged alertness if given after Mid-day
Methylphenidate	0.05–0.1 mg/kg/dose	PO	Q AM and Midday	Enhanced opioid analgesia; Inherent analgesia Therapy for opioid sedation	Addictive Prolonged alertness if given after Mid-day
Modafinil	Start at 1.5 mg/kg/dose 100–200 mg/dose in adults	PO	Q day	Obstructive sleep apnea, Therapy for opioid sedation	± Addictive
Diphenhydramine	0.5 mg/kg/dose	IV/PO	Q 4–6 h PRN	For itching and nausea	Sedating
Metoclopramide	0.1 mg/kg/dose	IV	Q4–6 h PRN	Nausea, gastric emptying;	Extrapyramidal effects possible
Nalbuphine	0.05 mg–0.1 mg/kg/dose	IV	Q4 h PRN	For severe pruritis	
Naloxone	1–1.5 mC cg/kg/h	IV	Continuous infusion	For itching, opioid side effects.	Pulmonary edema possible at higher doses, especially in pts receiving chronic mu opioids
	2–5 mg per dose	PO	TID	Constipation relief; laxation without reversal of analgesia	
Ondansetron	0.1–0.15 mg/kg/dose Max 4 mg	IV/PO	Q 4–6 h PRN	First line for nausea and vomiting	QT prolongation

"is a group of different medical and health care systems, practices, and products that are not presently considered to be part of conventional medicine (NCCAM 2010)." Complementary medicine is used in conjunction with conventional medicine while alternative medicine is used in place of conventional medicine. Integrative medicine is defined as treatment that combines conventional medicine with CAM therapies.

CAM therapies are used by 31–84% of children with cancer, both in and outside of clinical trials. The therapies used most often were prayer and spiritual practice (61%), relaxation (44%), faith and spiritual healing (42%), and nutritional supplements and vitamins (40%). CAM therapies are often used for the treatment of side-effects of cancer or cancer treatment and rarely for cure of the disease (Kelly 2004).

Spiritual healing is the most prevalent complementary therapy in the United States and includes prayer and meditation (Barnes et al. 2004). Spiritual healing is sometimes assigned under mind-body therapies and by others under the classification of bioenergetic therapies (NCCAM 2010). Eighty-two percent of Americans believe in the healing power of personal prayer, 73% believe that praying for someone else can help cure their illness. Enhanced immune system functioning has been observed. Prayer is used by more than 60% of parents for their children (Pitetti et al. 2001; Sawni-Sikand et al. 2002; Acupuncture, aromatherapy, homeopathy, hypnotherapy, massage, and reflexology are other accepted CAM therapies.

The Impact of Childhood Cancer on the Family

The Survivor

The Damocles Syndrome in Childhood Survivors

O'Malley and Koocher (1981) coined the term, "The Damocles Syndromes" and published their findings in a book of that same name, based on studies of 120 young people who developed cancer before the age of 18 and were disease-free

12 years later. The stress, anxiety, apprehension of an uncertain future, and fear of cancer recurrence was likened to the sword of Damocles in the Disputations of Cicero, "that there can be nothing happy for the person over whom some fear always looms" Everitt (2001). In the 1980s childhood cancer had a 50% survival rate and current 5-year survival is more than 70% yet, the Damocles Syndrome persists for many children and their families. Although this fear tends to subside with time, certain events such as follow-up medical visits, unexplained pain, or particular sights and smells associated with treatment can trigger bouts of anxiety and fear that are just as debilitating as those that occurred during active treatment. Family and individual counseling is recommended especially at critical time points of the cancer experience. Counseling would be helpful: at the time of diagnosis; at the onset of treatment; during negative physical reaction to treatment; when treatment is terminated; when the child re-enters school; during recurrence of the disease; at the time research treatments are given; and when the decision is made to end all treatment (Christ et al. 2002).

The quality of life for survivors of childhood cancer is improving, however, important variables include the type of cancer the child had and the emotional impact of treatment. A survey from the Cleveland Clinic, revealed that survivors of ALL and those who received radiation therapy of <25 Gy for CNS tumors were less likely to achieve higher educational goals thus, impairing their ability to improve social and economic status (Langeveld et al. 2002; Langeveld et al. 2004). Additionally, survivors have lower rates of marriage and parenthood and worry about their ability to procreate and/or about future health problems their children could encounter as a result of their cancer history. Most survivors are healthy physically and psychologically (Langeveld et al. 2002). Issues of job insecurity and difficulty in obtaining health insurance are major concerns of vulnerability.

The Sibling

It is critical for the well being of healthy siblings that they understand the effect cancer has for them. Because of parents' lack of attention to the healthy siblings, usually out of ignorance, the siblings are afflicted with behavioral, psychosocial, and physical problems (Spinetta et al. 1999). In a multi-center collaborative, structured interviews of 254 siblings of children with cancer identified significant sibling distress about issues of family separation from lack of parental presence at home due to hospital stays and clinic visits. The disruption of family schedules and home life frequently occurred. Focus of the family on the ill child, negative feelings in themselves and toward family members are causes for sibling distress (Sargent et al. 1995).

The same group of institutions undertook a collaborative study on the prevalence of sibling distress. Emotional/behavioral distress was worse in the healthy sibling at 6–42 months after the diagnosis of cancer. Twenty five percent of younger boys (4–11 years) and 15% of older girls (12–17 years) experienced greater distress than the general population with prevalence of 7.9 and 2.1%, respectively for comparable gender and age (Sahler et al. 1994). Anxiety regarding cancer treatments and their effects and fear of death were expressed by the healthy sibling.

The sibling may often feel marginalized in the family due to lack of attention. Organized educational interventions for parents has considerable effect on lessening sibling isolation compared with usual hospital care processes for family involvement of the sick child. Formal information equips parents with insight and methods for proper balance of attentiveness toward care concerns of the healthy sibling. Effective planning of care, support groups, attendance of sibling camps, and proper education play major roles in reducing stress and improving quality of life for siblings (Murray 2000 Murray 2001; Hashemi and Shokrpour 2010).

The Parents

Parental affective responses are likely to change from the acute stress of the diagnostic period to the chronic less intense period of the course of treatment and follow-up phase (Barbara et al. 1984; Dahlquist et al. 1993). Most studies focus on the

mother–child dyad since it is often the mother who is present for much of the care. But, the marital relationship can play a major role in the coping styles and emotional distress parents display during their child's illness. The literature does not support the misconception that divorce rates increase due to the impact of childhood cancer on family structure and function. Marital distress is predicted by state anxiety and depression and the degree of discrepancy in anxiety levels between the parents. Dahlquist studied 42 mother–father dyads using standardized assessments which included the Spielberger State-Trait Anxiety Inventory, the Beck Depression Inventory, and the Dyadic Adjustment Scale. She found that, state anxiety significantly decreased for mothers but not for fathers at 2 months after diagnosis (Dahlquist et al. 1996). However, fathers generally had lower state anxiety scores than those of their spouse. Also no change was evident in depression scores for fathers over time. Dahlquist found that parents who were already maritally distressed at the time of diagnosis did not become increasingly distressed. This is in contrast to other studies where marital distress increased with chronicity of stress (Gotlib et al. 1998). Poor health status of the child predicted a more positive attitude toward the marriage for fathers but not for mothers. This finding may be due to women having a broader social support base for stressful situations than men who may rely on the marriage for social support. Studies are needed on the impact of anxiety and marital distress on discrepancy in acceptance of pain management techniques.

Summary

The majority of cancer-associated pain can be managed by systemic analgesics, yet, less than 50% of all cancer patients have good pain control. Obstacles to care should be sought out and addressed. Cultural taboos and attitudes of the caregiver weigh heavily on effective treatment implementation. Treatment must be tailored for the individual; however, adherence to pain management principles is imperative. It should be reassuring to patients, families, and caregivers, alike that most patients' pain can be controlled with systemic analgesics. Invasive therapies for neurablation or externalized neuraxial catheters can enhance the quality of life, especially in the terminal phase where escalation of pain may occur and for those whom systemic analgesia is no longer feasible. However, with the increasing survivor rates of various malignancies, the controversial placement of implantable, closed system devices placed along the neuraxis of a growing child must have strong indications. The accessibility of our patients to pediatric interventional pain physicians is limited and many adult pain physicians choose not to see pediatric patients. Our charge is to ensure our patients access to responsible clinical care and expertise in pain management as we strive to improve their quality of life.

References

Aksnes, L. H., Bauer, H. C., Jebsen, N. L., Folleras, G., Allert, C., Haugen, G. S., et al. (2008). Limb-sparing surgery preserves more function than amputation: A Scandinavian sarcoma group study of 118 patients. *The Journal of Bone and Joint Surgery. British Volume, 90*(6), 786–794.

Bachanas, P. J., & Blount, R. L. (1996). The behavioral approach-avoidance and distress scale: An investigation of reliability and validity during painful medical procedures. *Journal of Pediatric Psychology, 21,* 671–681.

Baghdoyan, H. A. (2006). Hyperalgesia induced by REM sleep loss: A phenomenon in search of a mechanism. *Sleep, 29*(2), 137–139.

Bannister, K., & Dickenson, A. H. (2010). Opioid hyperalgesia. *Current Opinion in Supportive and Palliative Care, 4*(1), 1–5.

Barasch, A., Elad, S., Altman, A., Damato, K., & Epstein, J. (2006). Antimicrobials, mucosal coating agents, anesthetics, analgesics, and nutritional supplements for alimentary tract mucositis. *Supportive Care in Cancer, 14*(6), 528–532.

Barbara, F., Sabbeth, B. F., & Leventhal, J. M. (1984). Marital adjustment to chronic childhood illness: A critique of the literature. *Pediatrics, 73*(6), 762–768.

Barnes, P. M., Powell-Griner, E., McFann, K., & Nahin, R. L. (2004). Complementary and alternative medicine use among adults: United States 2002. *Advance Data, 343,* 1–19.

Bekkering, W. P., Vlieland, T. P., Koopman, H. M., Schaap, G. R., Schreuder, H. W., Beishuizen, A., et al. (2010). Quality of life in young patients after bone tumor surgery around the knee joint and comparison with healthy controls. *Pediatric Blood & Cancer, 54*(5), 738–745.

Bellin, S. L., & Selim, M. (1988). Cisplatin-induced hypomagnesemia with seizures: A case report and review of the literature. *Gynecologic Oncology, 30,* 104–113.

Berde C. B. & Sethna N. F. (2002). Analgesics for the treatment of pain in children. *The New England Journal of Medicine, 347*(14), 1094–103.

Berger, A., Henderson, M., Nadoolman, W., Duffy, V., Cooper, D., Saberski, L., et al. (1995). Oral capsaicin provides temporary relief for oral mucositis pain secondary to chemotherapy/radiation therapy. *Journal of Pain and Symptom Management, 10*(3), 243–248 [Erratum appears in J Pain Symptom Manage 1996 May;11(5):331].

Bieri, D., Reeve, R., Champion, G. O., Addicoat, L., & Ziegier, J. (1990). The Faces Pain Scale for the self-assessment of the severly of pain experienced by the children: Development, initial validation and preliminary investigation for ratio scale properties. *Pain, 41,* 139–150.

Blount, R. L., Corbin, S. M., Sturges, J. W., Wolfe, V. V., Prater, J. M., & James, L. D. (1989). The relationship between adult's behavior and child coping and distress during BMA/LP procedures: A sequential analysis. *Behavior Therapy, 20,* 585–601.

Blount, R. L., Bunke, V., Cohen, L. L., & Forbes, C. J. (2001). The Child-Adult Medical Procedure Interaction Scale-Short Form (CAMPIS-SF): Validation of a rating scale for children's and adults' behaviors during painful medical procedures. *Journal of Pain and Symptom Management, 22*(1), 591–599.

Chaudhry, V., Chaudhry, M., Crawford, T. O., et al. (2003). Toxic neuropathy in patients with pre-existing neuropathy. *Neurology, 60,* 337–340.

Chauvenet, A. R., Shashi, V., Selsky, C., Morgan, E., Kurtzberg, J., & Bell, B. (2003). Pediatric oncology group study. Vincristine-induced neuropathy as the initial presentation of charcot-marie-tooth disease in acute lymphoblastic leukemia: A pediatric Oncology group study. *Journal of Pediatric Hematology/Oncology, 25*(4), 316–320.

Cheng, K. K., Molassiotis, A., Chang, A. M., Wai, W. C., & Cheung, S. S. (2001). Evaluation of an oral care protocol intervention in the prevention of chemotherapy-induced oral mucositis in paediatric cancer patients. *European Journal of Cancer, 37,* 2056–2063.

Christ, G. H., Siegel, K., & Christ, A. E. (2002). Adolescent grief: "It never really hit me...until it actually happened". *The Journal of American Medical Association, 288*(10), 1269–1278.

Cleeland, C.S. (2009). *Brief pain inventory user's guide* (pp. 9–10). Last Accessed May 31, 2010, from www.mdanderson.org./education-and-research/departments

Collins, J. J., Grier, H. E., Kinney, H. C., & Berde, C. B. (1995). Control of severe pain in children with terminal malignancy. *Jornal de Pediatria, 126*(4), 653–657.

Collins, J. J., Grie, H. E., Sethna, N. F., Wilder, R. T., & Berde, C. B. (1996). Regional anesthesia for pain associated with terminal pediatric malignancy. *Pain, 65*(1), 63–69.

Collins, J. J., Devine, T. D., Dick, G. S., Johnson, E. A., Kilham, H. A., Pinkerton, C. R., et al. (2002). The measurement of symptoms in young children with cancer: The validation of the Memorial Symptom Assessment Scale in children aged 7-12. *Journal of Pain and Symptom Management, 23*(1), 10–16.

Conte, P. M., Walco, G. A., Sterling, C. M., Engel, R. G. & Kuppenheimer, W. G. (1999). Procedural pain management in pediatric oncology: a review of the literature. *Cancer Invest, 17*(6), 448–459

Cote, C. J. (2001). Why we need sedation guidelines. *Jornal de Pediatria, 138*(3), 447–448.

Coyle, N., & Foley, K. (1985). Pain in patients with cancer: Profile of patients and common pain syndromes. *Seminars in Oncology Nursing, 1*(2), 93–99.

Cummings, E. A., Reid, G. J., Finley, G. A., McGrath, P. J., & Ritchie, J. A. (1996). Prevalence and source of pain in pediatric inpatients. *Pain, 68*(1), 25–31.

Dahlquist, L. M., Czyzewski, D. I., Copeland, K. G., Jones, C. L., Tauh, E., & Vaughan, J. K. (1993). Parents of children newly diagnosed with cancer: Anxiety, coping, and marital distress. *Journal of Pediatric Psychology, 18*(3), 365–376.

Dahlquist, L. M., Czyzewski, D. I., & Jones, C. L. (1996). Parents of children with cancer: A longitudinal study of emotional distress, coping style, and marital adjustment two and twenty months after diagnosis. *Journal of Pediatric Psychology, 21*(4), 541–554.

Darbyshire, P. J., Weightman, N. C., & Speller, D. C. (1985). Problems associated with indwelling central venous catheters. *Archives of Disease in Childhood, 60*, 129–134.

de Jong, J. C. F., Paul, B., van den Berg, P. B., Hilde, T., & de Jong-van den Berg, L. T. W. (2003). Combined use of SSRIs and NSAIDs increases the risk of gastrointestinal adverse effects. *British Journal of Clinical Pharmacology, 55*(6), 591–595.

Dijkstra, P. U., Rietman, J. S., & Geertzen, J. H. (2007). Phantom breast sensations and phantom breast pain: A 2-year prospective study and a methodological analysis of literature. *European Journal of Pain, 11*(1), 99–108.

Dodd, M. J., Dibble, S. L., Miaskowski, C., Paul, S. M., MacPhail, L., Greenspan, D., et al. (2000). Randomized clinical trial of the effectiveness of 3 commonly used mouthwashes to treat chemotherapy-induced mucositis. *Oral Surgery, Oral Medicine, Oral Pathology, Oral Radiology & Endodontics, 90*, 39–47.

Dodd, M. J., Miaskowski, C., Dibble, S. L., Paul, S. M., MacPhail, L., Greenspan, D., et al. (2000). Factors influencing oral mucositis in patients receiving chemotherapy. *Cancer Practice, 8*(6), 291–297.

Dougherty, M., & DeBaun, M. R. (2003). Rapid increase of morphine and benzodiazepine usage in the last three days of life in children with cancer is related to neuropathic pain. *Jornal de Pediatria, 142*(4), 373–376.

Doyle, E., & Bowler, G. M. R. (1998). Pre-emptive effect of multimodal analgesia in thoracic surgery. *British Journal of Anaesthesia, 80*(2), 147–151.

Duflos, A., Kruczynski, A., & Barret, J. M. (2002). Novel aspects of natural and modified vinca alkaloids. *Current Medicinal Chemistry – Anti-Cancer Agent, 2*(1), 55–70.

Elad, S., Cohen, G., Zylber-Katz, E., Findler, M., Galili, D., Garfunkel, A. A., et al. (1999). Systemic absorption of lidocaine after topical application for the treatment of oral mucositis in bone marrow transplantation patients. *Journal of Oral Pathology & Medicine, 28*(4), 170–172.

Elisaf, M., Milionis, H., & Siamopoulos, K. C. (1997). Hypomagnesemic hypokalemia and hypocalcemia: Clinical and laboratory characteristics. *Mineral and Electrolyte Metabolism, 23*(2), 105–112.

Ellis, J. A., O''Connor, B. V., Cappelli, M., Goodman, J. T., Blouin, R., & Reid, C. W. (2002). Pain in hospitalized pediatric patients: How are we doing? *The Clinical Journal of Pain, 18*(4), 262–269.

El-Tahtawy, A., Kokki, H., & Reidenberg, B. E. (2006). Population pharmacokinetics of oxycodone in children 6 months to 7 years old. *Journal of Clinical Pharmacology, 46*, 433–442.

Everitt, A. (2001). *Cicero: The life and times of Rome's greatest politician.* New York: Random House. ISBN 0375507469.

Fall-Dickson, J. M., Ramsay, E. S., Castro, K., Woltz, P., & Sportes, C. (2007). Oral mucositis-related oropharyngeal pain and correlative tumor necrosis factor-alpha expression in adult oncology patients undergoing hematopoietic stem cell transplantation. *Clinical Therapeutics, 29*(Suppl), 2547–2561.

Fishman, B., Pasternak, S., Wallenstein, S. L., Houde, R. W., Holland, J. C., & Foley, K. M. (1987). The Memorial Pain Assessment Card. a valid instrument for the evaluation of cancer pain. *Cancer, 60*(5), 1151–1158.

Flor, H. (2008). Maladaptive plasticity, memory for pain and phantom limb pain: Review and suggestions for new therapies. *Expert Review of Neurotherapeutics, 8*(5), 809–818.

Froberg, M. K., Garg, U. C., Stroncek, D. F., Geis, M., McCollough, J., & Brown, D. M. (1999). Changes in serum osteocalcin and bone- specific alkaline phosphatase are associated with bone pain in donors receiving granulocyte colony–stimulating factor for peripheral blood stem and progenitor cell collection. *Transfusion, 39*(4), 410–414.

Galloway, K. S., & Yaster, M. (2000). Pain and symptom control in terminally ill children. *Pediatric Clinics of North America, 47*(3), 711–746.

Garrido, M. J., Habre, W., Rombout, F. & Troconiz, I. F. (2006). Population pharmacokinetic/pharmacodynamic modelling of the analgesic effects of tramadol in pediatrics. *Pharmacology Research, 23*(9), 2014–2023.

Gaur, A. H., Liu, T., Knapp, K. M., Daw, N. C., Rao, B. N., Nee, M. D., et al. (2005). Infections in children and young adults with bone malignancies undergoing limb-sparing surgery. *Cancer, 104*(3), 602–610.

Getter, L., & Trieger, N. (1996). Sedation – guidelines and controls. *Journal of the American Dental Association, 127*(1), 20–22.

Gotlib, I. H., Lewinsohn, P. M., & Seeley, J. R. (1998). Consequences of depression during adolescence: marital status and marital functioning in early adulthood. *Journal of Abnormal Psychology, 107*(4), 686–690.

Greco, M. A., Fuller, P. M., Jhou, T. C., Martin-Schild, S., Zadina, J. E., Hu, Z., et al. (2008). Opioidergic projections to sleep-active neurons in the ventrolateral preoptic nucleus. *Brain Research, 1245,* 96–107.

Grond, S., Radbruch, L., & Lehmann, K. A. (2000). Clinical pharmacokinetics of transdermal opioids: Focus on transdermal fentanyl. *Clinical Pharmacokinetics, 38*(1), 59–89.

Groninger, E., Meeuwsen-De Boe, G. J., De Graaf, S. S., Kamps, W. A., & De Bont, E. S. (2002). Vincristine induced apoptosis in acute lymphoblastic leukaemia cells: A mitochondrial controlled pathway regulated by reactive oxygen species? *International Journal of Oncology, 21*(6), 1339–1345.

Hanks, G. W. (1995). Cancer pain and the importance of control. *Anti-Cancer Drugs, 6*(supp 3), 14–17.

Hanowell, S. T., & Kennedy, S. F. (1979). Phantom tongue pain and causalgia: Case presentation and treatment. *Anesthesia and Analgesia, 58*(5), 436–438.

Harrison, L. B., Chadha, M., Hill, R. J., Hu, K., & Shasha, D. (2002). Impact of tumor hypoxia and anemia on radiation therapy outcomes. *The Oncologist, 7*(6), 492–508.

Hashemi, F., & Shokrpour, N. (2010). The impact of education regarding the needs of pediatric leukemia patients' siblings on the parents' knowledge and practice. *Health Care Manager, 29*(1), 75–79.

Hernandez-Diaz, S., & Rodriguez, L. A. (2001). Steroids and risk of upper gastrointestinal complications. *American Journal of Epidemiology, 153*(11), 1089–1093.

Hicks, C. L., von Baeyer, C. L., Spafford, P. A., van Korlaar, I., & Goodenough, B. (2001). The Faces Pain Scale-Revised: Toward a common metric in pediatric pain measurement. *Pain, 93*(2), 173–183.

Hirth, A., Pederse, P. H., Baardsen, R., Larsen, J. L., Krossnes, B. K., & Helgestad, J. (2003). Gamma-knife radiosurgery in pediatric cerebral and skull base tumors. *Medical and Pediatric Oncology, 40*(2), 99–103.

Hollingworth, P. (1993). The use of non-steroidal anti-inflammatory drugs in paediatric rheumatic diseases. *Rheumatology, 32*(1), 73–77.

Hosalkar, H. S., & Dormans, J. P. (2004). Limb sparing surgery for pediatric musculoskeletal tumors. *Pediatric Blood & Cancer, 42*(4), 295–310.

Ingram, J., Weitzman, S., Greenberg, M. L., Parkin, P., & Filler, R. (1991). Complications of indwelling venous access lines in the pediatric hematology patient: A prospective comparison of external venous catheters and subcutaneous ports. *American Journal of Pediatric Hematology/Oncology, 13*(2), 130–136.

Karmakar, M. K., Anthony, M. H., & Ho, A. M. H. (2004). Postthoracotomy pain syndrome. *Thoracic Surgery Clinics, 14,* 345–352.

Keefe, D. M., Brealey, J., Goland, G. J., & Cummins, A. G. (2000). Chemotherapy for cancer causes apoptosis that precedes hypoplasia in crypts of the small intestine in humans. *Gut, 47,* 632–647.

Kelly, K. M. (2004). Complementary and alternative medical therapies for children with cancer. *European Journal of Cancer, 40*(14), 2041–2046.

Kim, H. J., Chalmers, P. N., & Morris, C. D. (2010). Pediatric osteogenic sarcoma. *Current Opinion in Pediatrics, 22*(1), 61–66.

Klassen, A. F., Klaassen, R., Dix, D., Pritchard, S., Yanofsky, R., O'Donnell, M., et al. (2008). Impact of caring for a child with cancer on parents' health-related quality of life. *Journal of Clinical Oncology, 26*(36), 5884–5889.

Kocoglu, H., Pirbudak, L., Pence, S., & Balat, O. (2002). Cancer pain, pathophysiology, characteristics and syndromes. *European Journal of Gynaecological Oncology, 23*(6), 527–532.

Lambert, A. W., Dashfield, A. K., Cosgrove, C., Wilkins, D. C., Walker, A. J., & Ashley, S. (2001). Randomized prospective study comparing preoperative epidural and intraoperative perineural analgesia for the prevention of postoperative stump and phantom limb pain following major amputation. *Regional Anesthesia and Pain Medicine, 26*(4), 316–321.

Langeveld, N. E., Stam, H., Grootenhuis, M. A., & Last, B. F. (2002). Quality of life in young adult survivors of childhood cancer. *Support Care Cancer. 10*(8), 579–600.

Langeveld, N. E., Grootenhuis, M. A., Voute, P. A., de Haan, R. J., & van den Bos, C. (2004). Quality of life, self-esteem and worries in young adult survivors of childhood cancer. *Psychooncology, 13*(12), 867–881.

LeBaron, S., & Zeltzer, L. (1984). Assessment of acute pain and anxiety in children and adolescents by self-report, observer reports, and a behavior checklist. *Journal of Consulting and Clinical Psychology, 52,* 729–738.

Lee, S. S., Yosipovitch, G., Chan, Y.-H., & Goh, C.-L. (2004). Pruritus, pain, and small nerve fiber function in keloids: A controlled study. *Journal of the American Academy of Dermatology, 51*(6), 1002–1006.

Ljungman, G., Gordh, T., Srensen, S., & Kreuger, A. (1999). Pain in paediatric oncology: Interviews with children, adolescents and their parents. *Acta Paediatrica, 88*(6), 623–630.

Loeffler, J. S., Siddon, R. L., Siddon, R. L., Wen, P. Y., Nedzi, L. A., & Alexander, E., 3rd. (1990). Stereotactic radiosurgery of the brain using a standard linear accelerator: A study of early and late effects. *Radiotherapy and Oncology, 17*(4), 311–321.

Lothstein, L., Israel, M., & Sweatman, T. W. (2001). Anthracycline drug targeting: Cytoplasmic versus nuclear – a fork in the road. *Drug Resistance Updates, 4*(3), 169–177.

Mahaney, G. D., & Peeters-Asdourian (1998). Cancer pain management in: Pain Management. Vol.VI Abrams, SE. (Ed.), Current Medicine, Inc. London.

Marbach, J. J. (1996). Phantom tooth pain: Differential diagnosis and treatment. *Journal of the Massachusetts Dental Society, 44*(4), 14–18.

Marchese, V. G., Spearing, E., Callaway, L., Rai, S. N., Zhang, L., Hinds, P. S., et al. (2006). Relationships among range of motion, functional mobility, and quality of life in children and adolescents after limb-sparing surgery for lower-extremity sarcoma. *Pediatric Physical Therapy, 18*(4), 238–244.

Marulanda, G. A., Henderson, E. R,. Johnson, D. A., Letson, G. D., & Cheong, D. (2008). Orthopedic surgery options for the treatment of primary osteosarcoma. *Cancer Control, 15*(1), 13–20.

May, M. E., Harvey, M. T., Valdovinos, M. G., Kline, R. H., 4th, Wiley, R. G., & Kennedy, C. H. (2005). Nociceptor and age specific effects of REM sleep deprivation induced hyperalgesia. *Behavioural Brain Research, 159*(1), 89–94.

Megabane, B., Buisine, A., Jacobs, F., Resiere, D., Chevillard, L., Vicaut, E., & Baud, F. J. (2010). Prospective comparative assessment of buprenorphine overdose with heroin and methadone: clinical characteristics and response to antidotal treatment. *J Subst Abuse Treat. 38*(4), 403–407.

McGrath, P. A. (1996). Development of the World Health Organization Guideline on Cancer Pain Relief and Palliative Care in Children. *Journal of Pain and Symptom Management, 12*(2), 87–92.

McGrath, P. J., Walco, G. A., Turk, D. C., Dworkin, R. H., Brown, M. T., Davidson, K., et al. (2008). Core outcome domains and measures for pediatric acute and chronic/recurrent pain clinical trials: PedIMMPACT recommendations. *The Journal of Pain, 9*(9), 771–783.

Melzack, R. (1975). The McGill pain questionnaire: Major properties and scoring methods. *Pain, 1*(3), 277–299.

Mercadante, S. (2004). Cancer pain management in children. *Palliative Medicine, 18*(7), 654–662.

Mercadante, S., Girelli, D., & Casuccio, A. (2004). Sleep disorders in advanced cancer patients: Prevalence and factors associated. *Supportive Care in Cancer, 12*(5), 355–359.

Merskey, H., & Bogduk, N., (eds.). (1994). Task force on taxonomy of the international association for the study of pain: classification of chronic pain. Description of pain syndromes and definitions of pain terms. Seattle: IASP. p. 210– 213.

Miaskowski, C. (2004). Recent advances in understanding pain mechanisms provide future directions for pain management. *Oncol Nurs Forum.* 31(4 Suppl), 25–35.

Miser, A. W., McCalla, J., Dothage, J. A., Wesley, M., & Miser, J. S. (1987). Pain as a presenting symptom in children and young adults with newly diagnosed malignancy. *Pain, 29,* 85–90.

Moore, J. T., & Kelz, M. B. (2009). Opiates, sleep, and pain: The adenosinergic link. *Anesthesiology, 111*(6), 1175–1176.

Moran, H., Yaniv, I., Ashkenazi, S., Schwartz, M., Fisher, S., & Levy, I. (2009). Risk factors for typhlitis in pediatric patients with cancer. *Journal of Pediatric Hematology/ Oncology, 31*(9), 630–634.

Mullican, W. S., & Lacy, J. R. (2001). Tramadol/acetaminophen combination tablets and codeine/acetaminophen combination capsules for the management of chronic pain: A comparative trial. *Clinical Therapeutics, 23*(9), 1429–1445.

Murray, J. S. (2000). Understanding sibling adaptation to childhood cancer. *Issues in Comprehensive Pediatric Nursing, 23*(1), 39–47.

Murray, J. S. (2001). Self-concept of siblings of children with cancer. *Issues in Comprehensive Pediatric Nursing, 24*(2), 85–94.

National Institutes of Health (2010). National Center for Complementary and Alternative Medicine Web site. Accessed June 25, 2010, Available at: http://nccam. nih.gov

Nayak, S., Roberts, S., & Cunliffe, M. (2008). Management of intractable pain from a chronic dislocated hip in an adolescent. *Paediatric Anaesthesia, 18*(4), 357–8.

Nilsson, S., Finnstrom, B., & Kokinsky, E. (2008). The FLACC behavioral scale for procedural pain assessment in children aged 5–16 years. *Paediatric Anaesthesia, 18*(8), 767–774.

Nuamah, N. M., Goker, H., Kilic, Y. A., Dagmoura, H., & Cakmak, A. (2006). Spontaneous splenic rupture in a healthy allogeneic donor of peripheral-blood stem cell following the administration of granulocyte colony-stimulating factor (g-csf). A case report and review of the literature. *Haematologica, 91*(5 Suppl), ECR08.

Ocean, A. J., & Vahdat, L. T. (2004). Chemotherapy-induced peripheral neuropathy: Pathogenesis and emerging therapies. *Supportive Care in Cancer, 12*(9), 619–625.

O'Malley, J. J., & Koocher, G. P. (1981). Damocles syndrome. MGraw-Hill Education, New York 219pp.

Ozalevli, M., Unlugenc, H., Tuncer, Ü., Gunes, Y., & Ozcengiz, D. (2005). Comparison of morphone and tramadol by patent controlled analgesia for postoperative analgesia after tonsillectomy in children. *Paediatric Anaesthesia, 15*(11), 979–984.

Park, S. H., Bang, S. M., Nam, E., Cho, E. K., Shin, D. B., Lee, J. H., et al. (2008). A randomized double-blind placebo-controlled study of low-dose intravenous Lorazepam to reduce procedural pain during bone marrow aspiration and biopsy. *Pain Medicine, 9*(2), 249–252.

Peltier, A. C., & Russel, J. W. (2002). Recent advances in drug-induced neuropathies. *Current Opinion in Neurology, 15,* 633–638.

Pfefferbaum, B., Adams, J., & Aceves, J. (1990). The influence of culture on pain in Anglo and Hispanic children with cancer. *Journal of the American Academy of Child and Adolescent Psychiatry, 29,* 642–647.

Pitetti, R., Singh, S., Hornak, D., Garcia, S. E., & Herr, S. (2001). Complementary and alternative medicine use in children. *Pediatric Emergency Care, 17*(3), 165–169.

Plowman, P. N., Cooke, K., & Walsh, N. (2008). Indications for tomotherapy/intensity-modulated radiation therapy in paediatric radiotherapy: Extracranial disease. *The British Journal of Radiology, 81*(971), 872–880.

Portenoy, R. K., & Waldman, S. D. (1991). Recent advances in the management of cancer pain. Part 1: Pharmacologic approaches. *Pain Management, 4*(3), 10–25.

Portenoy, R. K., Neil, A., & Hagen, N. A. (1990). Breakthrough pain: Definition, prevalence and characteristics. *Pain, 41*(3), 273–281.

Portenoy, R. K., Payne, R., Coluzzi, P., Raschko, J. W., Lyss, A., Busch, M. A., et al. (1999). Oral transmucosal fentanyl citrate (OTFC) for the treatment of breakthrough pain in cancer patients: A controlled dose titration study. *Pain, 79*(2–3), 303–312.

Pratt, C. B., Goren, M. P., Meyer, W. H., Singh, B., & Dodge, R. K. (1990). Ifosfamide neurotoxicity is related to previous cisplatin treatment for pediatric solid tumors. *Journal of Clinical Oncology, 8*, 1399–1401.

Ramchandren, S., Leonard, M., Mody, R. J., Donohue, J. E., Moyer, J., Hutchinson, R., et al. (2009). Peripheral neuropathy in survivors of childhood acute lymphoblastic leukemia. *Journal of the Peripheral Nervous System, 14*(3), 184–189.

Reinoso-Barbero, F., & de Andres, I. (1995). Effects of opioid microinjections in the nucleus of the solitary tract on the sleep-wakefulness cycle states in cats. *Anesthesiology, 82*(1), 144–152.

Rocha, E. M., Marche, T. A., & von Baeyer, C. L. (2009). Anxiety influences children's memory for procedural pain. *Pain Research & Management, 14*(3), 233–237.

Rose, J. B., Finkel, J. C., Arquedas-Mohs, A., Himelstein, B. P., Schreiner, M., & Medve, R. A. (2003). Oral tramadol for the treatment of pain of 7–30 days' duration in children. *Anesthesia and Analgesia, 96*, 78–81.

Rubenstein, E. B., Peterson, D. E., Schubert, M., Keefe, D., McGuire, D., Epstein, J., et al. (2004). Clinical practice guidelines for the prevention and treatment of cancer therapy- induced oral and gastrointestinal mucositis. *Cancer, 100*(Suppl(9)), 2026–2046.

RxList (2010) Provigil. Accessed June 25, 2010, from www.RxList.com

Sahler, O. J., Roghmann, K. J., Carpenter, P. J., Mulhern, R. K., Dolgin, M. J., Sargent, J. R., et al. (1994). Sibling adaptation to childhood cancer collaborative study: Prevalence of sibling distress and definition of adaptation levels. *Journal of Developmental and Behavioral Pediatrics, 15*(5), 353–366.

Sargent, J. R., Sahler, O. J., Roghmann, K. J., Mulhern, R. K., Barbarian, O. A., Carpenter, P. J., et al. (1995). Sibling adaptation to childhood cancer collaborative study: Siblings' perceptions of the cancer experience. *Journal of Pediatric Psychology, 20*(2), 151–164.

Sawni-Sikand, A., Schubiner, H., & Thomas, R. L. (2002). Use of complementary/alternative therapies among children in primary care pediatrics. *Ambulatory Pediatrics, 2*(2), 99–103.

Schweizerhof, M., Stosser, S., Kurejova, M., Njoo, C., Gangadharan, V., Agarwal, N., et al. (2009). Hematopoietic colony-stimulating factors mediate tumor-nerve interactions and bone cancer pain. *Natural Medicines, 15*(7), 802–807.

Senturk, M., Ozcan, P. E., Talu, G. K., Kiyan, E., Camci, E., Ozyalcin, S., et al. (2002). The effects of three different analgesia techniques on long-term postthoracotomy pain. *Anesthesia and Analgesia, 94*(1), 11–15.

Shankar, S., & Hosking, D. J. (2006). Biochemical assessment of Paget's disease of bone. *J Bone Mineral Res, 21*(Suppl 2), 22–27.

Shih, A., Miaskowski, C., Dodd, M. J., Stotts, N. A., & MacPhail, L. (2003). Mechanisms for radiation induced oral mucositis and the consequences. *Cancer Nursing, 26*(3), 222–229.

Silvasti, M., Tarkkila, P., Tuominen, M., Svartling, N., & Rosenberg, P. H. (1999). Efficacy and side effects of tramadol versus oxycodone for patient-controlled analgesia after maxillofacial surgery. *European Journal of Anesthesiology, 16*(12), 834–839.

Simons, S. H., van Dijk, M., Anand, K. S., Roofthooft, D., van Lingen, R. A., & Tibboel, D. (2003). Do we still hurt newborn babies? A prospective study of procedural pain and analgesia in neonates. *Archives of Pediatrics & Adolescent Medicine, 157*(11), 1058–1064.

Sirkia, K., Hov, L., Pouttu, J., & Saarinen-Pihkala, U. M. (1998). Pain medication during terminal care of children with cancer. *Journal of Pain and Symptom Management, 15*, 220–226.

Smith, J., & Thompson, J. (1995). Phantom limb pain and chemotherapy in pediatric amputees. *Mayo Clinic Proceedings, 70*(4), 357–364.

Spinetta, J., Jankovic, M., Eden, T., Green, D., Martins, A. G., & Wandzura, C. (1999). Guidelines for assistance to siblings of children with cancer: Report of the SIOP working committee on psychosocial issues in pediatric leukemia. *Medical and Pediatric Oncology, 33*, 395–398.

Stevens, B., McGrath, P., Gibbins, S., Beyene, J., Breau, L., Camfield, C., et al. (2003). Procedural pain in newborns at risk for neurologic impairment. *Pain, 105*(1–2), 27–35.

Susman, E. (2005). Cancer pain management guidelines issued for children; adult guidelines updated. *Journal of the National Cancer Institute, 97*(10), 711–712.

Sutton, E. J., Tong, R. T., Gillis, A. M., Henning, T. D., Weinberg, V. A., Boddington, S., et al. (2009). Decreased aortic growth and middle aortic syndrome in patients with neuroblastoma after radiation therapy. *Pediatric Radiology, 39*(11), 1194–1202.

Tanner, K. D., Levine, J. D., & Topps, K. S. (1998). Microtubule disorientation and axonal swelling in unmyelinated sensory axons during vincristine-induced painful neuropathy in rat. *The Journal of Comparative Neurology, 395*, 481–492.

Tigue, C. C., McKoy, J. M., Evens, A. M., Trifilio, S. M., Tallman, M. S., & Bennett, C. L. (2007). Granulocyte-colony stimulating factor administration to healthy individuals and persons with chronic neutropenia or cancer: An overview of safety considerations from the Research on Adverse Drug Events and Reports project. *Bone Marrow Transplantation, 40*(3), 185–192.

Uman, L. S., Chambers, C. T., McGrath, P. J., & Kisely, S. (2008). A systematic review of randomized controlled trials examining psychological interventions for needle-related procedural pain and distress in children and adolescents: An abbreviated cochrane review. *Journal of Pediatric Psychology, 33*(8), 842–854.

Van Cleve, L., Johnson, L., Pothier, P. (1996). Pain responses of hospitalized infants and children to venipuncture and intravenous cannulation. *Journal of Pediatric Nursing, 11*(3), 161–168.

Varni, J. W., Burwinkle, T. M., & Katz, E. R. (2004). The PedsQL in pediatric cancer pain: A prospective longitudinal analysis of pain and emotional distress. *Journal of Developmental and Behavioral Pediatrics, 25*(4), 239–246.

Walco, G. A., Conte, P. M., Labay, L. E., Engel, R., & Zeltzer, L. K. (2005). Procedural distress in children with cancer: Self-report, behavioral observations, and physiological parameters. *The Clinical Journal of Pain, 21*(6), 484–490.

Wallace, M. S., Wallace, A. M., Lee, J., & Dobke, M. K. (1996). Pain after breast surgery: A survey of 282 women. *Pain, 66*(2–3), 195–205.

Westberg, J., & Gobel, B. H. (2004). Methylphenidate use for the management of opioid induced sedation. *Clinical Journal of Oncology Nursing, 8*(2), 203–205.

Whitelaw, G. L., Blasiak-Wal, I., Cooke, K., Usher, C., Macdougall, N. D., & Plowman, P. N. (2008). A dosimetric comparison between two intensity-modulated radiotherapy techniques: Tomotherapy vs dynamic linear accelerator. *The British Journal of Radiology, 81*(964), 333–340.

Wild, M. R., & Espie, C. A. (2004). The efficacy of hypnosis in the reduction of procedural pain and distress in pediatric oncology: A systematic review. *Journal of developmental and behavioral pediatrics, 25*(3), 207–213.

Wilkins, K. L., McGrath, P. J., Finley, G. A., & Katz, J. (1998). Phantom limb sensations and phantom limb pain in child and adolescent amputees. *Pain, 78*(1), 7–12.

Wittig, J. C., Bickels, J., Kellar-Graney, K. L., & Malawer, M. M. (2002). Osteosarcoma of the proximal humerus: Long-term results with limb-sparing surgery. *Clinical Orthopaedics and Related Research, 397*, 156–176.

Worthington, H.V., Clarkson, J.E., & Eden, O.B. (2006). Interventions for preventing oral mucositis for patients with cancer receiving treatment [Update in Cochrane Database Syst Rev. 2007;(4):CD000978; PMID: 17943748]. [Update of Cochrane Database Syst Rev. 2003;(3):CD000978; PMID: 12917895]. *Cochrane Database of Systematic Reviews, 2*, CD000978.

www.jcaho.org (2009). Standards on Moderate Sedation. Last accessed April 25, 2011.

Xu, X. J., Colpaert, F., & Wiesenfeld-Hallin, Z. (2003). Opioid hyperalgesia and tolerance versus 5-HT1A receptor-mediated inverse tolerance. *Trends in Pharmacological Sciences, 24*(12), 634–639.

Yamashita, S., Sato, S., Kakiuchi, Y., Miyabe, M., & Yamaguchi, H. (2002). Lidocaine toxicity during frequent viscous lidocaine use for painful tongue ulcer. *Journal of Pain and Symptom Management, 24*(5), 543–545.

Yeh, C. H., Lin, C. F., Tsai, J. L., Lai, Y. M., & Ku, H. C. (1999). Determinants of parental decisions on 'drop out' from cancer treatment for childhood cancer patients. *Journal of Advanced Nursing, 30*(1), 193–199.

Yeoh, A., Gibson, R., Yeoh, E., Bowen, J., Stringer, A., Giam, K., et al. (2006). Radiation therapy-induced mucositis: Relationships between fractionated radiation, NF-κB, COX-1 and COX-2. *Cancer Treatment Reviews, 32*, 645–651.

ZENIT (2004) *Slippery slope of Euthanasia for children.* http://www.zenit.org/english/visualizza.phtml?sid= 58462

Zernikow, B., Smale, H., Michel, E., Hasan, C., Jorch, N., & Andler, W. (2006). Paediatric cancer pain management using the WHO analgesic ladder - results of a prospective analysis from 2265 treatment days during a quality improvement study. *European Journal of Pain, 10*(7), 587–595.

John Curran, Ali Sephadari,
and Hariharan Shankar

Keywords
CRPS, use of imaging in • Sympathetic blockade • Back pain, in children
• Neuroimaging • PET in combination with CT

Introduction

Imaging plays a part in the workup and management of a large range of conditions in children and adults (Tables 14.1 and 14.2). A complete discussion of imaging as it relates to all conditions that cause chronic pain in children is beyond the scope of this chapter. Thus, we limit our discussion to a group of relatively common conditions, including complex regional pain syndrome, low back pain, headache, and cancer pain, with discussion of image-guided interventions when appropriate. We also briefly discuss basic interpretation of spine magnetic resonance imaging.

Complex Regional Pain Syndrome/ Reflex Sympathetic Dystrophy

Complex regional pain syndrome (CRPS) describes an intense, burning extremity pain that most commonly occurs following trauma or similar insult. CRPS is believed to relate to nerve injury. CRPS is

classified into two types; CRPS type I (formerly "reflex sympathetic dystrophy") which occurs without a definable nerve lesion, whereas CRPS type II (formerly "causalgia") occurs when a definable nerve lesion is present. This is discussed in greater depth in Chap. 23. The diagnosis is based on clinical criteria. Several diagnostic criteria have been proposed, including the commonly used Breuhl's criteria, but there is no consensus on optimal clinical diagnosis (Bruehl et al. 1999). As a result, much investigation has centered on the role of imaging in assisting with a diagnosis. Plain radiography, radionuclide bone scintigraphy, and magnetic resonance imaging (MRI) are modalities that have been studied in CRPS.

Plain Radiography

Sudek originally described in 1902 the radiographic findings of the disease that would come to be known as Reflex sympathetic dystrophy and later as CRPS Type 1. The primary radiographic findings are diffuse osteoporosis with severe patchy demineralization, most notably in the periarticular regions, with subperiosteal bone resorption. The findings are similar to those of disuse osteoporosis, though with a more marked and prolonged bone loss. Studies designed to

J. Curran (✉)
Director of Neuroradiology, Phoenix Children's Physician
Network, 1919 E. Thomas Road, Phoenix, AZ 85016, USA
e-mail: jcurran@phoenixchildrens.org

B.C. McClain and S. Suresh (eds.), *Handbook of Pediatric Chronic Pain:
Current Science and Integrative Practice*, DOI 10.1007/978-1-4419-0350-1_14,
© Springer Science+Business Media, LLC 2011

Table 14.1 Imaging techniques for diagnosis

Plain radiograph	CRPS
	Disc disease
CT scan	CRPS
	Headaches
	Facet disease
	Disc disease
MRI	CRPS
	Headaches
	Facet disease
	Disc disease

Table 14.2 Imaging for procedures

Plain X ray	Epidural injection
	Lumbar sympathetic block
	Stellate ganglion
CT scan	Lumbar sympathetic block
	Stellate ganglion
	Facet blocks
US guidance	Stellate ganglion block
	Facet block
	Lateral femoral cutaneous block
	Suprascapular block
	Ilioinguinal and iliohypogastric block

assess the sensitivity and specificity of radiography have shown inconsistent results (Schürmann et al. 2007a). The radiographic findings tend to appear late in the course of the disease, making radiography a poor screening tool and limiting its usefulness in early diagnosis of the condition.

Radionuclide Bone Scintigraphy

Radionuclide bone scan has been employed for several decades to diagnose CRPS. The characteristic finding of increased activity during the blood flow and blood pool phases, with increased periarticular uptake on the delayed static phase, are said to be pathognomonic for CRPS. Increased periarticular uptake on delayed static images is the most sensitive finding (Intenzo et al. 1989).

Most of the published data on this topic are retrospective. A handful of prospective studies have also been performed, but most are confounded by the selection criteria; only patients with clinical suspicion for CRPS were imaged, rather than all unselected post-trauma patients. A prospective study of 175 unselected trauma patients showed only a 16% sensitivity of triple phase bone scan, but a high specificity (Schürmann et al. 2007b). A meta-analysis of 19 articles showed a composite sensitivity of about 50% for radionuclide bone scan (Lee and Weeks 1995). The sensitivity of bone scan is related to the severity of disease, with mild disease often showing normal findings. It is believed to be more helpful in diagnosing non-traumatic CRPS than in CRPS following trauma.

Magnetic Resonance Imaging

MRI is a modality that allows for excellent contrast resolution among bone and soft tissue and has been an area of recent investigation. Skin thickening, tissue enhancement, and bone signal intensity changes in carpals and metacarpals, along with adjacent joint effusions, and are said to be related to the early findings of CRPS (Borre et al. 1995) cannot find. Several large studies have reported poor sensitivity with MRI, and found it to be no better than bone scan (Koch et al. 1991; Schürmann et al. 2007b). Oddly, some investigators have found that sensitivity increases with time following injury, while others have found that sensitivity decreases. Schweitzer et al. retrospectively studied MRI and found a sensitivity of 87% for CRPS Type 1 (termed "RSD" in their study) when using the finding of soft tissue enhancement. In their study, they did not use bone edema as a diagnostic criterion. The justification for this choice was that bone edema is a result of denervation, a late feature of the disease. They posited that earlier investigations that focused on the finding of bone marrow edema had erroneously grouped CRPS with transient osteoporosis of the hip and regional migratory osteoporosis on the basis that all diseases show similar clinical findings. However, Schweitzer et al. believe that the different pathogenesis of CRPS results in differences in the timing of bone edema (Schweitzer et al. 1995). Subsequent studies have retained bone marrow edema as a criterion for MR diagnosis of CRPS, and it is unclear if attempts have been made to validate Schweitzer et al.'s hypothesis. In a small series, Crozier et al. found soft tissue changes in only 3 of 15 patients (Crozier et al. 2003).

Overall we believe that MRI, much like radionuclide bone scan, is not sufficiently sensitive to exclude CRPS when it is clinically suspected and thus is best used as to exclude other diagnoses rather than to confirm or exclude CRPS.

The Role of Imaging in CRPS

While some advocate strongly for the use of imaging in diagnosing CRPS, particularly bone scan and to a lesser extent MRI, it is a widely held belief that these imaging studies are most useful for excluding some other orthopedic abnormality that may be causing neurovascular changes, and that CRPS remains a clinical diagnosis (Wilder 2006).

Imaging Guided Sympathetic Block

Optimal treatment of CRPS requires a multidisciplinary approach, and some experts advocate for greater emphasis on physiotherapy rather than pharmacologic and interventional procedures for management of CRPS in children.

Sympathetic blockade, achieved through percutaneous injection of long-acting anesthetic into prevertebral sympathetic ganglia, can be a valuable tool in managing CRPS, primarily through relieving pain sufficiently to allow the patient to participate in physical therapy. Lumbar sympathetic block and stellate ganglion block are used to treat CRPS symptoms referable to the lower extremities and upper extremities, respectively.

Techniques involving use of bony anatomic landmarks have been well described, and employed by a significant percentage of anesthesia pain practitioners according to a survey study of Canadian physicians performed in 2004. However, the prevailing opinion is that image guidance should be employed to maximize the safety and effectiveness of the procedure, particularly when

neurolysis is performed. Potential complications of lumbar sympathetic block relate to ureteral or renal hilum injury, lumbar somatic nerve injury, or direct consequences of neurolysis (Cherry and Rao 1982). Fluoroscopic guidance, CT guidance, or a combination of the two may be used to minimize these risks.

Lumbar Sympathetic block: The lumbar sympathetic ganglion cannot be directly visualized by CT or radiography, and thus cannot be directly targeted. Thus, sympathetic blockade is achieved by ensuring accurate needle placement in the retroperitoneal space. The L2, L3, or L4 level is typically targeted. The procedure is best performed with the patient prone, using a C-arm fluoroscopy unit. A 22 g spinal needle is most commonly used. The skin entry site is typically 6–10 cm off the midline. The needle tip is directed toward midline, and the optimal final position is 0.6–0.8 cm posterior to the anterior margin of the vertebral body and approximately 1 cm from midline. Injection of a small amount of contrast material will help confirm retroperitoneal needle position.

Recent literature has focused on CT guidance, with or without fluoroscopy, for performing lumbar sympathetic block, and there has been a recent report of a successful CT-guided lumbar block in a child (Nordmann et al. 2006). Direct visualization of the aorta and inferior vena cava virtually eliminate the risk of inadvertent vascular puncture. Patient positioning and needle path are typically the same for the CT-guided approach as for the fluoroscopic approach. Below are examples of optimal needle position:

Stellate Ganglion block: Stellate ganglion block is performed from an anterior approach with the patient in the supine position. A 25-G spinal needle is most commonly used. Under fluoroscopy, the C6 or C7 vertebral body is identified. The needle is directed at a 90° angle to the vertical toward the junction of the vertebral body and ipsilateral transverse process. Once the bone is reached, a small amount of contrast is injected to confirm location of the needle tip.

As with lumbar sympathetic block, CT-guided injection techniques have also been well described. CT guided technique typically requires a much smaller volume of anesthetic, typically no more than 1–2 mL, and has been described to have a higher efficacy as determined by skin temperature response. Ultrasound guidance has been used for performing; this is described at the end of this chapter in detail.

US guidance for Stellate ganglion block: More recently, an ultrasound-guided technique for the placement of stellate ganglion blocks has been described (Narouze et al. 2007). This technique is performed with the patient supine and with head extended. A curvilinear probe is placed and the transverse process is localized. The longus colli muscle is identified. The stellate ganglion is located above the longus colli and above the transverse process. After careful aspiration, 10 mL of local anesthetic solution is injected into the area of the stellate ganglion (Shibata et al. 2007).

Back Pain in the Pediatric Patient

Although less common than in adults, back pain is a vexing-presenting complaint in children. Back pain is usually related to muscle strains and sprains. Therefore, it is vital to identify those patients with more serious underlying conditions such as infection, neoplasm, or tethered cord. Early recognition of disk herniation and spondylolysis can also result in better management strategies and outcomes. It is beyond the scope of this chapter to discuss the imaging features of each of these diseases individually. This chapter will deal primarily with devising an appropriate imaging workup for back pain, with a more detailed discussion of disc disease and percutaneous pain management procedures.

Epidemiology

The exact prevalence and incidence of back pain in the pediatric population is unclear. Although it is typically described as "rare," the estimated prevalence in adolescents ranges from 17.6% to 26% in several European studies, while others show a 16–22% 1 year incidence of low back pain symptoms in 11–14 year-olds (Balagué et al. 1995; Salminen et al. 1992; Taimela et al. 1997; Watson et al. 2002). Retrospective chart reviews focused on emergency department and clinic visits suggest a much lower incidence (Selbst et al. 1999). These statistics would suggest that low back pain is in fact rather common, but that it does not typically cause disability that leads to clinical evaluation.

Low back pain is more common in girls than in boys, particularly in younger age groups. There is inconsistent evidence suggesting that tall height, BMI, and rapid growth in height are associated with low back pain (Jones and Macfarlane 2005). Young athletes playing at a competitive level, particularly in sports such as weightlifting, gymnastics, rowing, golf, and racket sports are at increased risk for low back pain (LBP). Likewise, sedentary children, particularly those with ≥2 h per day of television watching or video game playing, are at increased risk (Balagué et al. 1988). Schoolbag carrying likely does not play a role in the development of back pain, within the normal range of backpack weights. Psychological and psychosocial factors have also been shown to correlate with reporting of back pain in children.

Basic Workup

Initial workup should be aimed at effectively identifying patients at risk for significant pathology (e.g., tumor, infection, herniated nucleus pulposus, scheuermann kyphosis, spondylolysis, scoliosis) from those with nonspecific "benign" back pain syndromes (e.g., muscle sprain, overuse syndrome). Feldman et al. published a prospective analysis of outcomes in pediatric back pain patients treated according to a set of protocol aimed at making this distinction. A thorough history and physical examination are, as always, the first step in the workup. Key historical points may lead to a specific diagnosis (Table 14.3 reproduced from Bernstein and Cozen).

Table 14.3 Differential diagnosis of back pain

Presenting feature	Symptomatology	Differential Diagnosis
Acute pain	• Radiation to legs, positive straight leg raise • Other injuries, neurological deficits	• Herniation of disc, spondylolysis, slipped apophysis • Vertebral fracture
Chronic pain	• Rigid kyphosis • Morning stiffness, tenderness over the sacroiliac joints	• Scheuermann's kyphosis • Inflammatory spondyloarthropathies
Pain with fever	Malaise, weight loss, nocturnal pain	Tumor, Infection
Spinal flexion pain	Radicular pain, dull low back pain, local spinal tenderness, positive straight leg raise	Slipped apophysis, disc herniation, discogenic pain
Spinal extension pain	Negative straight leg raise, paraspinal tenderness, referred pain in the leg	Spondylolysis, spondylolisthesis, pedicle injury or lesion
Dull paraspinal pain	Local diffuse tenderness, fever, dysuria,	Pyelonephritis

Many investigators believe that children and adolescents without significant physical findings, short duration of pain, and a history of minor injury can be treated conservatively without radiographic or laboratory studies. A CBC, ESR, and plain radiographs are low cost, useful initial studies when these criteria are not met, and can provide evidence of underlying infection or leukemia. Plain radiographs sometimes lead to a specific diagnosis, obviating the need for further imaging. When plain radiographs are unrevealing, and when the history and physical exam are not reassuring (neurological exam abnormality, constant pain, night pain, radicular pain), noncontrast MRI is typically the next step. Feldman et al. found that 21/87 patients had a specific diagnosis on plain radiography (Feldman et al. 2006). In their series, an additional 10 patients had a specific diagnosis that was detected on MRI following negative plain radiographs. The 56 patients with reassuring history and physical, and with normal labs and plain film, were treated conservatively and after 3 years of follow-up showed no evidence of a serious condition missed at initial workup.

The literature on pediatric back pain is sparse, and the study by Feldman et al. is the only prospectively validated diagnostic algorithm identified. The remaining studies are retrospective chart reviews. The prevailing opinion is that back pain in the pediatric patient, while typically of benign etiology, should be worked up to assess for serious underlying pathology. AP and lateral radiographs are generally considered helpful and are the appropriate initial imaging studies, although it is noteworthy that Selbst et al. did not find them helpful in the emergency department setting (Selbst, et al. 1999). If additional imaging is necessary (i.e., if there are concerning history or physical exam findings), MRI is generally the next appropriate imaging study. If there is clinical concern for spondylolysis, oblique radiographs are easy to obtain and inexpensive. Radionuclide bone scintigraphy can be a useful troubleshooting tool for detecting developing spondylolysis in the contralateral side when there is an existing pars defect, but has too low sensitivity and specificity to use as a screening study alone.

Disc Disease in the Pediatric Patient

Disc diseases, including disc degeneration and nucleus pulposus herniation, are generally thought of as adult diseases. Although disc herniation is much less common in the pediatric population, with children accounting for less than 1% of all patients with disc herniation, it nevertheless occurs often enough to warrant consideration.

MRI is the imaging modality of choice to evaluate for disk herniation; it delivers no ionizing radiation, and has superior contrast between soft tissues, disc, and CSF. A full set of sagittal and axial T2- and T1-weighted sequences are necessary for diagnosing disk herniation. Axial images are acquired perpendicular to the long axis of the spine from T12 to L5. Angled axial images perpendicular to the long axis of the sacrum are obtained from L5 through the sacral segments. Over-reliance on the sagittal T2 sequence without similar attention to the axial sequences is a common cause of missed disc herniation, particularly lateral herniation. It is essential to obtain contiguous axial images rather than images only through the disc levels, as a migrated fragment can easily be missed this way. A linear high T2 signal focus can often be seen in the annulus fibrosis, indicating a tear.

Herniation typically occurs in degenerated discs, but it is unclear whether there is a causal relationship. Tertti et al. performed a well-designed cross-sectional case control study of children with back pain, with age-matched controls. Disc protrusion occurred at levels that showed degeneration, but age-matched controls without back pain had disc degeneration (as determined by MRI signal characteristics) at the same levels and at a similar frequency to those with back pain. The prevalence of disk signal abnormality was higher in this study than had been suggested in prior studies, and raises question as to whether an isolated finding of low disc signal should lead one to attribute low back pain to degenerative disc disease (Tertti et al. 1991).

Percutaneous Interventional Therapies

When conservative therapy for low back pain is unsuccessful, there are several percutaneous procedures which may be helpful for relieving symptoms. We discuss epidural injection and facet joint injection in the management of back pain. *Epidural Injection*: Patient selection for epidural injection is poorly described in the literature. Its use has been described for treatment of local pain or radiculopathy in the settings of documented disk herniation, central or foraminal stenosis, and absent imaging findings. The technique is usually used if rest has failed to relieve the symptoms or if the patient is considered a surgical candidate but does not desire to undergo surgery. The technique is infrequently used in acute situations. Various combinations of saline solution, local anesthetics, and steroids have been injected. Theories for explaining the method of relief include lysis of adhesions, change in relationship between the disk and the nerve root, anesthetic breaking the pain cycle, and reduction of inflammation and swelling.

Imaging guidance should be used for epidural injection, as there is a high rate of erroneous placement in the epidural space, even in experienced hands. Fluoroscopic and CT-guided approaches have been described. A commonly used fluoroscopic technique was initially described by El-Khoury et al. and has been detailed by Silbergleit et al. (el-Khoury et al. 1988; Silbergleit et al. 2001). With the patient prone on the fluoroscopy table, the sacral hiatus is palpated by feeling for the cornua on either side and by fluoroscopic localization. The skin over the hiatus is cleaned and 4 × 4 gauze pads are typically used to prevent dripping of topical antiseptic onto perineal structures. After administering local anesthetic, a 5-in. 22-gauge. spinal needle is advanced under fluoroscopic guidance through the sacral hiatus. Care is taken to keep the needle below the S2–3 level to minimize risk of intradural puncture. The needle is usually advanced primarily under lateral fluoroscopic guidance with intermittent frontal guidance. On a frontal projection, the needle should lie between the pedicles of the sacral segments. Having the patient cough with the stylet out will exclude intradural needle position. Epidurography is performed with injection of 3 mL of nonionic contrast material. The lumbosacral epidural space is usually opacified to the L4 level and occasionally higher. The images below demonstrate the schematic anatomy of the dural sac, with images.

Interlaminar ESI – L4-L5 – lateral view

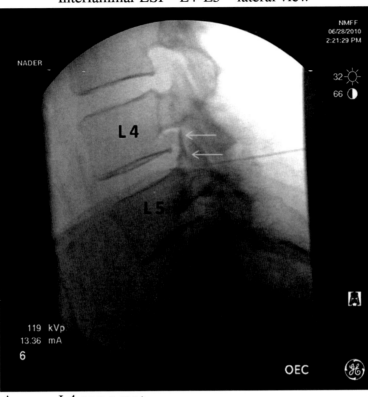

Arrow = L4 nerve root

Fig. 14.1   Epidural steroid injection; flouroscopic image AP view

A dorsal interlaminar approach has also been described for epidural injection. With the patient in the prone position, the needle is advanced into the epidural space, using a loss-of-resistance technique to confirm needle position. Absence of CSF flow is verified as above (Figs. 14.1 and 14.2).

Facet Blocks: Facet joints are heavily innervated, and studies have shown correlation between facet disease on radiography and positive response to injections (Helbig and Lee 1988). Facet joint injection can be performed under fluoroscopic or CT guidance. A newer technique with the use of ultrasound guidance has been described in adults (Greher et al. 2004a, b).

Fluoroscopy: When performed under fluoroscopic guidance, the patient is rotated into the prone oblique position to profile the facet joint of interest. A 22-gauge needle is then directed vertically into

the joint, and the patient is rolled into the lateral and frontal positions to confirm needle location.

CT-Guided facet blocks: Facet joint injections can also be performed under CT, typically with the patient in the prone position.

Imaging in Pediatric Headache

Headache is a common complaint, accounting for up to 4% of all outpatient visits with annual estimated direct and indirect costs exceeding 5.6 billion dollars (de Lissovoy and Lazarus 1994). The prevalence of headaches increases with age, rising from 37% to 51% during elementary school years up to 57–82% during the high school years (Deubner 1977; Sillanpää 1983a, b; Stewart et al. 1991). The etiology of headache is almost

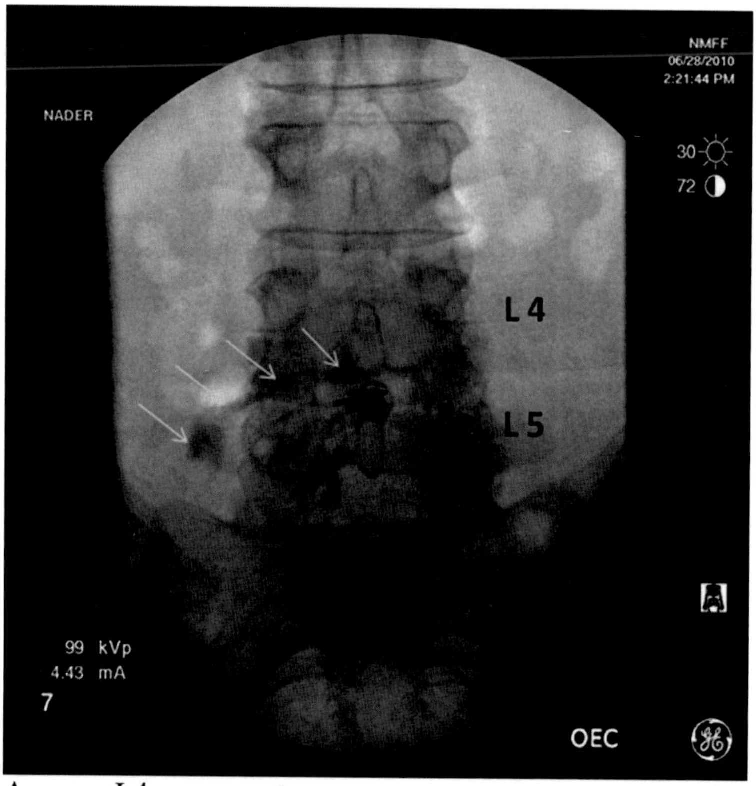
Interlaminar ESI – L4-L5 – AP view
NMFF
06/28/2010
2:21:44 PM
NADER
30
72
L4
L5
99 kVp
4.43 mA
7
OEC
Arrow = L4 nerve root

Fig. 14.2 Epidural steroid injection; fluoroscopic image, lateral view

always benign, and common causes include migraine, tension headache, cluster headache, and sinus headache. The challenge facing the clinical practitioner is in identifying the subset of patients who are at higher risk for having serious underlying conditions requiring treatment, such as intracranial neoplasm, benign intracranial hypertension (pseudotumor cerebri), or venous sinus thrombosis. This is not always a simple task. The difficulty of making a diagnosis of intracranial neoplasm is well illustrated in a large retrospective study that reported a mean time to diagnosis of more than 4 months (and a median time of about 2 months) for children with posterior fossa tumors.

The American Academy of Neurology's most recent published guidelines on the evaluation of headache in children and adolescents directly addresses the issue of when to image in cases of headache (Lewis et al. 2002). Their report reviews six studies on neuroimaging in pediatric headache. Based on those studies, their recommendations are as follows:

1. Imaging should not be performed routinely in patients with recurrent headaches and normal neurological examination.
2. Imaging should be considered in patients with abnormal neurologic examination or coexistent seizures.
3. Imaging should be considered in with recent onset of severe headache, change in type of headache, or features that suggest neurologic dysfunction.

In general, MRI is the preferred modality when the decision has been made to image a child with headache. In addition to its inherently superior contrast resolution, MR has the added advantage of avoiding the use of ionizing radiation and of superior imaging of the posterior fossa, where a high proportion of pediatric neoplasms occur. Dural venous sinus thrombosis is probably best detected with MR (assuming ideal conditions and techniques), and MR is also superior in detecting "benign" findings that have a known association with headache, including Chiari I malformation, arachnoid cyst, and pineal cyst. MRI can generally be performed without contrast, with a decision to administer contrast to better evaluate any abnormality.

For patients with a contraindication to MRI (e.g., cochlear implants), CT is also very sensitive and specific for detecting neoplasms, and is very sensitive for venous sinus thrombosis, for which it is likely the best modality if high-field MR is not available. In one series, CT was able to detect all surgical space occupying lesions that were seen on MR (Medina et al. 1997). Although MR is the preferred modality, a negative CT scan, performed without and with contrast, is adequate to exclude significant underlying pathology when MR is contraindicated.

Metastatic Cancer Pain

Tumors such as leukemia, neuroblastoma, lymphoma, and Ewing's sarcoma may be complicated by bony metastases causing bone pain. Careful clinical evaluation is necessary in any child presenting with pain to exclude metastatic bone pain as the underlying cause. In general, nonarticular pain or tenderness that is localized to bone is always worrisome. Significant night sweats, focal neurologic abnormalities, and bruising are also concerning clinical features. Plain radiography is a cost-effective and useful initial screening tool. For generalized symptoms, whole body nuclear medicine scan is an efficient way to evaluate the entire skeleton. Recently positron emission tomography scan (PET scan) in combination with CT has been used successfully in identifying patients with metastatic bone disease. Nuclear medicine also offers therapy for bone pain with bone targeting high-energy radionuclides such as strontium-89.

Neoplastic Brachial Plexopathy

Brachial plexopathy can occur secondary to neoplasm. In children, particularly those with neurofibromatosis, nerve sheath tumors are the most common cause of neoplastic brachial plexopathy. Neurofibroma, plexiform neurofibroma, schwannoma, and malignant nerve sheath tumor can all cause brachial plexopathy.

MR imaging is the preferred modality for evaluating nerve sheath tumors, due to inherently superior soft tissue contrast and avoidance of ionizing radiation, particularly as nerve sheath tumors are often followed longitudinally to assess for malignant transformation. For imaging nerve sheath tumors of the cervicothoracic spine, conventional spine MR can be performed. When the lesion is located more peripherally, however, it is important to modify the study and surface coil positioning to image the area appropriately. Nerve sheath tumors are typically hypo- to isodense on CT; contrast enhancement is more often seen with schwannomas than with conventional or plexiform neurofibromas. MRI usually shows low to intermediate signal T1 and intermediate to high signal T2, with nonuniform gadolinium enhancement. T1 hyperintensity precontrast represents hemorrhage and is seen with Antoni B type schwannoma. Malignant degeneration is seen in 15–30% of cases. In plexiform neurofibromatosis, the tumors form a network that often involves the contiguous soft tissue. Below is an example of a plexiform neurofibroma involving the brachial plexus.

Imaging the Spine: MRI 101

A classic approach to interpret imaging studies of the spine is the "ABCD" approach.

"A" refers to alignment: The cervical spine and lumbar spine should show a gentle lordotic curvature, and the thoracic spine should have a gentle kyphosis. Any abnormal curvature of the spine in a child should be viewed with caution. Note that in young children; the lumbar curvature is relatively straightened compared to adults.

"B" refers to bones: On plain radiographs, bone mineral density and vertebral body shape are important to assess. On MRI, marrow signal intensity should be assessed on both T1- and T2-weighted sequences. A rule of thumb is that marrow signal should be brighter than disc signal on T1, and darker than disc signal on T2. Deviations from this may represent a marrow replacing process such as hematologic malignancy or diffuse bony metastases, or may reflect marrow expansion as can be seen in hematologic diseases such as sickle cell anemia or thalassemia.

"C" Cord signal or CSF space or caudal equina: This refers to several structures, including the cord signal and morphology, CSF space, location of the conus medullaris, and the cauda equina. Cord signal should be uniformly dark, although faintly higher intensity can be seen in the gray matter relative to the white matter on heavily T2-weighted sequences. With the exception of a focal area of widening in the lower cervical cord, there should be a smooth tapering of the cord as it progresses caudally down the neural axis. The conus should lie at L2-3 or above, and the nerve roots of the cauda equina should be seen separately and distinctly on axial images. High intensity CSF should be seen ventral and dorsal to the cord throughout the entire spine.

"D" refers to the intervertebral discs: They should be assessed for signal and height, and for herniation of the nucleus pulposus. The annulus fibrosis is seen as a low signal ring surrounding the higher signal nucleus pulposus. In the setting of acute nucleus pulposus herniation, a linear focus of T2 bright signal can be seen in the annulus fibrosis. When nucleus pulposus herniation occurs, it is important to look at the levels above and below the herniation for migrated disc fragments, or for additional herniations.

In addition, a word of caution is appropriate regarding the naming of vertebral levels. Conventionally, there are 7 cervical, 12 rib-bearing thoracic, and 5 lumbar-type vertebra, each with fully formed intervertebral discs. The sacral vertebra is typically fused, and the last fully formed disc is at L5-S1. Vertebral body numbering quickly becomes more complicated when anatomic variations or segmentation anomalies occur. Lumbar spine imaging is complicated by the presence of either 11 or 13 rib-bearing vertebra or presence of a "sacralized" L5 segment or "lumbarized" S1 segment. This confusion can lead to interventions at the wrong level, or confusion when localizing a radiculopathy.

The most accurate way to number vertebral bodies is to count from C2 downward, which can be accomplished by using a full-spine counting localizer sequence (MR), or by cross-referencing with complete spine radiographs. This ensures that the named vertebral level is concordant with the nerve distribution.

Conclusion: The use of imaging for pediatric pain management is crucial in diagnosis and procedure performance. It is important to view all images prior to the appointment.

Ultrasound Guided Imaging and Interventions in Pediatric Pain Medicine

Introduction

The scope of diagnostic ultrasound imaging has increased tremendously in the recent past. It is being increasingly used for various pain medicine interventions for needle guidance and real time visualization of injectate (Gorthi et al. 2010). Its role in pediatric pain medicine is slowly increasing and is likely to be a major imaging modality in the future (Table 14.4). There are many advantages to using ultrasound guidance. It provides real time visualization without the risk of radiation. With newer portable devices, procedures can be performed at the bedside or in an office setting. Presently, the limitations of ultrasound imaging include the poor visualization of needles and the lack of demonstration of safety from intravascular and intraneuronal injections. In this section, the focus will be on the various pain interventions that lend itself to the use of ultrasound guidance. Recommendations applicable to all ultrasound-guided blocks include (1) all blocks are performed with adequate water soluble gel in a sterile transducer sheath and adopting sterile

Table 14.4 Ultrasound imaging for pediatric pain

Block	Transducer type	Indications	Complications
Greater occipital nerve	"Hockey stick" or linear array	Headache, occipital neuralgia	Intravascular injection, Hematoma,
Suprascapular nerve	Linear array	Shoulder pain	Pneumothorax, hematoma
Intercostal nerve	Linear array	Chest wall pain, post thoracotomy pain	Pneumothorax, hematoma
Lateral femoral cutaneous nerve	Hockey stick or linear array	Meralgia paraesthetica	Hematoma
Stellate ganglion	Hockey stick or linear array	Sympathetic pain of the upper extremity, CRPS	Pneumothorax, injury to esophagus, intravascular injection, hematoma,

precautions including antibacterial prep, (2) the choice of transducer depends on the body habitus and age, (3) a scout scan be regularly performed prior to the actual interventional scan to identify other structures in the vicinity of the target and finally, (4) with the poor visibility of the needle tip "hydro-localization" is recommended prior to local anesthetic solution injection to ensure appreciation of appropriate real time injectate spread.

Peripheral Nerve Blocks

Peripheral nerve blocks are traditionally performed using either landmarks or nerve stimulators. Landmark-based injections assume that human anatomy is similar in every human being. Individual variations in location of various nerves even between the two sides in the same individual are very well recognized. Because of these variations landmark-based injections are inherently destined to have failures. Nerve stimulators may aid in locating the nerves and provide an ability to deposit the injectate close to target. But it may involve multiple needle punctures for proper location. The good resolution images of ultrasound guidance allow accuracy in identifying and targeting adjacent to the nerve. Some of the commonly performed peripheral nerve injections include greater occipital nerve block for headache, suprascapular nerve block for shoulder pain especially in cancer pain, intercostal nerve block for chest wall pain, and lateral femoral cutaneous nerve block for meralgia paresthetica.

Greater Occipital Nerve Block
Pain in the distribution of the greater occipital nerve usually follows trauma, whip-lash injuries,

and myofascial pain syndrome. Greater occipital nerve is the posterior ramus of C2. It has a constant relationship with the superior surface of the obliquus capitis inferior before piercing the trapezius and exiting in a more superficial location. The obliquus capitis inferior is attached to the spinous process of C2 and the transverse process of C1.

The scanning technique for locating the greater occipital nerve starts with scanning longitudinally from the base of the cranium using a high frequency "hockey stick" transducer to identify the spinous process of C2 vertebra. Following identification, the transducer is rotated to a transverse view so that the bifid spinous process of C2 is visualized. Once the obliqus capitis inferior muscle is identified, the transducer is rotated on the lateral part to have a longitudinal view of the muscle with the spinous process medially (Greher et al. 2010). The cross sectional view of the nerve can be obtained over the superior surface of the muscle. An alternate technique has also been described to target it over the C2-3 facet joint (Figs. 14.3 and 14.4). Using either an in-plane or out of plane technique and a 25 G hypodermic needle, local anesthetic may be deposited around the nerve.

Suprascapular Nerve Block
Suprascapular nerve provides nerve supply to the supraspinatus and infraspinatus muscles besides an articular branch to the shoulder. It is usually a branch from C5 nerve root with variable contribution from the adjacent roots. It travels underneath the omohyoid and moves posteriorly to pass underneath the transverse scapular ligament in the suprascapular notch. After exiting from the

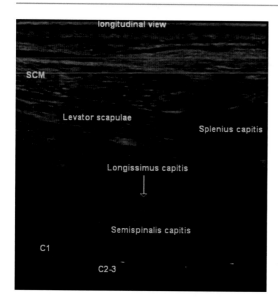

Fig. 14.3 Longitudinal view over the C2-3 facet joint showing the target for the greater occipital nerve block

notch, the nerve travels on the floor of the scapular spine on its way to the glenoid notch. Although the nerve could be blocked anywhere in the path, it is traditionally blocked in the floor of the spine or the notch (Gorthi et al. 2010; Harmon and Hearty 2007). Ultrasound-guided technique for this block uses a linear array transducer. Scanning technique starts from the acromion and moved medially along the superior border of the scapula. The glenoid notch is identified initially and then the floor of spine. At this point the transducer is rotated 90-degrees to visualize the suprascapular notch with the transverse scapular ligament overlying the notch. Color Doppler is used to identify the artery which runs over the ligament. The nerve may be approached either in plane or out of plane using a 25 G needle.(Figs. 14.5–14.7) It may be safer to approach from the anterior end to avoid the pleura. A newer anterior approach following the C5 nerve root as it bifurcates anteriorly into the suprascapular nerve has been attempted with good success.

Intercostal Nerve Block

Chest wall pain secondary to thoracotomy or cancer pain may be relieved by interventions to the intercostal nerve. This is used for persistent pain following thoracotomy as well as for some instances of costo-chondral pain (Byas-Smith and Gulati 2006). The intercostal nerve originates from the thoracic spinal roots and after passing through the paravertebral space travels between the innermost and inner intercostal muscles. Accompanied by the intercostal artery and vein, it travels under the lower margin of the rib until the angle of the rib at which point it may start to divide. The lateral cutaneous branch comes off anterior to the mid-axillary line. This makes it imperative that the nerve be targeted prior to its division.

Using a linear array transducer, the ribs are scanned in a transverse view from T12. The ribs appear hyperechoic and crescent-shaped with an acoustic shadow beneath it. This helps to identify the level. In the intercostal space the external and inner intercostal muscle layers are identified. The hyperechoic pleura can be seen to move with respiration. In addition it also displays "comet tail" artifacts when intact. The depth to pleura is measured using calipers on the US system. It may be difficult to identify the vessels unless the transducer is obliquely tilted to scan the under surface of the rib. Following this the transducer may be positioned longitudinal to the rib. The transducer is then slid down to the intercostal space when external and intercostal muscles may be more clearly visualized. The target is the internal intercostal muscles as the nerves are located within the muscle at this location posterior to the axillary line. Using an in-plane or out of plane approach with a 25-G needle, the intercostals nerve block is performed with great care to avoid the pleura (Figs. 14.8 and 14.9).

Lateral Femoral Cutaneous Nerve Block

Meralgia paraesthetica is an entrapment neuropathy of the lateral femoral cutaneous nerve seen in obesity, hypothyroidism, following surgery in the area and more recently with tight fitting garments. Pain relief may be provided by depositing steroids in the area of the nerve proximal to the compression. The nerve is a branch from the lumbar plexus with contributions from the roots of the L2 and L3 spinal nerves. It courses anterior to the sartorius muscle in the thigh before supplying

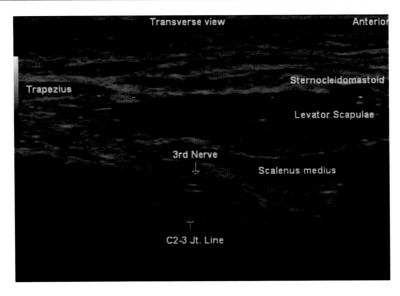

Fig. 14.4   Transverse view over the C2-3 facet joint showing the greater occipital nerve overlying the joint

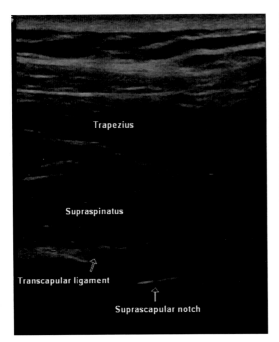

Fig. 14.5   Sonographic view of the suprascapular notch with the transducer tilted to align with the superior border of scapula

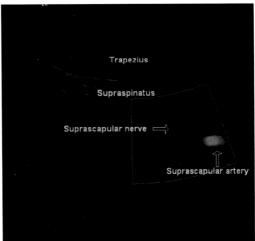

Fig. 14.6   Sonographic view over the suprascapular notch showing the suprascapular artery in the fossa

the anterolateral part of the thigh. The nerve is located by using a linear array transducer and scanning over the sartorius (Bodner et al. 2009). The nerve has a constant location in the fatty groove between the tensor fascia lata and the sartorius about 2 in. below the iliac crest (Fig. 14.10). From this area, the nerve may be traced upward to a location over the sartorius more close to the anterior superior iliac spine where it may be targeted. Like all peripheral nerves it appears hypoechoic with few hyperechoic fascicles within. An in-plane or an out of plane approach with a 25-G needle is used for targeting the nerve at this location.

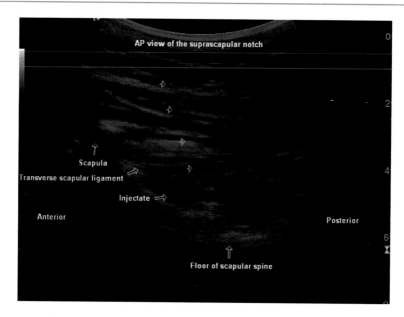

Fig. 14.7 Anteroposterior view of the scapula from the superior surface showing the floor of the scapular spine. The arrowheads point to the 25-G needle

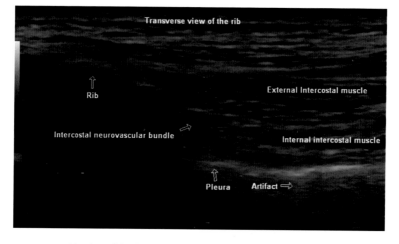

Fig. 14.8 Transverse sonographic view of the rib and the intercostal space with comet tail artifacts of the hyperechoic pleura

Sympathetic Nerve Blocks

Pain may be sympathetically mediated or non-sympathetically mediated. Sympathetically-mediated pain may be responsive to sympathetic blocks with local anesthetic or a combination of local anesthetic and steroids. One of the commonly performed sympathetic blocks for treatment of pain in the upper extremity is the stellate

ganglion block which is ideally performed under ultrasound guidance.

Stellate Ganglion Block

The stellate ganglion is a fusion of the inferior sympathetic ganglion and the T1 sympathetic ganglion. It is located over the transverse process of the T1 vertebra in proximity to major vessels and the dome of the pleura. Although the stellate

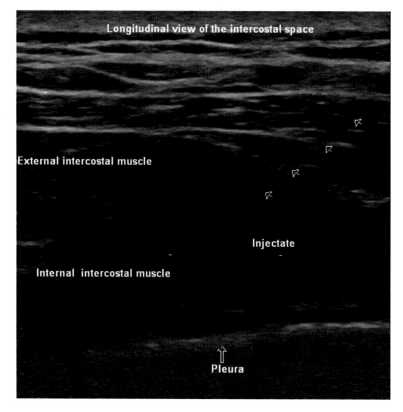

Fig. 14.9 Longitudinal view of the intercostal space. The arrowheads point to the 25-G needle

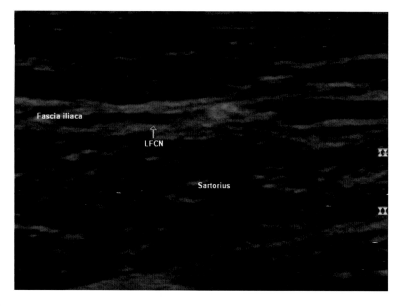

Fig. 14.10 Sonographic view of the lateral femoral cutaneous nerve over the Sartorius

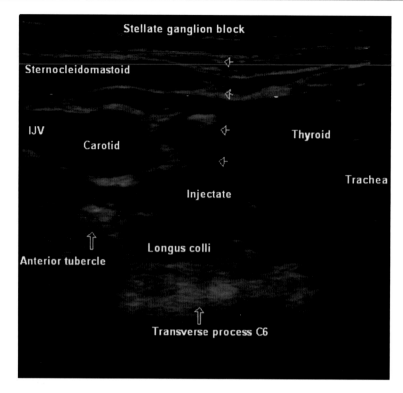

Fig. 14.11 Transverse sonographic view of the neck over the C6 transverse process. The arrow heads point to the 25-G needle. IJV- Internal jugular vein

ganglion itself may not be visualized, the longus colli muscle may be visualized. The ganglion is located underneath the fascia overlying the muscle and sometimes within the muscle belly (Fig. 14.11). The usual location for the block is over the transverse process of the C6 vertebra. The scanning sequence for the block is usually started from over the hyperechoic trachea with an air shadow beneath in a transverse view and moved laterally using a linear array transducer (Gofeld et al. 2009). The internal jugular vein and carotid artery are identified using color Doppler. The thyroid gland has a more granular appearance typical of most organs. As the scanning sequence is continued laterally, the anterior and medial scalene muscles and the brachial plexus in the scalene groove are located. Deeper to the scalenes, the transverse process is identified as a hyperechoic line. The longus colli muscle overlies the transverse process medially. The transverse process of C6 is usually the first cervical transverse process to have both anterior and posterior tubercles and

may be seen as a "double hump." It is important that a scout scan be performed especially in the left side to identify the hypoechoic esophagus which can be seen real time to "enlarge" with deglutition. The inferior thyroidal artery may be seen coursing inferior to the carotid close to the target and is a usual cause for hematoma. The trajectory is planned during the scout scan to avoid damage to any vital structures. Both in plane and out of plane approaches are possible and the injection is performed real time.

References

Balagué, F., Dutoit, G., & Waldburger, M. (1988). Low back pain in schoolchildren. An epidemiological study. *Scandinavian Journal of Rehabilitation Medicine, 20*(4), 175–179.

Balagué, F., Skovron, M., Nordin, M., Dutoit, G., Pol, L., & Waldburger, M. (1995). Low back pain in schoolchildren. A study of familial and psychological factors. *Spine (Phila Pa 1976), 20*(11), 1265–1270.

Bernstein, R. M., & Cozen, H. (2007). Evaluation of back pain in children and adolescents. *American Family Physician, 76*(11), 1669–1676.

Bodner, G., Bernathova, M., Galiano, K., Putz, D., Martinoli, C., & Felfernig, M. (2009). Ultrasound of the lateral femoral cutaneous nerve: Normal findings in a cadaver and in volunteers. *Regional Anesthesia and Pain Medicine, 34*(3), 265–268.

Borre, G. E., Borre, D. G., Hofer, B., & Vogeli, E., (1995). Sudeck's dystrophy of the hand. MR imaging. *Clin Imaging, 19*(3), 188–192.

Bruehl, S., Harden, R., Galer, B., Saltz, S., Bertram, M., Backonja, M., et al. (1999). External validation of IASP diagnostic criteria for Complex Regional Pain Syndrome and proposed research diagnostic criteria. International Association for the Study of Pain. *Pain, 81*(1–2), 147–154.

Byas-Smith, M. G., & Gulati, A. (2006). Ultrasound-guided intercostal nerve cryoablation. *Anesthesia and Analgesia, 103*(4), 1033–1035.

Cherry, D., & Rao, D. (1982). Lumbar sympathetic and coeliac plexus blocks. An anatomical study in cadavers. *British Journal of Anaesthesia, 54*(10), 1037–1039.

Crozier, F., Champsaur, P., Pham, T., Bartoli, J., Kasbarian, M., Chagnaud, C., et al. (2003). Magnetic resonance imaging in reflex sympathetic dystrophy syndrome of the foot. *Joint, Bone, Spine, 70*(6), 503–508.

de Lissovoy, G., & Lazarus, S. (1994). The economic cost of migraine. Present state of knowledge. *Neurology, 44*(6 Suppl 4), S56–62.

Deubner, D. (1977). An epidemiologic study of migraine and headache in 10–20 year olds. *Headache, 17*(4), 173–180.

el-Khoury, G., Ehara, S., Weinstein, J., Montgomery, W., & Kathol, M. (1988). Epidural steroid injection: A procedure ideally performed with fluoroscopic control. *Radiology, 168*(2), 554–557.

Feldman, D., Straight, J., Badra, M., Mohaideen, A., & Madan, S. (2006). Evaluation of an algorithmic approach to pediatric back pain. *Journal of Pediatric Orthopedics, 26*(3), 353–357. doi:01241398-200605000-00014 [pii] 10.1097/01.bpo.0000214928.25809.f9.

Gofeld, M., Bhatia, A., Abbas, S., Ganapathy, S., & Johnson, M. (2009). Development and validation of a new technique for ultrasound-guided stellate ganglion block. *Regional Anesthesia and Pain Medicine, 34*(5), 475–479.

Gorthi, V., Moon, Y. L., & Kang, J. H. (2010). The Effectiveness of ultrasonography-guided suprascapular nerve block for perishoulder pain. *Orthopedics, 33*, 238–241.

Greher, M., Kirchmair, L., Enna, B., Kovacs, P., Gustorff, B., Kapral, S., et al. (2004a). Ultrasound-guided lumbar facet nerve block: Accuracy of a new technique confirmed by computed tomography. *Anesthesiology, 101*(5), 1195–1200.

Greher, M., Scharbert, G., Kamolz, L. P., Beck, H., Gustorff, B., Kirchmair, L., et al. (2004b). Ultrasound-guided lumbar facet nerve block: A sonoanatomic study of a new methodologic approach. *Anesthesiology, 100*(5), 1242–1248.

Greher, M., Moriggl, B., Curatolo, M., Kirchmair, L., & Eichenberger, U. (2010). Sonographic visualization and ultrasound-guided blockade of the greater occipital nerve: A comparison of two selective techniques confirmed by anatomical dissection. *British Journal of Anaesthesia, 104*(5), 637–642.

Harmon, D., & Hearty, C. (2007). Ultrasound-guided suprascapular nerve block technique. *Pain Physician, 10*(6), 743–746.

Helbig, T., & Lee, C. (1988). The lumbar facet syndrome. *Spine (Phila Pa 1976), 13*(1), 61–64.

Intenzo, C., Kim, S., Millin, J., & Park, C. (1989). Scintigraphic patterns of the reflex sympathetic dystrophy syndrome of the lower extremities. *Clinical Nuclear Medicine, 14*(9), 657–661.

Jones, G. T., & Macfarlane, G. J. (2005). Epidemiology of low back pain in children and adolescents. *Archives of Disease in Childhood, 90*(3), 312–316.

Koch, E., Hofer, H., Sialer, G., Marincek, B., & von Schulthess, G. (1991). Failure of MR imaging to detect reflex sympathetic dystrophy of the extremities. *AJR. American Journal of Roentgenology, 156*(1), 113–115.

Lee, G., & Weeks, P. (1995). The role of bone scintigraphy in diagnosing reflex sympathetic dystrophy. *Journal of Hand Surgery. American Volume, 20*(3), 458–463. doi:10.1016/S0363-5023(05), 80107-8.

Lewis, D., Ashwal, S., Dahl, G., Dorbad, D., Hirtz, D., Prensky, A., et al. (2002). Practice parameter: evaluation of children and adolescents with recurrent headaches: Report of the Quality Standards Subcommittee of the American Academy of Neurology and the Practice Committee of the Child Neurology Society. *Neurology, 59*(4), 490–498.

Medina, L., Pinter, J., Zurakowski, D., Davis, R., Kuban, K., & Barnes, P. (1997). Children with headache: Clinical predictors of surgical space-occupying lesions and the role of neuroimaging. *Radiology, 202*(3), 819–824.

Narouze, S., Vydyanathan, A., & Patel, N. (2007). Ultrasound-guided stellate ganglion block successfully prevented esophageal puncture. *Pain Physician, 10*(6), 747–752.

Nordmann, G., Lauder, G., & Grier, D. (2006). Computed tomography guided lumbar sympathetic block for complex regional pain syndrome in a child: A case report and review. *European Journal of Pain. 10*(5), 409–412. doi:S1090-3801(05)00063-7 [pii] 10.1016/j.ejpain.2005.05.006.

Salminen, J., Pentti, J., & Terho, P. (1992). Low back pain and disability in 14-year-old schoolchildren. *Acta Paediatrica, 81*(12), 1035–1039.

Schürmann, M., Gradl, G., & Rommel, O. (2007a). Early diagnosis in post-traumatic complex regional pain syndrome. *Orthopedics, 30*(6), 450–456.

Schürmann, M., Zaspel, J., Löhr, P., Wizgall, I., Tutic, M., Manthey, N., et al. (2007b). Imaging in early posttraumatic complex regional pain syndrome: A comparison of diagnostic methods. *The Clinical Journal of Pain, 23*(5), 449–457.

Schweitzer, M., Mandel, S., Schwartzman, R., Knobler, R., & Tahmoush, A. (1995). Reflex sympathetic dystrophy revisited: MR imaging findings before and after infusion of contrast material. *Radiology, 195*(1), 211–214.

Selbst, S., Lavelle, J., Soyupak, S., & Markowitz, R. (1999). Back pain in children who present to the emergency department. *Clinical pediatrics, 38*(7), 401–406.

Shibata, Y., Fujiwara, Y., & Komatsu, T. (2007). A New Approach of Ultrasound-Guided Stellate Ganglion Block. *Anesthesia and Analgesia, 105*(2), 550–551.

Silbergleit, R., Mehta, B., Sanders, W., & Talati, S. (2001). Imaging-guided injection techniques with fluoroscopy and CT for spinal pain management. *Radiographics, 21*(4), 927–939. discussion 940–922.

Sillanpää, M. (1983a). Changes in the prevalence of migraine and other headaches during the first seven school years. *Headache, 23*(1), 15–19.

Sillanpää, M. (1983b). Prevalence of headache in prepuberty. *Headache, 23*(1), 10–14.

Stewart, W., Linet, M., Celentano, D., Van Natta, M., & Ziegler, D. (1991). Age- and sex-specific incidence rates of migraine with and without visual aura. *American Journal of Epidemiology, 134*(10), 1111–1120.

Taimela, S., Kujala, U., Salminen, J., & Viljanen, T. (1997). The prevalence of low back pain among children and adolescents A nationwide, cohort-based questionnaire survey in Finland. *Spine (Phila Pa 1976), 22*(10), 1132–1136.

Tertti, M., Salminen, J., Paajanen, H., Terho, P., & Kormano, M. (1991). Low-back pain and disk degeneration in children: A case-control MR imaging study. *Radiology, 180*(2), 503–507.

Watson, K., Papageorgiou, A., Jones, G., Taylor, S., Symmons, D., Silman, A., et al. (2002). Low back pain in schoolchildren: Occurrence and characteristics. *Pain, 97*(1–2), 87–92.

Wilder, R. (2006). Management of pediatric patients with complex regional pain syndrome. *The Clinical Journal of Pain, 22*(5), 443–448.

Regional Anesthesia for Chronic Pain Management in Children and Adolescents

15

Santhanam Suresh

Keywords

Regional anesthesia • Peripheral nerve blocks • Ultrasonography • Sympathetic blocks • Intravenous regional anesthesia (IVRA)

Introduction

The diagnosis of chronic pain in children and adolescents has often been overshadowed by the potential for malingering and school phobia. Nevertheless, with greater stride in the field of pediatric acute pain, there is greater emphasis on the diagnosis and management of pain due to the potential for significant bio-behavioral changes with untreated pain (Taddio et al. 1997). The purpose of this chapter is to look into the use of regional anesthesia techniques in pediatric chronic pain and provide an algorithmic approach to pain management.

The use of regional anesthesia can be divided into diagnostic and therapeutic. Most pediatric regional anesthesia techniques are performed both for diagnostic and therapeutic reasons. I will discuss in this chapter, several commonly used approaches for managing chronic pain in children (Table 15.1).

(a) Intravenous regional anesthesia: The Bier block was used commonly in adults and children for managing CRPS-type 1 (Taskaynatan et al. 2004). Multiple solutions have been used including bretylium, lidocaine, clonidine, and ketorolac for intravenous regional anesthesia. We have found IVRA with lidocaine and ketorolac as an ideal solution for providing pain relief in CRPS-Type 1 (Suresh et al. 2003).

(b) Central neuraxial blocks: The use of central neuraxial blocks including epidural catheter placement has been used for managing acute pain following the diagnosis of CRPS-type 1. We have used this as an opportunity to provide analgesia for pain control after the initial diagnosis of CRPS-Type 1 for initiating physical therapy.

(c) Peripheral nerve blocks: A variety of peripheral nerve blocks have been used for managing chronic pain in children. These include upper and lower extremity blocks with catheter placement (Dadure et al. 2005), ilioinguinal nerve blocks for groin pain (Suresh et al. 2008), and occipital nerve blocks for occipital neuralgia (Loukas et al. 2006). In addition, newer blocks including the transversus abdominis plane block (Pak et al. 2009) and intercostals blocks have been used

S. Suresh (✉)
Department of Pediatric Anesthesiology, Children's Memorial Hospital, 2300 Children's Plaza, 19, Chicago, IL 60614, USA
e-mail: ssuresh@childrensmemorial.org

B.C. McClain and S. Suresh (eds.), *Handbook of Pediatric Chronic Pain: Current Science and Integrative Practice*, DOI 10.1007/978-1-4419-0350-1_15,
© Springer Science+Business Media, LLC 2011

Table 15.1 Blocks used for chronic pain in children and adolescents

Block type	Indication	Local anesthetic	Volume
Bier block	CRPS-type 1	Lidocaine/ketorolac	20 mL(30 mgKetorolac)
Brachial plexus	CRPS-type 1	Bupivacaine (0.1%)	3 mL/h (catheter)
Lumbosacral plexus	CRPS-type 1	Bupivacaine (0.1%)	3–4 mL/h (catheter)
Sciatic nerve	CRPS-type 1	Bupivacaine (0.05%)	3 mL/h (catheter)
TAP block	Abdominal wall pain	Bupivacaine (0.05%)	5 mL/h
Ilioinguinal nerve	Inguinal neuralgia	Bupivacaine 0.25%	Single shot 2 mL
Intercostal nerve	Chest wall pain	Bupivacaine 0.25%	Single shot 2 mL
Supraorbital nerve	Headaches	Bupivacaine 0.25%	2 mL single shot
Occipital nerve	Occipital neuralgia	Bupivacaine 0.25%	2 mL single shot

for abdominal pain and chest wall pain. Ultrasonography has become popular for the placement of these blocks for all pain procedures.

(d) Sympathetic blocks: Although sympathetic blocks are used commonly in adults, the use of them in children has now decreased significantly. Stellate ganglion blocks for upper extremity CRPS-type 1 and lumbar sympathetic blocks for CRPS-type 1 of the lower extremity are now rarely preformed after peripheral nerve block catheters have been attempted.

(e) Intravenous local anesthetic infusions: Although rarely used, this technique is used in children as an adjuvant to other techniques used in children for pain management (Edwards 1999). Although the technique is rarely used now due to the potential for toxicity, intravenous lidocaine has been used for pain control in children and adolescents.

Intravenous Regional Anesthesia (IVRA)

This is used in children and adolescents as a first line interventional management for pain control in our clinics. The criteria for qualifying to attempt a trial of IVRA are based on the child's inability to either participate in active physical therapy and/or inability to mobilize the limb. An attempt is made to provide the IVRA with the child awake with minimal sedation. This allows

Table 15.2 Intravenous regional anesthesia

Intravenous regional anesthesia (Bier block)
22 G IV in affected extremity placed with LMX cream or EMLA cream (topical)
Tourniquet inflated to systolic pressure x 2 after elevating the limb for 5 min to facilitate venous drainage
Lidocaine (2 mg/kg) maximum dose 200 mg diluted in 10 mL saline (upper) 20 mL saline (lower) is injected
The tourniquet is kept inflated for 30 min. Careful when deflating the tourniquet
The patient is taken to the PACU to facilitate physical therapy

the child the ability to participate in physical therapy after the provision of the block. We feel that the use of IVRA provided at two-weekly intervals for a maximum of four blocks offers the best possible relief, we feel that more than four interventions does not offer greater relief and a secondary measure of intervention is then sought out (Suresh et al. 2003) (Table 15.2). Although guanethedine used as IVRA has been described for management of CRPS in adults, it is rarely used in children. Clonidine has been attempted for IVRA for CRPS; however the efficacy in children has not been proven to be effective.

Continuous Neuraxial Anesthesia

The use of continuous neuraxial anesthesia for management of chronic pain in children is generally performed to facilitate participation in physical therapy. Usually the use of lower concentrations of local anesthetic solution along with the use of adjuvants including clonidine or opioids is used in the neuraxial areas. It is often used for lower extremity CRPS although in rare occasions, the use of a cervical epidural catheter is used for upper extremity CRPS. These blocks are performed with strict observation of sterile techniques and the catheter is often tunneled to avoid accidental removal of the catheter while performing physical therapy (Table 15.3).

Peripheral Nerve Blocks

The use of peripheral nerve blocks for managing chronic pain in children and adolescents has now become even more popular with the introduction of ultrasound guidance. A variety of peripheral nerve blocks are performed including head and neck, upper, lower extremity, as well truncal blocks for managing chronic pain. A retrospective analysis of the use of peripheral nerve blocks in children and adolescents demonstrated improvement in symptoms after a continuous nerve block for a variable amount of time (Dadure et al. 2005).

(a) *Head and neck*: Patients presenting with a history of headaches particularly when they are non-migrainous can be treated with a variety of modalities (Fig. 15.1). Despite these modalities, there may be no resolution of symptoms. In these cases we have resorted to blocking the trigeminal nerve for frontal headaches and occipital nerves for occipital headaches for occipital neuralgia. In younger children especially in those under 8 years of age, we may resort to the use of mild sedation for provision of the blocks. We have been able to perform these blocks with topical anesthesia using either the EMLA cream or a 4% lidocaine cream (LMX) (Smith and Gjellum 2004). A newer modality using a gas-powered lidocaine pen (J-tip) is now used

Table 15.3 Continuous neuraxial catheter

Lumbar or cervical epidural catheter placed
Tunneling preferred for maintenance of the catheter
Local anesthetic solution plus alpha adrenergic blocker (clonidine) or opioid
Epidural catheter is left in place for at least a week

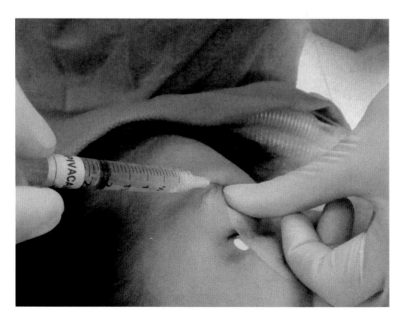

Fig. 15.1 Supraorbital nerve block: The supraorbital foramen is located at the midpoint of the supraorbital foramen and supplies the anterior portion of the forehead. A 30-G needle is placed subcutaneously to provide analgesia to the anterior portion of the forehead

routinely in our clinic for patients for performance of the blocks (Jimenez et al. 2006).

(i) *Supraorbital nerve blocks*: The first division of the trigeminal nerve, (the supraorbital and supratrochlear nerve), exits the supraorbital foramen to supply the sensory supply to the forehead. The nerve is easily accessed in the orbital rim and can be blocked easily using local anesthetic solution (Fig. 15.1). We prefer to block the nerve with local anesthetic solution only and perform the block every week for at least four blocks (Table 15.4). If there is no dramatic improvement of symptoms other modalities are used. More recently, peripheral nerve stimulators are used for providing continuous analgesia in adults (Amin et al. 2008). Although this technique has not been reported in children, it appears to have a potential especially for patients who may have significant neuropathic pain.

(ii) *Occipital nerve blocks*: Occipital neuralgia, although rare, is a debilitating entity in children- and adolescent-use of occipital nerve blocks, and has been described in great detail in the adult population (Loukas et al. 2006). However, this has been under-utilized in children. A retrospective review of our pain clinic database demonstrated the efficacy of this block in children. Besides its diagnostic and therapeutic efficacy in occipital neuralgia, the block is easy to perform and can be easily performed in the clinic space. There are multiple ways of performing this block and more recently the use of US guidance has been described for easy performance of this block (Eichenberger et al. 2006). This offers the ability to precisely perform the block with very little failure. However, this block is a surface landmark block and has an excellent response rate (Fig. 15.2) (Table 15.5).

(b) *Upper extremity blocks*: This is used mainly for managing CRPS-type 1 of the upper extremity. There are multiple approaches to the brachial plexus at the interscalene,

Table 15.4 Supraorbital nerve

Indicated for frontal headaches
The supraorbital foramen is palpated
Local anesthetic solution is placed subcutaneously over the foramen
Gentle massage is provided to distribute the local anesthetic solution

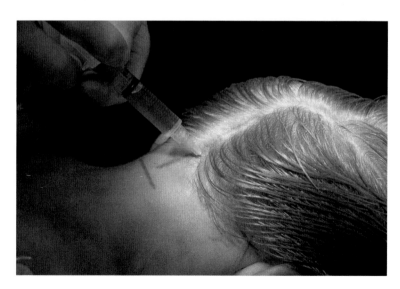

Fig. 15.2 Occipital nerve block: The occipital nerve is located lateral of the occipital artery inferior to the sub-nuchal line. A subcutaneous injection lateral of the midline provides analgesia to the posterior occipital area

Table 15.5 Occipital nerve block

Palpate the occipital protuberance
Palpate the occipital artery
The occipital nerve runs medial to the occipital artery inferiorly and laterally cranially
After palpation, inject 2 mL of 0.25% bupivacaine in a subcutaneous wheal spreading laterally
Massage the area after injection

Table 15.6 Upper extremity blocks

Indicated for neuropathic pain of the upper extremity
Brachial plexus catheter; Interscalene or infraclavicular
Sterile placement (gown and glove)
Tunneled catheter to be placed
An infusion of 0.1% bupivacaine with 2 mcg/mL of clonidine at a low infusion rate
Catheter is placed in situ for 5–7 days
Physical therapy is provided twice a day

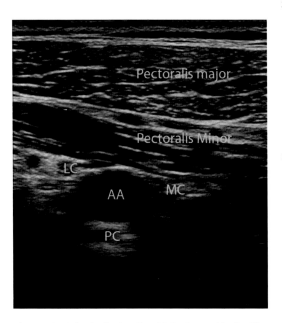

Fig. 15.3 Infraclavicular Brachial plexus block: The infraclavicular area is ideal for placing a catheter in the area of the cord of the brachial plexus; this is placed using ultrasound guidance which demonstrates the presence of the lateral, posterior, and medial cords around the second part of the axillary artery. Local anesthetic is deposited in the area of the posterior cord with an indwelling catheter that can be used to provide analgesia while allowing for physical therapy

supraclavicular, infraclavicular, and the peripheral branch area in the axillary area. Although each of the above areas are good for placement of single shot blocks, we feel that the use of the infraclavicular area seems ideal for placement of a catheter for an extended period of time (upto 7 days) for managing chronic pain (Fig. 15.3). The catheter is placed using sterile technique (gown and glove) in a sterile environment. The catheter is then tunneled for maintaining sterility. An infusion of 0.1% bupivacaine with 2 mcg/

mL of clonidine is our preferred solution for infusion (Table 15.6). We discharge the patients home and continue physical therapy on an outpatient basis. This seems to work best for upper extremity CRPS and in our experience is superior to a stellate ganglion block.

(c) *Lower extremity blocks*: Common pain blocks used for the lower extremity includes sciatic, lateral femoral cutaneous, and an obturator nerve block. These are usually provided with ultrasound guidance. A continuous catheter is preferred for the sciatic nerve while single shot blocks are performed for the lateral femoral cutaneous and the obturator nerves.

(i) *Sciatic nerve block*: the sciatic nerve is usually blocked at the level of the popliteal fossa for pain relief. The sciatic nerve usually blocked its bifurcation in the popliteal fossa. This is located approximately 6 cm above the popliteal crease. The nerve can be identified using a nerve stimulator or ultrasonography (Fig. 15.4). Once the nerve is identified, local anesthetic solution is injected followed by a catheter placement. We have preferred placing the nerve block and the catheter around the tibial nerve to avoid blocking the common peroneal leading to foot drop. The catheter is tunneled and we usually run a dilute local anesthetic solution with clonidine for pain control. It is not uncommon to see motor block even with low volumes and concentrations of local anesthetic solution hence it is important to recognize this early in the treatment phase to allow the patient participation in physical therapy (Table 15.7).

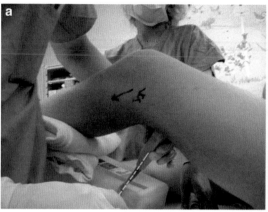
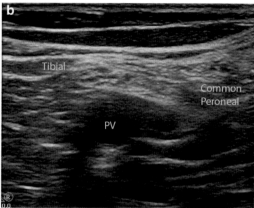

Fig. 15.4 (a) The sciatic nerve is blocked in the popliteal fossa using a linear ultrasound probe using an in-plane approach; the needle is inserted toward the tibial nerve and local anesthesia is injected around the nerve. A catheter can be also left in place to continue providing analgesia while getting the child involved in extensive physical therapy. (b) The ultrasound image of the popliteal fossa with a linear high frequency probe placed axially in the popliteal fossa. The tibial nerve is located medially and the common peroneal is located laterally, the nerves converge approximately 5 cm above the crease of the popliteal fossa, the biceps femoris is located lateral and superior to the sciatic nerve at the confluence of the two nerves in the popliteal fossa

Table 15.7 Sciatic nerve block

Indication: neuropathic pain of the lower extremity
Sterile technique using gown and gloves
US guidance with a linear probe is used for localizing the nerve
Catheter placed in the popliteal fossa area (more stable than more proximal)
The catheter will be tunneled
Catheter placed in the vicinity of the tibial nerve to prevent foot drop from blocking the peroneal nerve

(ii) *Lateral femoral cutaneous nerve*: The lateral femoral cutaenous nerve supplies the sensory area of the lateral portion of the thigh and is used for treatment of pain on the lateral side of the thigh. It is diagnostic and therapeutic for the management of pain associated with meralgia paresthetica (Edelson and Stevens 1994). The usual method to block the nerve is to find a point of entry of the needle two finger breaths below and medial to the anterior superior iliac crease, finding two pops as the facial planes are entered and the needle is located between the fascia lata and the

fascia iliaca. More recently, an US-guided technique is now used for this procedure with greater accuracy and better placement of the needle (Fig. 15.5). The sartorius and followed cephalad to its insertion and the fascial plane between the tensor fascia lata and the sartorius accommodates the lateral femoral cutaneous nerve. A 5 mL of 0.25% bupivacaine is injected with excellent results (Table 15.8). We have performed serial blocks using US guidance in the clinic with very good results.

(d) *Truncal blocks*: The common truncal blocks performed in children and adolescents include intercostals nerve blocks, ilioinguinal nerve blocks, and TAP blocks for chronic pain. These blocks have become more popular with the addition of US guidance for their performance.

Intercostal Nerve Block

The intercostals nerves are located in a plane between the inner intercostals and the innermost

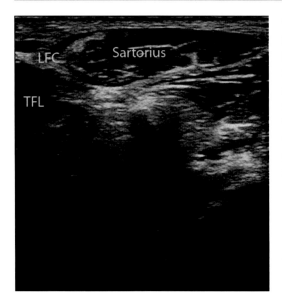

Fig. 15.5 The lateral femoral cutaneous nerve is located in the fascial plane between the fascia lata and the fascia iliaca in the groove between the tensor fascial lata and the insertion of the Sartorius. The ultrasound image demonstrates the fat pad that exits lateral of the insertion of the Sartorius that contains the lateral femoral cutaneous nerve. Local anesthetic injection in the area provides analgesia to the lateral portion of the thigh and can be used for diagnosis and management of meralgia paresthetica

Table 15.8 Lateral femoral cutaneous nerve block

Indicated for meralgia paresthetica
Using US guidance, the sartorius insertion point is obtained
The lateral femoral cutaneous nerve is lateral to the insertion in a fascial plane between the tensor fascia lata and the sartorius
Pain relief is obtained with injection of 5 mL of 0.25% bupivacaine
Instructions given to patient about the potential for weakness of the lower extremity

intercostal muscles. The nerves run in this plane to supply the anterior chest wall with the sensory innervation. This is used for providing pain relief for patients with costochondritis or rib cage pain following chest tube placement. A linear US probe is used for localizing the layers of the chest wall, using a 27-G needle, the skin, the outer and

the inner intercostals are pierced followed by placement of the needle in the space under the inner intercostals. Local anesthetic solution is injected into the area, accurate localization is seen with the displacement of the pleura (Fig. 15.6). These blocks can be repeated every week in a serial fashion for providing pain relief. Occasionally, if the patient continues to have persistent pain, cryoablation of the nerve is provided for sustained pain relief.

Ilioinguinal Nerve Blocks

The ilioinguinal and the iliohypogastric nerves are branches of the thoraco-lumbar nerve roots (L1) as they descend into the groin. The ilioinguinal nerve supplies the sensory supply to the groin area. Although this nerve can be easily accessed using a blind technique, the use of ultrasonography has made this technique easy and safer in children. We have demonstrated the value of this block in adolescents with persistent groin pain following inguinal hernia repair (Suresh et al. 2008). The patient is usually given mild sedation; the block is performed with the aid of a linear probe and a 27-G needle for placement of the block. The ilioinguinal nerve is located in the plane between the transversus abdominis and the internal oblique (Fig. 15.7). After aspiration, 2 mL of local anesthesia is injected into the plane, this provides adequate analgesia for pain relief. In certain instances with refractory pain, we have placed a continuous infusion catheter and if the pain is still refractory, we are likely to perform radiofrequency ablation of the nerve (Table 15.9).

Transversus Abdominis Plane (TAP) Block

The transversus abdominis plane is a potential space that exists between the internal oblique muscle and the transversus abdominis muscle. The thoracolumbar nerve roots (T8 to L1) pass in this plane to provide analgesia to the abdominal wall.

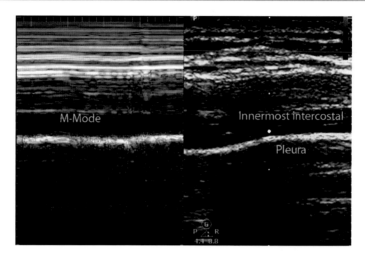

Fig. 15.6 Intercostal nerve is located in the fascial plane between the inner intercostal and the inner most intercostal muscles. Using a linear ultrasound probe, the muscles are visualized in the intercostal space; the pleura is identified and the parietal and visceral pleura can be seen. Using the M-mode, as demonstrated in the left panel of the figure, the demarcation between the pleura and the facial plane superior to it can be distinguished as the "sea shore line"; any infractions to the pleura results in the loss of the "sea shore" line

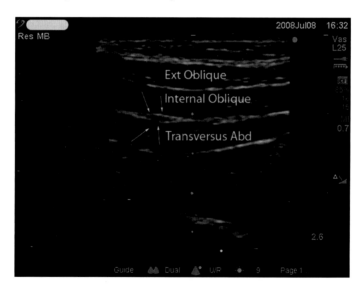

Fig. 15.7 The ilioinguinal nerve is blocked medial of the iliac crest as the L1 nerve runs into the groin; the nerve is located between the internal oblique and transversus abdominis muscle. The nerve can be visualized easily with a linear high frequency ultrasound probe medial of the anterior superior iliac spine, using an in-plane approach; local anesthetic solution is deposited between the two muscle layers

Table 15.9 Ilioinguinal nerve block

Indications: Persistent groin pain, ilioinguinal neuralgia
US guidance with a linear probe
The nerve is located between the transversus abdominis and the internal oblique
Local anesthetic solution (2 mL) is placed between the two layers
Spread of the potential space demonstrates adequate placement of the needle in the right space

This block can be used for patients with refractory abdominal pain following surgery or in patients with persistent neuropathic pain (Pak et al. 2009). Local anesthesia is injected into the space. Occasionally, we leave indwelling catheters in the space for a few days in the case of refractory abdominal pain. A linear US probe is used to recognize the space (Fig. 15.8) (Table 15.10).

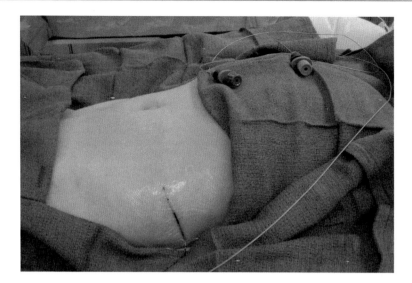

Fig. 15.8 The transversus abdominis plane (TAP) is located between the internal oblique and the transversus abdominis plane, this contains the thoraco-lumbar nerve roots run in this potential space. A linear high frequency ultrasound probe is used and the space can be accessed easily from the lateral aspect using an in-plane technique; 0.2 ml/kg of local anesthetic solution is injected into the space

Table 15.10 TAP block

US guidance is used for the block
A linear probe is placed to determine the various muscle layers
Once the space is accessed, local anesthesia is injected into the TAP space
Catheters can be left in this space for pain relief

Sympathetic Blockade

The use of sympathetic blocks in children and adolescents are commonly used for management of CRPS-Type 1. However, with the introduction of peripheral nerve block catheters and the introduction of more potent antiepileptic drugs including gabapentin, it has now become rare to use this block in children. A stellate ganglion block is used for upper extremity CRPS while a lumbar sympathetic block is used for lower extremity CRPS. Other sympathetic blocks including the celiac plexus or splanchnic plexus are very rarely used in children and adolescents. The introduction of ultrasound guidance has allowed the placement of stellate ganglion blocks with greater ease and without the aid of fluoroscopic techniques.

Stellate Ganglion Blocks

The cervical sympathetic chain is composed of the superior, middle, intermediate, and inferior cervical ganglia. The inferior cervical ganglia fuse with the first thoracic ganglion forming the stellate ganglion. It lies in close proximity to the seventh cervical vertebral body. Blockade of the stellate ganglion usually results in vasodilatation and a sympathetic blockade of the upper extremity leading to an improvement of symptoms associated with CRPS-type 1 of the upper extremity (Tong and Nelson 2000). This is usually performed with fluoroscopic guidance (Fig. 15.9). The introduction of US guidance has vastly improved the placement of these blocks in children. A linear probe is used and placed along the lower border of the transverse process of the sixth cervical vertebra (C6). This will allow the operator to visualize the longus colli muscle on top of which the stellate ganglion can be easily located (Table 15.11). The advantage of the use of US

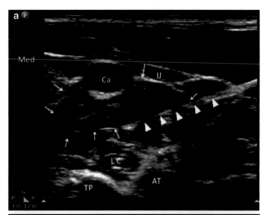

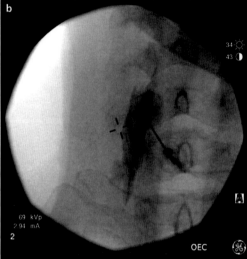

Fig. 15.9 (a) The stellate ganglion can be easily identified using a linear ultrasound probe in the neck. The stellate ganglion is located inferior of the thyroid, and on top of the longus colli muscle, it can be accessed easily using an in-plane approach at the C6 level. (b) The stellate ganglion can be blocked at the C6 level using conventional technique; the transverse process is identified and the needle is walked inferior of the transverse process. Local anesthetic spread is also identified using fluoroscopy as demonstrated in this image

Table 15.11 Stellate ganglion blocks

Used for upper extremity CRPS
Blind technique or fluoroscopic guided technique often used for performance of the block
US guidance is safer as it prevents vascular injury and esophageal puncture
Linear probe used and transverse process is identified
The longus colli muscle is identified and the stellate ganglion is located in close proximity to the muscle
Signs of an adequate block is ipsilateral Horner's syndrome and vasodilatation

guidance for the placement of this block is the avoidance of vascular injuries and hematoma formation and the potential for esophageal puncture as has been reported previously (Narouze et al. 2007).

Lumbar Sympathetic Block

The LSB is used for management of CRPS of the lower extremity. A cross over trial with an epidural catheter demonstrated the efficacy of the LSB for CRPS-type 1 (Meier et al. 2009). The block is performed using fluoroscopy with mild sedation or under general anesthesia in younger children. A linear spread of the local anesthetic solution along the sympathetic chain along with changes from a sympathectomy is usually indicators of a good blockade.

Conclusion

Regional anesthesia is used quite frequently for the management of chronic pain in children and adolescents. It is important to understand the indication and the application of these blocks in the pediatric population. Ultrasonography has provided a tremendous advantage in recognizing structures and providing a better and safer method of performing these blocks. With continued use and future prospective randomized controlled trials, we may be able to determine the efficacy of regional techniques in children and adolescents with chronic pain syndromes.

References

Amin, S., Buvanendran, A., Park, K. S., Kroin, J. S., & Moric, M. (2008). Peripheral nerve stimulator for the treatment of supraorbital neuralgia: A retrospective case series. *Cephalalgia, 28*(4), 355–359.

Dadure, C., Motais, F., Ricard, C., Raux, O., Troncin, R., & Capdevila, X. (2005). Continuous peripheral nerve blocks at home for treatment of recurrent complex regional pain syndrome I in children. *Anesthesiology, 102*(2), 387–391.

Edelson, R., & Stevens, P. (1994). Meralgia paresthetica in children. *The Journal of Bone and Joint Surgery. American Volume, 76*(7), 993–999.

Edwards, A. D. (1999). The role of systemic lidocaine in neuropathic pain management. *Journal of Intravenous Nursing, 22*(5), 273–279.

Eichenberger, U., Greher, M., Kapral, S., Marhofer, P., Wiest, R., Remonda, L., et al. (2006). Sonographic visualization and ultrasound-guided block of the third occipital nerve: Prospective for a new method to diagnose C2-C3 zygapophysial joint pain. *Anesthesiology, 104*(2), 303–308.

Jimenez, N., Bradford, H., Seidel, K. D., Sousa, M., & Lynn, A. M. (2006). A comparison of a needle-free injection system for local anesthesia versus EMLA for intravenous catheter insertion in the pediatric patient. *Anesthesia and Analgesia, 102*(2), 411–414.

Loukas, M., El-Sedfy, A., Tubbs, R. S., Louis, R. G., Jr., Wartmann, C. H., Curry, B., et al. (2006). Identification of greater occipital nerve landmarks for the treatment of occipital neuralgia. *Folia Morphologica (Warsz), 65*(4), 337–342.

Meier, P. M., Zurakowski, D., Berde, C. B., & Sethna, N. F. (2009). Lumbar sympathetic blockade in children with complex regional pain syndromes: A double blind placebo-controlled crossover trial. *Anesthesiology, 111*(2), 372–380.

Narouze, S., Vydyanathan, A., & Patel, N. (2007). Ultrasound-guided stellate ganglion block success fully prevented esophageal puncture. *Pain Physician, 10*(6), 747–752.

Pak, T., Mickelson, J., Yerkes, E., & Suresh, S. (2009). Transverse abdominis plane block: A new approach to the management of secondary hyperalgesia following major abdominal surgery. *Paediatric Anaesthesia, 19*(1), 54–56.

Smith, D. P., & Gjellum, M. (2004). The efficacy of LMX versus EMLA for pain relief in boys undergoing office meatotomy. *Journal d'Urologie, 172*(4 Pt 2), 1760–1761.

Suresh, S., Wheeler, M., & Patel, A. (2003). Case series: IV regional anesthesia with ketorolac and lidocaine: is it effective for the management of complex regional pain syndrome 1 in children and adolescents? *Anesthesia and Analgesia, 96*(3), 694–695.

Suresh, S., Patel, A., Porfyris, S., & Ryee, M. Y. (2008). Ultrasound-guided serial ilioinguinal nerve blocks for management of chronic groin pain secondary to ilioinguinal neuralgia in adolescents. *Paediatric Anaesthesia, 18*(8), 775–778.

Taddio, A., Katz, J., Ilersich, A. L., & Koren, G. (1997). Effect of neonatal circumcision on pain response during subsequent routine vaccination. *Lancet, 349*(9052), 599–603.

Taskaynatan, M. A., Ozgul, A., Tan, A. K., Dincer, K., & Kalyon, T. A. (2004). Bier block with methylprednisolone and lidocaine in CRPS type I: A randomized, double-blinded, placebo-controlled study. *Regional Anesthesia and Pain Medicine, 29*(5), 408–412.

Tong, H. C., & Nelson, V. S. (2000). Recurrent and migratory reflex sympathetic dystrophy in children. *Pediatric Rehabilitation, 4*(2), 87–89.

Complex Regional Pain Syndrome (CRPS)

16

Santhanam Suresh and Antoun Nader

Keywords

Complex regional pain syndrome (CRPS), types I and II • CRPS pathophysiology • Treatment goals of CRPS • Comorbidity in CRPS • Algorithm for management

Definition

The term Complex Regional Pain Syndrome (CRPS) is a pain disorder in which the pain is disproportionate to the initial inciting injury. The disorder is complex because it involves multiple organ systems with abnormal blood flow, sweating abnormalities, trophic changes, and fine motor impairment. The pain distribution tends to be regional (not dermatomal), and is not limited to the area initially affected (Rand 2009). The pathophysiology of CRPS is not entirely understood. The pain can be sympathetically-maintained (responsive to sympathetic interventions) or sympathetic-independent (Gibbs et al. 2008; Wilson 1999). The diagnosis is excluded by the presence of a condition that would otherwise account for the degree of pain and dysfunction. According to the International Association for the

Study of Pain (IASP), CRPS is divided into two categories based on the absence of a recognizable nerve injury (CRPS type I, formerly known as reflex sympathetic dystrophy) or the presence of a proximal nerve injury (complex regional pain syndrome type II, formerly known as causalgia) (Bruehl et al. 1999). It is often seen in teenage girls and has a greater predeliction for the lower extremity in children when compared to adults (Wilder et al. 1992). Unlike the adult population where there is workman's compensation etc., the main red flag in children is school absenteeism.

Clinical Features

1. *Somatosensory abnormalities*: Persistent pain is the essential feature of CRPS. It is characteristically disproportionate to the initiating event with often no dermatomal distribution to an individual nerve. It is frequently reported as a burning sensation, usually spontaneous, mostly felt at the distal extremity in the dependent

S. Suresh (✉)
Children's Memorial Hospital, Northwestern University's
Feinberg School of Medicine, Chicago, IL USA
e-mail: ssuresh@childrensmemorial.ori

B.C. McClain and S. Suresh (eds.), *Handbook of Pediatric Chronic Pain:*
Current Science and Integrative Practice, DOI 10.1007/978-1-4419-0350-1_16,
© Springer Science+Business Media, LLC 2011

position. Typically, joint movements and movement of the extremity exacerbate the pain. Mechanical and thermal allodynia (pain out of proportion to the inciting event) to cold more often than heat, and hyperalgesia are frequently present. In addition, 50% of patients with chronic CRPS Type I develop hypoesthesia and hypoalgesia in the same body quadrant or the whole half body of the affected site (van Bodegraven Hof et al. 2010) with increased mechanical and thermal threshold on the affected side. These patients have a longer period of illness, greater pain intensity, and a higher tendency to develop somatomotor changes (Walton et al. 2010). The pain can be described as sympathetic maintained (SMP) or sympathetic independent (SIP) based on the positive or negative effect of selective blockade of the sympathetic nervous system or blockade of adrenoreceptors. Therefore, SMP is a symptom in a subset of patients and is not essential for the diagnosis of CRPS.

2. *Autonomic and trophic abnormalities*: Autonomic abnormalities and trophic changes are present at some time during the course of the disease (Bruehl et al. 1999; Stanton-Hicks 2000). Swelling is found in almost all patients. It is usually exacerbated by evoked pain. Sudomotor abnormalities, frequently hyperhidrosis, are very common. Temperature asymmetry of more than 1° is present in 30–80% of patients. Three distinct vascular regulation patterns are identified in relation to the duration of the disorder.

    (a) In the early acute stage, the affected limb is usually warmer, skin perfusion values are higher, and norepinephrine concentrations in the venous effluent from the affected area are low. In addition, sympathetic vasoconstrictor neurons are difficult to activate.

    (b) In the intermediate stage, temperature and skin perfusion tests may be either high or low depending on the sympathetic activity.

    (c) In the chronic stage, the limb is colder, skin perfusion test values are low, and norepinephrine concentrations remain low in the affected side. Passing into the chronic stage, the edema resolves; and the limb atrophies with muscle contracture, constriction of the tendon sheaths and joint stiffness. Abnormal skin (thin, glossy), nail (brittle and discolored), and hair growth (fragile, uneven, curled) may be present. Bone involvement is frequent. Initially, increased isotope uptake on bone scanning is found. Later, there is rapid and profound bone loss with patchy demineralization. Although this is commonly seen in adults, this finding may not be commonly seen in children (Schurmann et al. 2007).

3. *Somatomotor abnormalities*: Motor symptoms, although not included in the definition, are frequently present and can be noted in the intermediate and the chronic phase of the disease. Weakness of all muscles in the affected area is present in approximately 70% of patients. In addition, patients may present with postural or action tremors and dystonia and myoclonus (Agrawal et al. 2009). Typically, small, precise movements are impaired. Nerve conduction studies may reveal sensory changes in over 46% of cases with chronic CRPS type1 (Rommel et al. 2001).

4. *Psychological abnormalities*: Most patients have a normal psychological profile although the incidence of fixed psychogenic dystonia has been described in adolescents (Majumdar et al. 2009). In addition, there is prone to be significant family dynamics that may alter the clinical scenario necessitating the need for family therapy in some instances. Most of the children with CRPS type I are athletic and have major impetus for improvement of symptoms to participate in their sport; this can also change the psychological milieu in these children. An association with previous psychological stress, however, has been noted. A low pain threshold, emotional lability, and depression are usually present.

Pathophysiology

A number of hypothetical mechanisms for the disease have been described. A recent study looking at fMRI (functional magnetic resonance imaging) in children who had active symptoms of CRPS when compared to children who did not have active symptoms revealed alterations in fMRI images when the children were in the active phase of CRPS suggesting that there may be altered neuronal circuits while in an active state of CRPS (Lebel et al. 2008). In the peripheral nervous system, the continuous barrage of noxious stimuli sensitizes the small polymodal A-δ and C-fibers, leading to hyperalgesia. In the spinal cord, there may be sensitization of the wide dynamic range neurons that occurs after intense peripheral stimulation of A-δ and C fibers. In addition, the activity of the low threshold A-β mechano-receptor fibers is altered, which may induce a state of hyperalgesia and allodynia. There is also growing evidence that the sympathetic nervous system is involved, especially when the pain or autonomic components are relieved using sympathetic blocks. In the acute stage of the syndrome, there is functional inhibition of cutaneous sympathetic vasoconstrictor activity leading to increased vascularity and hyperemia of the area. In the chronic stage, after the initial inhibition, secondary end-organ supersensitivity is manifested by increased vasoconstriction, reduced skin temperature, and enhanced sudomotor activity. The sympathetic-mediated pain may be maintained by pathologic coupling of sympathetic and afferent activity either in the periphery, between sympathetic fibers and C-fibers, or in the dorsal root ganglia. Central nervous system alterations, probably in the cortex and thalamus, may also play a role in CRPS, especially in patients with extensive sensory deficits; however it is not clear whether changes in the CNS are primary abnormalities or secondary to pain (Walton et al. 2010).

Treatment

Treatment of CRPS should be immediate and directed toward restoration of extremity function and rehabilitation (Hsu 2009). Treatment includes pain relief, mobilization, and mechanical desensitization of the affected extremity. The ultimate goal of any pharmacotherapy is to improve physical activity and functional ability of the patient. Movement phobia should be overcome, and phys-

ical therapy should be facilitated. A combination of analgesic and adjuvant drugs, including tricyclic antidepressants, anticonvulsants, membrane stabilizers, α-1 adreno-receptor antagonists, and α-2 adreno-receptor agonists are employed to help accomplish the above therapeutic goals. For the sake of this chapter, we will divide the treatment modalities to pharmacological and non-pharmacological approaches.

Non-pharmacological Approaches

Non-pharmacological approaches to the management of CRPS have been traditionally used in all instances. We use a variety of techniques including psychological interventions, biofeedback, hypnosis, and complementary interventions including massage and acupuncture.

Psychological measures: After a thorough psychological evaluation, the patients are evaluated for changes in family dynamics as well as the presence of any comorbid psychological problems including but not limited to anxiety and depression. We use several measures including visual-guided imagery as well as relaxation techniques in addition to other interventions including hypnosis for managing pain. Other techniques used for managing children and adolescents include the use of biofeedback therapy as an adjuvant to pain management (Linkenhoker 1983).

Physical therapy: Physical therapy measures including but not limited to active and passive motion and to facilitate recovery. This is the most important part of recovery from CRPS in children and adolescents. This has been addressed in this book in the chapter on interventional pain management. Other modalities in physical therapy that can help in managing pain in CRPS include heat therapy, ultrasound therapy, as well as the application of a TENS (Trancutaneous Electrical Nerve Stimulation) unit (Lee et al. 2002). A study in children demonstrated the efficacy of TENS in children with CRPS type 1 (Kesler et al. 1988). This is routinely introduced in children for managing pain

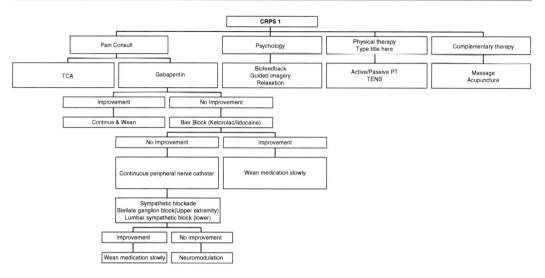

Fig. 16.1 Algorithm for management of CRPS in children

as an initial intervention for managing CRPS type 1 (Fig. 16.1).

Pharmacotherapy: Pharmacological management of CRPS type I is used commonly again to facilitate the ability to participate in physical therapy. The most common pharmacotherapy includes tricyclic antidepressants, anticonvulsants, as well as other interventions including SSRIs and SNRIs. This is still an evolving management therapy since the major side effects of pharmacotherapy especially sedation and somnolence are carefully avoided to allow the child to participate in regular activities.

(a) *Tricyclic antidepressants*: This is the most common pharmacological intervention used in children and adolescents. Clinical experience has demonstrated the efficacy of tricyclic antidepressants for the management of pain following CRPS in children and adolescents (Stanton-Hicks et al. 1998). Tricyclic antidepressants may have a propensity to prolong the QT interval, hence a screening EKG is obtained to rule out the potential for prolonged QT syndrome in which case the medication is avoided (Olgun et al. 2009). Amitriptyline may cause drowsiness especially in children who are school bound, hence we use nontriptyline which has less anticholinergic effects as well as possibly less sedation. Rarely imipramine and desimipramine are used in pain clinic settings.

(b) *Anticonvulsants(ACD)*: ACDs are used for managing pain in children and adolescents. Carbamezepine or oxycarbezine was used extensively in the past for managing neuropathic pain (Lalwani et al. 2005) until the gabalins were compounded. The introduction of voltage-gated calcium channel blockers like gabapentin as well as pregabalin has provided the clinician with a better modality for pain control. Side effects include potential for allergic reactions as well as the potential for weight gain with continued use of this drug.

(c) SSRI and SNRI: The use of SSRIs and SNRIs are controversial in the management of pain in children. Although there has been no direct correlation with potential benefits from the use of any of these drugs, there is an association with depression in these children and the beneficial effects may be the effect of these drugs on depression. In our own clinical setting, we have had great benefits from the use of duloxetine, an SNRI in the clinical setting of CRPS type I, we are able to provide pain control while we are able to decrease the incidence of weight gain (Meighen 2007).

(d) Opioids: Opioids are very rarely used in the setting of CRPS type.

Occasionally in patients with severe pain, opioids are used to facilitate physical therapy. However, with the introduction of nerve blocks, this therapy has been reserved for severely refractory CRPS type I.

Interventional Techniques

(a) *Intravenous Regional Anesthesia*: This is our first approach to the treatment of CRPS type 1. A combination of local anesthetic with a non-steroidal anti-inflammatory medication such as ketorolac has been shown to have significant advantages in children and adolescents with CRPS type 1 (Suresh et al. 2003). In our experience, we have noted that it may not be worthwhile performing more than four blocks. We often find that it is best to move down the algorithm to perform either a continuous peripheral nerve blocks or a sympathetic nerve block in this setting (Fig. 16.1).

(b) *Central neuraxial blocks*: The placement of central neuraxial catheters are placed for providing pain relief for pain control to provide analgesia for physical therapy. We resort to tunneling indwelling epidural catheters and leave the catheter in place for 7–10 days. This has demonstrated to be an effective mechanism for managing pain without the side effects of opioids etc. that can cause somnolence.

(c) *Peripheral nerve blocks*: The use of peripheral nerve blocks has now become the major first-line intervention in this setting. A study from France demonstrated the efficacy of continuous nerve blocks in CRPS type I (Dadure et al. 2005). We have demonstrated the efficacy of peripheral nerve catheters in children for pain control with a home management program. A dilute local anesthetic solution with the addition of an α-2 adrenergic agonist can be more effective in managing CRPS type I. Randomized controlled trials support the use of steroids, amitriptyline, and gabapentin. In addition, regional and neuraxial techniques play an important role in diagnosis as well as treatment, especially in sympathetically mediated pain (SMP). As discussed earlier, the diagnosis of SMP is established by determining the magnitude of pain relief achieved with an appropriate sympathetic block. However, the results of local anesthetic blocks should be interpreted with caution as the adequacy of the sympathetic block in SMP must be demonstrated simultaneously with the degree of pain relief obtained. Measuring changes in skin blood flow, skin temperature, or skin resistance on the involved extremity usually assesses the adequacy of a sympathetic block. This is especially important when the goal is diagnosis of SMP. Infection is the most feared complication of long-term catheter implantation. Infection, if it occurs, is usually local and is superficial to the deep fascia. It therefore readily responds to antibiotic treatment. If a spinal or paraspinous infection is suspected, the catheter should be removed and neurological consultation and spine imaging are required.

(d) *Sympathetic blocks*: Stellate ganglion blocks for upper extremity CRPS type 1 or lumbar sympathetic blocks for lower extremity CRPS type I are performed for managing pain (Nordmann et al. 2006; Yucel et al. 2009). Stellate ganglion blocks are placed using ultrasound guidance in children. This has been described in detail in the chapter on radiographic imaging for pain in this book. Lumbar sympathetic blocks are performed with the use of fluoroscopy or CT guidance.

(e) *Spinal Cord Stimulation*: Neuro-modulation in children is a much more uncommon intervention in children. This is something that we resort to as a later intervention in children and adolescents and not resorted to until all other modalities have failed. The use of neuromodulation especially for peripheral nerves may be a much more advantageous intervention than central neuromodulation. All these interventions need further recommendations after more controlled trials are performed in children (Olsson et al. 2008).

Conclusion

CRPS Type I and II are well recognized entities in children and adolescents. We feel that the current armamentariums for the management of CRPS has to be further researched. Multicenter prospective randomized trials should be performed in children and adolescents and future algorithms should be created for managing children with CRPS type-1.

References

Agrawal, S. K., Rittey, C. D., Harrower, N. A., Goddard, J. M., & Mordekar, S. R. (2009). Movement disorders associated with complex regional pain syndrome in children. *Developmental Medicine and Child Neurology, 51*(7), 557–562.

Bruehl, S., Harden, R. N., Galer, B. S., Saltz, S., Bertram, M., Backonja, M., et al. (1999). External validation of IASP diagnostic criteria for complex Regional Pain Syndrome and proposed research diagnostic criteria. International Association for the Study of Pain. *Pain, 81*(1–2), 147–154.

Dadure, C., Motais, F., Ricard, C., Raux, O., Troncin, R., & Capdevila, X. (2005). Continuous peripheral nerve blocks at home for treatment of recurrent complex regional pain syndrome I in children. *Anesthesiology, 102*(2), 387–391.

Gibbs, G. F., Drummond, P. D., Finch, P. M., & Phillips, J. K. (2008). Unravelling the pathophysiology of complex regional pain syndrome: focus on sympathetically maintained pain. *Clinical and Experimental Pharmacology & Physiology, 35*(7), 717–724.

Hsu, E. S. (2009). Practical management of complex regional pain syndrome. *American Journal of Therapeutics, 16*(2), 147–154.

Kesler, R. W., Saulsbury, F. T., Miller, L. T., & Rowlingson, J. C. (1988). Reflex sympathetic dystrophy in children: treatment with transcutaneous electric nerve stimulation. *Pediatrics, 82*(5), 728–732.

Lalwani, K., Shoham, A., Koh, J. L., & McGraw, T. (2005). Use of oxcarbazepine to treat a pediatric patient with resistant complex regional pain syndrome. *The Journal of Pain, 6*(10), 704–706.

Lebel, A., Becerra, L., Wallin, D., Moulton, E. A., Morris, S., Pendse, G., et al. (2008). fMRI reveals distinct CNS processing during symptomatic and recovered complex regional pain syndrome in children. *Brain, 131*(Pt 7), 1854–1879.

Lee, B. H., Scharff, L., Sethna, N. F., McCarthy, C. F., Scott-Sutherland, J., Shea, A. M., et al. (2002). Physical therapy and cognitive-behavioral treatment for complex regional pain syndromes. *Jornal de Pediatria, 141*(1), 135–140.

Linkenhoker, D. (1983). Tools of behavioral medicine: applications of biofeedback treatment for children and adolescents. *Journal of Developmental and Behavioral Pediatrics, 4*(1), 16–20.

Majumdar, A., Lopez-Casas, J., Poo, P., Colomer, J., Galvan, M., Lingappa, L., et al. (2009). Syndrome of fixed dystonia in adolescents–short term outcome in 4 cases. *European Journal of Paediatric Neurology, 13*(5), 466–472.

Meighen, K. G. (2007). Duloxetine treatment of pediatric chronic pain and co-morbid major depressive disorder. *Journal of Child and Adolescent Psychopharmacology, 17*(1), 121–127.

Nordmann, G. R., Lauder, G. R., & Grier, D. J. (2006). Computed tomography guided lumbar sympathetic block for complex regional pain syndrome in a child: a case report and review. *European Journal of Pain, 10*(5), 409–412.

Olgun, H., Yildirim, Z. K., Karacan, M., & Ceviz, N. (2009). Clinical, electrocardiographic, and laboratory findings in children with amitriptyline intoxication. *Pediatric Emergency Care, 25*(3), 170–173.

Olsson, G. L., Meyerson, B. A., & Linderoth, B. (2008). Spinal cord stimulation in adolescents with complex regional pain syndrome type I (CRPS-I). *European Journal of Pain, 12*(1), 53–59.

Rand, S. E. (2009). Complex regional pain syndrome in the adolescent athlete. *Current Sports Medicine Reports, 8*(6), 285–287.

Rommel, O., Malin, J. P., Zenz, M., & Janig, W. (2001). Quantitative sensory testing, neurophysiological and psychological examination in patients with complex regional pain syndrome and hemisensory deficits. *Pain, 93*(3), 279–293.

Schurmann, M., Zaspel, J., Lohr, P., Wizgall, I., Tutic, M., Manthey, N., et al. (2007). Imaging in early posttraumatic complex regional pain syndrome: a comparison of diagnostic methods. *The Clinical Journal of Pain, 23*(5), 449–457.

Stanton-Hicks, M. (2000). Complex regional pain syndrome (type I, RSD; type II, causalgia): controversies. *The Clinical Journal of Pain, 16*(2 Suppl), S33–S40.

Stanton-Hicks, M., Baron, R., Boas, R., Gordh, T., Harden, N., & Hendler, N. (1998). Complex Regional Pain Syndromes: guidelines for therapy. *The Clinical Journal of Pain, 14*(2), 155–166.

Suresh, S., Wheeler, M., & Patel, A. (2003). Case series: IV regional anesthesia with ketorolac and lidocaine: is it effective for the management of complex regional pain syndrome 1 in children and adolescents? *Anesthesia and Analgesia, 96*(3), 694–695.

van Bodegraven Hof, E. A., Groeneweg, G. J., Wesseldijk, F., Huygen, F. J., & Zijlstra, F. J. (2010). Diagnostic criteria in patients with complex regional pain syndrome assessed in an out-patient clinic. *Acta Anaesthesiologica Scandinavica, 54*(7), 894–9.

Walton, K. D., Dubois, M., & Llinas, R. R. (2010). Abnormal thalamocortical activity in patients with Complcx Regional Pain Pain (CRPS) Type I. *Pain, 150*(1), 41–51.

Wilder, R. T., Berde, C. B., Wolohan, M., Vieyra, M. A., Masek, B. J., & Micheli, L. J. (1992). Reflex sympa-

thetic dystrophy in children. *The Journal of Bone and Joint Surgery, 74,* 910–919.

Wilson, P. R. (1999). Complex regional pain syndrome-reflex sympathetic dystrophy. *Current Treatment Options in Neurology, 1*(5), 466–472.

Yucel, I., Demiraran, Y., Ozturan, K., & Degirmenci, E. (2009). Complex regional pain syndrome type I: efficacy of stellate ganglion blockade. *Operative Orthopadie und Traumatologie, 10*(4), 179–183.

Physical Therapy

17

Victoria Marchese, Kripa Dholakia, and Lori Brake

Keywords

Myofascial pain syndrome • Complex regional pain syndrome • Juvenile rheumatoid arthritis (JRA) • Physiologic cost index • Therapeutic exercise interventions

Introduction

Physical therapists diagnose and manage conditions that cause movement dysfunction which affect an individual's physical and functional ability. They work toward restoring, maintaining, and promoting not only optimal physical function, but optimal wellness, fitness, and quality of life as it relates to movement and health. Physical therapists provide interventions which prevent the onset and progression of impairments, activity limitations, and participation restrictions that may result from diseases, disorders, conditions, or injuries (Guide to Physical Therapist Practice, 2001). Physical therapists, as an integral part of a multidisciplinary team, collaborate with other members such as physicians, psychologists, dentists, nurses, social workers, occupational therapists, nutritionists, and speech language pathologists, to maximize patient outcomes. By implementing a

V. Marchese (✉)
Department of Physical Therapy, Lebanon Valley College, 101 North College Avenue, Annville, PA 17033, USA
and
Penn State Hershey College of Medicine at The Pennsylvania State University, Hershey, PA, USA
e-mail: marchese@lvc.edu

family-centered approach to determine the best plan of care, the physical therapist strives to improve the child's and family's quality of life.

Several common childhood disorders lead to the development of chronic pain with secondary musculoskeletal and neuromuscular complications that affect activity and participation; such as, cancer (Stevens, 2007), complex regional pain syndrome (Oerlemans et al. 2000; Sherry and Malleson, 2002), fibromyalgia (Siegel et al. 1998), neuropathic pain following an amputation (Nagarajan et al. 2002), sickle cell anemia (Bodhise et al. 2004), chronic arthritis including juvenile idiopathic arthritis (Klepper, 1999; Klepper, 2003; Klepper, 2007; Singh-Grewal et al. 2007; Singh-Grewal et al. 2006), and trauma (Saroyan et al. 2007). Children with chronic pain are not always referred to physical therapy early on in the treatment of their pain symptoms; however, as awareness among health care professionals regarding the various types of pediatric chronic pain is rising, children are being diagnosed early and receiving physical therapy earlier in the course of their treatment. Early referral plays a critical role in preventing secondary body function/structure impairments, activity limitations, and participation restrictions. Evidence has shown that there are limited documented treatment guidelines for chronic pain conditions but a multi-dimensional approach encompassing patient education, cognitive behavior therapy, physical therapy, and pharmacologic therapy have proven effective (Oerlemans et al. 2000; Guite et al. 2007; Stevens, 2007).

The physical therapist works with a child with chronic pain through a process of developing a physical therapy diagnosis derived from a thorough examination, and developing and implementing a plan of care, the effectiveness of which is monitored using outcome measures.

This chapter discusses the process involved in a physical therapy initial examination, determining a physical therapy diagnosis, developing an intervention plan, and finally provides a case study.

Brief Descriptions of Common Disorders that Require Physical Therapy Intervention for Pain

Fibromyalgia: At one time, fibromyalgia was considered an adult syndrome, but now this diagnosis is reported in children and adolescents (Yunus & Masi, 1989; Siegel et al. 1998). Fibromyalgia syndrome or juvenile primary fibromyalgia syndrome (FMS) is characterized by the following clinical features: numerous soft tissue tender points, diffuse pain, fatigue, stiffness, sleep disturbances, subjective swelling, headaches, paresthesias, irritable bowel syndrome, and normal findings on routine laboratory tests (Breau et al. 1999; Cedraschi et al. 2004; Siegel et al. 1998). The effectiveness of physical therapy intervention for children has not been well studied; however, in adults, programs that included education regarding pain, muscle physiology, aquatics, stretching, body awareness therapy, cognitive-behavioral strategies, and relaxation demonstrated significant improvements in pain compared before and after the programs (Havermark and Langius-Eklof 2006; Cedraschi et al. 2004; Hammond & Freeman 2006; Brown et al. 2001).

Myofascial Pain Syndrome: Travell and Simons (1983), define myofascial pain syndrome as "pain and/or autonomic phenomena referred from active myofascial trigger points with associated dysfunction." Myofascial trigger points are described as an area of hyperirritability located in a taut band of skeletal muscle that is associated with a hypersensitive palpable nodule which is painful on compression and can give rise to characteristic referred pain, motor dysfunction, and autonomic phenomena (Simons & Travell, 1981; Simons, Travell, & Simons, 1999). Dysesthesias, hyperalgesia, and referred pain are sensory disturbances and changes in skin temperature, sweating, and proprioceptive disturbances are some of the symptoms of a myofascial trigger point (Lavelle et al. 2007). Myofascial trigger points are described as either active or latent with an active trigger point producing symptoms with local or referred pain and a latent myofascial trigger point not producing pain symptoms unless the area is stimulated. Myofascial trigger points can cause muscle weakness and decreased ROM and therefore lead to limitation in functional mobility (Lucas et al. 2004). The presence of referred pain indicates that the patient may have myofascial pain syndrome versus fibromyalgia (Lavelle et al. 2007). Physical therapy intervention including home exercise programs, ischemic pressure relief, and sustained stretching have been reported to be effective in decreasing trigger point sensitivity and pain intensity (Hanten et al. 2000).

Complex Regional Pain Syndrome (CRPS): CRPS is categorized into two primary types. CRPS type I, previously known as reflex sympathetic dystrophy, is found to occur without any nerve injury. The clinical findings of type I include allodynia, regional pain, abnormalities in temperature, abnormal motor activity, swelling, and altered skin color following a history of a traumatic event. CRPS type II exists wherein a definable nerve lesion exists along with all the aforementioned symptoms (Low et al. 2007; Stanton-Hicks et al. 1998). The lower extremity is predominantly affected in 81–85% of the cases in children with CRPS type I as compared to the upper extremity (Kozin et al. 1977; Low et al. 2007; Sherry et al. 1999). The etiology of CRPS type I is unknown, however, psychological or

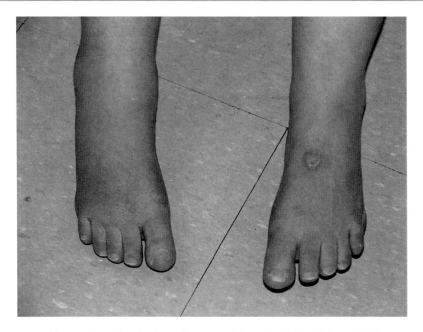

Image of a teenager with complex regional pain syndrome type I impacting bilateral feet and ankles

stress-related issues, and history of minor trauma have been seen to play a role (Carron et al. 1972; Sherry & Weisman, 1988; Stanton et al. 1993). Treatment of CRPS is a challenge, but physical therapy along with a strong multidisciplinary approach providing psychological support, has had promising outcomes (Bernstein et al. 1978; Sherry et al. 1999; Sherry et al. 1990; Stanton-Hicks et al. 1998; Wilder, 2005).

Juvenile idiopathic arthritis (JIA): Juvenile Idiopathic Arthritis is an umbrella term that encompasses all chronic arthritis in children 16 years of age or younger, including Juvenile rheumatoid arthritis (JRA), and is being adopted by the International League of Associations for Rheumatology (ILAR) (Haines, 2007). JRA is the most common rheumatic condition in children with a prevalence of approximately 30–150 per 100,000 and is defined as persistent arthritis in one or more joints lasting at least 6 weeks where certain exclusionary conditions have been eliminated. The disease subtype is defined through the clinical symptoms present in the first 6 months of disease (Ilowite, 2002). JRA is also further divided into three main subtypes based on symptoms present at disease onset. These are systemic, pauciarticular (less than five joints involved), and polyarticular (five or more joints involved) (Ilowite, 2002; Mason & Reed, 2005). Musculoskeletal impairments of JRA could include decreased ROM, joint tenderness, decreased bone mass, bone strength, and muscle mass (Felin et al. 2007) all leading to decreased physical function (Miller et al. 1999). Treatments for JRA may constitute the use of non-steroidal anti-inflammatory drugs, intra-articular corticosteroid administration, and when these two are deemend ineffective, methotrexate therapy has been employed (Haines, 2007). Physical therapy has shown to improve aerobic endurance without disease exacerbation and progression or pain amplification by employing a weight-bearing physical conditioning program (Klepper, 1999).

Sickle cell disease: Sickle cell disease (SCD) comprises of a disorder of hemoglobin wherein the red blood cells are damaged (hemolysis) and/ or deformed leading to anemia. These abnormally shaped red blood cells occlude blood vessels leading to vaso-occlusive conditions and recurrent pain. Several common forms of this disease are mentioned in the literature pertaining to the gene inheritance pattern and clinical presentation.

The SS type is the most common and severe form of the disease in which once sickle cell gene is inherited from each parent; the SC type is a milder form wherein one sickle cell gene is inherited from one parent and another "C" gene is inherited producing a different type of abnormal hemoglobin; S-beta thalassemia, wherein one sickle cell gene and another for beta thalessemia, is inherited. The sickle cell trait is identified when one has one sickle cell gene, but the other gene is normal categorizing them as a carrier (Crearym et al. 2007). SCD most commonly affects persons with origins in the Sub-Saharan Africa, Central or South America, the Caribbean Islands, and countries such as Turkey, Greece, Italy, India, and Saudi Arabia (Brawley et al. 2008). Multisystemic clinical signs and symptoms of this disease range from pain and ischemic organ damage due to occlusion; and/or fatigue, shortness of breath, and jaundice due to the anemia. Clinical signs are prophylactically managed with medications (Crearym et al. 2007). Most episodes of pain are acute, but when not treated adequately, can lead to the development of chronic pain (Ballas, 2007). There have been no randomized controlled studies investigating chronic pain arising from SCD (Dunlop & Bennett, 2006). The significance of physical therapy has been examined in the management of avascular necrosis of the hip in young adults (Neumayr et al. 2006). Studies on the role of physical therapy in addressing chronic pain in children with sickle cell disease is greatly lacking.

Cancer: Cancer and the medical treatment for cancer have both short- and long-term effects on the neuromuscular and musculoskeletal systems. With great improvements in survival rate from childhood cancers there have also been more studies examining the short- and long-term side-effects of treatments over the child's life span. These side effects depend on the type of cancer and location of cancer. Children who receive surgery such as limb-sparing or amputation from a solid tumor are at risk for limitations in ROM, neuropathic pain, decreased strength, endurance, and functional mobility (Nagarajan et al. 2002; Marchese et al. 2004a, b). Children

with leukemia are at risk for developing peripheral neuropathy, osteonecrosis, and bone fractures due to chemotherapy agents such as vincristine, corticosteroids, and methotrexate, respectively (Marchese et al. 2003; Marchese et al. 2004a, b; Marchese et al. 2008).

Physical Therapy Initial Examination

Frameworks such as the International Classification of Function, Disability, and Health (ICF) and the American Physical Therapy Guide to Practice are frequently utilized by physical therapists to perform examinations on children with complex medical histories or extensive disease processes. In addition, these frameworks provide organization and standardized language of practice (World Health Organization 2001; Guide to Physical Therapist Practice, 2001).

The ICF classifies function at the level of body part (body function/structure), whole person (activity), and whole person in social context (participation). Body structure and function represent the anatomical and physiological functioning of the body systems such as muscle strength and range of motion (ROM). The activity domain describes the execution of a task or action by an individual, for example walking, and the participation domain describes the ability of a person to be involved in life situations such as going to school and work. Also addressed are environmental factors (external and internal) that make up the physical, social, and attitudinal environment in which people live and conduct their lives such as age, gender, educational background, and past experience.

The Guide to Physical Therapist Practice (2001) includes a patient/client management model (examination, evaluation, diagnosis, prognosis, intervention, and re-evaluation) and specific practice patterns including musculoskeletal, neuromuscular, integumentary, and cardiopulmonary components (Table 17.1) that guide examinations and interventions. A thorough and comprehensive physical therapy examination is a crucial first step. Limitations identified following

Table 17.1 Recommended examination categories

Body function and structure		Activity	Participation
Musculoskeletal	*Integumentary*	• Locomotion & ambulation6	• Quality of life
• Range of motion	• Skin	• Developmental skills	• Community participation
• Strengthening	• Wounds	• Balance and coordination	
• Postural alignment	• Scar mobility	• Assistive devices	
Neuromuscular	*Cardiopulmonary*		
• Type of pain	• Endurance		
• Location of pain	• Visual exam		
• Muscle tone	• Heart rate		
• Vision	• Respiratory rate		
• Sensation			
• Sensory Integration			

the examination could range from being mild and not limiting functional activities, or could be severe wherein impairments include long-standing muscle atrophy, limitations in joint range of motion, sensitivity to touch, and dysesthesia, limited functional skills such as ambulation, which impose participation restrictions. The data gathered during the initial exam guides the physical therapy intervention, goal setting, and overall plan of care (Jett, 2006).

A detailed medical and social history is essential to any physical therapy evaluation. This includes onset of pain, evidence of trauma, type and location of pain, and activities that aggravate or relieve pain symptoms. Questions regarding possible stressors in the child's life and the child's coping strategies should be discussed with the child and family (Guite et al. 2007). In addition, the physical therapist gathers information as appropriate regarding the child's gross and fine motor development, social history including cultural beliefs, family resources, and social activities (school, work, sports, family); home, work, and school environments; and as appropriate the use of alternative interventions such as acupuncture or massage therapy.

Laboratory reports such as plain radiographs, magnetic resonance imaging, and/or bone scans are reviewed for evidence of osteoporosis or osteonecrosis that may have been caused by medical treatments including corticosteroids or methotrexate, or prolonged inactivity (Fletcher, 1997; Marchese et al. 2008; Mattano et al. 2000; Sherry & Malleson, 2002).

Body Structure and Function

Musculoskeletal

The physical therapy musculoskeletal examination provides the physical therapist with information pertaining to active and passive range of motion, joint play (accessory arthrokinematics), muscle strength, and posture/alignment. Range of motion limitation is a very common presentation resulting from a tendency to "protect" the limb or joint from activity or movement leading to progressive stiffness of the joint. The longer the limb is immobilized as a coping mechanism, surrounding joint structures become progressively stiff and immobile, causing a cascading effect of capsular tightness, muscle shortening, tendon contractures, progressive-dependent edema, or swelling from a failure of the muscle pump to push away fluid, eventually leading to complete immobility. Immobility also implies limited active muscle use which promotes progressive muscle weakness. In extreme cases, obvious muscle wasting is evident. Strength can be tested using manual muscle testing, utilizing dynamometers, or through the observation of movement and functional skills. Manual muscle testing or the use of a dynamometer provide objective values of muscle strength which thereafter guide intervention and also can monitor the effectives of interventions. The use of a dynamometer also provides for age and gender matched comparisons to be made with respect to isometric muscle force produced using documented normative data (Backman et al. 1989).

Examining strength through the observation of functional activities such as lifting up an object, transitioning sit to stand from a chair, stand to floor sit, squat to stand, or stair climbing provides the therapist with information regarding the child's functional strength.

Observation of movement also provides information regarding movement quality and any compensatory strategies that the patient may be utilizing (Butler et al. 1984). This may include an observation regarding deviations in postural alignment, which would necessitate a detailed examination of the child's posture. Observations of posture are made in various patient positions including supine, sitting, standing, and walking as well as in the act of performing functions in their natural environment such as carrying a school book bag or during a sports activity (Graumlich et al. 2001).

Neuromuscular

The neuromuscular examination includes the following: pain, sensation (neuropathic/nociceptive), vision, hearing, balance, and coordination. Pain is assessed using objective qualifiers regarding the intensity and location, as well as more subjective qualifiers such as its type and behavior. The physical therapist documents pain using age-appropriate pain assessment scales, Wong-Baker Faces pain scale, for children 3–7 years of age, visual analogue for children >5 years of age, verbal analogue for children and adolescents >9 years of age, CHEOPS (Children's Hospital of Eastern Ontario Pain Scale) for infants and children >1 year of age, and FLACC (Face, Legs, Activity, Cry, Consolability) for children <3 years of age or with limited cognition (Jensen et al. 1986; Wong et al. 2001). The visual analogue scale uses a 10-cm line with words at either end – "no pain" and "pain as bad as it could be," where a verbal analogue scale uses verbal descriptors such as no pain, mild pain, moderate pain, and severe pain. A numerical rating scale uses a set of numbers from 0 to 10 used to represent a range of pain from no pain to the worst pain ever experienced. To locate the areas of pain, a body schema diagram may be used upon which the child marks the areas and intensities of pain using colors and shades (Melzack, 1975; Scudds, 2001). Word descriptors also help to identify if the pain is neuropathic ("tingling") and nociceptive ("dull/achy") pain (Galer & Jensen, 1997). Neuropathic pain can also be described as burning, stabbing, tingling, shooting, or tight feeling, and may be caused by a chemotherapeutic agent such as vincristine, injury from surgery due to either cut or stretched nerve, by pressure from a tumor pressing on a nerve, or after an amputation causing phantom limb pain. Nociceptive pain, commonly described as dull aching or throbbing pain, may arise from disease, surgery, or side effects of treatment (i.e., mucositis) arising in the bone, joint, muscle, skin, or connective tissue. Allodynia is an exaggerated response to otherwise non-noxious stimuli (Singh et al. 2004) and is commonly seen in children with complex regional pain syndrome. Hyperesthesia is a condition that involves an abnormal increase in sensitivity to stimuli of the senses, including sound (auditory hyperesthesia), taste, and textures (tactile hyperesthesia). The presentation of pain may vary in conditions of varied etiologies. Children with juvenile rheumatoid arthritis may experience joint pain, while a child with fibromyalgia may experience pain at several tender points within the muscle. Pain can also be referred to other sites, from the original sources, and therefore the clinician must examine thoroughly to identify the primary source versus areas of referred pain.

Sensation is tested in the affected areas for light touch and or sharp/dull differentiation. Temperature changes in localized areas could also be observed, as in cases of children with complex regional pain syndromes, where autonomic signs such as increased localized perspiration and or coolness to touch, or a cold-blue extremity may be noted (Sherry & Malleson, 2002).

The physical therapist grossly examines a patient's vision and hearing as it pertains to their function. In some cases of childhood cancer, hearing loss may be a side effect of chemotherapy (Reddy & Witek, 2003). Balance and coordination are important to examine in children with chronic pain because some conditions such as fibromyalgia may cause the child to experience dizziness (Rusty et al. 1999). While in other instances, balance may be affected due to a somatosensory impairment, visual-perceptual deficits or a musculoskeletal issue such as tendency for decreased weight bearing on the involved extremity.

Integumentary

A close observation of the skin is made for localized or dispersed changes in skin color, appearance (glossy, blotchy discoloration), texture, temperature, hair loss, and edema. The physical therapist uses a tape measure to measure the surface area of change, and the size of the change in color/pigmentation. Bony landmarks or other birth marks help in describing the location for ease of reliable re-measurement. If available, a specialty camera with a pre-installed grid-lined paper can be used to monitor the area of involvement by regularly following the area with follow-up photographs. Edema is measured objectively by performing girth measurements using a standard tape measure using well documented landmarks and if appropriate, comparing with the uninvolved side.

Cardiovascular and Pulmonary

The cardiovascular and pulmonary examination evaluates the following elements: endurance, oxygenation capacity, and respiratory measures. Long periods of inactivity directly resulting from the pain and other complication from the disease process such as fatigue (Klepper, 2007), depression (Bodhise et al. 2004), and feelings of decreased self worth (Guite et al. 2007), may compromise a child's endurance abilities. The physical therapist observes for signs of increased or altered work of breathing; such as, the use of accessory muscles, nasal flaring, cervical and/or thoracic asymmetry, or belly breathing. In addition to testing the child's tolerance for and participation in functional activities, a variety of clinical tests may be used to examine a child's endurance and aerobic function (Health Related Physical Fitness: Test Manual, 1980; Grant et al. 1999; Jackson & Coleman, 1976; Steele, 1996; McArdle et al. 2000) (Table 17.2). Nene, (1993) and Chin et al. (1999) identified a significant correlation between physiologic cost index and oxygen uptake, indicating a close relationship between cardiopulmonary factors and energy consumption while walking.

Activity

Children with chronic pain are very likely to experience some level of decreased activity. Activity limitation could present as difficulty getting out of bed or rising from a chair to challenges with walking, negotiating stairs or avoidance of involved limb usage in any functional skills. The physical therapist examination focuses on activity measures that are age-appropriate for the child. Mobility is examined through a gait analysis using qualitative and quantitative gait parameters. The physical therapist examines gait

Table 17.2 Common clinical outcome measures for examining endurance

Measurement	Purpose
3, 6, 9, or 12-min walk/run tests	Measure distance covered in a period of time
Rate of perceived exertion	A subjective measure of the child's level of exertion or effort while performing an activity.
	The scale consists of numbers (6–20) and adjectives related to each of these numbers such as "very easy" to "somewhat hard" (Borg, 1971). The scale is presented during an activity and the participant is able to point to his or her RPE. The RPE has demonstrated the ability to estimate general fatigue
Physiologic cost index	is an objective measure of locomotor efficiency obtained by recording the participant's heart rate (HR) while walking, at rest, and the patient's average speed of walking (PCI = HR while walking – HR at rest/m/min)
Heart rate	An objective way to measure aerobic fitness and is a common method for measuring the amount of energy expended or economy of movement while performing a task.

characteristics such as arm-swing, gait speed, cadence, step length, and distance ambulated. Gait deviations also can arise from decreased weight-bearing abilities, joint immobility, or muscle weakness. In some cases, a child's gait may remain unaffected, but underlying impairments may higher level motor tasks such as running, jumping or stair negotiation.

Timed tests are frequently used in examining functional mobility. The Timed Up and Go (TUG) and Timed Up and Down Stairs (TUDS) are two examples of such tests that examine transitions from sit to stand, to walking, as well as, from ascending to descending stairs (Mathias et al. 1986; Marchese et al. 2003; Marchese et al. 2004a, b; Zaino et al. 2004; Habib & Westcott, 1998).

As a child's activity is linked to their developmental stage often developmental tests are utilized (Folio & Fewell, 2000). These measures are used to determine age-appropriate gross motor skills and higher developmental skills such as running speed and agility, balance, and coordination (Deitz et al. 2007). The age equivalents and percentile scores for these tests can also be used to objectively measure the effectiveness of a therapeutic intervention (Deitz et al. 2007) (Table 17.3).

Participation

The inability to be active and functional causes children to have a tendency to withdraw from school, social activities, and sports as compared to their peers (Sherry & Weisman, 1988; Eiser & Vance, 2002; Guite et al. 2007; Kashikar-Zuck et al. 2007). Reintegration back into the school with adequate supports should be included as part of every discharge planning process. Physical therapists select appropriate quality of life (QOL) questionnaires to objectively measure the level of participation of a child and their family in community, school, and sports (Ware et al. 2000; Varni et al. 1999; Varni et al. 2001). These questionnaires take less than 20 min to complete. These measures are frequently used to develop long-term goals and re-entry into the home and community which are both crucial to the rehabilitative process and the success of the outcome (Table 17.4).

Table 17.3 Common outcome measures utilized to examine developmental motor skills

Outcome measure	Purpose
Peabody Developmental Motor Scales-2 (PDMS-2)	An assessment tool designed to assess the motor skills of children from birth through 5 years of age, comprised of six subtests that measure interrelated motor abilities that develop early in life.
Bruininks-Oseretsky Test of Motor Proficiency-2 (BOT-2)	The BOT-2 is administered to children between the ages of 4 and 21. This test gives objective information on balance, fine and gross motor coordination, agility, and strength.

Table 17.4 Outcome measures to examine quality of life

Outcome measure	Purpose
Short-form 36 Health Survey version 2 (SF-36v2)	The questionnaire is a measure of quality of life specifically designed for use with a broad range of patient populations. The SF-36v2 consists of 36 items combined to form eight subscales. The SF-36v2 subscales can be scored individually to obtain specific domain scores; a physical component summary score emphasizes the physical subscales such as physical functioning, vitality, and physical role functioning; and a mental component summary score emphasizes social functioning, emotional role functioning, and mental health.
PedsQL	The PedsQL incorporates a generic core and disease/symptom-specific modular approach for pediatric chronic health conditions.

Physical Therapy Diagnosis, Prognosis, and Plan of Care

A physical therapy diagnosis involves labels that identify the impact of the condition on function at the level of the system (especially the movement system) and at the level of the whole person (Guide to physical therapists practice, 2001). The discrepancies between the level of function that is desired by the patient and the capacity of the patient to achieve this level, is identified through this diagnostic process. Once the diagnosis is established, the predicted optimal level of improvement in function is made by the physical therapist. The physical therapist then develops a plan of care that specifies anticipated goals and expected outcomes, the level of optimal improvement, the interventions to be used, proposed duration and frequency of treatment, and the expected outcomes (Guide to physical therapists practice, 2001).

The physical therapy diagnosis and prognosis for patients with chronic pain varies depending on the child's medical diagnosis, medical intervention, and family dynamics. The following physical therapy diagnoses are common for patients with chronic pain: pain (neuropathic/nociceptive), decreased tolerance to touch and textures, fatigue, decreased range of motion, decreased muscle strength and endurance, decreased cardio-pulmonary endurance, decreased functional mobility, and decreased participation in community activities. The formulation of a plan of care and goals requires individual consideration depending on the child's unique presentation of impairments pertaining to their primary diagnosis (Table 17.5). An open dialogue with the child and the family regarding their goals and expectations also play a crucial role in the formulation of the plan of care and goal development.

The frequency and duration of physical therapy provided for children with chronic pain ranges from intensive in-patient rehabilitation to an out-patient consultation. For example a child with severe complex regional pain syndrome experiencing significant body function impairments (decreased strength, range of motion, and pain), activity limitations (decreased mobility), and participation restrictions (unable to participate in social/school/family activities) may require physical therapy 5 days a week; however, as the child gains independence in mobility and diminished impairments, they may be transitioned to out-patient physical therapy with a home exercise program, with a frequency of one to two times a week. Once the child is independent with all mobility, independent with the home exercise program, and returned to school the physical therapist may provide consultative visits to address up-dating a home program if necessary.

Physical Therapy Intervention

Physical therapy intervention is the purposeful interaction of the physical therapist with the patient, family, and when appropriate other individuals involved in patient care to produce changes in the condition that are consistent with the diagnosis and prognosis, using various physical therapy procedures and techniques (Guide to Phys Therapy Practice, 2001).

Physical therapy interventions have the following components: coordination, communication, and documentation; patient-related instruction and procedural interventions. These procedural interventions include therapeutic exercise physical agents and mechanical modalities, including electrotherapeutic modalities and functional training; fabrication and application of devices and equipment.

In the pediatric population, physical therapy interventions are tailored to be age-appropriate and meaningful to the child and caregiver. Parents and caregivers have to be informed and trained to promote and optimize the outcomes of physical therapy services. Several factors influence the complexity, frequency, and duration of the intervention and the decision-making process may include one or more of the following: accessibility and availability of resources; adherence to the intervention program; age; anatomical and physiological changes related to growth and development; caregiver consistency or expertise; chronicity or severity of the present condition, cognitive status; co-morbidities; complications;

Table 17.5 Specific medical diagnosis and physical therapy evaluation considerations

Medical diagnosis	Physical therapy evaluation considerations
Complex regional pain syndrome	• Compromised weight-bearing • Altered sensitivity to touch • Edema • Loss of range of motion • Muscle weakness • Functional limitations • Decreased endurance
Fibromyalgia	• General muscle pain • Severe pain with tender points (occiput, low cervical, trapezius, supraspinatus, second rib, lateral epicondyle, gluteal, greater trochanter, and knee) • Soft tissue swelling with pain modulation by physical activities, weather factors, anxiety/stress, irritable bowel syndrome, chronic anxiety or tension, fatigue, poor sleep, numbness, chronic headaches • Decreased balance
Juvenile rheumatoid arthritis (pauciarticular, polyarticular, systemic)	• Age of onset <16 years of age • Joint swelling or effusion • Heat, decreased range of motion, pain with motion with symptoms lasting for at least 6 weeks • Bone pain due to possible fracture • Loss of range of motion (contractures) • Muscle weakness • Postural deviations • Pain • Gait deviations
Sickle cell anemia	• Decreased activity tolerance • Pain in joints and long bones leading to decreased ROM • Osteonecrosis, osteoporosis, skeletal deformities due to ischemia • Painful swelling and tenderness • Painful chest syndrome • Stroke and neurologic changes • Difficulty weight-bearing through the lower-extremities
Cancer	• Bone pain from build-up of blast cells • Joint pain due to osteonecrosis from corticosteroid • Bone pain due to fracture from methotrexate • Peripheral neuropathy due to chemotherapy agent, vincristine

or secondary impairments; decline in functional independence; level of impairment, level of physical function, living environment, potential discharge destinations, socioeconomic factors, social support, and stability.

Table 17.6 summarizes specific physical therapy interventions for certain medical diagnoses. A detailed and accurate examination, an in-depth knowledge of the disease process and the child's age guides the choice of interventions selected. Through collaboration among the patient, family, and therapist, ideas are generated on how the child and family can participate in activities together with the goal of enhancing the child's performance and functioning, and ultimately, his/her quality of life. A re-examination is performed at regular intervals to evaluate progress and modify or re-direct interventions.

Therapeutic Exercise

Therapeutic exercise interventions include range of motion, muscle strengthening, muscle endurance,

Table 17.6 Physical therapy intervention for specific medical diagnoses

Medical diagnosis	Specific physical therapy interventions
Complex regional pain syndrome	• Weight-bearing activities • Desensitization program • Functional skills • Compression • Strengthening and stretching • Endurance exercise • Aquatic therapy
Fibromyalgia	• Massage • Strengthening and stretching • Endurance exercises • Ice • Heat • Aquatics program
Neuropathic pain	• Compression stockings • Desensitization
Myofascial trigger points	• Vapocoolant spray and stretch • Ice massage • Deep pressure • Ultrasound • Transcutaneous nerve stimulation
Palliative care	• Education on positioning and transfer training • Provide appropriate assistive device • Massage • Heat • Cold
Juvenile rheumatoid arthritis	• Bracing/splinting • Active range of motion exercise • Avoid passive stretch during inflammation • Gravity assisted stretch • Isometric strengthening exercises in painful • Very light weight <1–2 lb if no pain • Guided imagery
Sickle cell anemia	• Mobility training with an assistive device • Active ROM exercises • Myofacial tender point release • Massage (Bodhise et al. 2004) • Breathing exercise during acute episodes • Strengthening

stretching, joint mobilization exercises, neuromuscular and postural control exercises, balance exercises, relaxation exercises, and cardiovascular/pulmonary aerobic endurance (Kisner & Colby, 2007). The aim of using therapeutic exercise is to not only improve body function/structure impairments, such as limitations in range of motion, strength, and endurance, but also to improve functional mobility and activity limitations, such as walking, running, and going up and down stairs.

Active and passive range of motion exercises are performed when a patient is at risk for developing, or has already developed, limitations due to inactivity, disease, or pain. In addition to range of motion exercises, a physical therapist may choose to perform manual soft tissue or joint mobility exercises with a patient. Depending on the desired outcome, various approaches to strengthening exercises are utilized including isotonic (dynamic) resistance exercise, performed concentrically or eccentrically, isokinetic (velocity is controlled) exercise, and isometric (static) exercise.

Stretching techniques may include manual passive stretch performed by the physical therapist or the patient themselves, or mechanical stretch produced by a machine or splinting device. Treadmill walking or any low-intensity activities such as dancing, riding a bike, swimming, and running drills – improve aerobic capacity. In all instances, the physical therapist incorporates these activities into fun, age-appropriate activities. An intensive therapeutic exercise program has demonstrated to be effective in children with CRPS, JRA, fibromyalgia, and cancer (Sherry et al. 1999; Klepper, 2007; Klepper, 1999; Singh-Grewal et al. 2006; Marchese et al. 2004a, b).

Aquatics

An interventional option for patients with pain, specifically fibromyalgia, CRPS, and JRA, is the use of aquatic physical therapy. The benefits of an aquatics program are decreased stress on weight-bearing joints through decreased compression, improved elasticity of muscle and connective tissue secondary to warm water temperatures in combination with stretching techniques, and strength gains from the ability to perform functional strengthening exercises in an un-weighted environment that one would otherwise not be able to perform in gravity-dependent environment (de Fernandes Melo Vitorino et al. 2006; Getz et al. 2006). The buoyancy of the water can be used to assist and/or resist functional movements to meet specific therapeutic goals such as increasing range of motion, strength, and functional abilities. Also, water can be a great tool for providing desensitization in children with amplified musculoskeletal pain. As with any exercise program goal-oriented creativity is utilized by the therapist to address specific patient needs and goals.

Desensitization

Children with musculoskeletal pain may experience hyper or hypo reactions to sensory stimulation

(Sherry and Malleson, 2002). Desensitization is used to assist in decreasing the patient's allodynia and tactile sensitivity through bombarding the area with various degrees of sensations. Various techniques and textures can be used, and can include one or many of the following: rubbing the areas with different textures, submerging the area in water-contrast baths, deep pressure, vibration, brushing, and weight bearing (Allen, 2006). Desensitization techniques are often not performed in isolation, but are incorporated into the therapeutic exercise program. Examples of this are standing barefoot on a roughly textured mat or rug for foot sensitivity. In several cases, wearing socks and shoes provides desensitization to the painful areas on their feet.

Therapeutic Heat

Therapeutic heat is delivered either through superficial thermal agents (moist hot pack, paraffin wax, electrical heating pads, hydrotherapy, fluidotherapy-dry heat) to heat the skin and superficial subcutaneous tissue or deeper tissue modalities, such as ultrasound. The primary therapeutic benefits of using heat as a modality is to increase local blood circulation to assist with healing, provide analgesia, decrease pain, relieve muscle-guarding spasms, increase elasticity, decrease joint stiffness, and increase flexibility (Michlovitz & Nolan, 2005; Allen, 2006). Contraindications to the use of superficial and deep heat include areas with a malignancy, decreased sensation, vascular insufficiency, acute inflammation, pregnancy, infection, and over the epiphyseal plates of undeveloped bones.

Cryotherapy

The therapeutic application of cryotherapy or cold modalities include ice massage, water baths, cold packs, cold compression units, vapocoolant sprays will lower local tissue temperature (Michlovitz & Nolan, 2005). These modalities are used for acute injury and chronic conditions (muscle spasms, myofascial pain syndrome, osteoarthritis, and rheumatoid arthritis) for the vasoconstriction properties to decrease bleeding, decrease inflammation, and decrease pain. For chronic conditions, cold modalities decrease muscle spasms and pain in an effort to increase mobility. Contraindications for the use of cold modalities include any circulatory compromise or peripheral vascular disease, cold intolerance or hypersensitivity, cold urticaria, cryoglobulinemia, Raynauds' phenomenon, and paroxysmal cold hemoglobinuria (Michlovitz & Nolan, 2005). Specifically, children with sickle-cell disease or any vaso-occlusive disease should not receive cryotherapy (Saleem & Rice, 2007).

Transcutaneous Electrical Nerve Stimulation

Transcutaneous Electrical Nerve Stimulation (TENS) relieves pain by employing the "pain gating" theory (Michlovitz & Nolan, 2005). Pain sensations are traditionally carried by the slow fibers, which are "gated" by the transmission of the electrical impulses, through the faster fibers, reaching the cortex of the brain earlier than the pain signals. In the author's experience, TENS is seldom used in the pediatric population as young children are usually fearful of the application, and if the child is able to tolerate the initial sensation, the intensity required to produce the desired clinical effect may not be reached due to anxiety or decreased tolerance to the sensation. There is a significant limitation of research on the use of TENS in the management of chronic pain in children (Näslund, 2001). Contraindications to TENS include decreased sensation, vascular insufficiency, pregnancy, hyper or hypotension, acute inflammation, history of seizures, obesity, or over a malignancy (Michlovitz & Nolan, 2005). The use of TENS should be made on an individual basis, thus the amplitude, duration, and frequency of the setting vary for each patient. For instance, the most commonly used setting is the conventional TENS because this setting tends to be more comfortable and accepted by the patient. The conventional setting uses short pulses (<150 microseconds), high frequency (>80 Hz) with a comfortable amplitude. The conventional setting typically provides a rapid onset of pain relief, but limited in duration. Acupuncture-like setting uses a long-pulse duration (>150 microseconds), a low frequency (<10 Hz), and comfortable to tolerable amplitude. Those settings tend to have a slow onset of relief, but a longer period of analgesia. The brief-intense setting of TENS uses a long-pulse duration (>150 microseconds), a high frequency (>80 Hz), and a comfortable to tolerable amplitude. These settings tend to have a rapid onset of relief with a longer period of analgesia (Belanger, 2002).

Massage

Physical therapists may choose to perform superficial and deep massage to increase local circulation and promote relaxation (Tsao, 2007). In children with JRA, massage therapy has been shown to reduce anxiety, decrease stress hormone levels, and after 30 days of nightly massage performed by the parents, it was shown to decrease pain and morning stiffness (Field et al. 1997). Massage techniques, such as "deep strokes" or ischemic compression therapy, where the pressure is maintained in a localized area, are used in patients experiencing pain due to trigger points or muscle spasms. The underlying neurophysiology of a trigger point release is the use of sustained pressure or ischemic compression on a localized hyper-irritable taught band within a muscle to increase blood flow to the area thus relieving the pain. Self management strategies that can be included in home exercise programs and discharge planning include the use of thera-canes, foam rollers, and towel rolls (Hanten et al. 2000).

Case Example

Past Medical History

Jessica is a 16-year-old Caucasian female who is in the 11th grade at a private high school taking college preparatory classes. She lives at home with both parents and is an only child. Two and one half years prior to admission,

Jessica injured her right shoulder while pitching in a softball game. She received physical therapy for her right shoulder twice weekly for 6 weeks and returned to playing softball. She re-injured the same shoulder twice and each time received physical therapy twice weekly for 6–8 weeks with a full recovery following the first injury; however, after the second injury she developed allodynia which did not resolve with the physical therapy. In February of the following year (9 months following initial injury), she was diagnosed as having complex regional pain syndrome in her arm and, subsequently, received multiple nerve blocks without relief and she did not receive physical therapy services. July of that year she reported to have injured her left foot; however, all radiographic imaging revealed no injury despite the ankle being edematous and painful. Throughout the remainder of that year, her pain spread to her left thigh, buttock, and entire right arm. She was hospitalized three times for medication infusions with no relief.

Physical Therapy Examination: Body Function/Structure

Musculoskeletal
Jessica arrived to her initial physical therapy session sitting in a wheelchair. She was not self-propelling her wheelchair due to upper extremity pain. The allodynia rendered her unable to tolerate resting her legs or feet on the leg rests of the chair. Her resting posture was kyphotic with arms positioned in internal rotation and flexed and her bilateral feet were plantar flexed, knees flexed with only her thighs supported on the wheelchair. She was able to correct her posture, when asked, into upright sitting posture, but was unable to hold the position for more than 10 s. Strength testing was performed and revealed weakness in bilateral lower and upper extremities with manual muscle testing scores 3 out of 5, while strength in neck and trunk were within normal limits. Due to the patient's pain level, decreased effort was put forth during all manual muscle testing. Range of motion was limited in all planes in both ankles, as well as flexion/

extension in right wrist. Active ankle range of motion measured as follows: dorsiflexion −7° on the left and −35° on the right; plantar flexion 25° on the left and 40° on the right; inversion 13° on the left and 20° on the right; eversion 5° on the left and 6° on the right. Right active wrist flexion range of motion was 40° and extension was 15°. All other range of motion was within normal limits.

Neuromuscular
Jessica rated her pain at 10/10 covering all areas of her body on a visual analog scale. Allodynia was present in both legs from mid thigh down to her toes, with variable borders and was severe enough that Jessica was not wearing pants or socks despite it being cold outside. She was found to have allodynia to her stomach and back as well, but was still able to tolerate wearing a bra and a shirt. Vision and hearing were normal.

Integumentary
Jessica had edema in both feet. Girth measurements were taken bilaterally and were measured as follows: around metatarsal heads, 24.5 cm on the right and 23.2 cm on the left; around maleoli, 29.0 cm on the right and 26.8 cm on the left; and 5 cm above maleoli, 25.5 cm on the right and 26.5 cm on the left. Also, bilateral feet were cool to touch and cyanotic with a waxy appearance to the skin.

Cardiovascular and Pulmonary
Jessica presented with brisk capillary refill in her bilateral upper extremities; however, bilateral feet were cyanotic in appearance and edematous. Resting heart rate, respiratory rate, and blood pressure were all within normal limits. Typically, the Bruce Treadmill Protocol is administered on the day of evaluation; however, due to Jessica's inability to stand it was not administered until the third day of the program. Due to reports of pain, she was only able to complete 40 s of the test. When performing transitional movements such as sit to stand or walking, she fatigued quickly and demonstrated shallow, rapid breathing with minimal chest expansion requiring frequent rest breaks.

Activity

Jessica arrived to her initial session in a wheelchair, and at the end of the session she was able to stand in parallel bars for 10 s with a 10/10 VAG scores in her entire body. Her score on the Functional Disability Index (FDI) was 39 (scale ranges 0–60 with 60 being least function). Jessica was able to sit at the edge of the mat without upper extremity support and without loss of balance, but was unable to stand without support. The Bruininks-Oseretsky Test of Motor Proficiency Version 2 was performed and she scored in the first percentiles in all the sections.

Participation

Per Jessica's report, she required minimal assistance for all activities of daily living (bathing, dressing, and toileting) and was attending school partial day for core subjects only. Outside of school, she was spending minimal time with friends and was unable to participate in leisure activities she typically enjoyed.

Physical Therapy Plan of Care

Jessica's personal goals for physical therapy were to participate in life activities without physical restrictions, as well as to drive and play softball again. Physical therapy short-term goals to be achieved in 6 weeks, as developed with Jessica, were as follows: (1) Full functional mobility without pain, (2) Complete 20 min of aerobic activity without pain, (3) Tolerate 20 min of desensitization without pain, (4) Wear her pants, socks, and shoes for an entire day, and (5) Demonstrate full bilateral upper-extremity active range of motion in order to be able to independently put hair in pony tail. Long-term goals, 3 month, were for Jessica to return to full function without limitations and return to school/leisure activities with zero reports of pain.

Physical Therapy Intervention

Jessica was seen in an inpatient rehabilitation setting due to the severity of her impairments. She received 3 hours of physical therapy and 2 hours of occupational therapy 5 days per week and 45 min of each on Saturday and Sunday. Additionally, a home program was provided including stretching, strengthening, desensitization, and aerobic exercise. She also received psychology and music therapy for 2 hours each week.

Day One

After her evaluation on day one, treatment was focused on weight bearing through bilateral lower extremities such as weight bearing on a scale, pedaling a bike, and therapeutic exercise. In her afternoon physical therapy session, Jessica was progressed to walking with a quad cane and wearing her shoes and socks for 30-min intervals.

Days Two and Three

Jessica walked with a quad cane for 50 ft and performed timed activities, such as, step-ups onto a bench ten times for three sets. She ambulated on the treadmill at 1.5 mph for 3 min, rode the bike for 5 min, and used the elliptical for 2 min. By the end of day 3, she completed standing activities without upper extremity support and did not require the use of the quad cane for ambulation; however, she performed these activities with pain behaviors such as crying and occasional screaming, thus requiring frequent rest breaks. She tolerated wearing shoes and pants throughout the day. Jessica moved very slowly through all activities. For example, she required 10 min and 30 s to complete a 60 ft crab walk which 1 week later she was able to complete in 34 s.

End of First Week

Jessica was ambulating without an assistive device and performed single leg stance for 5 s. She ambulated on the treadmill for 15 min at 1.7 mph. She ambulated on various surfaces such as foam and grass without loss of balance.

End of Week Two

Jessica ambulated for 20 min on the treadmill at 3.0 mph. Strengthening exercises included bilateral upper and lower-extremity and core strengthening such as, holding plank position, walking hands side to side while in plank position, lunges, single leg stance to perform skipping while reaching overhead, heel raises, hopping, jogging while holding weights, stepping forward and back over an object and heel raises on the edge of a step. Jessica presented with decreased edema in bilateral feet and ankles with color and temperature beginning to normalize. Jessica performed desensitization treatments such as vibration from an electronic massager on high for 10 min, wearing compression stockings on bilateral upper and lower extremities, towel, and lotion massages, and standing on rough textures such as plastic grass doormat, and a bumpy sensory disk. She was also wearing all forms of clothing and sneakers all day without pain behaviors.

End of Week Three

This week was focused on high-level activities. Rest periods between exercises were minimized and the number of consecutive activities was maximized to assist with increasing endurance. These exercises included power minutes where five exercises such as mountain climbers, jumping jacks, and repeated floor to stand are completed for 1 min each without rest between activities. She ambulated on the treadmill for 20 min at 3.5 mph. She performed single leg stance for 60 s, jumping on one leg, long jumping, and push-ups. Jessica increased self desensitization with various textures including soft and rough textures such as rubbing with scrub brush, massaging feet with lotion, and towel rubs.

End of Week Four and Discharge

During Jessica's last week in the in-patient rehabilitation facility, her physical therapy focused on incorporating sport-specific exercises and practicing her home exercise program. The physical therapist recommend Jessica perform her home exercise program daily which should take approximately 45 min to complete.

Prior to discharge Jessica presented with strength as measured by manual muscle testing as normal (5 out of 5) in her bilateral upper and lower-extremities, full active range of motion in all joints, pain score of three tenths in right foot, two tenths in bilateral upper and lower extremities and back with all other areas being pain free, performed all transitional movements (sit to stand) independently, ambulated independently on even and un-even surfaces, ascended/descended two flights of stairs independently, ambulated on the treadmill for 30 min at 5.0 mph. She no longer complained of fatigue and breathlessness during exercises. The color and temperature to Jessica's bilateral lower extremities was normal and absent of edema. She was independent with all activities of daily living. Her rating on the Functional Disability Index (FDI) was scored at 5 on a scale of 0–60 with 60 being least functional. She was expected to return to school full time the next day.

Clinic Follow-Up 3 Weeks Post Discharge

Upon return to see the pain clinic, her pain was rated at 3 out of 10 in bilateral heels and back, and 0 out of 10 in the remainder of her body. She presented with minimal allodynia in her heels and back and was encouraged to continue to exercise and follow through with her desensitization program. Her score on the Functional Disability Index was 0. She was fully functional and participating in all activities including attending school full time, taking driving lessons, and hanging out with friends.

References

Allen, R. J. (2006). Physical agents used in the management of chronic pain by physical therapists. *Physical Medicine and Rehabilitation Clinics of North America, 17*, 315–345.

American Alliance for Health, Physical Education, Recreation and Dance. (1980). *Health related physical fitness: Test manual*. Reston: American Alliance for Health, Physical Education, Recreation and Dance.

American Physical Therapy Association. (2001). A guide to physical therapist practice, second edition. *Physical Therapy, 81*, 9–746.

Backman, E., Odenrick, P., Henriksson, K. G., & Ledin, T. (1989). Isometric muscle force and anthropometric values in normal children aged between 3.5 and 15 years. *Scandinavian Journal of Rehabilitation Medicine, 21*, 105–114.

Ballas, S. K. (2007). Current issues in sickle cell pain and its management. *Hematology, 2007*, 97–105.

Belanger, A. (2002). *Evidenced-based guide to therapeutic physical agents*. Philadelphia: Lippincott Williams & Wilkins.

Bernstein, B. H., Singsen, B. H., Kent, J. T., Kornreich, H., King, K., Hicks, R., & Hanson, V. (1978). Reflex neurovascular dystrophy in childhood. *The Journal of Pediatrics, 93*, 211–215.

Bodhise, P. B., Dejoie, M., Brandon, Z., Simpkins, S., & Ballas, S. K. (2004). Non-pharmacologic management of sickle cell pain. *Hematology, 9*, 235–237.

Borg, G. (1971). The perception of physical performance. In R. J. Shephard (Ed.), *Frontiers of fitness* (pp. 280–294). Springfield: Charles C Thomas.

Brawley, O. W., Cornelius, L. J., Edwards, L. R., Gamble, V. N., Green, B. L., Inturrisi, C. E., James, A. H., Laraque, D., Mendez, M. H., Montoya, C. J., Pollock, B. H., Robinson, L., Scholnik, A. P., & Schori, M. (2008). NIH consensus development statement on hydroxyurea treatment for sickle cell disease: Draft. *NIH Consensus and State-of-the-Science Statements, 25*, 1–30.

Breau, L., McGrath, P. J., & Ju, L. H. (1999). Review of juvenile primary fibromyalgia and chronic fatigue syndrome. *Journal of Developmental and Behavioral Pediatrics, 20*, 278–288.

Brown, G. T., Delisle, R., Gagnon, N., & Sauve, A. E. (2001). Juvenile fibromyalgia syndrome: Proposed management using a cognitive-behavioral approach. *Physical & Occupational Therapy in Pediatrics, 21*, 19–36.

Butler, P., Engelbrecht, M., Major, R. E., Tait, J. H., Stallared, J., & Patrick, J. H. (1984). Physiological cost index of walking for normal children and its use as an indicator of physical handicap. *Developmental Medicine and Child Neurology, 26*, 607–612.

Carron, H., & McCue, F. (1972). Reflex sympathetic dystrophy syndrome in a ten year old. *The Southern Medical Journal, 65*, 631–632.

Cedraschi, C., Desmeules, J., Rapiti, E., Baumgartner, E., Cohen, P., Finckh, A., Allaz, A. F., & Vischer, T. L. (2004). Fibromyalgia: A randomized, controlled trial of a treatment programme based on self management. *Annals of the Rheumatic Diseases, 63*, 290–296.

Chin, T., Sawamura, S., Fujita, H., Nakajima, S., Ojima, I., Oyabu, H., Nagakura, Y., Otsuka, H., & Nakagawa, A. (1999). The efficacy of physiological cost index (PCI) measurement of a subject walking with an intelligent prosthesis. *Prosthetics and Orthotics International, 23*, 45–49.

Crearym, M., Williamson, D., & Kulkarni, R. (2007). Sickle cell disease: Current activities, public health implications, and future directions. *Journal of Womens Health, 16*, 575–582.

de Fernandes Melo Vitorino, D., de Bizari Coin Carvalho, L., & do Fernandes Prado, G. (2006). Hydrotherapy and conventional physiotherapy improve total sleep time and quality of life of fibromyalgia patients: Randomized clinical trial. *Sleep Medicine, 7*, 293–296.

Deitz, J. C., Kartin, D., & Kopp, K. (2007). Review of the Bruininks-Oseretsky test of motor proficiency, second edition (BOT-2). *Physical & Occupational Therapy in Pediatrics, 27*, 87–102.

Dunlop, R. J., & Bennett, K. C. L. B. (2006). Pain management for sickle cell disease. *Cochrane Database of Systematic Reviews, 2*, CD003350. DOI: 10.1002/14651858.CD003350.pub2.

Eiser, C., & Vance, Y. H. (2002). Implications of cancer for school attendance and behavior. *Medical and Pediatric Oncology, 38*, 317–319.

Felin, E. M. O., Prahalad, S., Askew, E. W., & Moyer-Mileur, L. J. (2007). Musculoskeletal abnormalities of the tibia in juvenile rheumatoid arthritis. *Arthritis and Rheumatism, 56*, 984–994.

Field, T., Hernandez-Reif, M., Seligman, S., Krasnegor, J., & Sunshine, W. (1997). Juvenile rheumatoid arthritis: Benefits from massage therapy. *Journal of Pediatric Psychology, 22*, 607–617.

Fletcher, B. D. (1997). Effects of pediatric cancer therapy on the musculoskeletal system. *Pediatric Radiology, 27*, 623–636.

Folio, R. M., & Fewell, R. R. (2000). *Peabody developmental motor scales* (2nd ed.). Austin, Texas: Pro-ed.

Galer, B. S., & Jensen, M. P. (1997). Development and preliminary validation of a pain measure specific to neuropathic pain: The neuropathic pain scale. *Neurology, 48*, 332–338.

Getz, M., Hutzler, Y., & Vermeer, A. (2006). Effects of aquatic interventions in children with neuromotor impairments: A systematic review of the literature. *Clinical Rehabilitation, 20*, 927–936.

Grant, S., Aitchison, T., Henderson, E., Christie, J., Zare, S., McMurray, J., & Dargie, H. (1999). A comparison of the reproducibility and the sensitivity to change of visual analogue scales, Borg scales, and likert scales in normal subjects during submaximal exercise. *Chest, 11*, 1208–1217.

Graumlich, S. E., Powers, S. W., Byars, K. C., Schwarber, L. A., Mitchell, M. J., & Kalinyak, K. A. (2001). Multidimensional assessment of pain in pediatric sickle cell disease. *Journal of Pediatric Psychology, 26*, 203–214.

Guite, J. W., Logan, D. E., Sherry, D. D., & Rose, J. B. (2007). Adolescent self-perception: Associations with chronic musculoskeletal pain and functional disability. *The Journal of Pain, 8*, 379–386.

Habib, A., & Westcott, S. (1998). Assessment of anthropometric factors on balance tests in children. *Pediatric Physical Therapy, 10*, 101–108.

Haines, K. A. (2007). Juvenile idiopathic arthritis: Therapies in the 21st century. *Bulletin of the NYU Hospital for Joint Diseases, 65*, 205–211.

Hammond, A., & Freeman, K. (2006). Community patient education and exercise for people with fibromyalgia: A parallel group randomized controlled trial. *Clinical Rehabilitation, 20*, 835–846.

Hanten, W. P., Olson, S. L., Butts, N. L., & Nowicki, A. L. (2000). Effectiveness of a home program ischemic pressure followed by sustained stretch for treatment of myofascial trigger points. *Physical Therapy, 80*, 997–1003.

Havermark, A. M., & Langius-Eklof, A. (2006). Long-term follow up of a physical therapy programme for patients with fibromyalgia syndrome. *Scandinavian Journal of Caring Science, 20*, 315–322.

Ilowite, N. T. (2002). Current treatment of juvenile rheumatoid arthritis. *Pediatrics, 109*, 109–115.

Jackson, A. S., & Coleman, A. E. (1976). Validation of distance run tests for elementary school children. *Research Quarterly, 47*, 86–94.

Jensen, M. P., Karoly, P., & Braver, S. (1986). The measurement of clinical pain intensity: A comparison of six methods. *Pain, 27*, 117–126.

Jett, A. (2006). Toward a common language for function, disability, and health. *Physical Therapy, 86*, 726–734.

Kashikar-Zuck, S., Lynch, A. M., Grahm, B., Sain, N. F., Mullen, S. M., & Noll, R. B. (2007). Social functioning and peer relationships of adolescents with juvenile fibromyalgia syndrome. *Arthritis and Rheumatism, 57*, 474–480.

Kisner, C., & Colby, L. A. (2007). *Therapeutic exercise: Foundations and techniques* (5th ed.). Philadelphia: F.A. Davis Company.

Klepper, S. (1999). Effects of an eight-week physical conditioning program on disease signs and symptoms in children with chronic arthritis. *Arthritis Care and Research, 12*, 52–60.

Klepper, S. (2003). Exercise and fitness in children with arthritis: Evidence of benefits for exercise and physical activity. *Arthritis and Rheumatism, 49*, 435–443.

Klepper, S. (2007). Making the case for exercise in children with juvenile idiopathic arthritis: What we know and where to go from here. *Arthritis and Rheumatism, 57*, 887–890.

Kozin, F., Haughton, V., & Ryan, L. (1977). The reflex sympathetic dystrophy syndrome in a child. *The Journal of Pediatrics, 90*, 417–419.

Lavelle, E. D., Lavelle, W., & Smith, H. S. (2007). Myofascial trigger points. *The Medical Clinics of North America, 91*, 229–239.

Low, A. K., Ward, K., & Wines, A. P. (2007). Pediatric complex regional pain. *Journal of Pediatric Orthopedics, 27*, 567–572.

Lucas, K. R., Plus, B. I., & Rich, P. S. (2004). Latent myofascial trigger points: Their effect on muscle activation and movement efficiency. *Journal of Bodywork Movement Therapy, 8*, 160–166.

Maltes, A. L. (1971). Reflex sympathetic dystrophy in a child: A case report. *Bulletin of the Hospital for Joint Diseases Orthopaedic Institute, 32*, 193–197.

Marchese, V. G., Chiarello, L. A., & Lange, B. J. (2003). Strength and functional mobility in children with acute lymphoblastic leukemia. *Medical and Pediatric Oncology, 40*, 230–232.

Marchese, V. G., Chiarello, L. A., & Lange, B. J. (2004a). Effects of physical therapy intervention for children with acute lymphoblastic leukemia. *Pediatric Blood & Cancer, 42*, 127–133.

Marchese, V. G., Ogle, S., Womer, R. B., Dormans, J., & Ginsberg, J. P. (2004b). An examination of outcome measures to assess functional mobility in childhood survivors of osteosarcoma. *Pediatric Blood & Cancer, 42*, 41–45.

Marchese, V. G., Connolly, B. H., Able, C., Booten, A. R., Bowen, P., Porter, B. M., Rai, S. N., Hancock, M. L., Pui, C.-H., Neel, M. D., & Kaste, S. C. (2008). Relationships among severity of osteonecrosis, pain, range of motion, and functional mobility in children, adolescents, and young adults with acute lymphoblastic leukemia. *Physical Therapy, 88*, 341–350.

Mason, T. G., & Reed, A. M. (2005). Update in juvenile rheumatoid arthritis. *Arthritis and Rheumatism, 53*, 796–799.

Mathias, S., Nayak, U. S., & Isaacs, B. (1986). Balance in elderly patients: the "get-up and go" test. *Archives of Physical Medicine and Rehabilitation, 67*, 387–389.

Mattano, L. A., Sather, H. N., Trigger, M. E., & Nachman, J. B. (2000). Osteonecrosis as a complication of treating acute lymphoblastic leukemia in children: a report from the Children's Cancer Group. *Journal of Clinical Oncology, 18*, 3262–3272.

McArdle, W. D., Katch, F. I., & Katch, V. L. (2000). *Essentials of exercise physiology* (2nd ed., pp. 200–201). Philadelphia: Lippincott Williams & Wilkins.

Melzack, R. (1975). The McGill Pain Questionnaire: Major properties and scoring methods. *Pain, 1*, 265–276.

Michlovitz, S. L., & Nolan, T. P. (2005). *Modalities for therapeutic intervention*. Philadelphia: F.A. Davis.

Miller, M. L., Kress, A. M., & Berry, C. A. (1999). Decreased physical function in juvenile rheumatoid arthritis. *Arthritis Care and Research, 12*, 309–313.

Nagarajan, R., Neglia, J. P., Clohisy, D. R., & Robison, L. L. (2002). Limb salvage and amputation in survivors of pediatric lower-extremity bone tumors: What are the long-term implications? *Journal of Clinical Oncology, 20*, 4493–4501.

Näslund, J. (2001). Modes of sensory stimulation: Clinical trials and physiological aspects'. *Physiotherapy, 87*, 413–423.

National Heart, Lung and Blood Institute, National Institute of Health. (2008). Sickle cell anemia: Who is at risk? Available at www.nhlbi.nih.gov/health/dci/Diseases/Sca/ SCA: Who Is At Risk.html.

Nene, A. V. (1993). Physiological cost index of walking in able-bodied adolescents and adults. *Clinical Rehabilitation, 7*, 319–326.

Neumayr, L. D., Aguilar, C., Earles, A. N., Jergesen, H. E., Haberkern, C. M., Kammen, B. F., Graber, N., Nancarrow, P. A., Padua, E., Milet, M., Stulberg, B. N., Williams, R. A., Orringer, E. P., Graber, N., Robertson, S. M., & Vichinsky, E. P. (2006). Vichinsky the national osteonecrosis trial in sickle cell anemia study group physical therapy alone compared with core decompression and physical therapy for femoral head osteonecrosis in sickle cell disease. Results of a multicenter study at a mean of three years after treatment. *Journal of Bone and Joint Surgery- American Volume, 88*, 2573–2582.

Oerlemans, H. M., Oostendorp, R. A. B., Boo, T., van der Lann, L., Severens, J. L., & Goris, J. A. (2000).

Adjuvant physical therapy versus occupational therapy in patients with reflex sympathetic dystrophy/complex regional pain syndrome type I. *Archives of Physical Medicine and Rehabilitation, 81*, 49–56.

Reddy, A. T., & Witek, K. (2003). Neurologic complications of chemotherapy for children with cancer. *Current Neurology and Neuroscience Reports, 3*, 137–142.

Rusty, L. M., Harvey, S. A., & Beste, D. J. (1999). Pediatric fibromyalgia and dizziness: Evaluation of vestibular function. *Journal of Developmental and Behavioral Pediatrics, 20*, 211–215.

Saleem, S., & Rice, L. (2007). Limb amputation in hemoglobin SC disease after application of ice and elevation. *American Journal of Hematology, 82*, 53–54.

Saroyan, J. M., Winfree, C. J., Schecter, W. S., Roye, D., & Gold, A. P. (2007). Sciatic neuropathy after lower-extremity trauma: Successful treatment of an uncommon pain and disability syndrome in an adolescent. *American Journal of Physical Medicine & Rehabilitation, 86*, 587–600.

Scudds, R. A. (2001). Pain outcome measures. *Journal of Hand Therapy, 14*, 86–90.

Sherry, D. D., & Malleson, P. N. (2002). The idiopathic musculoskeletal pain syndromes in childhood. *Rheumatic Disease Clinics of North America, 28*, 669–685.

Sherry, D. D., & Weisman, R. (1988). Psychologic aspects of childhood reflex neurovascular dystrophy. *Pediatrics, 81*, 572–578.

Sherry, D. D., McGuire, T., Mellins, E., Salmonson, K., Wallace, C. A., & Nepom, B. (1990). Psychosomatic musculoskeletal pain in childhood: Clinical and psychological analyses of 100 children. *Pediatrics, 88*, 1093–1099.

Sherry, D. D., Wallace, C. A., Kelley, C., Kidder, M., & Sapp, L. (1999). Short- and long-term outcomes of children with complex regional pain syndrome type I treated with exercise therapy. *The Clinical Journal of Pain, 15*, 218–223.

Siegel, D. M., Janeway, D., & Baum, J. (1998). Fibromyalgia syndrome in children and adolescents: Clinical features at presentation and status at follow-up. *Pediatrics, 101*, 377–382.

Simons, D. G., & Travell, J. (1981). Myofascial trigger points, a possible explanation. *Pain, 10*(1), 106–109.

Simons, D. G., (ed.). (1999). Travell and Simons' Myofascial Pain and Dysfunction. The Trigger Point Manual Volume 1&2.

Singh, G., Willen, S., Boswell, M. V., Janata, J., & Chelmisky, T. C. (2004). The value of interdisciplinary pain management in complex regional pain syndrome type I: A prospective outcome study. *Pain Physician, 7*, 203–209.

Singh-Grewal, D., Wright, V., Bar-or, O., & Feldman, B. M. (2006). Pilot study of fitness training and exercise testing in polyarticular childhood arthritis. *Arthritis and Rheumatism, 55*, 364–372.

Singh-Grewal, D., Schneiderman-Walker, J., Wright, V., Bar-or, O., Behyene, J., Selvadurai, H., Cameron, B., Laxer, R. M., Schneider, R., Silverman, E. D., Spiegle, L., Tse, S., Leblanc, C., Wong, J., Stephens, S., & Feldman, B. M. (2007). The effects of vigorous exercise training on physical function in children with arthritis: A randomized, controlled, single-blinded trial. *Arthritis and Rheumatism, 57*, 1202–1210.

Stanton, R. P., Malcom, J. R., Wesdock, K. A., & Singsen, B. A. (1993). Reflex sympathetic dystrophy in children: an orthopedic perspective. *Orthopedics, 16*, 773–779.

Stanton-Hicks, M., Baron, R., Boas, R., Gordh, T., Harden, N., Hendler, N., Koltzenburg, M., Raj, P., & Wilder, R. (1998). Complex regional pain syndromes: Guidelines for therapy. *Journal of Pediatric Orthopedics, 14*, 155–166.

Steele, B. (1996). Timed walking tests of exercise capacity in chronic cardiopulmonary illness. *Journal of Cardiopulmonary Rehabilitation, 16*, 25–33.

Stevens, B. (2007). Pain Assessment and management in infants with cancer. *Pediatric Blood & Cancer, 49*, 1097–1101.

Travell, J. G., & Simons, D. G. (1983). *Myofascial Pain and dysfunction: The trigger point manual*. Baltimore: Williams & Wilkins.

Tsao, J. (2007). Effectiveness of massage therapy for chronic, non-malignant pain: A review. *Evidence-Based Complementary and Alternative Medicine, 4*, 165–179.

Varni, J. W., Seid, M., & Rode, C. S. (1999). The PedsQL measurement model for the pediatric quality of life inventory. *Medical Care, 37*, 126–139.

Varni, J. W., Seid, M., & Kurtin, P. S. (2001). Reliability and validity of the pediatric quality of life inventory version 4.0 generic core scales in healthy and patient populations. *Medical Care, 39*, 800–812.

Ware, J. E., Snow, K. K., Kosinski, M., & Gandek, B. (2000). *Health survey manual and interpretation guide*. Lincoln: Quality Metric.

Wilder, R. T. (2005). Management of pediatric patients with complex regional pain syndrome. *The Clinical Journal of Pain, 22*, 443–448.

Wong, D. L., Wilson, D., Hockenberry-Eaton, M., Winkelstein, M. L., & Schwartz, P. (2001). *Wong's essentials of pediatric nursing* (6th ed.). St Louis: Mosby.

World Health Organization. (2001). *International classification of functioning, disability and health: ICF*. Geneva: World Health Organization.

Yunus, M. B., & Masi, A. T. (1989). Juvenile primary fibromyalgia syndrome: A clinical study of thirty-three patients and matched normal controls. *Arthritis and Rheumatism, 28*, 138–145.

Zaino, C. A., Gocha-Marchese, V., & Westcott, S. L. (2004). Timed up and down stairs test: Preliminary reliability and validity of a new measure of functional mobility. *Pediatric Physical Therapy, 16*, 90–98.

The Integrative Approach for Management of Pediatric Pain Acupuncture

18

Shu-Ming Wang

Keywords

Complementary and alternative medical (CAM) therapies • Naturopathic physicians • Cupping • Acupressure • Acupuncture • ST-36

An Overview

Chronic pain in the pediatric population is a significant problem. It is estimated that 15–20% of children were affected by chronic pain (Goodman and McGrath 1991). The common pediatric chronic pain symptoms include headache, abdominal pain, and complex-regional pain syndromes (type I and type II). Other pain syndromes can be cerebral palsy (spasticity), malignant tumors, scoliosis, benign tumor, cystic fibrosis, irritable bowel syndrome, fibromyalgia, flat feet, and vertebral and spinal cord abnormalities.Despite advances in understanding and treating chronic pain in pediatric patients, treatment is inadequate in many cases (Anand and Hickey 1987; Romej et al. 1996; Kemper et al. 2000; Howard 2003). The major reasons are several: (1) Pain is multifactorial and that requires patient care considerations beyond the use of analgesics. (2) Pain is a subjective expression that can be easily influenced by the child's developmental level, past experiences with

pain, coping skills, anxiety level, culture, family dynamics, and peer issues, as well as the level of fatigue, focus of attention, and the child's general state of well-being. (3) Since the treatment of pain relies on self-report, only children who have attained a certain degree of cognitive ability have been able to provide information. Several self-report pain scales/drawings, specifically designed for young children to understand and use, were developed. However, the sensitivity and specificity of these scales remain questionable and frequently rely on how a scale was presented to the child (McGrath et al. 1985). Objective measurements were developed such as behavioral observations, changes in physiologic characteristics, and/or combinations of these measures. Thus far, facial expression has been one of the most reproducible. However, this behavioral measurement is age related. Generally, the utility of physiologic measures is diminished because of the homeostatic mechanisms that tend to oppose such changes over time. Despite the fact that multiple scales have been developed, each having its advantages and limitations (such as more than 20 validated pain scales to assess the pain in infants), no individual scale has emerged as superior. The lack of a gold standard or a universally reliable indicator that can be used to accurately assess pain in pediatric

S.-M. Wang (✉)
Department of Anesthesiology and Perioperative Care,
University of California-Irvine School of Medicine,
New Haven, CT 06520, USA
e-mail: shuminw1@uci.edu

B.C. McClain and S. Suresh (eds.), *Handbook of Pediatric Chronic Pain:*
Current Science and Integrative Practice, DOI 10.1007/978-1-4419-0350-1_18,
© Springer Science+Business Media, LLC 2011

patients has limited the health-care providers' ability to treat pediatric pain adequately.

Broome and colleagues conducted a national survey to determine how health-care providers in US teaching hospitals assess and manage children's pain (Broome et al. 1996). The researchers reported that 227 questionnaires were sent and 113 were returned. Two thirds were from nurses and one third from physicians. Sixty percent of the respondents stated that they had standards of care or protocols for pain in their institutions, but only 25% of the respondents reported that the standards were followed 80% or more of the time. Use of formal pain-assessment tools was reported by 73% of the respondents. Respondents reported that the effectiveness of pain assessment and management was lower for infants and younger children. Only 35% of the respondents indicated that it was "likely" or "very likely" that parents would be involved in the planning prior to a painful event. Through this national survey, the respondents identified that the significant deficiencies in knowledge, attitudes, and resources are the major obstacles to adequate pain management in the pediatric patient population. Lastly, the lack of suitable research on which to firmly establish evidence-based care is likely to have contributed to the delay in translating the knowledge of safe and effective pediatric pain management to routine clinical practice (McGrath et al. 1985).

In spite of multiple limitations in assessing and treating pediatric pain, there are strong evidences supporting the so-called psychobiologic approach that consists of psychological, behavioral, and pharmacologic interventions as well as the use of complementary and alternative medical (CAM) therapies. This interdisciplinary team approach is accepted as a valuable practice in the comprehensive pain management for pediatric pain patients (Zeltzer et al. 1997). In this setting, "alternative" therapy practitioners work with physicians and other health-care providers as part of an interdisciplinary team. In 2001, at a symposium entitled "CAM Research in Children with Chronic Pain" in American Pain Society Annual Meeting, Michael Joseph, MD, from the University of California, Los Angeles (UCLA), began the session with a call to the medical community to move away from the concepts of alternative versus conventional medicine and toward an understanding of medicine as an integrative approach that evaluates all therapies independently, rather than stigmatizing some therapies as being off the mainstream." In 2005, 86% of the pediatric anesthesia fellowship programs, accredited by the Accreditation Council for Graduate Medical Education, offered one or more CAM therapies for their patients (Lin et al. 1999). CAM therapies are used as adjunctive therapies designed to treat the patient as well as the source of pain. All clinicians involved in providing care contribute information and services for the child's benefit. The use of Complementary and Alternative Medicine (CAM) continues to grow both in popular demand and in acceptance from the medical community.

In 1998, Congress established the National Center for Complementary and Alternative Medicine (NCCAM) at the National Institutes of Health (NIH). This center funds research on vitamins, therapeutic herbs, and practices such as acupuncture, chiropractics, hypnosis, massage, and traditional Eastern medicine. To date, there are some well-designed CAM studies with valid results, but many more studies with questionable results. Further research on the use of CAM in children with chronic pain is still lacking. Therefore, there is an urgent need to conduct well-designed and valid clinical studies in evaluating the use of CAM therapies in pediatric patients with chronic pain. Although there is limited clinical evidence to support the use of CAM in treating pediatric patients with chronic pain, several CAM therapies including herbs, hypnosis, acupuncture, and related techniques have been integrated into the comprehensive pain management for pediatric pain.

Naturopathic Intervention

A systematic audit of pediatric and adolescent case files was conducted in a large, college-based, Canadian naturopathic teaching clinic (Wilson and Keye 1989). Wilson and colleagues reviewed a total of 482 charts and found the mean age of patients was 6.5 years (95% confidence interval [CI]: 1.6–11.4 years). The ratio of female subjects to male subjects was 1.09:1 (248:227). The most common reasons for presentation were skin disorders (23%), gastrointestinal complaints (17%), and psychiatric/behavioral disorders (15%). Thirty-five percent of children were using CAM products at presentation (21.2% when both vitamins and minerals were excluded). Vitamins were the most commonly used products (34.6%), followed by herbal remedies (14.9%), oil blends/fats (7.2%), minerals (5.6%), probiotics (4.5%), and homeopathic remedies (3.7%). Weber and colleagues conducted a mailed survey of licensed naturopathic physicians residing in Washington State (Weber et al. 2007). Of 499 surveys delivered to providers, 251 surveys were returned for a response rate of 50.3%. Among the 204 naturopathic physicians currently practicing, only 31(15%) treated five children per week. For these pediatric naturopathic physicians (pedsNDs), pediatric visits constituted 28% of their office practice. Pediatric naturopathic physicians were more likely to be licensed midwives (19.4% vs 0.6%) and treated significantly more patients per week (41.6 vs 20.2) than naturopathic physicians who provided less pediatric care. Only 58% of the 31 pediatric naturopathic physicians returned data on 354 pediatric visits; 30.5% of the visits were by children <2 years old, and 58.5% were by those <6 years old. Within each age group, the five most common reasons for visiting a pedsND included health supervision visits, upper respiratory tract infection, allergies, skin disorders, and mental health conditions. In addition to the reasons noted above, 9.3% of visits by children <2 years old were for infant conditions (colic, teething, failure to thrive, or thrush). Immunizations were given during 18.6% of health supervision visits by children <2 years of age. Respiratory conditions (asthma or bronchitis) were recorded as the chief complaint for 6.1% of children ages 2–5 years. In this age group, immunizations were administered in 27.3% of health supervision visits. Oral antibacterial or antifungal prescriptions were prescribed in 6.1% of visits. However, no antibiotics were prescribed for children presenting with upper respiratory symptoms. Other reasons for visits of adolescents between the ages of 12 and 18 included 9% for

gastrointestinal complaints (diarrhea or irritable bowel syndrome) and 7.5% for gynecologic disorders (amenorrhea, vaginitis, or premenstrual syndrome). Overall, no antibiotics were prescribed for any of the 65 children presenting with upper respiratory symptoms. Similar to adults who are seen by NDs, 24% of the visits by pediatric patients to pedsNDs were for the treatment of chronic disorders, particularly those in which therapies provided by conventional practitioners are either controversial to some parents, such as with ADHD, or of limited benefit, as with autism. However, in this study, the two most common reasons for visits by children to pedsNDs were health supervision and URI symptoms. In addition, preschool-aged children made most of these visits. In conclusion, health supervision and URI symptoms are also the most common reasons that children see pedsNDs. Although limited numbers of children are cared for by pedsNDs, they provide the majority of care for preschool-aged children. Therefore, it is important to seek clinical evidence that supports the use of naturopathic interventions in pediatric patients.

To date, only two randomized, double-blinded, controlled trials tested a naturopathic herbal extract (NHE)[1] on ear pain associated with acute otitis media (AOM) (Sarrell et al. 2001). The first study was conducted on 103 children (age 6–8 years) with AOM. All children were randomized into two groups: one group received NHE ($n=61$) eardrops, and another group received anesthetic eardrops (AE)[2] ($n=42$). The first administration of the topical eardrops was during a clinic visit and the instructions were given to the parent of the child who administered the assigned eardrops for an additional 2 days as an "at-home" treatment. The level of pain and discomfort of these children was evaluated daily

---

[1] Natureopathic herb extract-Otikon Otic Solution (Healthy-On Ltd, Petach-Tikva, Israel), a naturopathic herbal extract containing *Allium sativum, Verbascum thapsus, Calendula flores, and Hypericum perforatum* in olive oil.
[2] Anesthetic ear drops (Vitamed Pharmaceutical Ltd, Benyamina, Israel), ear drops containing amethocaine and phenazone in glycerin.

by an independent physician. There was no difference in age, sex, or laterality of AOM. Children from both groups showed significant reduction in pain across time (Sarrell et al. 2001). Thus, the researchers suggested that an ear solution of herbal extracts applied in the affected ear canal may reduce ear pain associated with AOM, and that it is at least as effective as anesthetic ear drops. A second study also conducted by Sarrell and colleagues explored the therapeutic effect of NHE in children with otalgia (Sarrell et al. 2003). The researchers enrolled a total of 171 children between the ages 5 and 18 years who suffered from otalgia with clinical findings associated with middle-ear infection into this randomized, double-blinded, controlled trial. Once a child was enrolled, he/she was randomized to receive NHE 5 drops, three times daily, alone (group A); together with oral amoxicillin 80 mg/kg/d (maximum 500 mg/dose) divided into three doses (group B); a topical anesthetic alone 5 drops, three times daily (group C); or topical anesthetic with amoxicillin, 5 drops, three times daily (group D). These researchers found that children in each group had a statistically significant improvement in ear pain over the 3-day course. It is noteworthy that the effects of naturopathic extract in reducing ear pain were equivalent to that of anesthetic drops and also that antibiotics did not improve the effects of the extract or topical anesthetic drops on ear pain. The naturopathic extract used in these two studies has been found to have analgesic, anti-inflammatory, hygroscopic, and occlusive effects, as well as anti-infective properties.

Herbs and Dietary Therapies

Dysmenorrhea

Dysmenorrhea refers to the occurrence of painful menstrual cramps of uterine origin and is a common gynecological complaint (Klein and Litt 1981; Wilson and Keye 1989). Epidemiologic studies showed that at least 72.7% of female adolescents reported "pain or discomfort" during their period and almost 58.9% of them reported decreased activity and 45.6% reported school or work absenteeism. A small survey conducted among 88 female adolescents also found that the majority of the female adolescents identified dysmenorrhea and premenstrual symptoms as problems that significantly affected their academic performance and were responsible for school absenteeism. Thus, dysmenorrhea and premenstrual symptoms are common pediatric pain problems. Common treatment for dysmenorrhea is medical therapy such as nonsteroidal anti-inflammatories (NSAIDs) or oral contraceptive pills (OCPs). Both drug classes work by reducing myometrial activity (i.e., contractions of the uterus). The efficacy of conventional treatments such as NSAIDs is considerable; however, the failure rate is still often 20–25%. Many patients/parents are now seeking alternatives to conventional medicine. Research in dysmenorrhea and premenstrual symptoms suggests that nutritional intake and metabolism may play an important role in the cause and treatment of menstrual disorders. Therefore, herbal and dietary therapies are among the more popular complementary medicines. In the USA, since 1994, herbs and other phytomedicinal products have been legally classified as dietary supplements. Included in this category are vitamins, minerals, herbs or other botanicals, amino acids, and other dietary substances. In 2002, Proctor and colleagues did several electronic searches using search engines such as the Cochrane Menstrual Disorders and Subfertility Group Register of controlled trials, CCTR, MEDLINE, EMBASE, CINAHL, Bio extracts, and PsycLIT as well as the Cochrane Complementary Medicine Field's Register of controlled trials (CISCOM) to identify relevant randomized controlled trials (RCTs) (Proctor et al. 2002). Attempts were also made to identify trials from the National Research Register, the Clinical Trial Register, and the citation lists of review articles and included trials. In most cases, the first or corresponding author of each included trial was contacted for additional information. The inclusion criteria were RCTs of herbal or dietary therapies as treatment for primary or secondary dysmenorrhea versus each other, placebo, no treatment, or conventional treatment.

Interventions could include, but were not limited to, the following: vitamins, essential minerals, proteins, herbs, and fatty acids. Exclusion criteria were mild or infrequent dysmenorrhea or dysmenorrhea from an IUD. The results are summarized as follows:

(a) MAGNESIUM: Three small trials were included that compared magnesium and placebo. Overall magnesium was more effective than placebo for pain relief and the need for additional medication was less. There was no significant difference in the number of adverse effects experienced.

(b) VITAMIN B6: One small trial of vitamin B6 showed it was more effective at reducing pain than both placebo and a combination of magnesium and vitamin B6.

(c) MAGNESIUM AND VITAMIN B6: Magnesium was shown to be no different in pain outcomes from both vitamin B6 and a combination of vitamin B6 and magnesium by one small trial. The same trial also showed that a combination of magnesium and vitamin B6 was no different from placebo in reducing pain.

(d) VITAMIN B1: One large trial showed vitamin B1 to be more effective than placebo in reducing pain.

(e) VITAMIN E: One small trial comparing a combination of vitamin E (taken daily) and ibuprofen (taken during menses) versus ibuprofen (taken during menses) alone showed no difference in pain relief between the two treatments.

(f) OMEGA-3 FATTY ACIDS: One small trial showed fish oil (omega-3 fatty acids) to be more effective than placebo for pain relief.

(g) JAPANESE HERBAL COMBINATION: One small trial showed the herbal combination to be more effective for pain relief than placebo, and less consumption of pain medication by the treatment group.

Proctor and colleagues concluded that based on one large RCT, vitamin B1 is shown to be an effective treatment for dysmenorrhea taken at 100 mg daily (Proctor and Farquhar 2006). The data from the literature suggest that magnesium is a promising treatment for dysmenorrhea.

However, it is unclear what dose or regimen of treatment should be used as a result of variations in the included trials. Lastly, there is, overall, insufficient evidence to recommend the use of any of the other herbal and dietary therapies considered in this review for the treatment of primary or secondary dysmenorrhea.

Infantile Colic

Infantile colic is one of the most common problems within the first 3 months of life, affecting as many as 3–28% of newborn children (Wessel et al. 1954; Illingworth 1985). It is characterized by abdominal distention, excessive gas, excess stool output, and pulling up of legs, suggesting a gastrointestinal etiology as well as a behavioral syndrome characterized by paroxysmal, excessive, and inconsolable crying (Savino et al. 2007). Despite more than 40 years of research, the pathogenesis of infantile colic remains unclear (Barr 1991). Several etiologies were suggested including temperament, mother–infant bonding, milk allergy, etc. Most recently, the role of intestinal microflora has been growing in importance, and lower counts of intestinal lactobacillus were observed in colicky but otherwise healthy infants. This led to the hypothesis that infantile colic may be related to a deficiency in certain intestinal microflora. *Lactobacillus reuteri* is one of the few human endogenous intestinal *Lactobacillus* species and it has a long safety record as probiotic dietary supplement – yogurt. A recent study indicated that within one week of dietary supplementation with *Lactobacillus reuteri*, the symptoms of colic improved in infants and is as effective as Simethicone (Savino et al. 2007).

Arthritis

Extracts of *Tripterygium wilfordii* Hook F (TWHF) have been widely used in China to treat a broad spectrum of autoimmune and inflammatory diseases, including rheumatoid arthritis RA (RA), systemic lupus erythematosus (SLE), ankylosing spondylitis, psoriasis, and idiopathic

IgA nephropathy (Salahuddin et al. 2005; Tao et al. 2002). Although the active components responsible for the therapeutic and adverse effects of the preparations of TWHF have not been completely delineated, triptolide, a diterpenoid in TWHF, has been shown to be one of the major components responsible for its effects. A randomized, double-blinded, placebo trial was carried out in a group of patients with long-standing RA. Tao and colleagues enrolled a total of 35 patients with RA into a 20-week treatment program (Tao et al. 2002). These patients were randomized to extracts of TWHF or placebo. These investigators found that the ethanol/ethyl acetate extract of TWHF showed therapeutic benefit in patients with treatment-refractory RA. At therapeutic dosages, the TWHF extract was well tolerated by most patients in this study. In addition to the extract of TWHF, *Camellia sinensis* (green tea), *Uncaria tomentosa* (cat's claw), *Curcuma longa* (turmeric), and *Zingiber officinale* (ginger) are also found to decrease pain and inflammation as well as disability caused by RA or osteoarthritis in animal studies (Salahuddin et al. 2005). The American College of Rheumatology recommends the careful use of dietary supplements and herbal medicines during early stages of treatment or disease development to limit the degree of joint destruction. For example, the use of Cat's claw is not advised for women attempting pregnancy, during pregnancy and lactation, or for children <3 years of age. TWHF usage can lead to the development of *amenorrhea*, which is reversible if present for <2 years in patients <40 years of age. TWHF induced amenorrhea irreversible in perimenopausal women.

Acupuncture and Related Intervention

When practitioners think of acupuncture, they traditionally envision a medical practice that involves puncturing the skin sites (described as acupuncture points) with sharp objects. Actually the term "acupuncture" is used loosely in the literature that includes two major principles (traditional body acupuncture system and microsystem,

e.g., ear, hand, foot, tongue, scalp, and pulse) and a *family* of procedures involving stimulation of acupuncture points using a variety of techniques such as direct pressure, needles, laser, heat, low-voltage electrical current, and direct deposition of fluid/medication (acupoint injection) (Wang et al. 2008). Acupuncture has more than 4,000 years of history as a therapeutic procedure for prevention and treatment of pain and many medical illnesses in China. However, the use of acupuncture and related techniques did not become popular in the USA until after Nixon visited China in early 1970. The landmark event that brought the awareness of this ancient medical intervention was the front-page article written by Mr. James Reston. During his visit to China, Mr. Reston suffered from acute appendicitis and required surgery. After surgery, Mr. Reston's postoperative pain was resolved by the use of acupuncture. Three months afterward, the physicians who accompanied Mr. Nixon to China witnessed the acupuncture-assisted, open-heart surgery performed on a child. In 1997, a National Institute of Health consensus conference indicated that acupuncture may be useful as treatment for menstrual cramps, tennis elbow, and fibromyalgia. In addition, ample clinical experience, supported by some research data, suggests that acupuncture may be a reasonable option for a number of clinical conditions (NIH consensus 1998). Examples are postoperative pain and myofascial and low back pain. Examples of disorders for which research evidence is less convincing but for which there are some positive clinical trials include carpal tunnel syndrome, osteoarthritis, and headache. Since then, acupuncture has been considered as part of a comprehensive treatment program for pain symptoms in the adult population. However, the integration of acupuncture in pediatric pain management is much slower than its progression in adult pain management (Kemper et al. 2000). This is partly due to the perception that children are afraid of needles, acupuncture therapy involves only needles, and children and their families will not accept another therapy that requires needles besides immunization. There is a lack of familiarity in pediatrics regarding available interventions within the realm of acupuncture.

It takes great effort for pediatricians to consider acupuncture as a therapeutic option. Frequently, acupuncture is only recommended or accepted by parents and/or children as the "last effort" after all other interventions have failed to improve the child's condition or symptoms. Since 2000, the American Academy of Pediatrics has offered acupuncture workshops at national meetings to educate pediatricians about the concepts and practice of acupuncture.

The practice of acupuncture consists of two major systems, body and micro. Under these two major systems, different philosophies such as traditional Chinese, Korean, five elements, and meridian can be found in the literature. The techniques of acupuncture manipulation include pressure, needles, burning of herbs (moxibustion), electrical stimulation, cupping, and hydroinjection/topical medication application to the acupuncture points. Thus far, acupuncture and related techniques have only been tested in three pediatric-related pain problems as adjuvant treatment. The nomenclature used in the following section of this chapter describes assorted acupuncture practices that are used in clinical studies in the current literature. The results of various clinical studies are summarized as follows:

Dysmenorrhea

1. *Acupressure*: A randomized clinical trial to determine the effectiveness and safety of an acupressure garment (the Relief Brief®) in decreasing pain and symptom distress associated with dysmenorrhea (Taylor et al. 2002). Sixty-one young women with moderately severe primary dysmenorrheal were randomized and assigned to the standard treatment control group or the Relief Brief® acupressure device group. The researchers found that patients who received Relief Brief® have less pain and decreased use of pain medication ($P < 0.05$). The use of Relief Brief® was associated with at least a 50% decline in menstrual pain intensity in more than two thirds of the women. The researchers recommended that this acupressure device serves as an adjuvant

therapy to medication in more severe cases of dysmenorrhea.

2. *Needle Acupuncture*: Helm conducted a randomized control trial to study the effectiveness of acupuncture in managing the pain of primary dysmenorrhea. Forty participants were followed for 1 year. They were randomized into one of four groups: the real acupuncture group was given appropriate acupuncture, the placebo acupuncture group was given random point acupuncture on a weekly basis for three menstrual cycles, the standard control group was followed without medical or acupuncture intervention, and the visitation control group had monthly non-acupuncture visits with the project physician for three cycles. The investigator found that 10 of 11 (90.9%) participants in real acupuncture group, 4 of 11 (36.4%) in the placebo acupuncture group, 2 of 11 in the Standard Control group, and 1/11 in the visitation control group showed improvement (Helms 1987). There was a 41% reduction of analgesic medication used by the women in the real acupuncture group after their treatment series, and no change or increased use of medication seen in the other groups.

3. *Electrical stimulation*: Transcutaneous electrical nerve stimulation (TENS) and acupuncture have been used as adjunctive treatment for primary dysmenorrhea (Proctor et al. 2002). A Cochrane databases system–revealed overall high-frequency TENS was found to be more effective in reducing pain than placebo TENS. Low-frequency TENS was found to be more effective in reducing pain than placebo TENS. There were conflicting results regarding whether high-frequency TENS is more effective than low-frequency TENS. However, there is a paucity of data in the literature regarding the use of electroacupuncture as a treatment for dysmenorrhea. Thus, more clinical studies are needed to determine the efficacy of electroacupuncture as a treatment for dysmenorrhea.

4. *Medication at the acupuncture points*: Intramuscular injection of vitamin K_3 was evaluated as a treatment for primary dysmenorrhea

(Zhao et al. 2003). One hundred and eighty patients with history of dysmenorrhea or pelvic inflammatory diseases were enrolled in the study. All these patients had been treated ineffectively with Chinese or Western medicine. They were divided into three groups according to the history of their illness, pelvic examination, and ultrasonography: Group A consisted of 60 patients with primary dysmenorrhea, group B of 60 with chronic pelvic inflammation, and group C of 60 with endometriosis. These patients received intramuscular injection of a total 8 mg of vitamin K_3 (4 mg in each acupoint) into the spleen 6 acupuncture points. These patients were followed for three menstrual cycles. The researchers found that 95% of patients with primary dysmenorrhea had significant improvement in their pain and daily activities ($p<0.05$). Sixty-three percent and 65% of patients in groups B and C also had reduction in their pelvic pain. The researchers concluded that bilateral intramuscular injection of vitamin K_3 into spleen 6 is effective in decreasing the pain and dysfunction associated with primary dysmenorrhea.

Migraine Headache

Migraine is the most common cause of headaches in both children and adults. It affects 2.7% of children by age 7 and 10.6% by age 14. Forty-two percent of children were subject to one or more episodes each month that were severe enough to prevent the child from carrying on with his or her usual daily activities. An epidemiological study was conducted in 1999 through a validated, self-administered questionnaire that was mailed to a sample of 20,000 households in the USA (Lipton et al. 2001). This report was restricted to individuals 12 years and older. Of the 43,527 age-eligible individuals, 29,727 responded to the questionnaire for a 68.3% response rate. The prevalence of migraine was 18.2% among females and 6.5% among males. Approximately 23% of households contained at least one member suffering from migraines. Migraine prevalence was higher in whites than in

blacks and was inversely related to household income. Prevalence increased from age 12 years to about age 40 years and declined thereafter in both sexes. Fifty-three percent of respondents reported that their severe headaches caused substantial impairment in activities or required bed rest. Approximately 31% missed at least 1 day of work or school in the previous 3 months because of migraine; 51% reported that work or school productivity was reduced by at least 50%. The number of migraineurs has increased from 23.6 million in 1989 to 27.9 million in 1999 commensurate with the growth of the population and migraine-associated disability remains substantial and pervasive Migraine is an important target for public health interventions because it is highly prevalent and disabling. The etiology of migraine remains unclear. However, the mechanism of this central pain may be related to a dysfunction in the endogenous opioid antinociceptive system. Acupuncture may be beneficial in migraine treatment, as an ample number of studies in the acupuncture analgesia indicate that acupuncture modulates the pain perception through activating the release of endogenous opioids.

1. *Needle Acupuncture*: Pintov and colleagues conducted a randomized control study to test the effectiveness of acupuncture in childhood migraine (Pintov et al. 1997). A total of 22 children with migraine were randomly divided into two groups: a true acupuncture group (12 children) and a placebo acupuncture group (10 children) and 10 healthy children served as a control group. The investigators found that children in the true acupuncture treatment group experienced significant clinical reduction in both migraine frequency and intensity. At the beginning of the study, significantly greater opioid activity was evident in plasma of the control group than in plasma of the migraine group. The true acupuncture group showed a gradual increase in the opioid activity in plasma, which correlated with the clinical improvement. After the tenth treatment, the values of opioid activity of the true acupuncture group were similar to those of the control group. In addition, a significant increase in β-endorphin levels was observed

in the migraine patients who were treated in the true acupuncture group as compared with the values before treatment or with the values of the placebo acupuncture group. The results suggest that acupuncture may be an effective treatment in children with migraine headaches and that it leads to an increase in activity of the opioidergic system.

Postoperative Pain

1. *Topical application of medication to acupuncture point:* Kim and colleagues applied capsicum plaster on to ST-36 to reduce the postoperative pain in children undergoing hernia repair. One hundred and eight children were randomized into group Z-true capsicum plaster at ST-36 and sham plaster on the shoulder, group S-sham plaster on ST-36 and capsicum plaster on the shoulder point or group C-the placebo tape at both ST-36 and the shoulder point. These investigators found that children in the capsicum plaster at ST-36 group and the sham plaster group had significantly decreased postoperative pain and the opioid analgesic consumption during the first 24 h after surgery (Kim et al. 2006).

CAM has demonstrated effectiveness in a variety of medical and surgical pain conditions. The spectrum of acupuncture techniques currently available provides many methods of treatment that are well tolerated by all age groups. Further research into the potential role of CAM in pediatric pain management is warranted.

References

Anand, K., & Hickey, P. (1987). Pain and its effects in the human neonate and fetus. *New England Journal of Medicine, 317*(21), 1231–9.

Barr, R. (1991). Colic and Gas. In W. Walker, P. Durie, & J. Hamilton (Eds.), *Pediatric gastrointestinal disease: pathophysiology, diagnosis and management* (pp. 55–61). Philadelphia: Decker.

Broome, M., Richtsmeier, A., et al. (1996). Pediatric pain practices: a national survey of health professionals. *Journal of Pain Symptom and Management, 11*(5), 312–20.

Goodman, J., & McGrath, P. (1991). The epidemiology of pain in children and adolescents: a review. *Pain, 46*(3), 247–64.

Helms, J. (1987). Acupuncture for the management of primary dysmenorrhea. *Obstetrics Gynecology, 69*(1), 51–6.

Howard, R. F. (2003). Current status of pain management in children. *Journal of the American Medical Association, 290*(18), 2464–9.

Illingworth, R. (1985). Infantile colic revisited. *Archives Disease of in Childhood, 60*(10), 981–5.

Kemper, K., Sarah, R., et al. (2000). Complementary and alternative medicine: on pins and needles? Pediatric patients' experience with acupuncture. *Pediatrics, 105*(4), 941–7. Part 2.

Kim, K. S., Kim, D. W., et al. (2006). The effect of capsicum plaster in pain after inguinal hernia repair in children. *Paediatric Anaesthesthsia, 16*(10), 1036–41.

Klein, J., & Litt, I. (1981). Epidemiology of adolescent dysmenorrhea. *Pediatrics, 68*(6), 661–4.

Lin, Y., Lee, A. C., et al. (1999). Acupuncture services provided by pediatric pain treatment services in North America. Pediatric Academic Societies Meeting, May 3, San Francisco, CA.

Lipton, R., Stewart, W. S., et al. (2001). Prevalence and burden of migraine in the United States: data from the American migraine study II. *Headache, 41*(7), 646–57.

McGrath, P., Johnson, G., Goodman, J. T., Schillinger, J., Dunn, J., & Chapman, J. (1985). CHEOPS: A behavioral scale for rating postoperative pain in children. In In fields HI, R. Dubner, & F. Cerrero (Eds.), *Advances in pain research and therapy* (pp. 395–402). New York: Raven.

NIH consensus conference. Acupuncture. (1998). *Journal of the American Medical Association, 280*(17), 1518–1524.

Pintov, S., Lahat, E., et al. (1997). Acupuncture and the opioid system: implications in management of migraine. *Pediatric Neurology, 17*(2), 129–33.

Proctor, M., & Farquhar, C. (2006). Diagnosis and management of dysmenorrhea. *British Medical Journal, 332*(May 13), 1134–8.

Proctor, M. L., Smith, C. A., et al. (2002). Transcutaneous electrical nerve stimulation and acupuncture for primary dysmenorrheal. *Cochrane Database System Review, 1*, CD002123.

Romej, M., Voepel-lewis, T., et al. (1996). Effect of preemptive acetaminophen on postoperative pain score and oral fluid intake in pediatric tonsillectomy patients. *American Association of Nurse Anesthetists, 64*(6), 535–40.

Salahuddin, A., Jeremy, A., et al. (2005). Biological basis for the use of botanicals in osteoarthritis and rheumatoid arthritis: a review. *Evidence-based Complementary and Alternative Medicine, 2*(3), 301–30.

Sarrell, E., Cohen, H., et al. (2003). Naturopathic treatment for ear pain in children. *Pediatrics, 111*(5), e574–9.

Sarrell, E., Mandelberg, A., et al. (2001). Efficacy of naturopathic extracts in the management of ear pain associated with acute otitis media. *Archive Pediatric and Adolescence Medicine, 155*(7), 796–9.

Savino, F., Pelle, E., et al. (2007). Lactobacillus reuteri (American type culture collection strain 55730) versus simethicone in the treatment of infantile colic: a prospective randomized study. *Pediatrics, 119*(1), 1–30.

St James-Roberts, I. (1991). Persistent infant crying. *Achieve of Disease in Childhood, 66*(5), 653–5.

Tao, X., Younger, J., et al. (2002). Benefit of an extract of Tripterygium WI fordii Hook F in patients with rheumatoid arthritis. *Arthritis and Rheumatism, 46*(7), 1735–43.

Taylor, D., Miaskowski, C., et al. (2002). A randomized clinical trial of the effectiveness of an acupressure device (Relief Brief) for managing symptoms of dysmenorrhea. *Journal Alternative Complementary Medicine, 8*(3), 357–70.

Wang, S., White, P., & Kain, Z. (2008). Acupuncture analgesia (Part I): basic Mechanism. *Anesthesia and Analgesia, 106*(2), 602–10.

Weber, W., Taylor, J., et al. (2007). Frequency and characteristics of pediatric and adolescent visits in naturopathic medical practice. *Pediatrics, 120*(1), e142–146.

Wessel, M., Cobb, J., Jackson, E., et al. (1954). Paroxysmal fussing in infancy, sometimes called "colic". *Pediatrics, 14*(5), 421–434.

Wilson, C., & Keye, W. (1989). A survey of adolescent dysmenorrhea and premenstrual symptom frequency. A model program for prevention, detection, and treatment. *Journal Adolescent Health Care, 10*(4), 317–22.

Busse, W. K., Busse, J., et al. (2005). Characteristics of pediatric and adolescent patients attending a naturopathic college clinic in Canada. *Pediatrics, 115*(3), 3–43.

Zeltzer, L., Bush, J., et al. (1997). A psychobiologic approach to pediatric pain: part I. History, physiology, and assessment strategies. *Current Problems in Pediatrics, 27*(6), 221–53.

Zhao, W., Wang, L., et al. (2003). Clinical study of vitamin K3 acupoint injection in treating pelvic pain. *Chinese Journal Integrative Medicine, 9*(2), 136–138.

Clinical Hypnosis in Children

19

Haleh Saadat

Keywords

Hypnotic phases • Idiomotor activities • Magic Glove • Hypnotic techniques • Certification in hypnosis

Introduction

As with adults, pain in children is a multidimensional experience which varies significantly depending on previous experience with pain; personality, expectations, and cognitive maturation. Recent investigations reveal that pain in children correlates directly with more than just the degree of actual tissue damage (Goodman and McGrath 1991). Consequently, interventions that treat only the initial cause of the pain will not be completely successful. It is essential to address both psychological and physiological aspects when developing a pain management course for children.

In addition, children with chronic pain disorders undergo numerous invasive procedures for diagnostic, therapeutic, and supportive purposes during the course of their illness. The majority of these procedures have the potential to trigger stress and inflict more pain. Children often consider painful procedures to be the most difficult part of their illness (Broome et al. 1990). Hypnosis is a non-pharmacological technique that enables children to deal with pain by exploring and enhancing their abilities of self efficacy and self control.

Hypnosis can be integrated into a variety of medical interventions to improve outcome. Over the past few decades, hypnosis has been successfully utilized to assist children through acute painful medical treatment in the emergency room, a variety of invasive diagnostic procedures such as bone marrow aspiration and lumbar puncture, and management of post-operative pain. It has also been used successfully to treat pain associated with chronic disorders, such as cancer, asthma, rheumatoid arthritis, migraine headache, cystic fibrosis, sickle cell disease, and burns.

This chapter reviews the concept of hypnosis and hypnotherapy including the theories and scientific evidence that define how hypnosis works as well as the practical clinical applications in pediatric pain management.

History

The early history of hypnosis dates back several 1,000 years with evidence of use by the Greeks, Egyptians, Persians, and Indian Yogis (Braid 1844). Examining the ceremonies of primitive peoples, some tribes of whom still exist primarily

H. Saadat (✉)
Department of Anesthesiology, Yale University School of Medicine, New Haven, CT, USA
e-mail: Haleh.Saadat@Yale.Edu

B.C. McClain and S. Suresh (eds.), *Handbook of Pediatric Chronic Pain:*
Current Science and Integrative Practice, DOI 10.1007/978-1-4419-0350-1_19,
© Springer Science+Business Media, LLC 2011

in Africa and Australia, indicates the ability to accomplish induction of trance by rhythmic chanting and monotonous drum beats with strained eye fixation. Such primitive ceremonies contain the two essential components of hypnosis: the focus of attention and the relative suspension of the peripheral awareness.

Modern history of current hypnosis began with Franz Anton Mesmer (1734–1815), the first physician who introduced the phenomenon to the medical profession (Donaldson 2005). While studying medicine at the University of Vienna, Mesmer published in 1766 his doctoral dissertation entitled, *"De planetarum influxu in corpus humanum"* (On the Influence of the Planets on the Human Body). He moved to France in 1778, where he introduced and practiced his new theory and treated patients. Subsequent publications include, *"Memoirre Sur La Decouverte Du Magnetisme Animal"* in 1779, where, Mesmer discussed his theory regarding the influence of the moon and the planets on the human body and on illness (Mesmer 1779). He believed that the planets exuded power over humans through a subtle fluid. He called this phenomenon "animal magnetism," to highlight the similarities between this influence and magnetic properties. Mesmer thought that the even distribution of "universal fluids" was responsible for health and believed that the blockade of this flow caused illness. Despite Mesmer's success in treating patients in clinical practice, The Royal Faculty of Medicine rejected his proposals. In 1784, King Louis XVI appointed a commission to investigate Mesmer's theory. The commission concluded that there was no evidence for such a fluid and the cure was the result of patient's expectation and imagination (L'Imprimerie Royale 1784). Despite the commission's negative report, Mesmer's method spread throughout Europe.

The first recorded uses of hypnosis for analgesia and anesthesia occurred in France and the United States, independently in the 1820s. In the 1830s, John Elliotson, famous for introducing the stethoscope to England, published several reports of painless surgeries using Mesmerism. James Esdaile, an English surgeon, performed over 3,000 surgical procedures in a prison hospital in India between 1840 and 1850, with the use of Mesmerism as the solo anesthetic. Esdaile reported that with this method, his mortality rate dropped to 5%, at a time when surgical mortality ranged from 25 to 50%. James Braid (1795–1860), a Scottish surgeon, used Mesmerism for pain control during surgery. He subsequently wrote a book on the subject entitled *"Neurypnology" or, "The Rationales of Nervous Sleep,"* in which he redefined the concept of animal magnetism and created the term *"hypnosis"* from the Greek word *"hypnos"* meaning sleep. In his book, James Braid, rejected Mesmer's magnetism theory, and discussed that the phenomenon was based more on suggestibility. Later on, in order to distinguish the state of hypnosis from sleep, he tried to change the name, but the word "hypnosis" became popular and is used to this day (Braid 1846).

The mixed reception of hypnosis continued until the First World War, when it was used to treat shell shock victims with visible success. During the Second World War, it served a similar purpose in the treatment of post-traumatic stress disorder.

Clarke Hull (1884–1952), Milton Erickson (1901–1980), and Ernest Hilgard (1904–2001) were among the first investigators in the United States to undertake a modern, systematic approach to hypnosis research. The British Medical Association officially recognized the use of hypnosis in medicine in 1955 and endorsed the teaching of hypnosis in medical schools. In 1958, the American Medical Association (AMA) published and approved a report from a 2-year study by the Council of Mental Health that recognized the definite and proper use of hypnosis in medical and dental practice (American Medical Association 1958). The National Institutes of Health (NIH) issued a statement in 1996 that acknowledged the strong evidence of the use of hypnosis in alleviating pain associated with cancer (NIH Technology Assessment Panel 1996).

Definition

The American Psychological Association's Division of Psychological Hypnosis defines hypnosis as a "therapeutic procedure in which a health professional makes suggestions that will help a patient experience post-hypnotic alterations in perception, sensation, emotion, thought, and/or behavior" (Rhue et al. 1993). Hypnosis is further defined as a state of inner absorption, concentration, and focused narrowed attention. During the past two decades, multiple neuro-physiological studies demonstrated that the hypnotic state can effectively alter or modify several aspects of the person's psychological, physiological, and neurological function (Rainville et al. 1997, 1999, 2000; Crawford et al. 2000).

The term hypnosis is different from the term hypnotherapy, as hypnosis itself is not a treatment but rather a tool. Hypnotherapy, in contrast, is a term that describes the clinical use of specific *suggestions*, in order to achieve a specific therapeutic goal (e.g., alleviate pain) (Raz et al. 2002). Myths and misconceptions about hypnosis have limited its use in clinical settings. Eliminating these myths is essential to establishing a strong therapeutic alliance and a positive expectation for patients and their families, as well as clinicians.

Contrary to the myths, all hypnosis is self-hypnosis. There is no mind control. Hypnosis cannot force anyone to do anything against their will or values. During hypnosis, the patient remains aware of the process, and unless amnesia has been specifically suggested, he or she will remember most, if not all of the hypnosis session. Hypnotic subjects are not immobilized. In fact, during a session children frequently will wriggle, shift, have rapid eye movements, or open their eyes. Subjects hear the surrounding sounds; remain oriented as to person, place, and time; and can even hold a conversation while in trance.

Although the word hypnosis is derived from the name of the Greek god of sleep, Hypno, this modality is significantly dissimilar to sleep and is therefore experienced differently. Some people describe hypnosis as a deep, heavy restful feeling; while others may experience it as a light, floating sensation. Patients also vary in their hypnotizability and assessment scales are available to measure the depth of hypnosis attained (Rhue et al. 1993).

Clinicians can easily integrate hypnosis with appropriate positive suggestions within the limits of their professional expertise. The American Society of Clinical Hypnosis (ASCH), as well as the Society of Clinical and Experimental Hypnosis (SCEH) and the Society of Developmental and Behavioral pediatrics (SDBP) are among the organizations that offer recognized clinical hypnosis training workshops for health care professionals.

Hypnosis Components

Most experts agree that children are excellent hypnotic subjects because of their vivid imaginations, desire for mastery of new experiences, and the ease with which they intertwine fantasy and reality (Olness and Kohen 1996). In fact, children are capable of going into hypnosis spontaneously, without any help. There are much less clear distinctions between the phases of hypnosis in children, compared with adults. A typical hypnosis session in adults and adolescents consists of induction, deepening of the trance state, delivery of specific suggestions, and finally re-emergence. The induction phase assists to focus the patient's attention. The length and the manner that one achieves with this phase in children vary according to the nature of the problem, the child's developmental age, learning style, interests, and strengths. Parental cooperation, and that of the pain management team, is crucial to achieving success. Olness and Gardner believe that the most important role for the hypnotherapist is "to guide rather than control the child" (Olness and Gardner 1978).

In general, children respond to a large variety of hypnotic induction techniques. These methods and strategies include eye fixation and guided imagery, using visual images reminiscent of a favorite place, auditory images in the vein of a favorite song or movement images such as a flying blanket or sport activity. Additional techniques include storytelling, idiomotor activities such as arm levitation and progressive muscle relaxation.

Studies suggest that there is limited classic hypnotic ability in children less than 3 years of age, followed by a peak in hypnotic ability between the years of 7 and 14, after which there is a plateau. While children of different age groups frequently favor different induction techniques, there are no hard and fast rules. Skilled clinicians stay flexible and modify their technique to the individual child. Infant and toddlers usually respond to kinesthetic (i.e., rocking, moving) as well as auditory stimulation (e.g., music or singing) while early verbal children respond to story-telling, bubble blowing and pop-up books. Pre-school and early-school children enjoy imagining themselves in variety of imaginative situations, such as imagining of being a "mighty oak tree"; that can't be moved even with a strong wind. This image is usually very attractive to young children and can be employed in instances where the child's immobility is required (e.g., dressing changes, radiation therapy). A skilled clinician can ask the young child to imagine a "favorite place" or a "favorite activity" (playing with ball, blowing bubbles, etc.) while integrating pertinent suggestions during different stages of a painful procedure (Olness and Kohen 1996).

Alternatively, many middle school children like to use a videogame fantasy or pretend to be on a "flying blanket." Compared to adults, young children have a tendency to keep their eyes open, move and make spontaneous comments throughout hypnotic procedures. These acts simply show that the child is adopting the procedure into his/her own behavioral style and is not a sign of resistance.

Induction of hypnosis in adolescence can be achieved by asking patients to imagine being in a safe, favorite place or doing a favorite activity or sport. By using deep rhythmic breathing, counting down or shifting their focus toward the details in their favorite place, they can achieve a deeper state (Holroyd 1996). Although most experts believe that patterns of hypnotizability in children vary with age, children of the same age can also have vast differences in hypnotizability.

Hypnotizability Scales in Children

Hypnotic susceptibility is the degree of an individual's ability to experience specific feelings, sensations, and images in response to different suggestions. This responsiveness can be measured by standardized tests (Hilgard and Hilgard 1997; Hilgard 1973). The Stanford Hypnotic Scale for Children (SHCS-C) assesses a broad range of hypnotic behaviors and dimensions in children. The scale was developed by Morgan and Hilgard with two forms, one for young children (4–8 years) and one for older children (6–16 years). Although a relatively quick test for hypnotizability, some clinicians believe that this scale does not accurately reflect or predict a child's response to hypnotherapy (Olness and Kohen 1996). These investigators argue that hypnotic responsivity should be viewed from a developmental perspective that takes into consideration the social, behavioral, and verbal abilities of the child (Vandenberg 2002). Other investigators suggest that the capacity for hypnotic trance can be increased by teaching and increase motivation in individuals (Diamond 1984).

The Scientific Conceptual Framework

Theories

Traditionally, hypnosis is described as "*an altered state*" of concentration coupled with a relative suspension of peripheral awareness" (Spiegel and Moore 1997). This view is opposed by contemporary cognitive-behavioral theorists. In their view, a hypnotic phenomenon is *normal state of consciousness* that involves the focusing of attention and thinking along the therapist's suggestion (McConkey 1986; Kihlstorm 1985). This theory states that the result can also be produced by *suggestion* without hypnotic induction. From a cognitive-behavioral perspective, hypnosis simply provides a *context* in which various therapeutic interventions are suggested (Kirsch 1999, 2001; Benedetti 2002).

Neuro Imaging Correlates in Hypnotic Analgesia

Pain is a multi-dimensional experience with a *sensory dimension* that correlates to intensity of pain, and an *affective dimension* that correlates to the unpleasantness of the pain experience.

Multiple anatomic regions, (e.g., the primary and secondary somatosensory cortex, anterior cingulate cortex, basal ganglia, and anterior frontal cortex) are involved and communicate in perception of pain (William 2003). Psychological factors, such as "anticipation" and "context" have shown to be as important as the intensity of the stimulus in the experience of pain (Chen 2007). Neuro-imaging studies show that the mere *anticipation* of a painful stimulus, in spite of the absence of direct physical stimulus can activate various areas of the brain (Price 2002; Hsieh et al. 1999; Porro et al. 2002). The advancement of brain imaging techniques (e.g., functional magnetic resonance imaging [f-MRI]), positron emission tomography [PET] enabled neuroscientists to gain a better understanding of the effects of hypnosis on activating specific neural regions. Recent investigations show that hypnosis can modulate distinct neural settings in a variety of experimental and clinical settings (De Pascalis et al. 2002; Chaves and Dworkin 1997). The modulation of pain by hypnosis is different from relaxation, cognitive coping, or a placebo-like mechanism (Faymonville et al. 1997). This difference was documented by PET scan and electroencephalography (EEG) measurements (Rainville et al. 1997; DePascalis et al. 1987). Rainville et al. studied selective hypnotic suggestions to alter the unpleasantness of a painful stimulus without changing the perceived intensity using PET. The study showed significant changes in pain-evoked activity within the anterior cingulate cortex, consistent with the encoding of perceived unpleasantness, without any changes in primary somato-sensory cortex activation (Rainville et al. 1997). Rainville et al. also demonstrated that hypnosis is associated with a significant increase in occipital regional cerebral blood flow (rCBF) and EEG delta activity. Based on his findings, Rainville proposes that hypnosis is modulated by brain structures centrally involved in the regulation of consciousness (Rainville et al. 2002). Multiple investigations suggest that hypnosis is effective through modulation of cerebral structures within the frontal lobe and anterior cingulated cortex which are responsible for "attention" (Rainville and Price

2003; Davis et al. 1997; Davis et al. 2000). Data from PET studies corroborate the findings that hypnotic and post-hypnotic suggestions modulate cerebral structures that are involved in attention. In addition, there seems to be a positive correlation between dopamine levels (the main neurotransmitter responsible for attention) and measured hypnotizability (Swanson et al. 2000; Raz et al. 2002). These findings provide supporting evidence for the involvement of the thalamo-cortical attentional network in hypnosis (Quist et al. 2003; Raz et al. 2005; Raz and Shapiro 2003).

Hypnosis Applications in Pain Management

Hypnosis has been used both as a solo technique and as an adjunct to analgesic medications in variety of painful situations ranging from acute painful settings such as burns (Martin-Herz et al. 1986) and fractures (Iserson 1998) to chronic painful conditions including recurrent abdominal pain (Humphreys and Gevirtz 2000), migraine headache (Olness et al. 1987; Richter et al. 1986), and sickle cell disease (Dinges et al. 1997). Extensive randomized control trials in pediatric oncology confirm the efficacy of hypnosis in alleviating pain and anxiety during needle-related procedures as well as reducing the incident of chemotherapy-related nausea and vomiting (Uman et al. 2007; Genuis 1995). Hypnosis has also been successfully used during invasive painful procedures, such as the voiding cystourethrogram (VCUG), and for the management of post-operative pain (Butler et al. 2005; Huth et al. 2004; Lambert 1996).

Hypnosis in Children

It is important to note that natural, spontaneous hypnotic states are common in children. This state can be recognized by some physiological indicators such as fixed gaze with eyes open, staring without blinking, or closed eyes with fluttering eyelids followed by eye movement under closed eyelids, slowing of the respiratory rate, and a child's unsuggested stillness. Children in this state have focused attention and are absorbed in fantasy and imagination. During these states, whether spontaneous or induced by hypnosis, children are intensely focused on the clinician's communication and have a tendency to interpret each word in a literal manner. Children tend to move in and out of the hypnotic state effortlessly. Recognition of this fact as well as careful observation, positive rapport, and strong therapeutic alliances are essential for an effective therapeutic communication. The clinician must tailor the hypnotic strategies to meet the child's particular developmental level. Age is of less importance, since children of the same age may be in different developmental levels.

Introducing Hypnosis

A context is defined by the circumstances and the settings in which an event occurs. By learning hypnotic language and techniques, clinicians become aware of the context, the choice of language, and the timing and pacing of verbal and non-verbal communications. The clinician's confidence in the child's ability to overcome pain, the child's past experience, as well as the parents' and pain management team's perception and attitude toward the situation impact the outcome. These are examples of context that have significant effects on the outcome. Many skilled clinicians appear to instinctively recognize the value and the effect of context in the success of the patients' treatment (Di Blasi et al. 2001; Di Blasi et al. 2001).

The first step in developing any treatment plan is a medical evaluation for diagnosis. Patients with chronic pain conditions need to be frequently evaluated to update the course of the disease and the effect of treatment (Syrjala and Abrams 1996). Prior to using hypnotic intervention, the clinician must demystify the process for the patient and his or her family, addressing and correcting any misconceptions that may lead to avoidance or poor adherence. Parents should be involved in a positive manner early in the process as their conceptions regarding hypnosis may either impede or assist in their child's therapy. Parents should recognize that all hypnosis is self-hypnosis, and that the clinician's role is to guide the child during the intervention. In fact, their child's interest to learn the skill and the motivation to change are essential factors for successful treatment.

Frequently, parents can provide valuable information regarding their child's learning style, strengths, and weaknesses, which assists in the choice of an appropriate therapeutic plan. The clinician must also explain the plan to the child in appropriate language, tailored to the child's developmental level, learning style, and interests. Some adolescents require a lengthy descriptive explanation of pain pathways, whereas a brief explanation with pictures or videotape may be adequate for younger children.

The initial session for patients with chronic pain disorders may take between 45 and 60 min. Follow-up sessions are usually shorter and 20–30 min is usually adequate. It should be emphasized that in emergency situations, hypnosis in children can be achieved within minutes. The frequency of sessions needed depends on the nature of the condition and the patient response.

Induction of hypnosis may start as the clinician walks into the room and greets the child. Capturing the child's attention and evoking his curiosity can be easily accomplished by welcoming the child in a personal and direct manner. Clinicians should attempt to create an environment of expectancy for positive change with the use of both verbal and non-verbal communication. During the initial session, after the establishment of rapport and a comprehensive medical evaluation to establish diagnosis, it is essential to look for the meaning of the pain experience to the child and discover the child's own motivation to change before introducing hypnosis as a part of the treatment plan. For example, the clinician may explore if there are any activities in which the child fails to participate as a result of pain and whether this avoidance has a positive or negative effect in the child's outlook. The clinician may also inquire about prior situations, where the child did not experience any pain. Encouraging the child to describe the pain (location, frequency, quality, and severity) in their own language provides valuable information regarding the child's own understanding of the condition. This helps construct a therapeutic plan which is tailored to the individual child. Introducing the concept of self-hypnosis to children early in the treatment course will provide the child with the sense of control and mastery.

Hypnotic Induction Techniques

A clinician's ultimate goal in use of hypnosis is to alter the child from the relatively helpless and passive state, to a state of empowerment, self mastery, and control. Clinicians must avoid the temptation to impose their own imagery on the child. Instead they should use child's interests, strengths, and internal resources to solve problems. The therapist should encourage the child to practice the learned skills in hypnotic analgesia. Many different techniques may be successfully used in pain management.

The clinician may begin by asking the child, "*Do you want to learn a 'special way' to help yourself and feel better?*" It is important to use a positive language like, "*I can help you change how that knee feels.*" Versus a negative statement such as, "You won't feel any pain."

A comprehensive description of different hypnotic inductions and suggestions for a variety of medical disorders can be found in, "Hypnosis and Hypnotherapy with Children" by Dr. Karen Olness and Dr. Daniel Kohen. The following techniques are brief examples of some hypnotic induction techniques and analgesic suggestions used with children and are based on the above reference.

Imagery

Children do not have to close their eyes unless they wish to do so. They can be encouraged to talk during the imagery or to nod their head during the session. Younger children may want to move around during the hypnosis session, especially if they are imagining their favorite activity.

A. Favorite place: Imagine yourself in your favorite place…. Once you are there, take a good look around and see if there is anybody else there with you,…. your favorite friend or family or you are alone; …either way is fine…now see if you can see different colors… …and see if you can hear the sounds around your favorite place… some kids can even smell and taste the food that they had in their favorite place. …Take some time to enjoy being there and feel yourself in your own favorite place.

B. Favorite activity: I wonder what your favorite activity is. (Play ground, sports, playing musical instruments, etc.) ….now just imagine that you are right there in the middle of your activity and doing it better than ever…take your time to enjoy every minute of it…

C. Favorite song: imagine singing your favorite song in your favorite place,… you can imagine a music band of your own… enjoy doing that very well… sing as many songs as you like…

Idiomotor Techniques

A. Moving hands together; put your hands straight in front of you and imagine there are two powerful magnets in each palm…notice how your hands become closer to each other,… all by themselves,…without your help…. it is fun to see how much closer and closer they get…

B. Arm rigidity; Stretch one arm straight out to the side and make a tight fist….Imagine that your arm is as strong as a branch of a tree… Stronger …and stronger…and I can not push it down… when you are ready, I will try to move your powerful arm… Just like your favorite super-hero….

Progressive Relaxation

A. Concentration on breathing; let's pay attention to each time you breath out…every time you do that your shoulders go down automatically… isn't that interesting… and you get more and more comfortable in your chest…the comfort is just like a magical flow that goes to your tummy,…. moves to your legs….

B. Floppy raggedy Ann; pretend that you are floppy all over just like the Raggedy Ann doll…so loose and comfortable…let me check that floppy arm …it's fun to see how it flops down again…

Hypnotic *Suggestions* for Analgesia

Many analgesic suggestion options are available and effective, especially when the technique is tailored to the child's interests and internal resources. Once the patient has learnt hypnotic inductions and enjoys experiencing that favorite place or activity, then the clinician delivers the appropriate suggestions which have come to light during child's assessment.

Some examples of analgesic suggestions are described below.

Blocking the Pain through Suggestion of Numbness, Anesthesia, and Analgesia

Magic Glove

One of the hypnotic pain management techniques that aims to decrease a child's pain is the "Magic Glove" introduced by Jacobsen as an acute pain intervention for blood draws (Jacobsen 1974). The "Magic Glove" technique is especially helpful for children aged 3–12 years undergoing blood draws, intravenous catheter placement, vaccinations, or emergency room suture procedures. Prior to applying the magic glove, the clinician should start by saying, " …*Let's see how much you can feel in your hands without the magic gloves? …*" Then apply equal pressure by using the tip of a pencil to "test" the hands, and ask, "…*How does it feel? Do both hands feel the same?*" Next reinforce the suggestion by saying, "*pretty soon after the application of the magic glove …you feel much less.*" After the child relaxes their hand in the clinician's hand, he might ask, "*Where would you like the glove to begin and end?*" Once that is known, the clinician takes the magic glove out of his pocket and gently strokes upward over the designated area. More positive suggestions are given during the application of the magic glove, "*this will numb your hand, so you won't be bothered. This is a really special and strong glove.*" Gently pressure the top of the hand at the end of the application of magic glove indicates that "*the glove is now in place.*" By applying equal pressure with the tip of a pencil to each hand, the clinician can test the glove for the difference child feels in each hand. Children may describe the feeling as tingly or funny. After the procedure, the magic glove is removed. This method has been successfully used during invasive procedures in children.

(i.e., lumbar puncture, bone marrow aspirates, etc.). In those cases after application of the magic glove, the clinician can ask the child to, "Now *touch your back with that hand which has the magic glove and transfer the same comfortable numb sensation from your hand to your back.*"

Sensory Transformation (Zeig and Geary 2001; Evans 2001)

A. Take the pain description and present an image that can be modified as the pain changes. After describing the idea that pain is transmitted by the nerves to the brain, ask the child to, "*Imagine being inside your body looking for that nerve….Find out the color of the nerve which is sending the pain message and change its color to one that you like.*"

B. Changing the intensity of pain; "*see the pain scale from 0 to 10 in your mind… adjust it by lowering your pain's rating. Make your pain move down the scale. If it is 10, move it to 5.*"

C. "*See yourself in a cold artic place… where you can blow a refreshing cold artic air through that hot burning area…*"

D. The switchbox technique. After explaining the idea that pain is transmitted by the nerves to the brain, which then sends back a "pain message" back to the body, ask the child to, "*Imagine that you are so tiny that can go inside your body to take a trip around…you can go around in a boat or on a bike…you can visit your heart and see how strong it is…or you can go to your lungs…once done, you can go to that main computer we call the brain….see all those lights and switches….find the switch for that knee…,… … And turn it all the way down….*"

Distraction

A. "*Imagine yourself in your favorite place and see that with each step you leave some pain behind.*"

B. "*Imagine that you are on the flying blanket ….. As the flying blanket starts moving up, the physical discomfort gets smaller and smaller.*"

Transference (Zeig and Geary 2001)

A. Transferring the pain to a smaller or less vulnerable area is a technique that is useful for most age groups. "*Imagine putting all the discomfort of your head into your right little toe and from there let it float away.*"

Relaxation

Older children can benefit from a technique that focuses on breathing and relaxation. Next, shift their focus to the painful area with continued emphasis on the fact that it is changing. "*While in your favorite place,... concentrate on breathing in and out, and notice that every time you breathe out... you get rid of some of that discomfort... And you become more and more comfortable...*"

Storytelling

Children love stories. Any of the above hypnotic suggestions can be incorporated in to a story. Stories can be about another child, a teddy bear, a favorite doll, or animal that was able to successfully utilize a certain technique to overcome the discomfort. Details in the story fascinate children and focus their attention. Erickson's metaphoric storytelling with the use of indirect suggestions and reframing approach is one of the more valuable methods in children's pain management.

Teaching Self-Hypnosis

Self-hypnosis increases the child's sense of mastery and control and reinforces the desired behavior by repetition of the appropriate exercise. Encouraging the child to practice the learned skill is essential to a successful outcome. Self-hypnosis can be taught to the child during the first session. Gardner described an easy three step method for teaching self-hypnosis to children (Gardner 1981).

Step 1 After allowing time for the child to enjoy imagery, the clinician asks the child to count silently up to five, with eyes open at three and

fully alert at five. This way child learns to return to the alert state without help. This way clinician emphasizes that the child now knows how to return to alert state all by himself.

Step 2 The clinician asks the child to describe the preferred induction method that was most helpful to him. During this time, clinician may assist the child with the details and asks him to go to hypnosis to feel the same good feelings and return to the normal alert state. Problems are discussed as necessary.

Step 3 In this step, the child is asked to repeat step two except this time to experience it silently as he or she goes into hypnotic trance without assistance and returns to the alert normal state without talking. Any remaining problems or questions are then discussed. The child is now fully ready for full independent use of self-hypnosis.

An alternative way is to give the child a *cue* during hypnosis session. This cue is used as a signal for the child to go to hypnosis. For example the clinician might say, "*Now that you have learned so well how to get so comfortable ...you can be proud that your brain and body are learning to talk to each other....And congratulate yourself ...it is nice to know, before you finish, to remind yourself that you can choose a sign to return to this state every time you practice at home .... For example you can choose an 'OK' sign by putting your index finger and thumb together, that will be a reminder of how to get back to the same comfortable feeling as you are right now....That sign will help you to go to this comfortable state so effortlessly and experience the same good feeling.*" Once the child is alert the clinician asks the child to use the cue sign and observers the child. Any question or problem should be discussed and answered. Sometimes clinician prepares a recording of a session and encourages the child to use it during practice at home.

Training and Certification in Hypnosis

The Society for Clinical and Experimental Hypnosis (SCEH) and the American Society of

Clinical Hypnosis (ASCH), are the hypnosis societies which maintain a high level of standards and limit their training to health care providers. Both SCEH and ASCH hold workshops for intensive training in basic, intermediate, and advanced skills in hypnosis. Both societies hold annual scientific meetings to discuss recent developments in clinical and experimental research. Each society publishes a journal quarterly: The International Journal of Clinical and Experimental Hypnosis (SCEH) and the American Journal of Clinical Hypnosis (ASCH). In addition, the Society of Behavioral and Developmental Pediatrics (SDBP) offers clinical hypnosis workshops at three levels: introductory, intermediate, and advanced. This workshop provides training for physicians and other pediatric health care professionals in the use of hypnosis and its applications in clinical pediatric settings. More detailed information about training and publications can be obtained directly from the society's central offices and Web sites.

References

American Medical Association. (1958). Council on mental health: Medical use of hypnosis. *Journal of the American Medical Association, 9,* 86–189.

Benedetti, F. (2002). How the doctor's words affect the patient's brain. *Evaluation & the Health Professions, 25,* 369–386.

Braid, J. (1844). Magic, Mesmerism, Hypnotism; historically and physiologically considered. *The Medical Times, a Journal of the English and Foreign Medicine, 11,* 203–224.

Braid, J. (1846). The power of the mind over the body: An experimental inquiry into the nature and cause of the phenomena. *The Medical Times, 14*(350), 214–216.

Broome, M. E., Bates, T. A., Lillis, P. P., & McGahee, T. W. (1990). Children's medical fears, coping behaviors, and pain perceptions during a lumbar puncture. *Oncology Nursing Forum, 17,* 361–367.

Butler, L. D., Symons, B. K., Henderson, S. L., Shortliffe, L. D., & Spiegel, D. (2005). Hypnosis reduces distress and duration of an invasive medical procedure for children. *Clinical Trials.* Journal article. Randomized controlled trial. Research support, Non-U.S. Gov't. *Pediatrics, 115,* e77–e85.

Chaves, J. F., & Dworkin, S. F. (1997). Hypnotic control of pain: Historical perspectives and future prospects. *International Journal of Clinical and Experimental Hypnosis, 45*(4), 356–376.

Chen, L. M. (2007). Imaging of pain. *International Anesthesiology Clinics, 44,* 39–57.

Crawford, H. J., Horton, J. E., Harrington, G. S., Hirsch Downs, T., Fox, K., Daugherty, S., & Downs, III, H. (2000). *Attention and dis-attention (hypnotic analgesia) to noxious somatosensory TENS stimuli: fMRI differences in low and highly hypnotizable individuals.* Poster presented at sixth annual meeting of the organization for Human Brain Mapping, San Antonio, TX.

Davis, K. D., Taylor, S. J., Crawley, A. P., Wood, M. L., & Mikulis, D. J. (1997). Functional MRI of pain and attention related activations in the human cingulate cortex. *Neurophysiology, 77,* 3370–3380.

Davis, K. D., Hutchison, W. D., Lozano, A. M., Tasker, R. R., & Dostrovsky, J. O. (2000). Human anterior cingulate cortex neurons modulated by attention demanding tasks. *Journal of Neurophysiology, 83,* 3575–3577.

De Pascalis, V. F. S., Chiaradia, C., & Carotenuto, E. (2002). The contribution of suggestibility and expectation to placebo analgesia phenomenon in an experimental setting. *Pain, 3,* 393–402.

DePascalis, V., Marucci, F. S., Penna, P. M., & Pessa, E. (1987). Hemispheric activity of 40 Hz EEG during recall of emotional events: Differences between low and high hypnotizables. *International Journal of Psychophysiology, 5,* 167–180.

Di Blasi, Z., Harkness, E., Ernst, E., Georgiou, A., & Kleijnen, J. (2001). Influence of context effects on health outcomes: A systematic review. *Lancet, 357,* 757–762.

Diamond, M. (1984). It takes two to tango: The neglected importance of the hypnotic relationship. *The American Journal of Clinical Hypnosis, 26,* 1–13.

Dinges, D. F., Whitehouse, W. G., Orne, E. C., Bloom, P. B., Carlin, M. M., Bauer, N. K., Gillen, K. A., Shapiro, B. S., Ohene-Frempong, K., Dampier, C., & Orne, M. T. (1997). Self-hypnosis training as an adjunctive treatment in the management of pain associated with sickle cell disease. Clinical trial. Comparative study. *The International Journal of Clinical and Experimental Hypnosis, 45,* 417–432.

Donaldson, I. M. L. (2005). Mesmer's 1780 proposal for a controlled trial to test his method of treatment using 'Animal Magnetism'. The James Lind Library (www.Jameslindlibrary.org). Accessed 10 Oct 2009.

Evans, F. J. (2001). Hypnosis in chronic pain management, in international handbook of clinical hypnosis (eds G. D. Burrows, R. O. Stanley and P. B. Bloom), John Wiley & Sons, Ltd, Chichester, UK.Evans, F. J. 17, 247–260.

Faymonville, M. E., Mambourg, P. H., Joris, J., et al. (1997). Psychological approaches during conscious sedation: Hypnosis versus stress reducing strategies: A prospective randomized study. *Pain, 73,* 361–367.

Gardner, G. G. (1981). Teaching self-hypnosis to children. *International Jornal of Clinical Hypnosis, 29,* 300–312.

Genuis, M. L. (1995). The use of hypnosis in helping cancer patients control anxiety, pain, and emesis: A review of recent empirical studies. *The American Journal of Clinical Hypnosis, 37*, 316–325.

Goodman, J. E., & McGrath, P. J. (1991). The epidemiology of pain in children and adolescents: A review. *Pain, 46*, 247–264.

Hilgard, E. R. (1973). The domain of hypnosis with some comments on alternative paradigms. *The American Psychologist, 28*, 972–982.

Hilgard, E. R., & Hilgard, J. R. (1997). *Hypnosis in the relief of pain*. New York: Brunner/Mazel. Rev sub edition.

Holroyd, J. (1996). Hypnosis treatment of clinical pain: Understanding why hypnosis is useful. *International Journal of Clinical and Experimental Hypnosis, 44*, 33–51.

Hsieh, J. C., Stone-Elander, S., & Ingvar, M. (1999). Anticipatory coping of pain expressed in the human anterior cingulate cortex: A positron emission tomography study. *Neuroscience Letters, 262*, 61–64.

Humphreys, P., & Gevirtz, R. N. (2000). Treatment of recurrent abdominal pain: Components analysis of four treatment protocols. *Journal of Pediatric Gastroenterology and Nutrition, 31*, 47–51.

Huth, M. M., Broome, M. E., & Good, M. (2004). Imagery reduces children's postoperative pain. *Pain, 110*, 439–448.

Integration of behavioral and relaxation approaches into the treatment of chronic pain and insomnia. (1996). NIH technology assessment panel on integration of behavioral and relaxation approaches into the treatment of chronic pain and insomnia. *Journal of the American Medical Association, 276*, 313–318.

Iserson, K. V. (1998). Hypnosis for pediatric fracture reduction. *The Journal of Emergency Medicine, 17*, 53–56.

Jacobsen, E. (1974). Progressive Relaxation: A Physiological & Clinical Investigation of Muscular States & Their Significance in Psychology & Medical Practice, Chicago University Press, Chicago Midway Reprint.

Kihlstorm, J. F. (1985). Hypnosis. *Annual Review of Physiology, 47*, 119–127.

Kirsch, I. (1999). Hypnosis and placebos: Response expectancy as a mediator of suggestion effects. *Anales de Psicología, 15*, 99–110.

Kirsch, I. (2001). The response set theory of hypnosis: Expectancy and physiology. *The American Journal of Clinical Hypnosis, 44*, 69–73.

Lambert, S. A. (1996). The effects of hypnosis/guided imagery on the postoperative course of children. *Journal of Developmental and Behavioral Pediatrics, 17*, 307–310.

Rapport des commissaires chargés par le Roi, de l'examen du magnétisme animale. (1784). Imprimé par ordre du Roi. Paris: L'Imprimerie Royale.

Martin-Herz, S. P., Thurber, C. A., & Patterson, D. R. (1986). Psychological principles of burn wound pain in children. II: treatment applications. Journal article. Research support, U.S. Gov't, P.H.S. *Journal of Burn Care & Rehabilitation 21*, 458–472.

McConkey, K. M. (1986). Opinions about hypnosis and self hypnosis before and hypnotic testing. *International Journal of Clinical and Experimental Hypnosis, 34*, 311–319.

Mesmer, F. A. (1779). Mémoire sur la découverte du magnétisme animal. Par M. Mesmer, Docteur en Médecine de la Faculté de Vienne. Geneva (and Paris): Didot le Jeune.

Olness, K., & Gardner, G. G. (1978). Some guidelines for uses of hypnotherapy in pediatrics. *Pediatrics, 62*, 228–233.

Olness K., & Kohen, D. (1996) Correlates of child hood hypnotic responsiveness in Hypnosis and hypnotherapy with children, 3rd ed. New York, NY: Guilford. 4(33–52).

Olness, K., MacDonald, J. T., & Uden, D. L. (1987). Comparison of self-hypnosis and propranolol in the treatment of juvenile classic migraine. *Pediatrics, 79*, 593–597.

Porro, C. A., Baraldi, P., & Pagnoni, G. (2002). Does anticipation of pain affect cortical nociceptive systems? *The Journal of Neuroscience, 22*, 3206–3214.

Price, D. D. (2002). Central neural mechanisms that interrelate sensory and affective dimensions of pain. *Molecular Interventions, 2*, 392–403.

Quist, J. F., Ball, C. L., Schachar, R., Roberts, W., & Malone, M. (2003). Receptor gene and attention deficit hyperactivity disorder. *Molecular Psychiatry, 8*, 98–102.

Rainville, P., & Price, D. D. (2003). Hypnosis phenomenology and the neurobiology of consciousness. *International Journal of Clinical and Experimental Hypnosis, 51*, 105–129.

Rainville, P., Duncan, G. H., Price, D. D., Carrier, B., & Bushnell, M. C. (1997). Pain affect encoded in human anterior cingulate but not somatosensory cortex. *Science, 277*(3528), 968–971.

Rainville, P., Hofbauer, R. K., Paus, T., Duncan, G. H., Bushnell, M. C., & Price, D. D. (1999). Cerebral mechanisms of hypnotic induction and suggestion. *Journal of Cognitive Neuroscience, 11*, 110–125.

Rainville, P., Hofbauer, R. K., Bushnell, M. C., Duncan, G. H., & Price, D. D. (2000). *Hypnosis modulates the activity in cerebral structures involved in arousal and attention*. Poster presented at Cognitive Neuroscience Society, San Francisco, CA.

Rainville, P., Hofbauer, R. K., Bushnell, M. C., Duncan, G. H., & Price, D. D. (2002). Hypnosis modulates activity in brain structures involved in the regulation of consciousness. *Journal of Cognitive Neuroscience, 14*, 887–901.

Ray, W. J., & Pascalis, V. F. S. (2003). Temporal aspects of hypnotic processes. *International Journal of Clinical and Experimental Hypnosis, 51*, 147–165.

Raz, A., & Shapiro, T. (2003). Hypnosis and neuroscience: A crosstalk between clinical and cognitive research. *Archives of General Psychiatry, 59*, 85–90.

Raz, A., Shapiro, T., & Fan, J. (2002). Hypnotic suggestion and the modulation of stroop interference. *Archives of General Psychiatry, 59*, 1155–1161.

Raz, A., Fan, J., & Posner, M. I. (2005). Hypnotic suggestion reduces conflict in the human brain. *Proceedings of the National Academy of Science, 102*, 9978–9983.

Rhue et al. (1993) Executive Committee of the American Psychological Association Division of Psychological Hypnosis. The Bulletin of Division 30. (http://psychologicalhypnosis.com/info/the-official-division-30-definition-and-description-of-hypnosis) Accessed 21 March 2011

Richter, I. L., McGrath, P. J., & Humphreys, P. J. (1986). Cognitive and relaxation treatment of paediatric migraine. *Pain, 25*, 195–203.

Spiegel, D., & Moore, R. (1997). Imagery and hypnosis in the treatment of cancer patients. *Oncology, 1*, 1179–1195.

Syrjala, K. L., & Abrams, J. R. (1996). Hypnosis and imagery in the treatment of pain. In: Gatchel RJ, Turk DC (eds.) *Psychological Approaches to Pain Management: A Practitioners' Handbook*. New York: Guilford Publications 231–258.

Swanson, J. M., Flodman, P., Kennedy, J., Spence, M. A., Moyzis, R., Schuck, S., Murias, M., Moriarity, J., Barr, C., Smith, M., & Posner, M. (2000). Dopamine, genes and ADHD. *Neuroscience and Biobehavioral Reviews, 24*, 21–25.

Uman, L. S., Chambers, C. T., McGrath, P. J., & Kisely, S. (2007). Psychological interventions for needle-related procedural pain and distress in children and adolescents. The Cochrane database of systematic reviews, the Cochrane Library, the Cochrane Collaboration.

Vandenberg, B. (2002). Hypnotic responsivity from a developmental perspective; insight from young children. *International Journal of Clinical and Experimental Hypnosis, 50*, 229–247.

Zeig, J., & Geary, B. (2001). Ericksonian approaches to pain management in The Handbook of Ericksonian psychotherapy, Milton H. Erickson Foundation Press. 252–285.

Pharmacology of Chronic Pain Management

20

Benjamin Howard Lee

Keywords

Bioavailability • Biotransformation of drugs • Cyclooxygenase (COX) • Opioid analgesics • Co-analgesics • Adjuvant analgesics

Pharmacokinetics and Pharmacodynamics of Analgesics and Adjuvants in Infants, Children, and Adolescents

Developmental Pharmacology

Developmental Considerations in Children

Rational and effective administration of medications for children requires a fundamental understanding and integration of the role of ontogeny in the disposition and actions of drugs. Dosing of analgesic medications for pediatric patients is dependent on the interplay between pharmacokinetics (PK), pharmacodynamics (PD), and pharmacogenomics (PG). There is much debate concerning the methodology employed to adjust PK parameters to body size. Traditionally, empirical approaches to drug dosing have been based on using either body weight or body surface area. However, the use of linear per kilogram and surface area models have generally been considered inappropriate for scaling small children to adults, and a non-linear relationship between weight and drug elimination capacity is now widely accepted. The consideration of accurate pharmacological and pharmacokinetic data for pediatric dosing may involve the use of cumbersome mathematical analysis in order to obtain a rational, safe, and effective dose. However, the log of basal metabolic rate plotted against the log of body weight in all species studied produces a straight line with a slope of 0.75, and the use of dosing equations has largely been replaced by adjustment (or normalization) of the drug dose for either body weight or body-surface area (Anderson and Holford 2008; Anderson and Meakin 2002).

The pharmacokinetics and pharmacodynamics of analgesics change during development with profound changes over the first few months of life (Table 20.1). Most current age-specific dosing requirements are based on the known influence of ontogeny on the disposition of drugs. Developmental changes in physiology produce many of the age-associated changes in the absorption, distribution, metabolism, and excretion of drugs that culminate in altered pharmacokinetics and thus serve as the determinants of age-specific dose requirements (Berde and Sethna 2002).

B.H. Lee (✉)
Johns Hopkins Medical Institutions, 600 North Wolfe Street/Blalock 904A, Baltimore, MD 21287, USA
e-mail: blee31@jhmi.edu

B.C. McClain and S. Suresh (eds.), *Handbook of Pediatric Chronic Pain: Current Science and Integrative Practice*, DOI 10.1007/978-1-4419-0350-1_20, © Springer Science+Business Media, LLC 2011

Table 20.1 Developmental considerations for pharmacology

System	Age-related changes	Affect on pharmacology
Body composition/ physiologic spaces	Larger extracellular and total body water spaces in neonates; Adipose stores with higher ratio of water to lipid.	Lower plasma levels of drugs in these compartments when given in weight-based dosing regimen.
Plasma protein binding	Decrease in quantity of total plasma proteins (albumin and α1-acid glycoprotein in neonate and young infant. Presence of fetal albumin and increase in bilirubin and free fatty acids.	Increased free traction of drug and availability of active moiety in drugs that are highly-protein bound. Potential for overdose or toxicity.
GI absorption	Relatively elevated intragastric pH (>4) and less gastric secretion in the neonate. Immature passive and active intestinal transport immature until age 4 months. Immature conjugation and transport of bile salts. Greater number of high-amplitude pulsatile rectal contractions.	Altered bioavailability of drugs given enterally. Enhanced expulsion of rectally administered drugs leading to decreased absorption.
Hepatic drug-metabolizing activity	Delayed maturation of hepatic drug-metabolizing enzyme activity. Immature expression of phase I enzymes (cytochrome P_{450} isozymes) and phase II conjugation enzymes (e.g., glucuronosyltransferases) in neonates and infants.	Decreased metabolic clearance of agents. Decreased infusion rates or an increase in the dosing interval (decreased frequency of dosing).
Skeletal muscle	Reduced skeletal muscle blood flow and inefficient muscular contractions in the neonate. Higher density of skeletal muscle capillaries.	Reduced rate of intramuscular (IM) absorption vs. higher rate of absorption via capillaries leads to relatively more efficient IM absorption in neonates.
Renal function	Decreased glomerular filtration rate, renal blood flow, and tubular secretion in the neonate and young infant.	Accumulation of renally-excreted drugs or active metabolites. Decreased infusion rates or increased dosing intervals (decreased frequency of administration).

Little information exists about the effect of human ontogeny on interactions between drugs and receptors and the consequence of these interactions (i.e., pharmacodynamics of agents).

Age-associated changes in body composition and organ function are dynamic and can be discordant during the first decade of life. Generally, the rate at which most drugs are absorbed is slower in neonates and young infants (<3 months of age) than in older children; thus, the time required to achieve maximal plasma levels of most drugs is prolonged in the very young. Age-dependent changes in body composition alter the physiologic spaces into which a drug is distributed. The relatively larger extracellular and total-body water spaces in neonates and young infants as compared with adults, coupled with adipose stores with a higher ratio of water to lipid, result in lower plasma levels of drugs in these compart-

ments when the drugs are administered in a weight-based fashion (Kearns et al. 2003).

The composition and amount of circulating plasma proteins (e.g., albumin and a_1-acid glycoprotein) are also likely to influence the distribution of highly protein-bound drugs. A reduction in the quantity of total plasma proteins (including albumin) in the neonate and young infant increases the free fraction of drug, thereby influencing the availability of the active moiety (Berde and Sethna 2002). The presence of fetal albumin (which has reduced binding affinity for weak acids) and an increase in endogenous substances (e.g., bilirubin and free fatty acids) capable of displacing a drug from albumin binding sites during the neonatal period may also contribute to the higher free fractions of highly protein-bound drugs in neonates. Age-related changes in the protein-binding of drugs and in the lipid content of the brain may alter the cerebrospinal fluid–brain and blood–brain concentration ratios and drug partitioning independent of the permeability of the blood–brain barrier(Berde and Sethna 2002).

During the neonatal period, intragastric pH is relatively elevated (>4) consequent to reductions in both basal acid output and the total volume of gastric secretions. Gastric emptying and intestinal motility are the primary determinants of the rate at which drugs are presented to and dispersed along the mucosal surface of the small intestine. Both passive and active transport are fully mature in infants by approximately 4 months of age. Developmental differences in the activity of intestinal drug-metabolizing enzymes that can markedly alter the bioavailability of drugs are incompletely characterized. Immature conjugation and transport of bile salts into the intestinal lumen result in low intraduodenal levels despite the presence of blood levels that exceed those of adults (Kearns et al. 2003).

Reduced skeletal-muscle blood flow and inefficient muscular contractions may reduce the rate of intramuscular absorption of drugs in neonates, off-set by the relatively higher density of skeletal-muscle capillaries in infants than in older children. Thus, the evidence supports the concept that intramuscular absorption of specific agents (e.g., amikacin) is more efficient in neonates and infants than in older children. The bioavailability of extensively metabolized compounds administered rectally may be enhanced in neonates and very young infants due to developmental immaturity of hepatic metabolism rather than to enhanced mucosal translocation. However, infants have a greater number of high-amplitude pulsatile contractions in the rectum than do adults, which can enhance the expulsion of solid forms of drugs, effectively decreasing the absorption of drugs such as acetaminophen (Kearns et al. 2003).

Delayed maturation of drug-metabolizing enzyme activity may account for the marked toxicity of drugs in infants and young children. Important developmental changes in the biotransformation of drugs prompt the need for age-appropriate dose regimens for many drugs commonly used in children. The developmental expression of phase I enzymes, such as the

P_{450} cytochromes, changes dramatically during early childhood (Lacroix et al. 1997; Sonnier and Cresteil 1998). The ontogeny of the conjugation reactions (i.e., those involving phase II enzymes) is less well established than the ontogeny of reactions involving phase I enzymes. Individual isoforms of glucuronosyltransferase (UGT) have unique maturational profiles. The glucuronidation of acetaminophen (a substrate for UGT1A6 and, to a lesser extent, UGT1A9) is decreased in newborns and young children as compared with adolescents and adults (Miller et al. 1976). Glucuronidation of morphine (a UGT2B7 substrate) can be detected in premature infants as young as 24 weeks of gestational age (Barrett et al. 1996). The clearance of morphine from plasma is positively correlated with post-conceptional age and increases fourfold between 27 and 40 weeks post-conceptional age, thereby necessitating corresponding increases in the dose of morphine to maintain effective analgesia (Scott et al. 1999).

A consistent observation in clinical studies of drugs metabolized in the liver is an age-dependent increase in plasma clearance in children younger than 10 years of age, which necessitates relatively higher weight-based dosing. The mechanisms underlying these age-related increases in plasma drug clearance are largely unknown. This higher rate of drug metabolism has been historically attributed to the larger liver mass/kg body weight (Blanco et al. 2000); however, it is unlikely that the greater drug clearance in infants and young children can be attributed solely to a disproportionate increase in liver mass, given that the weight of the liver as a percentage of total body mass reaches a maximum between 1 and 3 years of age and declines to adult values during adolescence (Kearns et al. 2003).

Maturation of renal function is a dynamic process that begins during fetal organogenesis and is complete by early childhood. The glomerular filtration rate, renal blood flow, and tubular secretion increase rapidly during the first 2 weeks of life and then rises steadily until adult values are reached at 8–12 months of age (Berde and Sethna 2002). Developmental changes in renal function can dramatically alter the plasma clearance of compounds with extensive renal elimination and thus constitute a major determinant of the age-appropriate selection of a dose regimen in young children.

Pharmacological Agents for Chronic Pain Management

Nonopioid Primary Analgesics [Acetaminophen, Salicylates, and Nonsteroidal Anti-inflammatory Drugs (NSAIDs)]

The peripheral and centrally acting primary nonopioid analgesics are medications that are useful for the management of acute, recurrent pain and chronic pain (Table 20.2). These agents may be used for postsurgical pain, trauma, arthritis, headache, and cancer-related pain. There is a wide variety of variability of response to these medications between individuals, and the benefits/risks of these agents for chronic use is an area of evolving research (Munir et al. 2007).

Acetaminophen

Acetaminophen (APAP) is a very popular analgesic for infants and children and is commonly used for the management of acute and chronic pain in adults and children. It is generally well-tolerated with demonstrated analgesia compared to placebo. The primary mechanism of action is the central inhibition of the cyclooxygenase enzymes in the central nervous system leading to an inhibition of prostaglandin synthesis. There is no clinically relevant inhibition of prostaglandin synthesis in the peripheral nervous system; hence, acetaminophen has no significant anti-inflammatory or hematological (platelet) effects. The analgesic and antipyretic potency of APAP is similar to aspirin. Acetaminophen suppresses neuronal excitability both centrally and peripherally (Anderson 2008; Graham and Scott 2005).

The route of administration determines the dose to be given with oral dosing of 10–15 mg/kg every 4–6 h to a maximum dose of 100 mg/kg/day or 4,000 mg/day. Acetaminophen is available as a rectal suppository (180, 325, and 650 mg); however, rectal absorption can often be erratic and the effective dose for analgesia is higher than with oral dosing (20–35 mg/kg rectally vs. 10–15 mg/kg orally) (Birmingham et al. 1997). Acetaminophen does not cause gastric mucosal irritation and is well-tolerated orally. It also has no hematological side-effects (no anti-platelet activity). The major pathway for the metabolism of acetaminophen is via glucuronidation or sulfation in the liver; the minor pathway for metabolism is the mixed function oxidases. There is a toxic intermediate metabolite which is inactivated by conjugation with glutathione. Use of acetaminophen in large doses may deplete glutathione stores resulting in accumulation of this toxic metabolite potentially resulting in centrilobular hepatic necrosis (a potentially fatal disease); therefore recommended daily maximum doses should not be exceeded (James et al. 2008; Mortensen 2002). APAP is a common ingredient in many prescription and nonprescription analgesics and caution should be exercised to avoid concomitant use and potential overdose.

ASA (Acetylsalicyclic Acid-[aspirin]) and Salicylate Salts

Invented in 1897, aspirin is one of the oldest nonopioid analgesics. It was very commonly used for children and adults; however, use as an analgesic has been largely replaced by nonsteroidal anti-inflammatory drugs (NSAIDs) and acetaminophen. Pediatric dosing is 10–15 mg/kg orally every 4–6 h. The potential association between aspirin use and Reye syndrome in young children with a concomitant viral illness has led to avoidance of this drug for routine use in children (Cron et al. 1999). In 2003, the US Food and Drug Administration ordered the placement of warning labels on all salicylates describing the potential for the development of Reye syndrome with use.

The salicylate salts, choline magnesium trisalicylate and salsalate, are compounds related to aspirin and are used as analgesics in the setting of patients with potential for the development of coagulopathies. Therapeutic doses of these agents do not effect bleeding time or platelet aggregation tests (Stuart and Pisko 1981; Sweeney and Hoernig 1991). Therefore, these medications are often useful in patients with oncologic diseases

Table 20.2 Peripherally acting nonopioid analgesics

Agent	Pediatric dose	Adult dose	Maximal daily adult dose (mg)	Plasma half-life (h)	Comments
Acetaminophen[a]	10–15 mg/kg q 4–6 h	500–1,000 mg q4–6 h	4,000	2–3	Do not exceed 100 mg/kg/day. Available as rectal suppository.
Salicylates					
Aspirin[a]	10–15 mg/kg q 4–6 h	500–1,000 mg q4–6 h	4,000	0.25	Do not use for children under 12 years of age with possible viral illness due to potential for Reye syndrome. Available as rectal suppository.
Choline magnesium trisalicylate	25 mg/kg BID	1,000–1,500 mg q12 h	2,000–3,000	9–17	Aspirin-like compound that does not increase bleeding time.
NSAIDs					
Ibuprofen[a]	5–10 mg/kg q6 h	200–400 mg q4–6 h	2,400	2–2.5	Most commonly used NSAID in the USA. Also available as 100 mg/5 mL suspension.
Naproxen[a]	5–10 mg/kg BID	500 mg load f/b 275 mg q6–8 h	1,500	12–15	Also available as 125 mg/5 mL suspension.
Indomethacin[a]	2–4 mg/kg q8 h	25 mg q8–12 h	200	2	GI and CNS side effects are common.
Oxaprozin[a]	10–20 mg/kg daily	600 mg q12–24 h	1,200	2–69	
Meloxicam[a]	0.125–0.25 mg/kg daily	7.5–15 mg q24 h	15	15–20	7.5 mg/ 5 mL suspension.
Piroxicam	0.2–0.4 mg/kg/day (max 15 mg/day)	20–40 mg q24 h	40	50	
Diclofenac	1–2 mg/kg/dose	50 mg q8 h	150		
Etodolac[a]	15–20 mg/kg/day q12 h	300–400 mg q8–12 h	1,000	–	
Celecoxib[a]	50 mg BID (for children 10–25 kg, 100 mg BID for children >25 kg.	200–400 mg q12–24 h	400	11	Selective COX-2 inhibition.

BID twice a day, *NSAIDs* nonsteroidal anti-inflammatory drugs, *COX* cyclo-oxygenase
[a]FDA-approved drugs for children

and pain in which the patient may benefit from analgesia without potential for further coagulopathies from medication. Choline magnesium trisalicylate is sometimes used for pediatric patients with oncologic disease, and the typical pediatric dosing regimen is 25 mg/kg given twice daily.

Nonsteroidal Anti-inflammatory Drugs (NSAIDs)

The nonsteroidal anti-inflammatory drugs (NSAIDs) are effective analgesics for chronic pain that is associated with inflammation as these agents have pharmacological properties that are both analgesic and anti-inflammatory. These agents have been shown in many clinical trials to be moderately effective for analgesia versus placebo. These agents are most effective for mild pain and often used in combination with opioids for moderate pain. These agents are structurally distinct with three major families of agents (carboxylic acids, pyrazoles, and oxicams) but exhibit a similar mechanism of action; NSAIDs are often referred to as peripherally acting nonopioid analgesics. All of the NSAIDs inhibit the enzyme cyclooxygenase (COX) resulting in a decreased production of prostaglandins, agents involved in the peripheral response to a noxious stimulus and the inflammatory and nociceptive events which accompany injury and disease, thereby suppressing neuronal excitability peripherally (Tobias 2000; Vane 1971).

There are two isoforms of the COX enzyme: COX-1, which is found constitutively in platelets, kidneys, the GI tract, and other tissues, and the COX-2 isozyme, which is found constitutively in the kidneys and central nervous system and whose formation is induced in the peripheral tissues by noxious stimuli that cause inflammation and pain (Morita 2002). Most of the NSAIDs are nonselective inhibitors of the COX isozymes and may vary in their relative COX-1 and COX-2 selectivity. While these agents principally are peripherally acting analgesics, there is evidence of a central mechanism of action (in the brain and spinal cord) as well involving the inhibition of prostaglandin synthesis, activation of endogenous opioid peptides, and serotonergic-mediated events (Malmberg and Yaksh 1992).

These agents have a widely varying chemical composition and are structurally distinct from one another; however, there is good clinical evidence that nonselective NSAIDs are comparable in efficacy to each other. There may be a great interpatient variability in the analgesic response to a particular NSAID, but no structure–activity relationship exists, so the efficacy of one agent for a particular patient vs. another cannot be fully understood at present. Thus, a patient who does not respond to a NSAID from one chemical class is just as likely to respond to another NSAID from the same chemical class as a NSAID from another chemical class. Therefore, when considering the use of a NSAID for chronic pain, if the patient does not respond to a particular agent, then the provider should consider a trial with an alternative NSAID agent.

The use of NSAIDs is limited by the analgesic ceiling effect of these medications in which there is no additional analgesic effect but an increase in toxicity with dose escalation. These agents do not produce physical or psychological dependence with use and are also antipyretic (Munir et al. 2007). NSAIDs are the mainstay of treatment for pain associated with pediatric rheumatic diseases

such as juvenile idiopathic arthritis (Kimura and Walco 2007). They provide effective analgesia in many patients and are commonly used as first-line agents. NSAIDs that are approved by the US FDA for use in pediatric patients include ibuprofen, naproxen, oxaprozin, etodolac SR, meloxicam, indomethacin, and celecoxib (Kimura and Walco 2007). Ibuprofen remains the most commonly used NSAID for pediatric pain; it is available as a 100 mg chewable tablet, 200 mg tablet, and 100 mg/5 cc oral suspension, and the routine dose for children is 5–10 mg/kg orally every 6 h with a recommended maximum dose of 40 mg/kg or 2,400 mg/day.

There are many potentially significant adverse events that may occur with prolonged use of NSAIDs. Patients may develop gastrointestinal (dyspepsia, bleeding, and peptic ulcer formation through inhibition of protective prostaglandin formation) and hematologic [platelet inhibition due to reversible inhibition of thromboxane synthesis (Niemi et al. 1997)] adverse events. Dyspepsia may occur early in therapy, and the provider should strongly encourage the patient to take these medications with food to minimize this potential effect. GI ulceration, bleeding, or perforation can occur at any time during therapy with NSAIDs, often without any warning symptoms (Garcia Rodriguez and Barreales 2007). Children receiving NSAIDs as treatment for chronic pain and disease are less likely than adults to have GI adverse effects.

NSAIDs may also lead to inability for platelets to aggregate due to reversible inhibition of thromboxane synthesis, and use of anticoagulants, coagulopathy, and thrombocytopenia is a relative contraindication for the use of NSAIDs. These agents may also be associated with bone marrow suppression (Nuki 1990). Renal dysfunction may occur with NSAID use due to inhibition of prostaglandin-mediated intrarenal vasodilatation during hypovolemia or reduced renal blood flow (Munir et al. 2007). NSAIDs can produce liver damage, and this is usually detected as an elevation in liver enzymes. Monitoring of liver enzymes, bilirubin, and markers of kidney function should be considered with prolonged use of these agents for chronic pain conditions. Liver disease or elevated liver function tests (LFTs) are relative contraindications for the use of NSAIDs (Rubenstein and Laine 2004). Bronchospastic NSAID-exacerbated respiratory disease (ERD) has been reported in children and adults, and NSAID ERD is a concern in one of three teenagers with severe asthma and coexisting nasal disease (Sturtevant 1999). Pseudoporphyria has been associated with the chronic use of NSAIDs in some children (Lang and Finlayson 1994).

Opioid Analgesics

Opioid analgesics are very commonly used in the analgesic management of children of all ages, from neonates to adolescents. These agents are often added to nonopioid analgesics to manage cancer-related pain and potentially noncancer chronic pain. Opioid analgesics will decrease or modify the perception of pain in the central nervous system, and these medications are titrated to effect as they have no ceiling effect for dose. Opioids provide analgesia principally via the mu (μ), kappa (κ), and delta (δ) opioid receptors by mimicking the actions of the endogenous opioid peptides resulting in membrane hyperpolarization and analgesia. These receptors are principally located in the brain and spinal cord, but they can also be found in peripheral nerve cells and immune cells (Snyder and Pasternak 2003). Endogenous and exogenous opioid compounds will bind to these receptors. Inter-individual variability in the response to opioids may be due in part to genetic polymorphisms that effect opioid binding and efficacy. The opioids that are most commonly used in the management of chronic pain in children are mu agonists; these agents include morphine, hydromorphone, fentanyl, meperidine, and methadone (Table 20.3). Mixed agonist–antagonists agents are used much less commonly; most of these drugs act as agonists or partial agonists at the kappa and sigma receptors but are antagonists at the mu receptor. Mixed agonist/antagonist agents in common use include butorphanol, buprenorphine, and nalbuphine.

Opioid receptors are found both presynaptically and postsynaptically, and are coupled to guanine nucleotide (GTP) binding regulatory proteins (G proteins). These receptors regulate via transmembrane signaling mechanisms of the inward K+ current, resulting in membrane hyperpolarization as well as decreased cyclic adenosine monophosphate production (cAMP), increased nitric oxide (NO) synthesis, and the production of 12-lipoxygenase metabolites. The opioid-sparing effect of concomitant use of NSAIDs is likely due to the blockade of prostaglandin synthesis leading to greater availability of 12-lipoxygenase metabolites (Pasternak 2005; Zelcer et al. 2005). Some of the adverse effects of opioids may result from the opioid binding to stimulatory G-proteins and is antagonized by ultra-low dose naloxone infusions (Ganesh and Maxwell 2007; Maxwell et al. 2005).

Most of the opioids are biotransformed by the liver prior to excretion by the kidneys. In the liver, most of the metabolism of the opioids occurs via glucuronidation or by the microsomal mixed-functions oxidases which use the cytochrome P_{450} system. The cytochrome P_{450} is not fully developed at birth and does not reach maturity until approximately 3 months of age; it is likely that the immaturity of this system is responsible for the prolonged effect of a dose of an opioid in a neonate and young infant. Opioid drugs should be used cautiously in patients with significant liver or kidney disease as the metabolism and excretion will be altered potentially leading to accumulation of drug. Prodrugs (such as codeine), which are inactive and require metabolism by the liver for activity, may be ineffective in patients with liver disease.

Side effects due to the opioid agents are often dose-dependent and may involve sedation and respiratory depression in some patients. Thus, patients who are taking opioid medications for pain need to be monitored regularly for efficacy and adverse effects. There is no evidence that one opioid is more effective clinically than another, and the choice of opioid is individualized with respect to the patient's clinical state, previous responses to the agent, and potential for side effects. Across all age groups, there is significant variability in the dose of an opioid needed to provide adequate analgesia, even in patients who are opioid-naïve. Polymorphisms in the genes that

Table 20.3 Commonly used opioid drugs

Agent	Equianalgesic dosing (mg)		Initial oral dose		Bioavailability (%)	Duration (h)	Comments
	Oral	Parenteral	Adult [>50 kg](mg)	Children (mg/kg)			
Mu (μ) agonist drugs							
Codeine	200	NA	30–60	0.5–1	15–80	3–4	Oral use only. Prescribed with APAP as tablet or elixir. Nausea/constipation very common. ~10% of people lack enzyme to make codeine to active morphine agent.
Hydrocodone		NA	5–10	0.1–0.2	60–80	3–4	Oral use only. Usually prescribed with APAP.
Oxycodone	15–20 mg	NA	5–10	0.1–0.2	60–80	3–4	Oral use only. Sustained-release tablet is available. Usually prescribed with APAP.
Morphine	30 mg (short term)/60 mg (single dose)	10 mg	20–50	0.3	20–40	3–4	"Gold Standard" for pain treatment. Available as sustained-release tablet (8–12, 24 h duration) and as liquid formulation (2–20 mg/mL). Inexpensive. May cause histamine release and vasodilation.
Hydromorphone	6–8 mg	1.5–2 mg	2–4	0.04–0.08	50–70	3–4	Often used when morphine causes intolerable side effects. Less itching and nausea usually compared to morphine. Useful in patients with decreased renal clearance.
Fentanyl	NA	0.1 mg (100 μg)	NA	NA		0.5–1	Very effective for short painful procedural pain. Oral transmucosal dose is 10–15 μg/kg. May cause nausea/vomiting (20–30%), bradycardia or chest wall rigidity-Rx with naloxone or muscle relaxants.
Meperidine	300 mg	75–100 mg	100–150 mg	2–3 mg/kg	40–60	3–4	Metabolite (normeperidine) may cause CNS excitation and seizures. Potential fatal interaction with MAO inhibitors. May cause tachycardia and is a negative inotrope. Not recommended for routine use.
Methadone	10–20 mg	10 mg	5–10 mg	0.1–0.2 mg/kg	70–100	12–36	Available as liquid preparation. Long duration of action. See text for dosing when pt is on chronic opioid use (varies [4–20X] due to incomplete cross tolerance). May prolong QT interval and some advocate ECG prior to starting therapy and regularly while on therapy.
Weak mu (μ) agonist-monoamine reuptake inhibitor							
Tramadol			50–100	1–3	68 (first dose), 90–100 (multiple doses)	3–6	Maximum dose is 400 mg/day or 8 mg/kg/day. Available as extended-release tablet. May lower seizure threshold in patients susceptible. Rarely associated with serotonergic syndrome.

APAP acetaminophen, *MAO* monoamine oxidase

control the mu-receptor and the melanocortin-1 receptor, as well as genes that regulate the agents of opioid metabolism (e.g., the cytochrome P_{450} 2D6 isozyme) are likely to account for some of this variability (Pasternak 2001; Pasternak 2005). It is important to obtain a pain medication history to elicit information on the efficacy and adverse effects of opioids used previously. Some patients will respond better to one opioid than another, even when the two opioids are from the same class; therefore, serial trials of opioids should be used to determine the most effective agent for the patient who is experiencing partial pain relief or significant adverse effects. Providers should administer opioid agents at regular intervals according to the predicted pharmacokinetics of the drug with "rescue" dosing for breakthrough pain. The typical "rescue" dose is 5–10% of the daily requirement of the opioid which can be given as frequently as every one hour for unrelieved pain. Escalation of dosing with incorporation of the breakthrough doses is encouraged to titrate to effect or side effects. Key concepts for the use of opioids for pain management include titration to effect, a goal for steady state analgesia, anticipation and treatment of side effects, and use of equianalgesic doses when switching opioids in patients who are opioid-naïve.

Codeine, hydroxycodone, and oxycodone are commonly used oral opioids to treat pain in children. The sustained-released formulations of oxycodone, hydromorphone, and morphine, as well as methadone, are more commonly used to treat chronic pain in children. Often, codeine, hydrocodone, and oxycodone are administered in combination with acetaminophen (Tylenol® with Codeine #1-#4, Tylenol® with codeine elixir, Vicodin®, Lortab®, Percocet®, and Tylox®). These agents will have similar efficacy (analgesia, cough suppression) and adverse effects (sedation, nausea, vomiting, constipation, respiratory depression) when given at equipotent dosing. Codeine, hydroxycodone, and oxycodone have an oral bioavailability of approximately 60%, and achieve analgesic efficacy within 20 min after oral dosing. The elimination half-life of these agents is 2.5–4 h so they are often prescribed every 4–6 h for pain control.

Codeine has a variable bioavailability (15–80%) but also is an inactive prodrug that has analgesic efficacy only via metabolism to morphine. This metabolism is dependent on the mixed function oxidases with the cytochrome P_{450} 2D6 enzyme isomer. There are slow metabolizers of codeine (Caucasian 10%, Chinese 30%), and the drug is ineffective for these patients while 5% of the population will be ultra-rapid metabolizers with increased concentrations of morphine (Williams et al. 2001). Typically, codeine is prescribed at a dose between 0.5 and 1 mg/kg/dose. Tylenol with codeine elixir contains 120 mg of acetaminophen and 12 mg of codeine in each 5 ml (1 tsp). Tylenol #1-#4 tablets contain acetaminophen with varying amounts of codeine per tablet: Tylenol #1 (7.5 mg), #2 (15 mg), #3 (30 mg), #4 (60 mg). The acetaminophen (APAP) will potentiate the analgesia and allows, through the opioid-sparing effects, a lower dose of opioid. However, these agents, if used beyond the recommended dose, may lead to acetaminophen toxicity, and the FDA is considering the removal of all combination APAP/opioid drugs from the US market to avoid this potential hazard.

Hydrocodone is prescribed at a dose of 0.1–0.2 mg/kg/dose and is available as an elixir or tablet combined with acetaminophen. Each 5 ml of the elixir contains 2.5 mg of hydrocodone and 167 mg of APAP. Tablets are available which contain between 2.5 and 10 mg of hydrocodone and 500–650 mg of APAP. Oxycodone is a semi-synthetic opioid with mu and kappa-receptor activity which is also prescribed at a dose between 0.1–0.2 mg/kg/dose and is most commonly available as a tablet combined with acetaminophen; Percocet® contains APAP 325 mg with 5 mg oxycodone, and Tylox® contains APA P 500 mg with 5 mg oxycodone. Oxycodone is available as an elixir (without acetaminophen) with a concentration of 1 mg/ml or 20 mg/ml. Oxycodone is also available with acetaminophen as a sustained-released tablet (OxyContin®) for use with patients with chronic pain. This sustained-release formulation allows for BID or TID dosing and should only be used for opioid-tolerant patients. If the tablet is crushed or chewed, large doses of the agent can be released resulting in potentially serious respiratory or cardiovascular injury.

Tramadol is a synthetic 4-phenyl-piperidine analog of codeine which is a racemic mixture of (+) and (−) entantiomers that is a weak mu-receptor opioid agonist and norepinephrine/serotonin reuptake inhibitor used for mild to moderate pain. It has been used in Europe for many decades and is becoming more popular in the USA. The opioid activity of tramadol results from low affinity binding of the (+) entantiomer to mu-opioid receptors. Tramadol has no affinity for the delta or kappa-opioid receptors. The (+) entantiomer inhibits serotonin uptake and has a direct serotonin-releasing action while the (−) entantiomer is an inhibitor of norepinephrine reuptake.

It is metabolized in the liver to O-desmethyltramadol by the cytochrome P_{450} system (cytochrome P_{450} 2D6 and cytochrome P_{450} 3A4 isozymes). The drug undergoes extensive first-pass metabolism in the liver. Tramadol is largely eliminated by the kidney (90%) and has nausea/vomiting, dizziness, constipation, and sedation as common side effects. It should be used cautiously in patients with a history of seizure disorder or with medications that potentially lower the seizure threshold. It has also been associated with serotonergic syndrome in some patients with concomitant risk factors (Bozkurt 2005). The use of 5-HT_3 antagonists (e.g., ondansetron) may decrease the efficacy of tramadol via the 5-HT_3 receptor (De Witte et al. 2001).

In adults, oral tramadol has a bioavailability of 68% after the first dose and 90–100% after multiple doses. The time to onset is 30–60 min and the time to peak concentration is 2 h. Tramadol is supplied as a 50 mg oral tablet or as an extended-release tablet (Ultram ER®-100, 200, or 300 mg). It can be used as a compounded liquid with stability of 30 days. The typical dose for children <50 kg is 1–3 mg/kg/dose given every 3–6 h [max dose 8 mg/kg/day] or 50–100 mg every 3–6 h in patients weighing ≥50kg [max dose 400 mg/day]. It is recommended as a potential analgesic in step 2 of the World Health Organization's guidelines for the treatment of patients with cancer pain (Leppert and Luczak 2005). In a study by Rose et al. for the treatment of chronic pain in children, tramadol had good efficacy and was well tolerated (Rose et al. 2003).

Potent opioids are used for the treatment of moderate to severe pain. Oral dosing is the most common route of administration; however, intravenous, subcutaneous injection/infusion, rectal dosing, and transdermal dosing options are used as needed. Morphine is the "gold standard" for pain management and is often the first-choice opioid prescribed for chronic cancer pain due to the long track record of safe use, the availability of the agent in various formulations, and its hydrophilicity. Morphine, of all the opioid agents, has been studied the most extensively in children. Morphine is metabolized in the liver principally by uridine diphosphate glucuronosyltransferases (UDPGT) into two compounds; morphine-6-glucuronide (M6G, a potent analgesic and respiratory depressant) and morphine-3-glucuronide (M3G, which antagonizes the action of morphine and M6G). Morphine and its metabolites are excreted via the kidneys so it should be used cautiously in the presence of renal disease/failure. Morphine has poor oral bioavailability (20–30%), has histamine release associated with its use, and may cause vasodilatation with hypotension in hypovolemic patients. Morphine is a very hydrophilic compound and does not cross the blood–brain barrier very well. The clearance and elimination half-life of morphine are shorter in children than adults, and a smaller dosing interval may be necessary to achieve adequate pain control (Hain et al. 1999; Hunt et al. 1999). Immediate-release morphine should be prescribed with a dosing frequency of every 2–4 h.

Hydromorphone is a morphine analog with similar pharmacokinetic and pharmacodynamic properties but is 5–7.5 times more potent than morphine with minimal active metabolites so it may be useful in patients with renal disease. Systematic reviews in adult patients have not demonstrated any differences between morphine and hydromorphone with respect to analgesic efficacy, adverse effects, or patient preference (Quigley and Wiffen 2003). Fentanyl is a highly lipid-soluble synthetic opioid with a rapid onset of action. It is 50–100 times more potent than morphine and has no active metabolites. Tolerance and dependence may occur rapidly, and fentanyl is available as a transdermal patch for patients with chronic pain. The transdermal fentanyl is absorbed across the skin and is stored in the upper layers of the skin providing a secondary reservoir of agent which contributes to the prolonged action of the drug even after removal of the patch. Transdermal fentanyl should only be used for opioid-tolerant individuals for chronic pain. The fentanyl patch is available in the following sizes: 12.5 mcg/h, 25 mcg/h, 50 mcg/h, 75 mcg/h, and 100 mcg/h. The patches cannot be physically cut into smaller pieces so must be placed intact on the skin (Finkel et al. 2005; Zernikow et al. 2007). Fentanyl is also available as a buccal transmucosal oralet (Actiq®) for use for procedural pain or as an agent for breakthrough pain. The fentanyl is placed in a candy matrix such that buccal absorption occurs with subsequent rapid systemic absorption of agent (10–20 min). The typical dose of transmucosal fentanyl is 10–15 mcg/kg and will last for approximately 2 h. The major adverse effects of transmucosal fentanyl are nausea and vomiting with a prevalence of 20–33%. A new, rapidly dissolving buccal tablet, Fentora®, is also available for the treatment of breakthrough pain; the tablets are available in the following doses: 100, 200, 400, 600, and 800 mcg), and approximately 50% of the total dose is absorbed transmucosally and 50% is swallowed with slow absorption via the GI tract (Messina et al. 2008; Weinstein et al. 2009). There is only anecdotal use of this agent in children.

Methadone is a unique synthetic, long-acting opioid agonist that is a racemic mixture of two isomers. The drug is a μ-receptor opioid agonist with some activity also at the δ and κ receptors; it is also a *N*-methyl-D-aspartate (NMDA) receptor antagonist. The NMDA receptor is associated with central sensitization, wind-up phenomenon, opioid-induced hyperalgesia, and the development of tolerance; thus, methadone may prevent these detrimental effects via antagonism of the NMDA receptor (Ebert et al. 1998; Gorman et al. 1997). The L-isomer of methadone inhibits serotonin and norepinephrine reuptake as well. Methadone may be administered by the oral, rectal, intravenous, or nasal route. The drug is lipophilic with high oral bioavailability (80–90%) and is slowly metabolized in the liver. The metabolites of methadone

are not pharmacologically active. This agent has a long and unpredictable elimination half-life ranging from 12 to 200 h. A single dose of methadone may provide 12–36 h of analgesia (Gourlay et al. 1984). The analgesic efficacy is much shorter than the elimination half-life. The potency of methadone is roughly equal for opioid-naïve patients; however, the potency of methadone is 4–20 times that of oral morphine with opioid-tolerant patients. The conversion of oral morphine to methadone is dose-dependent and is as follows (Houlahan et al. 2006):

Oral morphine (mg/24 h)	Oral morphine/ oral methadone ratio
<100 mg	4:1
101–300 mg	8:1
301–600	10:1
601–1,000	15:1
>1,000	20:1

The practitioner must use caution when switching from another opioid to methadone. After using the table to calculate equianalgesic dose of methadone, the calculated dose should be decreased by 50%, because of methadone inhibition of NMDA receptor. The agent is usually given as BID or TID dosing. Methadone is also a potent blocker of the delayed rectifier potassium ion channel with can result in prolongation of the QT interval, torsade de pointes, and ventricular tachycardia in susceptible individuals (Andrews et al. 2009). The effect of methadone on the QT interval may be enhanced by hypokalemia or the concomitant use of CYP 3A4 inhibitors such as fluoxetine, Valproate, or clarithromycin (Andrews et al. 2009; Ehret et al. 2006). Some practitioners are advocating routine ECG prior to initiation of therapy with methadone and regular ECG assessment during therapy.

Adverse effects due to opioids are not uncommon, and constipation is a predictable side effect with prolonged use. It occurs in virtually all cases, so a prescription to treat constipation should be administered as soon as an opioid is started. Sedation with opioid use is common and can significantly impact the child and the family's quality of life. If sedation doesn't dissipate after a few days, add an adjuvant drug and decrease the opioid dose, give the patient a stimulant such as methylphenidate or dextroamphetamine, or consider switching to a different opioid. Nausea and/ or vomiting may occur with opioid use and can be treated by opioid rotation, the use of selective 5-HT_3 receptor antagonists such as ondansetron, the addition of a bowel stimulant such as metoclopramide (Watcha and White 1992), or the use of an ultra-low dose naloxone infusion (0.25–1 mcg/kg/h) in patients with IV access (Maxwell et al. 2005). Pruritis is treated by opioid rotation, use of adjuvants to decrease opioid dose, or antipruretics such as naloxone (Maxwell et al. 2005), nalbuphine (Kendrick et al. 1996), or diphenhydramine. Respiratory depression is another potential side effect of opioids and is often cited by practitioners as a reason for not prescribing opioid analgesics for pain. However, an opioid-induced respiratory depression is less common than many practitioners believe and can largely be avoided with standard dosage titration and frequent monitoring in at-risk patients. Respiratory depression, if it does occur, is treatable with an opioid antagonist, stimulation, and bag/mask ventilation if necessary. Unless the patient is experiencing severe respiratory depression with hypoxia, small doses of naloxone (1–2 mcg/kg/dose) given every few minutes will often improve sedation without reversing the analgesic effects of the opioid. The patient will usually develop tolerance to the analgesic efficacy and the adverse effects of opioids with prolonged use with the exception of constipation. Frequent monitoring for efficacy and the development of adverse effects is needed, and, if the patient is developing tolerance to the medication, then the provider should consider opioid rotation. Switching to another agent will take advantage of the phenomenon of incomplete cross-tolerance in which lower doses vis-à-vis the recommended equianalgesic dose can be used with analgesic efficacy.

Co-analgesics/Adjuvant Analgesics

These are a diverse group of medications that may enhance the effects of nonopioid or opioid analgesics, have independent analgesic activity in certain pain syndromes or conditions, or counteract the side effects of analgesics. They represent multiple drug classes including the following: antidepressants, anticonvulsants, local anesthetics, corticosteroids, antispasmodic agents, benzodiazepines, alpha-2 adrenergic agents, NMDA-receptor antagonists, stimulants, skeletal muscle relaxants, bisphosphonates, calcitonin, radionucleotides, and cannabinoids. For many of these agents, their primary indication is for conditions other than pain. These adjuvant agents are especially useful for the treatment of neuropathic pain which may be a common problem in many chronic pain conditions; in fact, approximately 40–50% of adults with cancer have neuropathic pain, usually in combination with nociceptive pain (Manfredi et al. 2003). These medications are very commonly added to opioids to improve pain relief, manage refractory pain, or allow lower doses of opioids to reduce side effects. As with any medications, the use of these agents to treat chronic pain involves the weighing of potential benefit of the therapy compared to the risks and adverse effects of the therapy. Many of these medications may be safely used in children if the dose is adjusted for the weight of the patient; however, most of these medications do not have FDA approval for use in children. The efficacy and safety of these agents may not have been adequately evaluated in well-designed clinical trials in children (Table 20.4).

Antidepressants

Antidepressants are useful agents in the management of chronic pain (Saarto and Wiffen 2007). There are a variety of potential mechanisms of action for these drugs including the following: monoamine modulation, interactions with opioids, affecting the descending inhibitory pathways for pain expression, and ion-channel blocking. These agents block the presynaptic reuptake of serotonin and/or norepinephrine in the CNS, stabilize neuronal membranes through inhibition of sodium channels, and inhibit neuronal hyperexcitability through NMDA antagonist-like effects (Sindrup et al. 2005). They also provide improved pain control and well-being by their beneficial treatment of depressive symptoms and insomnia that often occur concomitantly with chronic pain.

Table 20.4 Adjuvant analgesics for chronic pain management

Class of agent	Usual effective adult		Pediatric dose	Comments
	Initial adult dose	Dose		
Antidepressants				
Tricyclic antidepressants (TCAs)				
Amitriptyline	10–25 mg qhs	50–150 mg qhs	Initial dose 0.2–0.3 mg/kg qhs or BID Titrate: 0.25 mg/kg (10–25 mg) every 5–7 days Maintenance: 0.2–3 mg/kg (10–150 mg)	Obtain ECG prior to therapy to rule out cardiac dysrhythmias, escalate dose over days to weeks, very sedating, anticholinergic side effects, drug levels are available. Analgesic effects typically seen with doses lower than usually needed to treat depression and response often seen within 5–7 days. Max dose is 150 mg for adults or 3 mg/kg/day in children.
Nortriptyline	10–25 mg qhs	50–150 mg qhs	As above for amitriptyline.	Fewer anticholinergic side effects and less sedating than amitriptyline, drug levels available, agent available as elixir (10 mg/5 mL), common first line Max dose is 150 mg for adults or 3 mg/kg/day in children. Agent for neuropathic pain.
Desimpramine	10–25 mg qhs	50–150 mg qhs	Safety	Fewer side effects than amitriptyline. Rare case reports of sudden death in children. Max dose is 150 mg for adults or 3 mg/kg/day in children.
Serotonin norepinephrine reuptake inhibitors (SNRIs)				
Venlafaxine	37.5 mg qd	150–225 mg qd	Safety and efficacy not determined for pediatric patients. 1–2 mg/kg as divided doses	Structurally similar to tramadol. Modulates allodynia and hyperalgesia in experimental pain models. Better tolerated than TCAs with no anticholinergic or antihistaminergic side effects. 5% of pts will develop ECG changes so monitoring suggested.
Duloxetine	20 mg qd	60 mg qd	Safety and efficacy not determined for pediatric patients.	FDA-approved for Rx of painful diabetic neuropathies.
Selective serotonin reuptake inhibitors (SSRIs)				
Paroxetine	10–20 mg qd	20–40 mg qd	Safety and efficacy not determined for pediatric patients.	SSRIs block metabolism of TCAs via inhibition of cytochrome P$_{450}$ 2D6 and may increase TCA blood levels. Relatively ineffective as analgesics but useful for concurrent depression and anxiety.
Citalopram	10–20 mg qd	20–40 mg qd	Safety and efficacy not determined for pediatric patients.	More selective SSRI that does not interact with TCAs via the P450 system.
Antiepileptic drugs (AEDs)				
Calcium-channel a$_2$-δ ligands				
Gabapentin	100–300 mg qhs	300–1,200 mg TID	Initial dose 2 mg/kg/day. Titrate to 5–30 mg/kg/day as TID dosing	Typically used as first line agent for neuropathic pain. May have opioid-sparing effect for cancer pain. Low toxicity profile and very few drug interactions. Does not act on GABA receptors or sodium channels. Available as oral solution 250 mg/5 mL.

(continued)

Table 20.4 (continued)

Class of agent	Usual effective adult Initial adult dose	Dose	Pediatric dose	Comments
Pregabalin	75–150 mg qd	300–600 mg daily as BID dosing	Not FDA-approved for use in children.	Weight gain occurs with some patients. Faster titration than gabapentin with faster pain relief.
Sodium-channel blockers				
Carbamazepine	100–200 mg qd	300–800 mg qd	Initial: 10 mg/kg/day as BID/TID dosing. Titrate by 100 mg/day at weekly intervals as needed. Do not exceed 800 mg or 30 mg/kg/day.	Many drug–drug interactions. Monitor hematological function (CBC) prior to and during therapy. Side effects common and include hematologic, CNS, and cardiac. Oral suspension (100 mg/5 mL) is available. Drug levels available.
Other anticonvulsants not commonly used				
Lamotrigine	25 mg qd	100–200 mg BID	Seizure dosing: 0.15 mg/kg/day (rounded to nearest whole tablet) in 1–2 divided doses for 2 weeks, and then 0.3 mg/kg/day (rounded to nearest whole tablet) in 1–2 divided doses. Increase to usual maintenance dose of 1–5 mg/kg/day (max 200 mg).	Adverse effects include somnolence, dizziness, and ataxia. Rarely associated with Stevens-Johnson syndrome.
Topiramate	25 mg qd	100–200 mg BID	1–3 mg/kg/day qhs for 1 week, then increase dose by 1–3 mg/kg/day (as BID dosing) at 1–2 week intervals to usual 25–400 mg/day	May cause hyperchloremic non ion gap metabolic acidosis so periodic measurement of sodium bicarb levels during Rx is recommended.
Valproate	250 mg TID	500–1,000 mg TID	Initial dose of 10–15 mg/kg/day. Titrate to maximum of 30–60 mg/kg/day as TID dosing.	Approved as migraine prophylaxis in adults but not for children.
a₂-adrenergic agents				
Clonidine	0.1 mg po qd	Variable	2–5 µg/kg/day po as TID/QID dosing or as 0.1 mg transdermal patch. Epidural dosing is 1–2 µg/kg loading dose with continuous epidural infusion of 0.02–0.1 µg/kg/h to maximum epidural dose of 0.2 µg/kg/h).	Side effects include bradycardia, hypotension, and sedation which limit clinical utility.

NMDA-receptor antagonists

Ketamine	0.2–0.5 mg/kg IV loading dose	0.2–0.5 mg/kg IV loading dose over 30 min f/b continuous infusion between 0.14 and 0.5 mg/kg/h	Not FDA-approved for use in children <16 years of age.	Elevates pain threshold and is used as co-analgesic with opioids. Useful for neuropathic pain as well as attenuation of opioid-induced hyperalgesia. Oral ketamine has poor bioavailability (20%).
Dextromethorphan	15–20 mg TID	Unknown		Not commonly used as analgesic.
Memantine	5 mg qd	10 mg BID	Safety and efficacy not established for children.	Safely used for the treatment of autism spectrum disorders in children.

Membrane stabilizers/local anesthetics

lidocaine IV	2 mg/kg over 2 min	2–5 mg/kg	1–5 mg/kg IV administered over 15–60 min depending on total dose	Measure plasma level every 8–12 h and maintain 2–5 µg/mL.
Topical 5% lidocaine patch	1 patch 12 h/24 h	1–3 patches 12 h/24 h	Cut to fit no more than 1 patch for 12 h/24 h	FDA-approved for PHN and useful for many neuropathic pain syndromes in adults. Cut patch as needed without loss of agent and can be used over multiple areas topically. Minimal systemic effects and plasma concentrations.
Mexiletine	150 mg qd	100–300 mg TID	Initial dose: 2–3 mg/kg (or 150–200 mg) po qd to TID. Titrate 0.5 mg/kg (or 25–50 mg) every 2–3 weeks. Maintenance dose: 2–8 mg/kg (150–400 mg) po qd to TID. Max dose 1,800 mg/day	Frequent side effects limit the utility of this agent and include nausea/vomiting, sedation, ataxia. IV lidocaine trial may predict success of this agent. Drug levels available.

Corticosteroids

Dexamethasone	4 mg BID	Variable	0.02–0.03 mg/kg/day as TID/QID dosing	Indication for use is rapidly escalating pain with significant functional impairment. Side effects include weight gain, edema, dyspepsia, osteoporosis, Cushing's syndrome, psychosis.

BID twice a day, *TID* three times a day, *QID* four times a day, *PHN* postherpetic neuralgia

Antidepressants have analgesic effects that are independent of their antidepressant effects.

Several systematic reviews and meta-analyses have determined that tricyclic antidepressants (TCAs) are effective for many neuropathic pain syndromes [postherpetic neuralgia (PHN), painful peripheral diabetic neuropathy, central post-stroke pain, and trigeminal neuralgia]; however, they do not appear to be useful in the treatment of HIV-related neuropathies (Saarto and Wiffen 2007; Sindrup et al. 2005). TCAs are inexpensive, effective, and usually require once-daily dosing (potentially improving compliance with treatment); thus, they are often first-line medications for the treatment of neuropathic pain. Secondary amine TCAs (nortriptyline and desimpramine) are better tolerated than the tertiary amines (amitriptyline/imipramine) and are equally efficacious. Nortriptyline has less anticholinergic side effects than amitriptyline, and is a common first-line agent used in the treatment of neuropathic pain. Nortriptyline is available in liquid form (10 mg/5 ml solution) for use in young children or given via gastrostomy tube in patients unable to take medications orally. Common side effects include sedation, dry mouth, orthostatic hypotension, constipation, urinary retention, and tachycardia (Knotkova and Pappagallo 2007; Kong and Irwin 2009).

A small number of patients who have received TCAs have had sudden death attributed to dysrhythmia (Amitai and Frischer 2006). It is unknown whether these children had a preexisting conduction disturbance, and these drugs have been used safely in children for decades. A baseline ECG should be obtained to rule out rhythm disturbances prior to starting a TCA and also when escalated to a full antidepressant dose range (Dworkin et al. 2007). These drugs should be used with extreme caution in patients with preexisting rhythm disturbances or cardiomyopathy. There is no established correlation between plasma concentration of TCAs and analgesic efficacy; therefore, routine measurement of plasma drug levels is useful only to determine patient compliance, optimization of dose before aborting a therapeutic trial, or to identify patients that need dosing modification based on metabolism of the drug (i.e., those patients who may need $b.i.d.$ dosing). If the drug needs to be discontinued for any reason, the dosing should be tapered over 1–2 weeks to avoid irritability and agitation.

Other antidepressants have been used for neuropathic pain but have not provided similar efficacy compared to the tricyclic antidepressants. Serotonin and norepinephrine reuptake inhibitors (SNRIs) such as duloxetine (Cymbalta®) and venlafaxine (Effexor®) do not possess the anticholinergic and antihistaminergic effects of the TCAs. Venlafaxine has been demonstrated to modulate allodynia and hyperalgesia in human models and to relieve neuropathic pain associated with breast cancer (Grothe et al. 2004; Rowbotham et al. 2004). Duloxetine has been recently approved by the FDA for the treatment of pain associated with diabetic neuropathy (Fishbain et al. 2006; Wernicke et al. 2006; Wernicke et al. 2007). In a study by Meighen, duloxetine was shown to be effective in the treatment of chronic pain and co-morbid depressive disorders in two adolescents (Meighen 2007). The selective serotonin reuptake inhibitors (SSRI) such as paroxetine and fluoxetine are relatively ineffective as analgesics but are helpful with associated depression, sleep disturbance, and anxiety (Max et al. 1992).

Anticonvulsant Drugs (AEDs)

Anticonvulsant or antiepileptic agents are a diverse group of agents with varied mechanisms of action to treat pain. These drugs are often first-line agents for the treatment of neuropathic pain and other painful chronic or recurrent pain conditions such as migraine headaches. The primary mechanism of action of these agents is to reduce the ectopic, spontaneous firing of cortical neurons which cause seizures leading to a dampening or attenuation of the neuronal excitability. It is presumed that these agents also reduce the ectopic, spontaneous firing of sensory neurons in the spinal dorsal horn or dorsal root ganglion (DRG) leading to the up-regulation of Na^+ and Ca^{++} after nerve injury which may lead to the onset of neuropathic pain and sensitization.

The calcium-channel α-2-δ ligands [gabapentin (Neurontin®)/pregabalin (Lyrica®)]

have established efficacy in the treatment of neuropathic pain and are common first-line agents in adults, and gabapentin is commonly used in pediatric pain management (Butkovic et al. 2006; Dayioglu et al. 2008). There are few studies of the use of pregabalin in pediatric patients for pain management (Vondracek et al. 2009). Gabapentin and pregabalin do not act on the γ-aminobutyric acid (GABA) receptors or sodium channels. These agents modulate the cellular calcium influx into nociceptive neurons by binding to the voltage-gated calcium channel (especially the $\alpha_2\delta$ subunit) resulting in decreased release of glutamine, norepinephrine, and substance P. Calcium-channel alpha-2-delta ligands such as gabapentin and pregabalin have been shown to be useful for the treatment of phantom limb pain, neuropathic cancer pain, and peripheral neuropathies. There are a few case reports describing the utility of gabapentin and pregabalin for the treatment of neuropathic pain in children (Butkovic et al. 2006; Carrazana and Mikoshiba 2003; Dayioglu et al. 2008; Lauder and White 2005; Vondracek et al. 2009).

Gabapentin has become the first-line drug for the treatment of postherpetic neuralgia (PHN), painful diabetic peripheral neuropathy, phantom limb pain, Guillian-Barré syndrome, neuropathic cancer pain, and chronic spinal cord injury; multiple randomized controlled trials have shown greater pain relief vs. placebo in these conditions. Improved sleep, mood, and health-related quality of life (HRQOL) has also been reported in some of these studies. Gabapentin may also be associated with an opioid-sparing effect for patients with cancer-associated pain. The typical adult dose is 100–300 mg qhs with titration every 3 days to effective doses (usually 1,800–3,600 mg/day as TID dosing). The typical pediatric dose is 2 mg/kg/day titrated to 5–50 mg/kg/day as TID dosing. The drug is available as 100, 300, and 400 mg capsules; 600 and 800 mg film-coated tablets, and 250 mg/5 ml oral solution. The capsules may be opened and mixed with liquid or food, but they are bitter-tasting. Gabapentin has a low toxicity profile and does not usually interact with other medications. If adverse effects occur, it is usually early in the course of treatment.

Typical side effects seen with gabapentin include dizziness, somnolence, ataxia, fatigue, myalgias, impaired concentration, and peripheral edema. Dosing frequency is greater for these medications compared to the tricyclic antidepressants, and common adverse effects include sedation and ataxia.

Pregabalin is the first FDA-approved medication for the treatment of fibromyalgia and has strong evidence of analgesic efficacy. The efficacy of pregabalin has been demonstrated in multiple randomized controlled trials in adults for the treatment of various neuropathic pain syndromes such as PHN, painful peripheral diabetic neuropathy, mixed neuropathic pain, and spinal cord injury pain. As with many agents, pregabalin is not FDA-approved for use in children. One open-label study in 30 pediatric oncology patients with neuropathic pain demonstrated a significant improvement in symptoms with very infrequent adverse effects (Vondracek et al. 2009).

Carbamazepine (Tegretol®) is the most widely studied anticonvulsant drug for the management of neuropathic pain, especially in the treatment of lancinating neuropathic pain from nerve root injury. It is very effective for the treatment of trigeminal neuralgia. The mechanism of action is blockade of voltage-dependent sodium channels, reducing ectopic nerve discharges. The number needed to treat (NNT) for neuropathic pain is 2.5. This agent has a less favorable side effect profile and requires monitoring of hematological function (CBC prior to therapy and every 3–6 months while receiving the agent) so clinicians are not using this agent as a first-line therapy very often. Adult dosing is 100–200 mg daily with titration to 300–800 mg BID. The recommended pediatric dosing is 10 mg/kg/day as BID or TID dosing initially with titration by 100 mg weekly as needed [max dose 30 mg/kg/day]. A suspension of 100 mg/5 cc is available for use. Common adverse effects are hematologic (aplastic anemia, agranulocytosis), cardiovascular (CHF, syncope, dysrhythmias), CNS (sedation, dizziness, fatigue, slurred speech, ataxia), and hepatitis (Lussier et al. 2004). Oxcarbazepine (Trileptal®) is the keto-analog of carbamazepine, and its mechanism of action is to inhibit voltage-sensitive sodium channels as well as high-voltage-activated calcium channels. Recent open-label studies have shown potential efficacy in the treatment of painful peripheral diabetic neuropathy (Carrazana and Mikoshiba 2003), and a case report in the literature showed improvement in pain control in a child with complex regional pain syndrome (CRPS) refractory to other treatments (Lalwani et al. 2005). At this time, without evidence of efficacy and safety, routine use of this agent is not recommended.

Several newer anticonvulsant drugs (lamotrigine, topiramate, zonisamide, and levetiracetam) have been studied for efficacy in a variety of pain conditions in adults, especially primary headache management. Despite the broad use of these agents for the treatment of neuropathic pain, no trials have been conducted in the pediatric population. Thus, at this time, there is inadequate evidence to recommend the use of these agents for the treatment of neuropathic pain in children. Topiramate and valproate are approved for migraine prophylaxis in adults; however, no AEDs have been approved for migraine prophylaxis in children. Open-label studies and chart reviews have supported the use of valproate for this purpose, and topiramate and levetiracetam have been evaluated for pediatric migraine prophylaxis with promising results. However, currently no AED is formally recommended for migraine prophylaxis in children and adolescents.

α_2 – Adrenergic Agents

The α_2-adrenergic agents, clonidine, tizanidine, and dexmedetomidine, are agents used for analgesia and sedation; the mechanism of action of these agents is by modulation of norepinephrine by the α_2 receptor subtype in the spinal cord leading to analgesia. Clonidine is a well-known agent that has been used clinically to treat neuropathic pain associated with diabetes. Clonidine can be administered via the oral, transdermal, or epidural route. Clonidine is known to potentiate the analgesic effect of opioids. Clonidine increases the release of acetylcholine at the spinal dorsal horn and activates spinal acetylcholine receptors enhancing the sensory and motor block of C fibers and A-δ fibers by local anesthetics. The epidural

administration of clonidine results in a peak analgesic effect within 60 min and a duration of effect as long as 6 h. Most pediatric studies of clonidine have focused on the epidural use in post-operative pain management. Extrapolation of adult dosing has led to a recommended loading dose of 1–2 mcg/kg with a continuous epidural infusion of 0.02–0.1 mcg/kg/h titrating to a maximum dose of 0.2 mcg/kg/h.

Transdermal clonidine has been demonstrated to be useful for some patients with painful peripheral diabetic neuropathy, and oral clonidine has been effective in the treatment of postherpetic neuralgia in a clinical trial in adults (Byas-Smith et al. 1995). Clonidine is given as 2–5 mcg/kg/day orally as every 6–8 h dosing (TID/QID) or as a 0.1 mg transdermal patch. The analgesic benefits of clonidine are only supported with limited data, and the side effect profile (bradycardia, hypotension, and sedation) limits its usefulness in some situations. Thus, it is not a first-line agent for chronic pain. Tizanidine is principally used for the management of spasticity and is reported to be useful for the treatment of some neuropathic pain disorders, chronic daily headache, migraine prophylaxis, and chronic back pain in adults (Semenchuk and Sherman 2000).

NMDA-Receptor Antagonists

Central and peripheral NMDA receptors may have a role in the management of hyperalgesia and chronic pain. NMDA receptors in the spinal cord are activated by repeated stimuli in nociceptive afferent nerves leading to central sensitization of dorsal horn cells resulting in perpetuation of pain sensation and reduced opioid sensitivity. NMDA antagonists may reduce pain by two mechanisms: reduction in central sensitization and reduction in opioid tolerance. The NMDA receptor is associated with the development of tolerance and hyperalgesia from opioids so NMDA receptor antagonists have been used to attenuate or reverse these effects. The N-methyl-D-aspartate (NMDA) receptor antagonists (ketamine, methadone, dextromethorphan, memantine, and amantadine) would theoretically have utility for the management of hyperalgesic neuropathic pain that is poorly responsive to opioids.

Ketamine is an NMDA-receptor antagonist that is used as an analgesic adjuvant in poorly controlled pain (Finkel et al. 2007). Ketamine is a mixture of two entantiomers, and the S (+) entantiomer has 4X the potency of the R (−) entantiomer. It is a noncompetitive antagonist of the NMDA receptor. Ketamine is also an opioid-receptor agonist and a serotonin/norepinephrine reuptake inhibitor. It elevates the pain threshold and is used as a co-analgesic with opioids. Subtherapeutic dosing of 0.25–0.5 mg/kg loading dose over 30 min followed by a continuous infusion between 0.14 and 0.5 mg/kg/h may be useful for neuropathic pain as well as attenuation of opioid-induced hyperalgesia (Tsui et al. 2004). NMDA-receptor blocking agents such as ketamine have been shown to decrease opioid requirements and improve pain control in a few case reports (Finkel et al. 2007; Grande et al. 2008).

The onset of action of ketamine is within 1–3 min of dosing due to the drug's lipophilicity and small size. Ketamine likely provides an additive analgesic effect as well as reversing opioid tolerance. Ketamine is metabolized to norketamine which has 1/3rd of the potency of the parent compound. Ketamine has a short elimination half-life of approximately 3 h so steady-state would be achieved in 12–15 h from the initial administration of the agent. Oral ketamine has poor oral bioavailability (20%) with 80% of the dose metabolized to norketamine at the first-pass. Adverse effects from ketamine include hypertension, tachycardia, increased muscle tone, increased ICP, pyschomimetic effects (alterations in body image and mood, floating sensations, vivid dreams, hallucinations, delirium, and drowsiness). Rarely, respiratory depression may occur with use of ketamine.

Other NMDA-antagonists such as dextromethorphan and memantine have not been commonly used for children with neuropathic pain. Memantine is a relatively newer NDMA-antagonist that is FDA approved for the treatment of dementia in moderate to severe Alzheimer disease. Studies to date with this drug for neuropathic pain has led to equivocal results (Rogers et al. 2009) with some investigators reporting successful treatment with CRPS (Sinis et al. 2007) while others have reported no analgesic efficacy with chronic phantom limb pain (Wiech et al. 2004). One study suggested that early use of memantine after surgical amputation was effective in reducing phantom limb pain (Schley et al. 2007). There are no studies to support the use of memantine for the treatment of chronic pain in children although the drug has been shown to be safely used in pediatric patients for the treatment of autism spectrum disorders (Chez et al. 2007). Studies of the use of dextromethorphan as an analgesic in children have produced mixed results (Dawson et al. 2001; Rose et al. 1999), and it is not commonly used as an analgesic in children.

Membrane Stabilizers/Local Anesthetics
Both animal and human studies demonstrate that injured nerves develop abnormal, spontaneously active sodium channels at the site of nerve injury, along the damaged nerve, and at the dorsal root ganglion of the injured nerve. Local anesthetics will suppress the spontaneous firing of these aberrant sodium channels without affecting normal nerve conduction or cardiac impulse conduction. Membrane-stabilizing agents (lidocaine, mexiletine) are potentially useful in the treatment of neuropathic pain (Ferrini 2000; Kastrup et al. 1987; Tremont-Lukats et al. 2006). Lidocaine is a local anesthetic that is a nonselective sodium channel blocker which may be useful in the treatment of neuropathic pain; however, it is not a first-line agent in the treatment of chronic, neuropathic pain. Small studies have established that lidocaine is effective in the treatment of postherpetic neuralgia and painful peripheral diabetic neuropathy; it was shown to be more effective than placebo in the treatment of neuropathic pain and is generally well tolerated. There is conflicting data as to the effectiveness of lidocaine for cancer-related pain. A therapeutic response to lidocaine may predict a similar response to mexiletine, an oral congener of lidocaine that is an antiarrhythmic agent. Multiple dosing regimens have been reported for use, but the typical loading dose is 1–5 mg/kg IV administered over 15–60 min depending on the total dose. The time to analgesic effect is between 1 and 45 min.

If the patient has a therapeutic response to the lidocaine test, then the patient may be given a continuous infusion over hours or days if needed (e.g., palliative care).

Lidocaine is rapidly and extensively metabolized in the liver and is excreted by the kidneys. Serum lidocaine levels should be followed at steady state (elimination half-life is approximately 100 min so 3–5 half-lives would be 5–8 h; the target serum plasma level is 2–5 mg/mL. Adverse effects are related to dose of agent and can occur when serum levels are >5 mg/mL. Myoclonus will occur with serum levels at 8 mg/mL, seizures at >10 mg/mL, and cardiovascular collapse at levels >25 mg/mL.

The use of lidocaine infusion of opioid-refractory pain was reported by Sharma et al. In this phase II randomized, placebo-controlled crossover study of refractory cancer pain in 50 patients, an improvement in pain relief and decrease in analgesic use was seen with a 60-min infusion of lidocaine. The effect of treatment persisted for an average of 9 days and with minimal tolerable side effects of therapy (Sharma et al. 2009). In a study by Schwartzman et al. of 49 patients with CRPS who were given a 5-day IV infusion of lidocaine titrated to 5 ml/L, the majority of patients reported a significant reduction in pain and signs/symptoms of CRPS that persisted for approximately 3 months (Schwartzman et al. 2009). There are a few case reports of the use of lidocaine infusion for neuropathic pain in children. Massey et al. reported a successful treatment of a 5-year-old child with terminal cancer pain using a continuous lidocaine IV infusion between 35 and 50 mcg/kg/min over 4 days with excellent pain relief and no side effects (Massey et al. 2002). There is another case report of an 11-year old with erythromelalgia with numerous pain episodes daily (20–30/day), who was successfully treated with IV lidocaine infusion that was transitioned to oral mexiletine with significant decrease in the intensity and frequency of the pain episodes and greatly improved function (Nathan et al. 2005). Mexiletine was originally used as an oral cardiac antiarrhythmic analog of lidocaine, and it has been used to treat neuropathic pain which is responsive to lidocaine infusion. Mexiletine has been used in doses as high as 10 mg/kg daily to treat diabetic neuropathy as well as pain associated with peripheral nerve injuries. There is no pharmacokinetic or pharmacologic difference in the absorption or metabolism of mexiletine between adults and children. This agent is associated with frequent side effects which limit its utility as an analgesic for chronic pain; these adverse effects include nausea/vomiting, sedation, confusion, difficulty concentrating, diplopia, and ataxia.

More commonly, the 5% transdermal lidocaine patch is used for neuropathic pain. The topical lidocaine 5% patch (Lidoderm®) is FDA-approved for the treatment of PHN and is associated with a reduction in pain in a variety of neuropathic pain syndromes in adults, including painful peripheral diabetic neuropathy, CRPS, post-mastectomy pain, and HIV-associated neuropathy. It is applied for 12 h/day with a maximum use of three patches at one time in the adult patient. The patch may be cut to size without loss of agent and used over multiple areas topically. There are minimal systemic effects and plasma concentrations (1/10 for cardiac effects and 1/32 for toxicity). In a study of five adolescents with chronic neuropathic pain, the use of 5% lidocaine patches were associated with improved analgesia in 80% of patients (Nayak and Cunliffe 2008).

Other Adjuvant Agents

Corticosteroids (e.g., dexamethasone or prednisone) are effective for the treatment of inflammatory neuropathic pain associated with peripheral nerve injury, pain associated with bone metastasis, pain associated with bowel obstruction, and headache pain associated with increased intracranial pressure (Shih and Jackson 2007). The analgesic effect of corticosteroids has been described for a broad range of doses. Indication for the use of corticosteroids is usually rapidly escalating pain with significant functional impairment. Common adverse effects of corticosteroids when used chronically or at high doses include weight gain, edema, dyspepsia, osteoporosis, Cushing's syndrome, psychosis, and rarely GI bleeding (Knotkova and Pappagallo 2007).

Bisphosphonate therapy is useful for pain related to bone metastases and has been used for the treatment of pain due to complex regional pain syndrome (CRPS) (Cortet et al. 1997; Varenna et al. 2000). In a study by Simm et al., bisphosphonates were used to treat five patients with chronic recurrent multifocal osteomyelitis with an 80% response rate (Simm et al. 2008). Pamidronate was used to treat intractable, chronic neuropathic pain in two adolescents with no evidence of improvement in pain or function (Brown et al. 2005). Thus, there are a few conflicting reports concerning the potential efficacy of bisphosphonates for children with chronic pain. Adverse effects from use of bisphosphonates include electrolyte abnormalities, GI symptoms (dyspepsia, reflux, nausea, and abdominal pain), and osteonecrosis of the jaw.

Cannabinoids have been shown to have analgesic properties in animal models and clinical observations. The mechanism of action for analgesia is via a peripheral anti-inflammatory action (Knotkova and Pappagallo 2007). Cannabinoids have been reported to be helpful in the management of neuropathic pain associated with multiple sclerosis (Rog et al. 2005). Good evidence for the efficacy of cannabinoids is lacking; however, there is a report of the effective use of the synthetic cannabinoid CT-3 (1',1'-dimethylheptyl-Δ8-tetrahydrocannabinol-11-oic acid) for the treatment of chronic neuropathic pain (Karst et al. 2003). In a case report by Rudich et al., dronabinol (Marinol®) was reported to be effective in the treatment of chronic intractable neuropathic pain in two adolescents (Rudich et al. 2003). Adverse effects include cognitive impairment, psychosis, and sedation.

FDA and Pediatric Drugs

Although only 15% of drugs listed in the *Physicians' Desk Reference* have labeled indications for children, it is common practice that providers prescribe medications off-label for children. These off-label prescriptions include not only dose adjustments (often by weight or body surface area) via the labeled route for adult patients, but also use for illness or conditions not included in labeling, and use via routes of administration not included in the product label (e.g., nasal fentanyl or midazolam, and clonidine for regional nerve blockade). A recent review of the literature suggests that the pharmacokinetics and pharmacodynamics of medications in neonates and children may not be well predicted by adult values, and that children may likely require significant adjustments in dose or interval for optimal efficacy and to minimize side effects. The United States Congress has enacted several laws intended to directly promote drug development for children, and these measures have increased the amount of information on the safe and efficacious use of drugs for children. The Food and Drug Administration Modernization Act (FDAMA) was passed in 1997 (Food And Drug Administration 1997), and offered pharmaceutical companies a 6-month period of marketing exclusivity if they performed studies in pediatric patients in response to a written request issued by the FDA. Marketing exclusivity incentives were attached to a period of existing patent protection or exclusivity and have been effective in prompting industry to conduct needed pediatric trials for drugs with existing patent protection or exclusivity. However, this program did not provide any incentivization for the study of off-patent, mostly generic, drugs due to the costs and risks of performing pediatric medication trials. Often by the time a pediatric trial has been conceived or performed, the drug is nearing its patent expiration and the trials cannot be completed in time to provide an adequate return on investment for the sponsor. With the common practice of off-label use and the paucity of available data concerning pediatric patients, the US Congress passed the Best Pharmaceuticals for Children Act (BPCA) in 2002. This legislation empowered the US Food and Drug Administration (FDA) and the National Institutes of Health (NIH) to fund studies of generic pharmaceuticals in children in which the sponsors would not support the study because of costs, risks, and lack of economic incentives. The Pediatric Research Equity Act (PREA) in 2003 codified the authority of the FDA to require pediatric studies of certain drugs and biologic agents (108th Congress 2009).

With the passage of these three laws, there has been a greater emphasis on the study of medications in the pediatric population in order to determine effectiveness and safety of therapeutic agents. Trials of pharmaceuticals with potential use for children have recently begun to evaluate agents in common use.

Computerized Provider Order Entry and Pediatric Patients

Medication errors are the most common type of medical error with significant potential for adverse events (ADE) (Bates et al. 1995b; Institute of Medicine and Committee on Quality Health Care in America 2000). According to the Committee on Quality Health Care in America, a medication error is any preventable event that occurs in the process of ordering or delivering a medication, regardless of whether an injury occurred or the potential for injury was present (Bates et al. 1995b; Institute of Medicine and Committee on Quality Health Care in America 2000). While human mistakes play an important role, over half of medication errors are preventable (Kelly 2001) and occur as a result of system flaws. Medication errors may occur at any step in the process but provider errors are common.

Most safety research has centered on medication errors and their prevention in adult patients. For adults, the reported incidence of medication errors is 1 in 20 written orders (Bates et al. 1995a). In a 2005 study in adult primary care practices, the medication error rate was 7.6% in a center with a basic computerized prescribing system which lacked dose and frequency checking. (Gandhi et al. 2005) In pediatrics, the error rate has been reported to be as high as one in six orders for inpatients with 31% associated with harm or death (Marino et al. 2000). Children are at a higher risk for ADEs, estimated as nearly triple that of adults.

In a study from my institution examining prescribing medication error rates for analgesics in children being discharged from the hospital, we found the process to be error-prone with approximately 3% of prescriptions with the potential for causing an adverse drug event (ADE) (Lee et al. 2009). Because of the complexity of medication dosing in the pediatric patient, pediatric patients are at higher risk than adults for dosing error and errors involving controlled substances (or narcotics) are the most dangerous. We developed a web-based controlled substance prescription writer that included weight-based dosing logic and alerts. We implemented the web-based program and evaluated the error reduction, behavior modifications, and attitudes toward the use of the application. We found that the web-based controlled substance prescription writer prevented analgesic medication errors by alerting users that their doses exceeded hard limits for weight-based dosing. The use of alerts changed prescriber behavior and prevented the potential for future medication errors as demonstrated by the increased likelihood of abandoned prescription attempts with alerts (Zimmer et al. 2008).

Even with limited data, it is empirically evident that pediatric patients are at higher risk for error due to several key factors. Most drug doses in pediatrics are weight-or body surface area-based and may be modified by other factors including age (Wong et al. 2004). Weight-based medication orders have a dosing error rate of 10.3% compared to 5.9% for non-weight-based drugs (Herout and Erstad 2004). A substantial proportion of providers make mistakes while calculating drug doses, (Rowe et al. 1998) often by an order of magnitude. Process factors, including the need for individualized dilution of stock medications and fluids, place children at increased risk for dispensing errors. Pharmacokinetic factors, including age based variability in absorption, metabolism, and excretion of drugs as compared with adults, expose special vulnerabilities to the adverse effects of overdosing (Lehmann and Kim 2005; Kanter et al. 2004).

Given the prevalence of prescribing errors, there is a need for systematic changes to reduce the likelihood of errors. Computerized provider order entry (CPOE) with clinical decision support (CDS) has been shown to be one of the most effective strategies for reducing errors in adult inpatients (Bates et al. 1998; Leape et al. 1999;

Leape et al. 1993). However, much of the arguments for CPOE in children are based on extrapolation of results from adult studies (Bates et al. 1999; Bates et al. 1998; Chamberlain et al. 2004; Johnson and Davison 2004; Lehmann and Kim 2006) The most common type of medication error in pediatrics is a dosing error at the ordering stage.(Crowley et al. 2001; Leape et al. 1995; Vincer et al. 1989) The use of computerized provider order entry (CPOE) has been advocated as a response to the high rates of medication errors that have been documented in many studies. CPOE has been endorsed by the Institute of Medicine in the report *To Err is Human* (Institute of Medicine 1999) and by organizations such as the Leapfrog Group (Leapfrog Group 2009). The use of CPOE is one of many recommendations made by the IOM to improve patient safely by providing safer patient care and improved outcomes by decreasing the potential for medication errors.

Most of the published studies concerning the use of CPOE have come primarily from academic and government medical centers. The use of CPOE in an academic emergency department demonstrated significant reductions in prescription errors and the need for pharmacist clarification (Bizovi et al. 2002). Adverse drug events (ADEs) due to medication errors were common and many occurred at the stage of prescribing and ordering medications. In one estimate, 64.4% of errors (including 43% of potentially harmful errors) were considered preventable by the use of CPOE (with clinical decision support [CDS]) (Lehmann and Kim 2006).

Despite government and health care industry endorsements and published evidence that CPOE will improve patient safety and prevent or reduce medical errors, successful adoption is not yet widespread in the United States. By 2002, only 9.6% of a sample of United States hospitals reported complete CPOE availability, with 6.5% reporting partial availability (Ash et al. 2004). Reasons for low adoption may include issues of local feasibility. Nonalignment of user incentives and disagreements on institutional priorities may impede local adoption. Technically, the expertise needed to achieve the safety and quality benefits of CPOE while maintaining operations may exceed the capabilities and resources of the institution. Financially, the initial costs of adoption and ongoing costs of maintenance of CPOE may be prohibitive to institutions in a competitive market (Lehmann and Kim 2006). The implementation of CPOE/CDS will directly connect:

- Prescribers to data (patient records, drugs, and laboratory or radiology test results)
- Prescribers to other health professionals (nurses and pharmacists)
- Information systems to one another (patient records, drug and laboratory databases)
- Departments to one another (patient care units, physician offices, pharmacies)

On a technical level, CPOE and CDS reduce variation and provide decision support by:

- Improving legibility
- Reducing transcription errors
- Using standard names, catalogues, and dictionaries
- Linking patient-specific data and information
- Providing evidence-based order sets
- Automating calculations
- Providing alerts and reminders
- Monitoring for adherence to best practice
- Screening populations at risk

There is an assumption that a decrease in medication error rates alone is sufficient to determine the efficacy of CPOE; this endpoint does not necessarily imply improved patient outcomes and safety. In a study by King et al., the introduction of CPOE into the hospital resulted in a 40% decrease in medication error rates; however, there was no evidence to demonstrate any effect from CPOE on actual or potential patient harm (King et al. 2003). Han et al. reported an increase in the mortality rate in a pediatric ICU (from 2.8 to 6.6%) after the introduction of CPOE, likely due to delays in medication administration and less nursing time at the patient's bedside (Han et al. 2005). In a study by Del Beccaro et al., there was no effect on mortality rates in the PICU with the introduction of CPOE (Del Beccaro et al. 2006). Clearly, there are complexities with an examination of the effects or process on patient outcomes; however, research is needed to discern the actual impact of CPOE on patient outcomes.

Summary

Chronic pain in children may be nociceptive, neuropathic, or a mixed pain etiology. The treatment of pain and suffering of children should be an important element of care. Knowledge of the developmental issues related to pharmacokinetics and pharmacodynamics will guide the clinician to a rational approach to pharmacological pain management. A thorough understanding of the mechanism of action of the pharmacologic agents will provide a safe and effective use of drugs for the treatment of chronic pain. More research is needed to determine the appropriate dosing of agents and likely efficacy for children, and the FDA is encouraging more studies in the pediatric population. The use of CPOE and clinical decision support analysis will hopefully lead to a safer system to provide analgesics to children.

References

108th Congress (2009). Pediatric Research Equity Act of 2003. S 650. Ref Type: Bill/Resolution.

Amitai, Y., & Frischer, H. (2006). Excess fatality from desipramine in children and adolescents. *Journal of the American Academy of Child and Adolescent Psychiatry, 45,* 54–60.

Anderson, B. J. (2008). Paracetamol (Acetaminophen): Mechanisms of action. *Paediatric Anaesthesia, 18,* 915–921.

Anderson, B. J., & Holford, N. H. (2008). Mechanism-based concepts of size and maturity in pharmacokinetics. *Annual Review of Pharmacology and Toxicology, 48,* 303–332.

Anderson, B. J., & Meakin, G. H. (2002). Scaling for size: Some implications for paediatric anaesthesia dosing. *Paediatric Anaesthesia, 12,* 205–219.

Andrews, C. M., Krantz, M. J., Wedam, E. F., Marcuson, M. J., Capacchione, J. F., & Haigney, M. C. (2009). Methadone-induced mortality in the treatment of chronic pain: Role of QT prolongation. *Cardiology Journal, 16,* 210–217.

Ash, J. S., Gorman, P. N., Seshadri, V., & Hersh, W. R. (2004). Computerized physician order entry in U.S. hospitals: Results of a 2002 survey. *Journal of the American Medical Informatics Association, 11,* 95–99.

Barrett, D. A., Barker, D. P., Rutter, N., Pawula, M., & Shaw, P. N. (1996). Morphine, morphine-6-glucuronide and morphine-3-glucuronide pharmacokinetics in newborn infants receiving diamorphine infusions. *British Journal of Clinical Pharmacology, 41,* 531–537.

Bates, D. W., Boyle, D. L., Vander Vliet, M. B., Schneider, J., & Leape, L. (1995a). Relationship between medication errors and adverse drug events. *Journal of General Internal Medicine, 10,* 199–205.

Bates, D. W., Cullen, D. J., Laird, N., Petersen, L. A., Small, S. D., Servi, D., et al. (1995b). Incidence of adverse drug events and potential adverse drug events. Implications for prevention. ADE Prevention Study Group. *Journal of the American Medical Association, 274,* 29–34.

Bates, D. W., Leape, L. L., Cullen, D. J., Laird, N., Petersen, L. A., Teich, J. M., et al. (1998). Effect of computerized physician order entry and a team intervention on prevention of serious medication errors. *Journal of the American Medical Association, 280,* 1311–1316.

Bates, D. W., Teich, J. M., Lee, J., Seger, D., Kuperman, G. J., Ma'Luf, N., et al. (1999). The impact of computerized physician order entry on medication error prevention. *Journal of the American Medical Informatics Association, 6,* 313–321.

Berde, C. B., & Sethna, N. F. (2002). Analgesics for the treatment of pain in children. *The New England Journal of Medicine, 347,* 1094–1103.

Best Pharmaceuticals for Children Act (2002). 115 Stat 1408 (2002). 107–109. Ref Type: Bill/Resolution.

Birmingham, P. K., Tobin, M. J., Henthorn, T. K., Fisher, D. M., Berkelhamer, M. C., Smith, F. A., et al. (1997). Twenty-four-hour pharmacokinetics of rectal acetaminophen in children: An old drug with new recommendations. *Anesthesiology, 87,* 244–252.

Bizovi, K. E., Beckley, B. E., McDade, M. C., Adams, A. L., Lowe, R. A., Zechnich, A. D., et al. (2002). The effect of computer-assisted prescription writing on emergency department prescription errors. *Academic Emergency Medicine, 9,* 1168–1175.

Blanco, J. G., Harrison, P. L., Evans, W. E., & Relling, M. V. (2000). Human cytochrome P450 maximal activities in pediatric versus adult liver. *Drug Metabolism and Disposition, 28,* 379–382.

Bozkurt, P. (2005). Use of tramadol in children. *Paediatric Anaesthesia, 15,* 1041–1047.

Brown, S. C., Jeavons, M., & Stinson, J. (2005). Effectiveness of pamidronate for treating intractable chronic neuropathic pain: Case report of two adolescents. *The Clinical Journal of Pain, 21,* 549–552.

Butkovic, D., Toljan, S., & Mihovilovic-Novak, B. (2006). Experience with gabapentin for neuropathic pain in adolescents: Report of five cases. *Paediatric Anaesthesia, 16,* 325–329.

Byas-Smith, M. G., Max, M. B., Muir, J., & Kingman, A. (1995). Transdermal clonidine compared to placebo in painful diabetic neuropathy using a two-stage 'enriched enrollment' design. *Pain, 60,* 267–274.

Carrazana, E., & Mikoshiba, I. (2003). Rationale and evidence for the use of oxcarbazepine in neuropathic pain. *Journal of Pain and Symptom Management, 25,* S31–S35.

Chamberlain, J. M., Slonim, A., & Joseph, J. G. (2004). Reducing errors and promoting safety in pediatric emergency care. *Ambulatory Pediatrics, 4,* 55–63.

Chez, M. G., Burton, Q., Dowling, T., Chang, M., Khanna, P., & Kramer, C. (2007). Memantine as adjunctive therapy in children diagnosed with autistic spectrum disorders: an observation of initial clinical response and maintenance tolerability. *Journal of Child Neurology, 22*, 574–579.

Cortet, B., Flipo, R. M., Coquerelle, P., Duquesnoy, B., & Delcambre, B. (1997). Treatment of severe, recalcitrant reflex sympathetic dystrophy: assessment of efficacy and safety of the second generation bisphosphonate pamidronate. *Clinical Rheumatology, 16*, 51–56.

Cron, R. Q., Sharma, S., & Sherry, D. D. (1999). Current treatment by United States and Canadian pediatric rheumatologists. *The Journal of Rheumatology, 26*, 2036–2038.

Crowley, E., Willaims, R., & Couisns, D. (2001). Medication errors in children: a descriptive summary of medication error reports submitted to the United States Pharmacopia. *Current Therapeutic Research, 26*, 627–640.

Dawson, G. S., Seidman, P., & Ramadan, H. H. (2001). Improved postoperative pain control in pediatric adenotonsillectomy with dextromethorphan. *The Laryngoscope, 111*, 1223–1226.

Dayioglu, M., Tuncer, S., & Reisli, R. (2008). Gabapentin for neurophatic pain in children· A case report. *Agri, 20*, 37–40.

De Witte, J. L., Schoenmaekers, B., Sessler, D. I., & Deloof, T. (2001). The analgesic efficacy of tramadol is impaired by concurrent administration of ondansetron. *Anesthesia and Analgesia, 92*, 1319–1321.

Del Beccaro, M. A., Jeffries, H. E., Eisenberg, M. A., & Harry, E. D. (2006). Computerized provider order entry implementation: No association with increased mortality rates in an intensive care unit. *Pediatrics, 118*, 290–295.

Dworkin, R. H., O'Connor, A. B., Backonja, M., Farrar, J. T., Finnerup, N. B., Jensen, T. S., et al. (2007). Pharmacologic management of neuropathic pain: Evidence-based recommendations. *Pain, 132*, 237–251.

Ebert, B., Thorkildsen, C., Andersen, S., Christrup, L. L., & Hjeds, H. (1998). Opioid analgesics as noncompetitive N-methyl-D-aspartate (NMDA) antagonists. *Biochemical Pharmacology, 56*, 553–559.

Ehret, G. B., Voide, C., Gex-Fabry, M., Chabert, J., Shah, D., Broers, B., et al. (2006). Drug-induced long QT syndrome in injection drug users receiving methadone: High frequency in hospitalized patients and risk factors. *Archives of Internal Medicine, 166*, 1280–1287.

Ferrini, R. (2000). Parenteral lidocaine for severe intractable pain in six hospice patients continued at home. *Journal of Palliative Medicine, 3*, 193–200.

Finkel, J. C., Finley, A., Greco, C., Weisman, S. J., & Zeltzer, L. (2005). Transdermal fentanyl in the management of children with chronic severe pain: results from an international study. *Cancer, 104*, 2847–2857.

Finkel, J. C., Pestieau, S. R., & Quezado, Z. M. (2007). Ketamine as an adjuvant for treatment of cancer pain in children and adolescents. *The Journal of Pain, 8*, 515–521.

Fishbain, D., Berman, K., & Kajdasz, D. K. (2006). Duloxetine for neuropathic pain based on recent clinical trials. *Current Pain and Headache Reports, 10*, 199–204.

Food And Drug Administration (1997). FDA Modernization Act of 1997. 111 Stat 2296. 107–109. Pub L 105. Ref Type: Bill/Resolution.

Gandhi, T. K., Weingart, S. N., Seger, A. C., Borus, J., Burdick, E., Poon, E. G., et al. (2005). Outpatient prescribing errors and the impact of computerized prescribing. *Journal of General Internal Medicine, 20*, 837–841.

Ganesh, A., & Maxwell, L. G. (2007). Pathophysiology and management of opioid-induced pruritus. *Drugs, 67*, 2323–2333.

Garcia Rodriguez, L. A., & Barreales, T. L. (2007). Risk of upper gastrointestinal complications among users of traditional NSAIDs and COXIBs in the general population. *Gastroenterology, 132*, 498–506.

Gorman, A. L., Elliott, K. J., & Inturrisi, C. E. (1997). The d- and l-isomers of methadone bind to the non-competitive site on the N-methyl-D-aspartate (NMDA) receptor in rat forebrain and spinal cord. *Neuroscience Letters, 223*, 5–8.

Gourlay, G. K., Willis, R. J., & Wilson, P. R. (1984). Postoperative pain control with methadone: Influence of supplementary methadone doses and blood concentration–response relationships. *Anesthesiology, 61*, 19–26.

Graham, G. G., & Scott, K. F. (2005). Mechanism of action of paracetamol. *American Journal of Therapeutics, 12*, 46–55.

Grande, L. A., O'Donnell, B. R., Fitzgibbon, D. R., & Terman, G. W. (2008). Ultra-low dose ketamine and memantine treatment for pain in an opioid-tolerant oncology patient. *Anesthesia and Analgesia, 107*, 1380–1383.

Grothe, D. R., Scheckner, B., & Albano, D. (2004). Treatment of pain syndromes with venlafaxine. *Pharmacotherapy, 24*, 621–629.

Hain, R. D., Hardcastle, A., Pinkerton, C. R., & Aherne, G. W. (1999). Morphine and morphine-6-glucuronide in the plasma and cerebrospinal fluid of children. *British Journal of Clinical Pharmacology, 48*, 37–42.

Han, Y. Y., Carcillo, J. A., Venkataraman, S. T., Clark, R. S., Watson, R. S., Nguyen, T. C., et al. (2005). Unexpected increased mortality after implementation of a commercially sold computerized physician order entry system. *Pediatrics, 116*, 1506–1512.

Herout, P. M., & Erstad, B. L. (2004). Medication errors involving continuously infused medications in a surgical intensive care unit. *Critical Care Medicine, 32*, 428–432.

Houlahan, K. E., Branowicki, P. A., Mack, J. W., Dinning, C., & McCabe, M. (2006). Can end of life care for the pediatric patient suffering with escalating and intractable symptoms be improved? *Journal of Pediatric Oncology Nursing, 23*, 45–51.

Hunt, A., Joel, S., Dick, G., & Goldman, A. (1999). Population pharmacokinetics of oral morphine and its glucuronides in children receiving morphine as immediate-release liquid or sustained-release tablets for cancer pain. *Jornal de Pediatria, 135*, 47–55.

Institute of Medicine. (1999). *To err is human: Building a safer health system*. Washington DC: National Academy Press.

Institute of Medicine & Committee on Quality Health Care in America. (2000). *To err is human: Building a safer health system* (Report of the Institute of Medicine). Washington DC: National Academy Press.

James, L. P., Capparelli, E. V., Simpson, P. M., Letzig, L., Roberts, D., Hinson, J. A., et al. (2008). Acetaminophen-associated hepatic injury: evaluation of acetaminophen protein adducts in children and adolescents with acetaminophen overdose. *Clinical Pharmacology and Therapeutics, 84*, 684–690.

Johnson, K. B., & Davison, C. L. (2004). Information technology: Its importance to child safety. *Ambulatory Pediatrics, 4*, 64–72.

Kanter, D. E., Turenne, W., & Slonim, A. D. (2004). Hospital-reported medical errors in premature neonates. *Pediatric Critical Care Medicine, 5*, 119–123.

Karst, M., Salim, K., Burstein, S., Conrad, I., Hoy, L., & Schneider, U. (2003). Analgesic effect of the synthetic cannabinoid CT-3 on chronic neuropathic pain: A randomized controlled trial. *Journal of the American Medical Association, 290*, 1757–1762.

Kastrup, J., Petersen, P., Dejgard, A., Angelo, H. R., & Hilsted, J. (1987). Intravenous lidocaine infusion–a new treatment of chronic painful diabetic neuropathy? *Pain, 28*, 69–75.

Kearns, G. L., Bdel-Rahman, S. M., Alander, S. W., Blowey, D. L., Leeder, J. S., & Kauffman, R. E. (2003). Developmental pharmacology – drug disposition, action, and therapy in infants and children. *The New England Journal of Medicine, 349*, 1157–1167.

Kelly, W. N. (2001). Potential risks and prevention, Part 4: Reports of significant adverse drug events. *American Journal of Health-System Pharmacy, 58*, 1406–1412.

Kendrick, W. D., Woods, A. M., Daly, M. Y., Birch, R. F., & DiFazio, C. (1996). Naloxone versus nalbuphine infusion for prophylaxis of epidural morphine-induced pruritus. *Anesthesia and Analgesia, 82*, 641–647.

Kimura, Y., & Walco, G. A. (2007). Treatment of chronic pain in pediatric rheumatic disease. *Nature Clinical Practice. Rheumatology, 3*, 210–218.

King, W. J., Paice, N., Rangrej, J., Forestell, G. J., & Swartz, R. (2003). The effect of computerized physician order entry on medication errors and adverse drug events in pediatric inpatients. *Pediatrics, 112*, 506–509.

Knotkova, H., & Pappagallo, M. (2007). Adjuvant analgesics. *The Medical Clinics of North America, 91*, 113–124.

Kong, V. K. F., & Irwin, M. G. (2009). Adjuvant analgesics in neuropathic pain. *European Journal of Anaesthesiology, 26*, 96–100.

Lacroix, D., Sonnier, M., Moncion, A., Cheron, G., & Cresteil, T. (1997). Expression of CYP3A in the human liver – evidence that the shift between CYP3A7 and CYP3A4 occurs immediately after birth. *European Journal of Biochemistry, 247*, 625–634.

Lalwani, K., Shoham, A., Koh, J. L., & McGraw, T. (2005). Use of oxcarbazepine to treat a pediatric patient with resistant complex regional pain syndrome. *The Journal of Pain, 6*, 704–706.

Lang, B. A., & Finlayson, L. A. (1994). Naproxen-induced pseudoporphyria in patients with juvenile rheumatoid arthritis. *Jornal de Pediatria, 124*, 639–642.

Lauder, G. R., & White, M. C. (2005). Neuropathic pain following multilevel surgery in children with cerebral palsy: A case series and review. *Paediatric Anaesthesia, 15*, 412–420.

Leape, L. L., Lawthers, A. G., Brennan, T. A., & Johnson, W. G. (1993). Preventing medical injury. *QRB. Quality Review Bulletin, 19*, 144–149.

Leape, L. L., Bates, D. W., Cullen, D. J., Cooper, J., Demonaco, H. J., Gallivan, T., et al. (1995). Systems analysis of adverse drug events. ADE Prevention Study Group. *Journal of the American Medical Association, 274*, 35–43.

Leape, L. L., Cullen, D. J., Clapp, M. D., Burdick, E., Demonaco, H. J., Erickson, J. I., et al. (1999). Pharmacist participation on physician rounds and adverse drug events in the intensive care unit. *Journal of the American Medical Association, 282*, 267–270.

Leapfrog Group (2009). Web page [On-line]. Available: http://www.leapfroggroup.org.

Lee, B. H., Lehmann, C. U., Jackson, E. V., Kost-Byerly, S., Rothman, S., Kozlowski, L., et al. (2009). Assessing controlled substance prescribing errors in a pediatric teaching hospital: an analysis of the safety of analgesic prescription practice in the transition from the hospital to home. *The Journal of Pain, 10*, 160–166.

Lehmann, C. U., & Kim, G. R. (2005). Prevention of medication errors. *Clinics in Perinatology, 32*, 107–123. vii.

Lehmann, C. U., & Kim, G. R. (2006). Computerized provider order entry and patient safety. *Pediatric Clinics of North America, 53*, 1169–1184.

Leppert, W., & Luczak, J. (2005). The role of tramadol in cancer pain treatment–a review. *Supportive Care in Cancer, 13*, 5–17.

Lussier, D., Huskey, A. G., & Portenoy, R. K. (2004). Adjuvant analgesics in cancer pain management. *The Oncologist, 9*, 571–591.

Malmberg, A. B., & Yaksh, T. L. (1992). Antinociceptive actions of spinal nonsteroidal anti-inflammatory agents on the formalin test in the rat. *The Journal of Pharmacology and Experimental Therapeutics, 263*, 136–146.

Manfredi, P. L., Gonzales, G. R., Sady, R., Chandler, S., & Payne, R. (2003). Neuropathic pain in patients with cancer. *Journal of Palliative Care, 19*, 115–118.

Marino, B. L., Reinhardt, K., Eichelberger, W. J., & Steingard, R. (2000). Prevalence of errors in a pediatric hospital medication system: Implications for error proofing. *Outcomes Management for Nursing Practice, 4*, 129–135.

Massey, G. V., Pedigo, S., Dunn, N. L., Grossman, N. J., & Russell, E. C. (2002). Continuous lidocaine infusion for the relief of refractory malignant pain in a terminally ill pediatric cancer patient. *Journal of Pediatric Hematology/Oncology, 24*, 566–568.

Max, M. B., Lynch, S. A., Muir, J., Shoaf, S. E., Smoller, B., & Dubner, R. (1992). Effects of desipramine, amitriptyline, and fluoxetine on pain in diabetic neuropathy. *The New England Journal of Medicine, 326*, 1250–1256.

Maxwell, L. G., Kaufmann, S. C., Bitzer, S., Jackson, E. V., Jr., McGready, J., Kost-Byerly, S., et al. (2005). The effects of a small-dose naloxone infusion on opioid-induced side effects and analgesia in children and adolescents treated with intravenous patient-controlled analgesia: A double-blind, prospective, randomized, controlled study. *Anesthesia and Analgesia, 100*, 953–958.

Meighen, K. G. (2007). Duloxetine treatment of pediatric chronic pain and co-morbid major depressive disorder. *Journal of Child and Adolescent Psychopharmacology, 17*, 121–127.

Messina, J., Darwish, M., & Fine, P. G. (2008). Fentanyl buccal tablet. *Drugs Today (Barc.), 44*, 41–54.

Miller, R. P., Roberts, R. J., & Fischer, L. J. (1976). Acetaminophen elimination kinetics in neonates, children, and adults. *Clinical Pharmacology and Therapeutics, 19*, 284–294.

Morita, I. (2002). Distinct functions of COX-1 and COX-2. *Prostaglandins & Other Lipid Mediators, 68–69*, 165–175.

Mortensen, M. E. (2002). Acetaminophen toxicity in children. *American Family Physician, 66*, 734.

Munir, M. A., Enany, N., & Zhang, J. M. (2007). Nonopioid analgesics. *Anesthesiology Clinics, 25*, 761–774. vi.

Nathan, A., Rose, J. B., Guite, J. W., Hehir, D., & Milovcich, K. (2005). Primary erythromelalgia in a child responding to intravenous lidocaine and oral mexiletine treatment. *Pediatrics, 115*, e504–e507.

Nayak, S., & Cunliffe, M. (2008). Lidocaine 5% patch for localized chronic neuropathic pain in adolescents: Report of five cases. *Paediatric Anaesthesia, 18*, 554–558.

Niemi, T. T., Taxell, C., & Rosenberg, P. H. (1997). Comparison of the effect of intravenous ketoprofen, ketorolac and diclofenac on platelet function in volunteers. *Acta Anaesthesiologica Scandinavica, 41*, 1353–1358.

Nuki, G. (1990). Pain control and the use of non-steroidal analgesic anti-inflammatory drugs. *British Medical Bulletin, 46*, 262–278.

Pasternak, G. W. (2001). The pharmacology of mu analgesics: From patients to genes. *The Neuroscientist, 7*, 220–231.

Pasternak, G. W. (2005). Molecular biology of opioid analgesia. *Journal of Pain and Symptom Management, 29*, S2–S9.

Quigley, C., & Wiffen, P. (2003). A systematic review of hydromorphone in acute and chronic pain. *Journal of Pain and Symptom Management, 25*, 169–178.

Rog, D. J., Nurmikko, T. J., Friede, T., & Young, C. A. (2005). Randomized, controlled trial of cannabis-based medicine in central pain in multiple sclerosis. *Neurology, 65*, 812–819.

Rogers, M., Rasheed, A., Moradimehr, A., & Baumrucker, S. J. (2009). Memantine (Namenda) for neuropathic pain. *The American Journal of Hospice & Palliative Care, 26*, 57–59.

Rose, J. B., Cuy, R., Cohen, D. E., & Schreiner, M. S. (1999). Preoperative oral dextromethorphan does not reduce pain or analgesic consumption in children after adenotonsillectomy. *Anesthesia and Analgesia, 88*, 749–753.

Rose, J. B., Finkel, J. C., Rquedas-Mohs, A., Himelstein, B. P., Schreiner, M., & Medve, R. A. (2003). Oral tramadol for the treatment of pain of 7 – 30 days' duration in children. *Anesthesia and Analgesia, 96*, 78–81. table.

Rowbotham, M. C., Goli, V., Kunz, N. R., & Lei, D. (2004). Venlafaxine extended release in the treatment of painful diabetic neuropathy: A double-blind, placebo-controlled study. *Pain, 110*, 697–706.

Rowe, C., Koren, T., & Koren, G. (1998). Errors by paediatric residents in calculating drug doses. *Archives of Disease in Childhood, 79*, 56–58.

Rubenstein, J. H., & Laine, L. (2004). Systematic review: The hepatotoxicity of non-steroidal anti-inflammatory drugs. *Alimentary Pharmacology & Therapeutics, 20*, 373–380.

Rudich, Z., Stinson, J., Jeavons, M., & Brown, S. C. (2003). Treatment of chronic intractable neuropathic pain with dronabinol: Case report of two adolescents. *Pain Research & Management, 8*, 221–224.

Saarto, T., & Wiffen, P. J. (2007). Antidepressants for neuropathic pain. *Cochrane.Database.Syst.Rev.,* CD005454.

Schley, M., Topfner, S., Wiech, K., Schaller, H. E., Konrad, C. J., Schmelz, M., et al. (2007). Continuous brachial plexus blockade in combination with the NMDA receptor antagonist memantine prevents phantom pain in acute traumatic upper limb amputees. *European Journal of Pain, 11*, 299–308.

Schwartzman, R. J., Patel, M., Grothusen, J. R., & Alexander, G. M. (2009). Efficacy of 5-day continuous lidocaine infusion for the treatment of refractory complex regional pain syndrome. *Pain Medicine, 10*, 401–412.

Scott, C. S., Riggs, K. W., Ling, E. W., Fitzgerald, C. E., Hill, M. L., Grunau, R. V., et al. (1999). Morphine pharmacokinetics and pain assessment in premature newborns. *Jornal de Pediatria, 135*, 423–429.

Semenchuk, M. R., & Sherman, S. (2000). Effectiveness of tizanidine in neuropathic pain: An open-label study. *The Journal of Pain, 1*, 285–292.

Sharma, S., Rajagopal, M. R., Palat, G., Singh, C., Haji, A. G., & Jain, D. (2009). A phase II pilot study to evaluate use of intravenous lidocaine for opioid-refractory pain in cancer patients. *Journal of Pain and Symptom Management, 37*, 85–93.

Shih, A., & Jackson, K. C. (2007). Role of corticosteroids in palliative care. *Journal of Pain & Palliative Care Pharmacotherapy, 21*, 69–76.

Simm, P. J., Allen, R. C., & Zacharin, M. R. (2008). Bisphosphonate treatment in chronic recurrent multifocal osteomyelitis. *Jornal de Pediatria, 152*, 571–575.

Sindrup, S. H., Otto, M., Finnerup, N. B., & Jensen, T. S. (2005). Antidepressants in the treatment of neuropathic pain. *Basic & Clinical Pharmacology & Toxicology, 96*, 399–409.

Sinis, N., Birbaumer, N., Gustin, S., Schwarz, A., Bredanger, S., Becker, S. T., et al. (2007). Memantine treatment of complex regional pain syndrome: a preliminary report of six cases. *The Clinical Journal of Pain, 23*, 237–243.

Snyder, S. H., & Pasternak, G. W. (2003). Historical review: Opioid receptors. *Trends in Pharmacological Sciences, 24*, 198–205.

Sonnier, M., & Cresteil, T. (1998). Delayed ontogenesis of CYP1A2 in the human liver. *European Journal of Biochemistry, 251*, 893–898.

Stuart, J. J., & Pisko, E. J. (1981). Choline magnesium trisalicylate does not impair platelet aggregation. *Pharmatherapeutica, 2*, 547–551.

Sturtevant, J. (1999). NSAID-induced bronchospasm – a common and serious problem. A report from MEDSAFE, the New Zealand Medicines and Medical Devices Safety Authority. *New Zealand Dental Journal, 95*, 84.

Sweeney, J. D., & Hoernig, L. A. (1991). Hemostatic effects of salsalate in normal subjects and patients with hemophilia A. *Thrombosis Research, 61*, 23–27.

Tobias, J. D. (2000). Weak analgesics and nonsteroidal anti-inflammatory agents in the management of children with acute pain. *Pediatric Clinics of North America, 47*, 527–543.

Tremont-Lukats, I. W., Hutson, P. R., & Backonja, M. M. (2006). A randomized, double-masked, placebo-controlled pilot trial of extended IV lidocaine infusion for relief of ongoing neuropathic pain. *The Clinical Journal of Pain, 22*, 266–271.

Tsui, B. C., Davies, D., Desai, S., & Malherbe, S. (2004). Intravenous ketamine infusion as an adjuvant to morphine in a 2-year-old with severe cancer pain from metastatic neuroblastoma. *Journal of Pediatric Hematology/Oncology, 26*, 678–680.

Vane, J. R. (1971). Inhibition of prostaglandin synthesis as a mechanism of action for aspirin-like drugs. *Nature: New Biology, 231*, 232–235.

Varenna, M., Zucchi, F., Ghiringhelli, D., Binelli, L., Bevilacqua, M., Bettica, P., et al. (2000). Intravenous clodronate in the treatment of reflex sympathetic dystrophy syndrome. A randomized, double blind, placebo controlled study. *The Journal of Rheumatology, 27*, 1477–1483.

Vincer, M. J., Murray, J. M., Yuill, A., Allen, A. C., Evans, J. R., & Stinson, D. A. (1989). Drug errors and incidents in a neonatal intensive care unit. A quality assurance activity. *American Journal of Diseases of Children, 143*, 737–740.

Vondracek, P., Oslejskova, H., Kepak, T., Mazanek, P., Sterba, J., Rysava, M., et al. (2009). Efficacy of pregabalin in neuropathic pain in paediatric oncological patients. *European Journal of Paediatric Neurology, 13*, 332–336.

Watcha, M. F., & White, P. F. (1992). Postoperative nausea and vomiting. Its etiology, treatment, and prevention. *Anesthesiology, 77*, 162–184.

Weinstein, S. M., Messina, J., & Xie, F. (2009). Fentanyl buccal tablet for the treatment of breakthrough pain in opioid-tolerant patients with chronic cancer pain: A long-term, open-label safety study. *Cancer, 115*, 2571–2579.

Wernicke, J. F., Pritchett, Y. L., D'Souza, D. N., Waninger, A., Tran, P., Iyengar, S., et al. (2006). A randomized controlled trial of duloxetine in diabetic peripheral neuropathic pain. *Neurology, 67*, 1411–1420.

Wernicke, J. F., Wang, F., Pritchett, Y. L., Smith, T. R., Raskin, J., D'Souza, D. N., et al. (2007). An open-label 52-week clinical extension comparing duloxetine with routine care in patients with diabetic peripheral neuropathic pain. *Pain Medicine, 8*, 503–513.

Wiech, K., Kiefer, R. T., Topfner, S., Preissl, H., Braun, C., Unertl, K., et al. (2004). A placebo-controlled randomized crossover trial of the N-methyl-D-aspartic acid receptor antagonist, memantine, in patients with chronic phantom limb pain. *Anesthesia and Analgesia, 98*, 408–413. table.

Williams, D. G., Hatch, D. J., & Howard, R. F. (2001). Codeine phosphate in paediatric medicine. *British Journal of Anaesthesia, 86*, 413–421.

Wong, I. C., Ghaleb, M. A., Franklin, B. D., & Barber, N. (2004). Incidence and nature of dosing errors in paediatric medications: A systematic review. *Drug Safety, 27*, 661–670.

Zelcer, S., Kolesnikov, Y., Kovalyshyn, I., Pasternak, D. A., & Pasternak, G. W. (2005). Selective potentiation of opioid analgesia by nonsteroidal anti-inflammatory drugs. *Brain Research, 1040*, 151–156.

Zernikow, B., Michel, E., & Anderson, B. (2007). Transdermal fentanyl in childhood and adolescence: A comprehensive literature review. *The Journal of Pain, 8*, 187–207.

Zimmer, K. P., Miller, M. R., Lee, B. H., Yaster, M., Miller, R., & Lehmann, C. U. (2008). Electronic narcotic prescription writer: Use in medical error reduction. *Journal of Patient Safety, 4*, 98–105.

Opioid Tolerance

21

Sarah E. Rebstock, Jill M. Eckert,
and Claude Abdallah

Keywords

Tolerance phenomena • Opioid action • Pseudoaddiction • Addiction
• Opioid induced hyperalgesia (OIH) • Opioid weaning

Introduction and History of Opioid Tolerance

Information regarding opioid tolerance in the pediatric population is limited, and the information for treating pediatric opioid tolerance is extrapolated from the adult population (Shapiro et al. 1995). The majority of the literature on withdrawal syndromes and tolerance comes from the adult literature and is associated with opioid-addicted patients (Collett 1998; Anand and Arnold 1994). Opioid dependence and withdrawal was first described in the pediatric literature after babies were born to drug-addicted mothers in the late 1970s and early 1980s (Tobias 2000a; Landau 2006; Margas et al. 2007; Zhang et al. 2005; Finnegan et al. 1975). It was these initial findings and description of Neonatal Abstinence Syndrome (NAS) that led to valuable information still used today in our treatment of children requiring long-term opioid therapy for pain management or sedation (Finnegan et al. 1975). The origin of scoring

S.E. Rebstock (✉)
Department of Anesthesiology,
Penn State Milton S. Hershey Medical Center,
P.O. Box 850/500, University Drive,
Hershey, PA 17033, USA
e-mail: srebstock@hmc.psu.edu;

systems to quantify symptoms of withdrawal and the pharmacologic treatment of children experiencing physiological withdrawal came from these early papers (Finnegan et al. 1975). It was not until 1990 that problems associated with dependency and withdrawal were identified in the PICU population in 37 neonates requiring extracorporeal membrane oxygenation (ECMO) for profound respiratory failure (Tobias 2000a; Arnold et al. 1991; Tobias 2005). These babies were on long-term intravenous fentanyl for sedation and pain management. Although the study goal was to look for signs and symptoms of NAS, upon examining these babies' requirements for adequate sedation; the criteria for adequate sedation being that the child could be aroused, but was sedate otherwise; it was observed that the fentanyl dose requirement dramatically increased throughout their clinical course. Thus, tolerance was first described in the pediatric literature. Their mean fentanyl requirements rose from 11.6±6.9 mcg/kg/h on day 1 to 52.5±19.4 mcg/kg/h on day 8 of their opioid therapy. In this same study, plasma fentanyl levels were measured in five babies, this revealed an increase in plasma fentanyl levels to maintain the same desired level of sedation. Tolerance was labeled as a pharmacodynamic process based on this information and the risk factors for development of tolerance, physical

B.C. McClain and S. Suresh (eds.), *Handbook of Pediatric Chronic Pain:*
Current Science and Integrative Practice, DOI 10.1007/978-1-4419-0350-1_21,
© Springer Science+Business Media, LLC 2011

dependency, and NAS were identified. They further went on to study a population of neonates requiring sedation with fentanyl for mechanical ventilation that did not require ECMO (Tobias 2000a; Arnold et al. 1991; Tobias and Deshpande 1996; Arnold et al. 1990). In this second study, the development of NAS was linked to total fentanyl dose and duration of fentanyl infusion with significant results. These studies showed that risk factors between the development of NAS was a cumulative dose of fentanyl greater than 1.6 mg/kg or an ECMO duration greater than 5 days. During this same time frame Tobias et al. (1990), described using methadone to prevent opioid withdrawal in an older PICU population with varying clinical disease processes and courses.

Definition of Tolerance

Understanding the terminology associated with opioid management, physical dependence, and tolerance is important for effective communication between clinicians and families. It is important when talking to other clinicians, or parents of children requiring opioid pain management, that we define tolerance clearly, and that clinicians take on an educator's role when discussing issues of tolerance, withdrawal, and addiction because of the powerful social stigma associated with this terminology (Anand and Arnold 1994).

Tolerance is defined by some as an attenuated response to opioids with repeated exposure (Zhao et al. 2007); other authors define the term tolerance as a decrease in the effect of a drug (opioids) over time requiring an increase in drug to achieve the same physiological response (Anand and Arnold 1994; Tobias and Deshpande 1996). There are two general forms of tolerance that develop in the cerebral nervous system, isolated tissues, and cells: one is at the level of the opioid receptor, where effector coupling is reduced, and the second is at the cellular, synaptic, and network levels, where counteradaptive changes occur to bring about normal function despite the continued activity of the drug. Another results from development of counteradaptations is that once

the drug is removed a sequence of rebound signs and symptoms are manifested. Long-term adaptations induced by chronic opioid treatment are expressed in the absence of the triggering drug and indicate long-lasting change in the functioning of specific neural systems. Tolerance can also be broken down into the types of tolerance, and this is discussed below (Collett 1998; Tobias 2000a). No matter how tolerance is defined, the opioid dose required to achieve analgesia increases with exposure to that opioid, and this phenomena can cause challenges to the clinician managing a patient requiring sedation or pain management over long periods of time.

How and why the tolerance phenomena occurs has created some debate and unanswered questions since tolerance in children was first described with NAS (Finnegan et al. 1975). Some refer to tolerance as an alteration in the drugs effect at the receptor or cellular transmission level, and others refer to genetics (innate tolerance), pharmacokinetics, pharmacodynamics, or learned behaviors when talking about tolerance (Collett 1998; Tobias 2000a; Lutfy and Yoburn 1991). Most authors would agree that the process of opioid tolerance is complex and that we have only just begun to understand the various mechanisms involved in the development of opioid tolerance (Anand and Arnold 1994; Tobias 2000a).

Initial Steps of Opioid Action

Agonists and antagonists exist to the opioids receptors μ, κ, and δ (Goldstein and Naidu 1989). The widespread anatomical and cellular distribution of opioid receptors indicates that opioids have the potential for affecting multiple systems, both nervous and hormonal. Activation of any of the opioid receptor subtypes produces common cellular actions. The most commonly reported actions include inhibition of adenylyl cyclase, activation of potassium conductance, inhibition of calcium conductance, activation of protein kinase C, release of calcium from extracellular stores, and activation of the mitogen-activated protein kinase cascade.

At the cellular level, opioids exert their effects at the cell surface through specific receptors. Of these receptors, four primary opioid agonist receptor types have been identified in the central nervous system (CNS), Mu, Kappa, Delta, Sigma. This receptor classification is only the tip of the iceberg in the complexity of opioid receptor subtypes and the development of tolerance that the last 25 years of research has established in the area of opioid pain management (Lutfy and Yoburn 1991; Hovav and Weinstock 1987; Katz et al. 1994; Coulbault et al. 2006; Compton et al. 2003). The Mu, Kappa, and Delta receptors all inhibit the transmission of synaptic information in the central nervous system (CNS) by way of a similar set of chemical changes. An opioid binds to a receptor on the cell surface and there is a conformational change of the proteinaceous receptor leading to activation of G-protein in the cell which further alters the concentration of cyclic adenosine monophosphate (AMP), ions such as Ca 2+, K+, and Na+, and enzyme cascades including the phospholipase A2 and C system (Tobias 2000a). The end result of these chemical changes is a decrease in excitatory neurotransmitters released into the synaptic clefts and hyperpolarization of nociceptive neural pathways (Sim-Selley et al. 2007).

Chronic Morphine Treatment and Cellular Adaptations

Cellular adaptations and neural processes after chronic exposure to opioids are responsible for tolerance and physical dependence. The desensitization/downregulation mechanisms involved in tolerance are passive and do not engage the rebound mechanisms that could underlie maintenance of drug dependence and the opioid withdrawal syndrome. Two phases of development of and recovery from tolerance can be distinguished in humans: a rapid phase of tolerance occurs within minutes and dissipates with a time course approximating the elimination of opioids. It involves acute desensitization, but counteradaptations can also play a role. The slowly developing phase dissipates over several weeks regardless of the opioid used (Cox et al. 1975). It involves long-term desensitization and counteradaptations of intracellular signaling mechanisms and in neuronal circuitry. These mechanisms involved and identified for μ-receptor desensitization and

downregulation have important implications in determining the extent of tolerance development.

Counteradaptations involved in withdrawal include acute and long-term desensitization of opioid receptor to effector coupling and internalization or downregulation of receptors. Counteradaptations of intracellular signaling mechanisms in opioid-sensitive neurons; and within the neuronal circuitry also occur.

It remains unclear at the cellular level whether tolerance and dependency are issues of decrease in the number of receptors, binding affinity, or a change in the chemistry of the receptor interactions with the g-protein system and/or the intracellular enzyme systems as mentioned above. The response of receptors to different opioids is also an enigma in this puzzle as naturally occurring and synthetic opioids bind with different affinities and exhibit different effects on the individual receiving opioids long term. In some studies, this even affected the development of tolerance (Drake et al. 2004).

The Mu receptor has been further classified into Mu1 and Mu2 receptor subtypes. The Mu1 being responsible for supraspinal analgesia, while the Mu2 subtype for respiratory depression, gastrointestinal immotility, and spinal analgesia. The delta and kappa receptors have also been subclassified, and others will follow as research into nociceptive mechanisms continues. With the advent of Polymerase Chain Reaction (PCR) DNA amplification, and the identification of the human genome, single nucleotide polymorphisms (SNPs) have been discovered in the coding for the Mu receptor in particular. Single nucleotide polymorphisms (SNPs) are naturally occurring alleles coding for slightly different genetic make up (ergo protein coding) of a functioning gene that may or may not alter function at the cellular level. There are over 118 different SNPs for the Mu opioid receptor alone, further leading to the extreme complexity of the opioid receptor function and extrapolation of how tolerance develops, and why (Landau 2006; Coulbault et al. 2006; Lotsch and Geisslinger 2006; Lotsch et al. 2005; Landau, et al. 2004). This complexity may partially help explain why some patients develop innate tolerance defined as genetic lack of sensitivity to a drug. For example, the genetic make up of a receptor

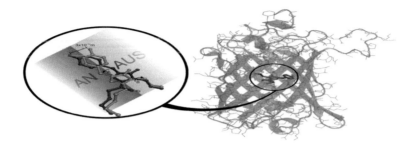

Fig. 21.1 OPRM1 with A118G Allele Carrier. MOR1 A118G SNP illustrating the possibility for conformational change in the morphine Mu receptor due to a single amino acid base that is naturally occurring in the population, and thus potential differences in the development of tolerance

may be slightly modified by an SNP, or naturally occurring allele, or set of multiple alleles, coding for the opioid receptor, thereby changing the conformation of the active site, and thus exhibit attenuation of the response to an opioid at the cellular level (see Fig. 21.1) (Margas, et al. 2007; Zhang et al. 2005; Sim-Selley et al. 2007). This is a simplified explanation for a complex biochemical process that is, of yet, not well understood.

Pharmacokinetic tolerance is the decrease in drug effect due to changes in distribution or metabolism of the opioid used. In the PICU, polypharmacy is often necessary to treat critical illness. Many of these necessary life saving drugs, or combinations of drug therapies, up-regulate microsomal enzyme systems, affecting opioid metabolism and creating pharmacokinetic tolerance to opioids (Collett 1998; Tobias 2000a; Nielsen et al. 2000).

Pharmacodynamic tolerance relates to the change in drug effect to spite maintaining the same opioid drug level in the plasma. Long-term opioid use is common practice in the PICU for sedation and analgesia during critical illness, and as such, pharmacodynamic tolerance has been demonstrated in multiple case reports and studies of opioid tolerance (Collett 1998; Tobias 2000a; Drake et al. 2004; Wheeler and Tobias 2006; Cho et al. 2007; Turner 2005; Crawford et al. 2006).

Learned tolerance is also a factor in opioid tolerance in children that can also not be overlooked. Learned tolerance is the tolerance to opioids from learned behavior allowing compensation for the opioids' usual effects (Tobias 2000a; Tobias and Deshpande 1996). Family dynamics, coping mechanisms, as well as social behaviors can play a role in learned tolerance. It is very important in this context to keep parents and clinicians informed about the different forms of tolerance as they present to help parents feel part of the pain management and healing process, and to prevent misunderstanding. In the pediatric forum, supplying support not only to the patient, but also for the family under duress will help clinicians work through issues of tolerance, withdrawal, dependence, and with opioid weaning (Collett 1998).

Physical and Psychological Dependence, Withdrawal, Pseudoaddiction, and Addiction Defined

In children, the difference between physical and psychological dependence must be well defined between clinicians and families to prevent confusion, and misconceptions as mentioned previously. Clinicians must also have a particularly unified front on adequate pain and sedation management. Psychological dependence in children is extremely rare, and thus the fear of psychological abuse, tolerance, withdrawal, or addiction should not prevent adequate treatment of acute pain, and/or adequate sedation, in children experiencing pain from acute or long-term disease states (Tobias 2000a). Psychological dependence refers to the need to continue opioid medication to perpetuate the feelings of euphoria, where as physical dependence on opioid medication is the need to continue opioids to prevent the symptoms of withdrawal. The signs and symptoms of withdrawal differ with the agent used, patient's age, cognition, and disease state, as well as the abruptness of opioid cessation in a patient who is already been on long-term opioid therapy and is thereby physically dependent (Tobias and Deshpande 1996).

Pseudoaddiction was first introduced in the late 1980s to describe the iatrogenic syndrome of abnormal behavior that develops in direct consequence to inadequate pain management (Weissman and Haddox 1989). By definition, the patient mimics behaviors that are commonly associated with addiction in order to get adequate pain relief. It usually occurs after an acute insult, and particularly when acute pain is overlaid on a chronic illness.

Three phases include inadequate prescription of analgesics to meet the primary pain stimulus. Next, escalation of analgesic demands by the patient associated with excessive behavioral changes to convince others of the pain's severity. Due to this, often times a climate of mistrust develops between the patient and the healthcare team. The patient must exhibit more and more dramatic behaviors and demands in order to have their pain alleviated, entering the third phase known as the crisis phase (Weissman 1994). By definition, the aberrant drug-related behaviors abate once the patient is adequately treated if the patient is truly pseudoaddicted (Collett 1998). Pseudoaddiction is a controversial issue. As in many areas of medicine physicians do not agree that pseudoaddiction is a true medical illness as described by Weissman (Weissman and Haddox 1989). Never-the-less, it is important to understand the psychology of pain management and have basic knowledge of what the literature describes as an enhanced pain state. As a result of inadequately treated pain, these patients are continually asking for more pain medication even at doses that would usually be more than adequate in a "normal" child with the same injury. The patients who have chronic disease states often know which opioid best treats their pain, and may even ask for it by name. The clinicians perceive their specific and continual requests for more opiates excessive, and become suspicious of these patients as exhibiting psychological dependence or addictive behaviors. The distrust and communication breakdown between the patient and the clinicians leads to more inadequately treated pain and a patient who often displays exaggerated pain behaviors to obtain the adequate pain relief. The vicious cycle continues with the staff becoming more suspicious of the patient, and the patient sometimes suffering isolation, and even neglect because of their inadequately treated pain and iatrogenically provoked drug-seeking behaviors.

True opioid addiction is psychological dependence accompanied by repetitive pathological behaviors to obtain and use opioids. These behaviors are very complex and are contiguous with criminal and/or antisocial behavior as part of accessing the opioid. These patients' lives revolve around their next dose of opioid and how to access the drug unrelated to a pain state. True addiction has a high incidence of relapse even after intense rehabilitation (Collett 1998; Tobias 2000a).

Withdrawal Symptoms

When a decision is made to wean an infant or child from opioid medication, careful weaning along with meticulous standardized monitoring for withdrawal symptoms is the key to the success of the weaning process. Clinical conditions and serious new onset illnesses that can be associated with the signs and symptoms of withdrawal must be ruled out prior to attributing new clinical presentations to withdrawal. Critically ill children can manifest central nervous system insults or infections, ICU psychosis, metabolic abnormalities, hypoxia, hypercarbia, and cerebral hypoperfusion with signs and symptoms similar or identical to those of withdrawal (Collett 1998; Anand and Arnold 1994; Tobias 2000a; Tobias et al. 1994). These signs and symptoms include: central nervous system activation; GI disturbances; and sympathetic hyperactivity. Irritability, increased wakefulness, tremulousness, hyperactive deep tendon reflexes, clonus, inability to concentrate, frequent yawning, sneezing, delirium, and hypertonicity are all manifestations of central nervous system withdrawal, with exaggerated Moro reflex, GI upset, and a high pitched cry being those symptoms most often seen in neonates and infants (Osborn et al. 2005; Kuschel 2007; Tenenbein et al. 1996;

Tobias 2006; Tobias 2007). Seizures as well as visual and auditory hallucinations have also been described in association with opioid withdrawal (Katz et al. 1994).

Opioid-Induced Hyperalgesia

Opioids have been used to treat acute and cancer-related pain for decades, and they are the foundation for treatment of moderate to severe pain. Clinicians have always been concerned with the adverse effects of opioids prior to placing a patient on these medications: nausea, vomiting, general GI upset, tolerance, and/or withdrawal. These adverse effects alone can give a physician pause prior to prescribing an opioid. Another possible side effect that can not be ignored is opioid induced hyperalgesia (OIH). More recently, opioids have gained popularity in treating chronic nonmalignant pain, and clinicians may need to rethink using opioids for long-term chronic pain syndromes because of the potential for development of OIH. OIH is a paradoxical problem related to opioid pain management. OIH presents itself when opioids are given to a patient to ameliorate pain, and the opioid medication paradoxically increases the intensity of painful stimulus, and/or exaggerates a pre-existing pain state. In OIH, opioids may provide initial analgesic and antihyperalgesic effects, but over time create symptoms of hyperalgesia, and this may point toward a process of upregulation in compensatory pronociceptive pathways in the spinothalamic axis (Angst and Clark 2006). Tolerance and OIH are distinct entities. Exposure to opioids can create the need to increase the dose over time to maintain the same level of analgesia in the development of opioid tolerance. This is a right shift of the dose effect relationship, or a loss of the potency of the opioid. OIH is an increase in pain sensitivity and a downward shift of the dose versus effect relationship. Tolerance appears to reflect a desensitization of the opioid antinociceptive pathways, whereas OIH or hyperalgesia is the sensitization of pronociceptive pathways (Angst and Clark 2006). Though both OIH and tolerance function via separate mechanisms, they both share the net effect of an increase in opioid dose requirements. An early observational indication of sig-

nificant changes that could be seen in neuronal systems during opioid therapy was recorded in the seventeenth century in an essay from Rossbach (1880), hyperesthesia (increased sensitivity to pain) was described as a symptom of opioid dependence, "when opioid dependence becomes an illness of itself," with pain described as one of the sequelae to opioid use. Pain is one of the current criteria used to evaluate a patient suspected of being in opioid withdrawal, and most of the research in OIH has been concentrated in the area of addiction and withdrawal. More recent studies have focused on OIH in the context of acute pain management. This newer research angle was started in response to animal studies in the 1970s suggesting that opioid administration may in fact increase sensitivity to new painful stimulus, or aggravate pre-existing pain (Angst and Clark 2006). The studies done in humans do point to OIH as a real phenomenon in opioid use. The data collected in human studies involve three clinical scenarios according to the review by Angst and Clark (2006): (1) former opioid addicts maintained on methadone, (2) patients undergoing surgical stimulus, and (3) in human volunteers modeling varied types of pain. Based on the current literature, opioid mechanisms originating in the spinothalamic and cortical axis can counteract analgesia and enhance pain sensitivity. What clinicians need to take from the current data is that aggressive opioid titration and management may cause increased pain sensitivity and/or aggravate preexisting pain. Discussing OIH with a patient's family, as a potential adverse side of effect of opioid therapy, might be taken into consideration prior to starting opioid management of pain, particularly when opioids are being used in the chronic pain setting. In addition, if opioid treatment is coinciding with a decrease in opioid effect, particularly in the face of increased pain, it should alert the clinician to the possible development of OIH. In this scenario, opioid weaning and detoxification in conjunction with alternative analgesics and therapies should be contemplated. Recommendations for the management of patients at risk of developing OIH are available in the literature in the context of acute pain, but some brief recommendations include: (1) management with multimodal analgesia, (2) avoidance of aggressive opioid titration with careful monitoring of same, and (3) the avoidance of periods of opioid abstinence (Angst and Clark 2006). Human studies involving OIH and chronic pain are lacking, and the evidence of OIH in other pain paradigms may suggest that clinicians need to carefully examine the risks of opioid use in the auspices of chronic pain treatment.

Neonatal Abstinence Syndrome
It is unfortunate that individuals of reproductive age have the highest prevalence of drug use in the population (Rayburn 2007). This presents a challenge for clinicians working with women ages 15–44 who are opioid-dependent or addicted and become pregnant. The care of women who are using opioids during pregnancy is very complex, difficult, and demanding at best due to the complexity of opioid dependency and addiction. Some women are not identified as being opioid-dependent until an infant is born and then the infant exhibits signs of neonatal opiate withdrawal in the first 48–120 h after birth. In the 1970s Finnegan et al. was one of the first groups to identify dependence and withdrawal in infants of opioid-addicted mothers (Finnegan et al. 1975). The phrase neonatal abstinence syndrome (NAS) was coined to describe a constellation of physical signs and symptoms associated with neonatal withdrawal from any volatile substance, but in particular, from the opioid class of drugs. Neonatal Opiate withdrawal (NOW) was termed later and is more specific for the purposes of opiate tolerance discussion (Coyle et al. 2002). Neonatal abstinence syndrome (NAS) is important for a clinician to recognize and treat because it can disrupt the mother–infant relationship, cause sleep–wake abnormalities, feeding difficulties, weight loss, and seizures. The morbidity of NAS can cause prolonged hospital stay and effect maternal–infant outcome, and thereby increase long-term health care outcomes and costs. NAS due to opiate withdrawal in the newborn infant is associated with a number of signs and symptoms including high pitched crying, insomnia, tremor, and myoclonic jerks. They can also experience vomiting, diarrhea, and poor weight gain; as previously mentioned NAS can be more deleterious in those infants born prematurely to a drug-dependent/addicted mother and are therefore, by definition, at high to extremely high risk for increased morbidity and mortality related to their prematurity alone. In high-risk patients like those mentioned above, identifying risk factors for developing withdrawal and starting appropriate treatment prior to its manifestation allows for withdrawal prevention and thereby protection from increased morbidity and mortality in an already high-risk group. Some of the risk factors identified for developing withdrawal have been studied and include total dose of opiate used as well as the duration of infusion (Tobias and Deshpande 1996; Katz et al. 1994). For example, a fentanyl dose of greater than or equal to 1.5 mg/kg, or duration of infusion greater than or equal to 5 days was associated with 50% incidence of withdrawal (Katz et al. 1994). These risks remain the same regardless of the opiate used; however, the dose and time interval may change slightly depending on the pharmacology of the opiate being given. Finnegan et al. identified the signs and symptoms with volatile substance withdrawal, and constructed an objective and comprehensive scoring system to evaluate an infant exhibiting the signs and symptoms of NAS (Finnegan et al. 1975). Other scoring systems are available to provide a measure for withdrawal although the Finnegan score is more comprehensive (Anand and Arnold 1994; Kahn et al. 1969). The Finnegan score helps clinicians and researchers objectively identify an infant in withdrawal and it also helps to evaluate the effectiveness of withdrawal ameliorating therapy once withdrawal has been identified (Tobias and Deshpande 1996). Some of the components of the Finnegan score are: excessive or continuous crying, time sleeping after feeding (1–3 h), exaggerated or hyperactive Moro reflex, tremors etc (Table 21.1).

Each of the criteria of the Finnegan score is assigned a numerical point value. The points are then added for objective classification of the severity of infant withdrawal and thereby also the efficacy of treatment modalities used to treat that infant. Point score 0–7 is the score for an infant in

Table 21.1 Table of common symptoms of Neonatal Abstinance Syndrome (NAS) and their frequency

Symptoms[a]	Frequency (%)
Common	
Tremors	
• Mild/disturbed	96
• Mild/undisturbed	95
• Marked/disturbed	77
• Marked/undisturbed	67
High-pitched cry	95
Continuous high-pitched cry	54
Sneezing	83
Increased muscle tone	82
Frantic sucking of fists	79
Regurgitation	74
Sleeps less than 3 h after feeding	65
Sleeps less than 2 h after feeding	66
Sleeps less than 1 h after feeding	58
Respiratory rate greater than 60/min	66
Poor feeding	65
Hyperactive Moro reflex	62
Loose stools	51
Less common	
Sweating	49
Excoriation	43
Mottling	33
Nasal stuffiness	33
Frequent yawning	30
Fever less than 101°F (39.3°C)	29
Respiratory rate greater than 60/min and retractions	28
Markedly hyperactive Moro reflex	15
Projectile vomiting	12
Watery stools	12
Fever less than 101°F (39.3°C)	3
Dehydration	1
Generalized convulsions	1

[a] http://depts.washington.edu/nicuweb/NICU-WEB/nas. stm#symptoms_RETURN#symptoms_RETURN

mild withdrawal, 8–11 indicates moderate withdrawal, and 12–15 severe withdrawal (Table 21.2 – Finnegan scoring).

The awareness of opioid dependency and withdrawal created by the description of NAS in the late 1960s and early 1970s by Kahn and Finnegan et al., along with the scoring system of Finnegan et al. triggering a series of different clinical trials and retrospective studies (Finnegan et al. 1975; Kahn et al. 1969). These studies examined the

prevalence of neonatal volatile substance withdrawal, maternal neonatal outcomes, withdrawal in the PICU after prolonged sedation or analgesic treatments, as well as the effectiveness of withdrawal treatment modalities (Osborn et al. 2005; Kuschel 2007; Tenenbein et al. 1996; Tobias 2006; Rayburn 2007; Coyle et al. 2002; McCarthy et al. 2005; Burns and Mattick 2007; Langenfeld et al. 2005; Sarkar and Donn 2006; Leeuwenburgh-Pronk et al. 2006; Kracke et al. 2005; Kaltenbach and Finnegan 1986; Osborn et al. 2002; Autret et al. 2004; Coghlan et al. 1999). Morphine, tincture of opium, phenobarbitone, diazepam, chlorpromazine, clonidine, dexmedetomidine, supportive care only, and a combination of multiple treatment modalities, all present themselves in the literature as treatments for NAS and neonatal opiate withdrawal (NOW) in various study paradigms. There is continued debate about the choice of method for treating neonatal opioid withdrawal, although clinicians would agree that once the decision is made to wean an opiate-dependent child from opiates, or to prevent NOW in an opiate exposed neonate, close observation and an objective scoring method is necessary to screen for and to assess a child for the development of withdrawal, as well as to assess the efficacy of the treatment modality. The main way to prevent opioid withdrawal is to slowly wean the opioid by tapering i.v. opioid infusion therapy 10–15% every 6–8 h. This method is only effective in children who have been on a short course of opiate analgesia or sedation. The patient's withdrawal response is the clinical guide to weaning a child. Parental concerns about symptoms should also be taken into account in the weaning process, as parents often notice the subtle changes in their child prior to their recognition by the clinical staff Coghlan et al. 1999.

Opioid weaning strategies in 2007 (Cho et al. 2007)

1. Reduction of opioid dose by 5–10% daily[a] (slowly over the course of a day depending on withdrawal score)
2. Initial reduction of opioid by 20–40% followed by a 10% reduction once or twice daily depending on the withdrawal response[a]

[a] Note: the longer a patient is administered an opioid medication, the slower and more conservative the wean

Table 21.2 Modified Finnegan Score 1996

SYSTEM	SIGNS & SYMPTOMS	SCORE							
CENTRAL NERVOUS SYSTEM DISTURBANCES	High-Pitched Cry	2							
	Continuous High-Pitched Cry	3							
	Sleeps < 1 hour after feeding	3							
	Sleeps < 2 hours after feeding	2							
	Sleeps < 3 hours after feeding	1							
	Mild Tremors Disturbed	1							
	Mod-Severe Tremors Disturbed	2							
	Mild Tremors Undisturbed	3							
	Mod-Severe Tremors Undisturbed	4							
	Increased Muscle Town **(= Tone)**	2							
	Excoriation (Specify Area)	1							
	Myoclonic Jerks	3							
	Generalised Convulsions	5							
METABOLIC/VASOMOTOR/ RESPIRATORY DISTURBANCES	Sweating	1							
	Fever (37.5° - 38.0°C)	1							
	Fever (38.4°C and higher)	2							
	Frequent Yawning (>3-4 times)	1							
	Nasal Stuffiness	1							
	Sneezing (>3-4 times)	1							
	Nasal Flaring	2							
	Respiratory Rate > 60/min	1							
	Respiratory Rate > 60/min with Retractions	2							
GASTROPOINTESTINAL DISTURBANCES	Excessive Sucking	1							
	Poor Feeding	2							
	Regurgitation	2							
	Projectile Vomiting	3							
	Loose Stools	2							
	Watery Stools	3							
	Total Score								
	Scorer's Initials								

DATE AND TIME IN HOURS

Consider Treatment if score >8

Auckland Healthcare
Te Toka Oranga O Tamaki Makau Rau

NAME:
DATE OF BIRTH:
WARD/UNIT:
HOSP. No
Please attach patient label here

NEONATAL SCORING CHART

CR421

9/96

It is important to note that these are only guidelines for weaning opioid medication. The longer a child has been on an opioid medication, the slower and more conservative the weaning process must be to avoid withdrawal symptoms; the wean must be tailored to each patient individually using a standardized scale as mentioned previously. It is also important to train clinicians on how to properly and objectively score the NAS, and treat accordingly.

Children who are difficult to wean are those children who have been on opiates for more than 5 days (Tobias 2000a; Tobias and Deshpande 1996; Tobias 2006; Tobias 2007). This group of patients includes opiate-dependent neonates of opiate-dependent mothers; children ventilated in the ICU for a prolonged period of time; and children having disease states requiring chronic opioid use. In these instances, opiate weaning can take 2 weeks to 1 month and require maintenance of a peripheral IV. This requires IV management in an inpatient setting to wean over this prolonged period. Prolonging hospital stays in our current health care environment is cost prohibitive. For these patients the opiate dose required can be converted into an oral or subcutaneous dosing regimen while monitoring the patient in the PICU. After the efficacy and safety of the enteral or subcutaneous opioid weaning regimen has been established in a monitored environment, the patient can be transferred to the floor where enteral opioid weaning can be continued with the ultimate goal of transitioning to sending the patient home and managing weaning and withdrawal in the outpatient setting. These oral or subcutaneous doses can be weaned slowly over an appropriate period of time monitoring for withdrawal symptoms (see Tables 21.1 and 21.3) (Tobias and Deshpande 1996; Cho et al. 2007; Jacobi et al. 2002; Brown et al. 2000). A caveat to this weaning process is that prior to converting to an enteral opioid dose, several factors must be considered and the Internet provides several conversion websites that can help with these conversions. The opioid conversion websites can automatically account for the following, IV to Oral, opioid dosing factors and can be of help in this process (Tobias et al. 1994). Caution is recommended

Table 21.3 Conversion factors for IV to oral opioid dosing

Potency of IV vs. oral medications
The drug half life
Oral bioavailability and liver first pass effects
Other medications or low protein nutritional states that can enhance opioid potency
1. Calculate current drug 24-h dose (dose times and number of times given per day).
2. Multiply this current 24-h dose times the ratio of 24-h equivalent dose of new drug over 24-h equivalent of old drug. This gives 24-h dose of new drug (equivalent doses from table above).
3. After determining the equianalgesic dose, start at one-half to two-thirds of the equianalgesic dose to account for incomplete cross-tolerance.
4. Divide new 24-h drug dose by number of times drug to be given per day. This gives new individual drug dose.
5. Order new individual drug dose to be divided per the dosing interval determined above. This is the target dose.

Note: This is only a guideline for clinicians. A full clinical evaluation and assessment must be performed to account for patient variability

when calculating doses using a website and checking calculations against recommendations in the literature is advised. When converting from one opioid to another, the amount of residual drug in the system has a large impact on how much new basal drug is to be started. Overdose can occur when the target dose of a new opioid is initiated without taking conversion factors (listed below) and residual drug into consideration, especially when long-acting opioids are in the mix (Hallenbeck 2003; Nielsen et al. 2000). The initial opioid conversion should be implemented in a monitored pediatric environment.

Once the transition has been made from IV to oral, subcutaneous, or transcutaneous opioids safely, the weaning process can continue in a less monitored environment with preparation for discharge and subsequent home opioid management. Parents usually know their children well; they are good monitors for their children and can be educated on the signs and symptoms of withdrawal and its subsequent safe treatment in the outpatient setting.

Liver Maturity and Opioids

Most medications have a different pharmacodynamic and pharmacokinetic spectrum when used in the pediatric population. This is most evident between adults and neonates. Pediatric patients have altered protein binding, a larger volume of distribution, smaller proportion of fat and muscle stores, as well as immature renal and hepatic function, and even an immature blood–brain barrier as seen in neonates ("Smith's Anesthesia," 2006). All of these physiologic differences are reasons for different drug response in the pediatric population. There can be a reduced drug metabolism or a delay in drug elimination based on these differences and a developing liver. The liver is an extremely important organ. It is responsible for glucose homeostasis, cholesterol synthesis and triglyceride production, coagulation factor production, hemoglobin metabolism, drug metabolism, urea production from nitrogen wastes, blood cell production in first trimester fetus, vitamin and mineral storage (B12, copper, and iron to name a couple), and osmolar plasma albumin production ("A Practice" 2001; "Liver Disease" 2007).

The liver develops into a well-differentiated organ with bile secretion by 12 weeks of gestation. It develops from progenitor cells from the embryo to fetus stage of human development. At birth, the liver cells are already specialized and have two surfaces of function: (1) liver sinus side exposed to liver blood flow from the portal vein that contain nutrients and oxygen as well as, (2) the bile surface that delivers bile and conjugated and metabolized products to the caniculi and bile ductules. The maturation of the liver after delivery is complex and involves normal gene expression in genes responsible for amino acid transport and insulin growth factors. Once the umbilical blood supply is terminated at delivery, the initiation of liver functions including transamination, glutamyl transferase, coagulation factor synthesis, bile production, and transport are stimulated at a rapid rate. To spite this rapid organ development and induction of function, full maturity of liver functions can take up to 2 years after the birth of a child ("A Practice 2001; Liver Ddisease in Cchildren 2007). This is particularly apparent into neonatal period during which the development of toxic drug levels and kernicterus is a real risk due to immature liver function at birth.

Morphine is a drug with high hepatic extraction coefficient. What this means is that morphine clearance is determined by hepatic blood flow. Morphine in particular is inactivated by liver N-demethylation and glucuronidation. The drug metabolites formed as a result of liver metabolism are morphine 6-glucuronide and morphine 3-glucuronide that are both excreted by the kidney. In the adult human, morphine is 30–35% protein bound in adults and 18–22% in neonates. Age-related changes in the pharmacokinetics of morphine have been observed, but there is some controversy in the literature with regard to age-related changes in the neonatal period ("Smith's Anesthesia" 2006; Bhat et al. 1990; Chay et al. 1992). The pharmacokinetics of morphine can be changed by disease. Renal and liver disease can change elimination half lives and have in part unpredictable pharmacokinetic effects on morphine. Awareness of disease states and their possible effects can be of particular advantage in weaning a child from opiate therapy and maintaining a safely monitored environment for changing from an IV to an oral, or transcutaneous opioid medication.

Clinical Implications of Opioid Tolerance

Cellular Mechanisms of Tolerance

As previously described, the four receptors in the central nervous system include the mu, kappa, delta, and sigma receptors. The development of tolerance and dependency are influenced by the "occupancy of the receptor by an agonist and the specificity or the degree of binding of the agonist to the receptor." "Despite the obvious development of clinical tolerance, the exact cellular mechanisms responsible for tolerance and dependency remain poorly defined." The mechanism may be alterations of the interactions between the receptor and regulatory proteins and enzyme systems instead of an actual decrease in receptor number or binding affinity (Lutfy et al. 1991).

"Abrupt discontinuation of the opioid with decreased receptor occupancy results in increased afferent activity to the central nervous system with activation of the reticular activating system as well as sympathetic centers such as the locus ceruleus with increased efferent sympathetic activity resulting in autonomic effects including hypertension and tachycardia" (Tobias 2000a).

Time for Development of Opioid Tolerance

The development of opioid tolerance is affected by the duration of opioid receptor occupancy and seems to develop more quickly with continuous IV infusion versus intermittent dosing. The major factor in the development of opioid tolerance is the "duration of opioid receptor occupancy" (Tobias and Deshpande 1996). It has also been suggested that "tolerance develops more rapidly with the continuous vs. intermittent administration of sedative and analgesic agents (Tobias 2000a; Tobias and Deshpande 1996). Patients receiving synthetic opioids may develop tolerance more quickly than those receiving natural occurring opioids such as morphine. Crawford et al. compared postoperative morphine requirements in pediatric patients receiving a continuous infusion of remifentanil versus intermittent boluses of morphine during scoliosis surgery (Crawford et al. 2006). Postoperatively, the patients that received a remifentanil infusion had a "30% greater morphine consumption" compared to those that received intermittent morphine (Crawford et al. 2006). Arnold et al. described changes in neonatal pharmacodynamic response to fentanyl infusion. The mean infusion rate greater than doubled from day 1 to day 6, suggesting the rapid development of tolerance to the sedating effects of fentanyl (Arnold et al. 1991). Arnold et al. reviewed 37 neonates who had required extracorporeal membrane oxygenation (ECMO). They received IV fentanyl for sedation and it was noted that from day 1 to day 8, an increase in plasma fentanyl concentration was required to achieve the same effect.

The development of withdrawal after continuous infusions of fentanyl is both duration-dependent and dose-dependent. Katz et al. studied the occurrence of withdrawal in critically ill children who had received a continuous fentanyl infusion. They found that a "duration of infusion greater than 9 days or a total fentanyl dose of 2.5 mg/kg was 100% predictive of withdrawal" (Katz et al. 1994). In light of these findings, the potential for tolerance and its effects must be weighed against the potential benefit of improved analgesia with continuous vs. intermittent bolusing in addition to effective control of stress and vasomotor tone of the pulmonary vasculature with synthetic opioids versus other agents.

When tolerance does develop, there are a few treatment options. Because opioids do not have a ceiling effect, an increase in the dose required to provide relief or desired effect may be performed gradually and slow enough to prevent intolerable side effects. Another option is opioid rotation rather than dose escalation. Because of incomplete cross tolerance, upon converting from one opioid to another, it is important to know the conversion factors of the different opioids, their pharmacokinetics, pharmacodynamics, and amount of incomplete cross-tolerance. To account for incomplete cross tolerance during opioid switching conversions, it is recommended to determine the equianalgesic conversion and start at one-half to two-thirds of the equianalgesic dose especially when converting from one opioid class to another.

Adjuvant Medications and Therapies

Another consideration is the use of adjuvant medications to attenuate the effect of tolerance/withdrawal symptoms. The use of adjuvant medications can attenuate the need for the escalating doses of opioid medications when tolerance does develop. Depending on the type of pain, various adjuvant medications may be of use. Some patients may be a candidate for the use of nonsteroidal anti-inflammatory medication; topical formulations are also available. The use of neuropathic pain medications such as gabapentin, pregabalin, antidepressants may be of use in some patients, remembering that most of the studies done in these drugs are in the adult population and some caution and monitoring is recommended. This does not deter their usefulness in complex cases where pain management and tolerance have become difficult, if not seemingly impossible to manage. The literature does support using adjuvant medications in specific pediatric cases of pain management and tolerance (Tobias 2006; Tobias 2007; Tobias and Berkenbosch 2001; Suresh and Anand 2001; Tobias 2000b; Hoder et al. 1981). The risks of these adjuvants must be weighed against their benefits, and involving families in the decision to use these adjuvants is prudent if not necessary, especially from a medical legal perspective. This is particularly true when using medications not FDA approved for their use in pain management, or approved for their use to treat infants, children, or neonates, without guidelines for specific medical indications. NMDA receptor antagonists such as ketamine have been used for sedation and in the perioperative setting, and may be of use in the PICU environment.

Alpha-adrenoreceptor agonists, such as Clonidine, may be of use and has been used for years to assuage withdrawal from opioids. Dexmedetomidine is an alpha-2 adrenergic receptor agonist that has a shorter half-life and more alpha-2 specificity than clonidine. Infusions of dexmedetomidine have been used in the pediatric population for sedation in the perioperative and intensive care setting. It has also been used for withdrawal prevention following opioid and/or benzodiazepine administration (Tobias 2007).

In the appropriate clinical setting, some patients may be candidates for neuraxial analgesia including epidural catheter infusions. Peripheral nerve blocks or continuous infusions via catheter may also be a helpful alternative to providing pain relief. These methods are often underused in the clinical setting of opioid tolerance, particularly outside the surgical forum because they require skilled anesthesia personnel and are relatively time intensive to place and manage. The potential adverse events associated with neuraxial and regional anesthesia may not be overlooked and a risk benefit scenario examined prior to their use. Again, in appropriate situations this does not contraindicate their use in complex patients that have become tolerant to opioid medications, where their utility may be invaluable (Tobias 2000c; Tobias 2004). Other pain management strategies that can be useful to treat opioid tolerance/withdrawal symptoms are massage therapy, relaxation techniques, biofeedback training, music therapy, distraction techniques, and child life resources. These alternate treatment modalities can be invaluable in the opioid weaning process, and their utility should not be dismissed or overlooked.

Outpatient Therapy

Tobias et al. described case reports of patients that required prolonged sedation in the pediatric intensive care unit. Conversion to oral agents and discharge with an oral taper schedule was performed which allowed the patient to be discharged earlier and to not require intravenous access (Tobias et al. 1994). Recommendations in the literature vary significantly regarding rate of dose reduction. As a general rule, the longer that a patient is on opioids and higher the dosages, the slower the weaning. Opioid weaning decreases opioids by 10–20% every 3–7 days. Drake et al. performed a retrospective study to determine the "therapeutic value" of opioid rotation for pediatric cancer patients (Drake et al. 2004). They found that opioid rotation had a "positive impact" on managing side effects or tolerance to the medication (Drake et al. 2004).

Summary

As pain management in the pediatric population becomes more sophisticated, and more aggressive approaches are chosen to manage pediatric pain, so must our recognition and treatment of opioid-induced side effects. Tolerance, Opioid Hyperalgesia, Withdrawal, and Addiction must be clearly defined, identified, and managed early in the care of patients requiring opioid medication for pain management and sedation. In addition, knowing how to treat tolerance and withdrawal with opioid rotation and preventative weaning strategies for withdrawal is critical to adequate management of the above opioid seque-lae. To do this, comprehensive, valid pain scoring and weaning scales should be used by trained personnel to ensure adequate and early treatment of tolerance and its closely related, but different cohorts. As a rule, the longer a patient has been on opioid therapy, the greater the chance of developing tolerance and the slower the opioid wean will have to be to prevent withdrawal symptoms. A patient that has been given opioid medication for less than 5 days can generally be weaned faster than a patient on opioids greater than 5 days. This rule varies from patient to patient and withdrawal scoring becomes essential in opioid weaning. We discussed a couple of weaning strategies in this chapter keeping in mind that more or less conservative weaning strategies must be used on a patient to patient basis. Generally a patient can be weaned from an opiate 10–15% daily by way of a slow decrease in dose over the course of a day with careful monitoring for signs and symptoms of opiate withdrawal. Another option is to initially wean the opioid by 20–40%, and then decrease the opioid dose 10% once or twice daily depending on their withdrawal score. In the event that a patient requires a long opioid wean over weeks, the initial conversion from intravenous opioid therapy to oral or subcutaneous longer acting opioids, is best implemented in a monitored environment to prevent unrecognized hypopnea. Once this initial switch has been safely achieved, continued weaning can take place in the inpatient ward or at home with parental preparation and education prior to discharge. Finally when it has been established that tolerance is developing in a patient or an opioid conversion or rotation is necessary, it is essential that clinicians know the potency of a medication (IV vs. Oral), the drug half life, and the bioavailability of the opioid and liver first pass effect to accurately calculate the dose. Clinicians should recognize their arsenal of adjuvant therapies for pain management, become familiar with their profile, as well as their risks and benefits to be better able to contend with the consequences of opioid therapy.

References

A practice of anesthesia for infants and children. (2001). Philadelphia: Saunders.

Anand, K. J., & Arnold, J. H. (1994). Opioid tolerance and dependence in infants and children. *Critical Care Medicine, 22*, 334–342.

Angst, M. S., & Clark, J. D. (2006). Opioid-induced hyperalgesia: a qualitative systematic review. *Anesthesiology, 104*, 570–587.

Arnold, J. H., Truog, R. D., Orav, E. J., Scavone, J. M., & Hershenson, M. B. (1990). Tolerance and dependence in neonates sedated with fentanyl during extracorporeal membrane oxygenation. *Anesthesiology, 73*, 1136–1140.

Arnold, J. H., Truog, R. D., Scavone, J. M., & Fenton, T. (1991). Changes in the pharmacodynamic response to fentanyl in neonates during continuous infusion. *Jornal de Pediatria, 119*, 639–643.

Autret, F., Mucignat, V., De Montgolfier-Aubron, I., Blond, M. H., Duerocq, S., Lebas, F., & Gold, F. (2004). Use of diazepam in the treatment of opioid neonatal abstinence syndrome. *Archives of Pediatrics, 11*, 1308–1313.

Bhat, R., Chari, G., Gulati, A., Aldana, O., Velamati, R., & Bhargava, H. (1990). Pharmacokinetics of a single dose of morphine in preterm infants during the first week of life. *Jornal de Pediatria, 117*, 477–481.

Brown, C., Albrecht, R., Pettit, H., McFadden, T., & Schermer, C. (2000). Opioid and benzodiazepine withdrawal syndrome in adult burn patients. *The American Surgeon, 66*, 367–370. discussion 370–371.

Burns, L., & Mattick, R. P. (2007). Using population data to examine the prevalence and correlates of neonatal abstinence syndrome. *Drug and Alcohol Review, 26*, 487–492.

Chay, P. C., Duffy, B. J., & Walker, J. S. (1992). Pharmacokinetic-pharmacodynamic relationships of morphine in neonates. *Clinical Pharmacology and Therapeutics, 51*, 334–342.

Cho, H. H., O'Connell, J. P., Cooney, M. F., & Inchiosa, M. A., Jr. (2007). Minimizing tolerance and withdrawal to prolonged pediatric sedation: Case report and review of the literature. *Journal of Intensive Care Medicine, 22*, 173–179.

Coghlan, D., Milner, M., Clarke, T., Lambert, I., McDermott, C., McNally, M., Beckett, M., & Matthews, T. (1999). Neonatal abstinence syndrome. *Irish Medical Journal, 92*, 232–233. 236.

Collett, B. J. (1998). Opioid tolerance: The clinical perspective. *British Journal of Anaesthesia, 81*, 58–68.

Compton, P., Geschwind, D. H., & Alarcon, M. (2003). Association between human mu-opioid receptor gene polymorphism, pain tolerance, and opioid addiction. *American Journal of Medical Genetics. Part B: Neuropsychiatric Genetics, 121*, 76–82.

Coulbault, L., Beaussier, M., Verstuyft, C., Weickmans, H., Dubert, L., Tregouet, D., Descot, C., Parc, Y., et al. (2006). Environmental and genetic factors associated with morphine response in the postoperative period. *Clinical Pharmacology and Therapeutics, 79*, 316–324.

Cox, B. M., Ginsburg, M., & Willis, J. (1975). The offset of morphine tolerance in rats and mice. *British Journal of Pharmacology, 53*(3), 383–391.

Coyle, M. G., Ferguson, A., Lagasse, L., Oh, W., & Lester, B. (2002). Diluted tincture of opium (DTO) and phenobarbital versus DTO alone for neonatal opiate withdrawal in term infants. *Jornal de Pediatria, 140*, 561–564.

Crawford, M. W., Hickey, C., Zaarour, C., Howard, A., & Naser, B. (2006). Development of acute opioid tolerance during infusion of remifentanil for pediatric scoliosis surgery. *Anesthesia and Analgesia, 102*, 1662–1667.

Drake, R., Longworth, J., & Collins, J. J. (2004). Opioid rotation in children with cancer. *Journal of Palliative Medicine, 7*, 419–422.

Finnegan, L. P., Connaughton, J. F., Jr., Kron, R. E., & Emich, J. P. (1975). Neonatal abstinence syndrome: Assessment and management. *Addictive Diseases, 2*, 141–158.

Goldstein, A., & Naidu, A. (1989). Multiple opioid receptors: ligand selectivity profiles and binding site signatures. *Mol Pharmacology, 36*(2), 265–272.

Hallenbeck, J. (2003). *Palliative care perspectives*. New York: Oxford University Press.

Hoder, E. L., Leckman, J. F., Ehrenkranz, R., Kleber, H., Cohen, D. J., & Poulsen, J. A. (1981). Clonidine in neonatal narcotic-abstinence syndrome. *The New England Journal of Medicine, 305*, 1284.

Hovav, E., & Weinstock, M. (1987). Temporal factors influencing the development of acute tolerance to opiates. *The Journal of Pharmacology and Experimental Therapeutics, 242*, 251–256.

Jacobi, J., Fraser, G. L., Coursin, D. B., Riker, R. R., Fontaine, D., Wittbrodt, E. T., Chalfin, D. B., Masica, M. F., et al. (2002). Clinical practice guidelines for the sustained use of sedatives and analgesics in the critically ill adult. *Critical Care Medicine, 30*, 119–141.

Kahn, E. J., Neumann, L. L., & Polk, G. A. (1969). The course of the heroin withdrawal syndrome in newborn infants treated with phenobarbital or chlorpromazine. *Jornal de Pediatria, 75*, 495–500.

Kaltenbach, K., & Finnegan, L. P. (1986). Neonatal abstinence syndrome, pharmacotherapy and developmental outcome. *Neurobehavioral Toxicology and Teratology, 8*, 353–355.

Katz, R., Kelly, H. W., & Hsi, A. (1994). Prospective study on the occurrence of withdrawal in critically ill children who receive fentanyl by continuous infusion. *Critical Care Medicine, 22*, 763–767.

Kracke, G. R., Uthoff, K. A., & Tobias, J. D. (2005). Sugar solution analgesia: the effects of glucose on expressed mu opioid receptors. *Anesthesia and Analgesia, 101*, 64–68. table of contents.

Kuschel, C. (2007). Managing drug withdrawal in the newborn infant. *Seminars in Fetal & Neonatal Medicine, 12*, 127–133.

Landau, R. (2006). One size does not fit all: Genetic variability of mu-opioid receptor and postoperative morphine consumption. *Anesthesiology, 105*, 235–237.

Landau, R., Cahana, A., Smiley, R. M., Antonarakis, S. E., & Blouin, J. L. (2004). Genetic variability of mu-opioid receptor in an obstetric population. *Anesthesiology, 100*, 1030–1033.

Langenfeld, S., Birkenfeld, L., Herkenrath, P., Muller, C., Hellmich, M., & Theisohn, M. (2005). Therapy of the neonatal abstinence syndrome with tincture of opium or morphine drops. *Drug and Alcohol Dependence, 77*, 31–36.

Leeuwenburgh-Pronk, W. G., de Vries, M. C., & Clement-de Boers, A. (2006). A multidisciplinary approach is necessary in the neonatal withdrawal syndrome. *Nederlands Tijdschrift voor Geneeskunde, 150*, 761–765.

Liver disease in children (2007). New York: Cambridge University Press.

Lotsch, J., Freynhagen, R., & Geisslinger, G. (2005). Are polymorphisms in the mu-opioid receptor important for opioid therapy? *Schmerz, 19*(378–382), 384–385.

Lotsch, J., & Geisslinger, G. (2006). Relevance of frequent mu-opioid receptor polymorphisms for opioid activity in healthy volunteers. *The Pharmacogenomics Journal, 6*, 200–210.

Lutfy, K., Chang, S. C., Candido, J., Jang, Y., Sierra, V., & Yoburn, B. C. (1991). Modification of morphine-induced analgesia and toxicity by pertussis toxin. *Brain Research, 544*, 191–195.

Lutfy, K., & Yoburn, B. C. (1991). The role of opioid receptor density in morphine tolerance. *The Journal of Pharmacology and Experimental Therapeutics, 256*, 575–580.

Margas, W., Zubkoff, I., Schuler, H. G., Janicki, P. K., & Ruiz-Velasco, V. (2007). Modulation of Ca2+ channels by heterologously expressed wild-type and mutant human micro-opioid receptors (hMORs) containing the A118G single-nucleotide polymorphism. *Journal of Neurophysiology, 97*, 1058–1067.

McCarthy, J. J., Leamon, M. H., Parr, M. S., & Anania, B. (2005). High-dose methadone maintenance in pregnancy: Maternal and neonatal outcomes. *American Journal of Obstetrics and Gynecology, 193*, 606–610.

Nielsen, C. K., Ross, F. B., & Smith, M. T. (2000). Incomplete, asymmetric, and route-dependent cross-tolerance between oxycodone and morphine in the Dark Agouti rat. *The Journal of Pharmacology and Experimental Therapeutics, 295*, 91–99.

Osborn, D. A., Cole, M. J., & Jeffery, H. E. (2002). Opiate treatment for opiate withdrawal in newborn infants. *Cochrane Database of Systematic Reviews*, CD002059.

Osborn, D. A., Jeffery, H. E., & Cole, M. J. (2005). Sedatives for opiate withdrawal in newborn infants. *Cochrane Database of Systematic Reviews*, CD002053.

Rayburn, W. F. (2007). Maternal and fetal effects from substance use. *Clinics in Perinatology, 34*, 559–571.

Sarkar, S., & Donn, S. M. (2006). Management of neonatal abstinence syndrome in neonatal intensive care units: A national survey. *Journal of Perinatology, 26*, 15–17.

Shapiro, B. A., Warren, J., Egol, A. B., Greenbaum, D. M., Jacobi, J., Nasraway, S. A., Schein, R. M., Spevetz, A., & Stone, J. R. (1995). Practice parameters for intravenous analgesia and sedation for adult patients in the intensive care unit: An executive summary. Society of critical care medicine. *Critical Care Medicine, 23*, 1596–1600.

Sim-Selley, L. J., Scoggins, K. L., Cassidy, M. P., Smith, L. A., Dewey, W. L., Smith, F. L., & Selley, D. E. (2007). Region-dependent attenuation of mu-opioid receptor-mediated G-protein activation in mouse CNS as a function of morphine tolerance. *British Journal of Pharmacology, 151*, 1324–1333.

Smith's anesthesia for infants and children. (2006). Philadelphia: Mosby Elsevier.

Suresh, S., & Anand, K. J. (2001). Opioid tolerance in neonates: A state-of-the-art review. *Paediatric Anaesthesia, 11*, 511–521.

Tenenbein, M., Casiro, O. G., Seshia, M. M., & Debooy, V. D. (1996). Neonatal withdrawal from maternal volatile substance abuse. *Archives of Disease in Childhood. Fetal and Neonatal Edition, 74*, F204–207.

Tobias, J. D. (2000a). Tolerance, withdrawal, and physical dependency after long-term sedation and analgesia of children in the pediatric intensive care unit. *Critical Care Medicine, 28*, 2122–2132.

Tobias, J. D. (2000b). Weak analgesics and nonsteroidal anti-inflammatory agents in the management of children with acute pain. *Pediatric Clinics of North America, 47*, 527–543.

Tobias, J. D. (2000c). Applications of intrathecal catheters in children. *Paediatric Anaesthesia, 10*, 367–375.

Tobias, J. D. (2004). A review of intrathecal and epidural analgesia after spinal surgery in children. *Anesthesia and Analgesia, 98*, 956–965. table of contents.

Tobias, J. D. (2005). Sedation and analgesia in the pediatric intensive care unit. *Pediatric Annals, 34*, 636–645.

Tobias, J. D. (2006). Dexmedetomidine to treat opioid withdrawal in infants following prolonged sedation in the pediatric ICU. *Journal of Opioid Management, 2*, 201–205.

Tobias, J. D. (2007). Dexmedetomidine: applications in pediatric critical care and pediatric anesthesiology. *Pediatric Critical Care Medicine, 8*, 115–131.

Tobias, J. D., & Berkenbosch, J. W. (2001). Tolerance during sedation in a pediatric ICU patient: Effects on the BIS monitor. *Journal of Clinical Anesthesia, 13*, 122–124.

Tobias, J. D., & Deshpande, J. K. (1996). *Pediatric pain management for primary care.* Philadelphia: Mosby-Yearbook.

Tobias, J. D., Deshpande, J. K., & Gregory, D. F. (1994). Outpatient therapy of iatrogenic drug dependency following prolonged sedation in the pediatric intensive care unit. *Intensive Care Medicine, 20*, 504–507.

Tobias, J. D., Schleien, C. L., & Haun, S. E. (1990). Methadone as treatment for iatrogenic narcotic dependency in pediatric intensive care unit patients. *Critical Care Medicine, 18*, 1292–1293.

Turner, H. N. (2005). Complex pain consultations in the pediatric intensive care unit. *AACN Clinical Issues, 16*, 388–395.

Weissman, D. E. (1994). Understanding pseudoaddiction. *Journal of Pain and Symptom Management, 9*, 74.

Weissman, D. E., & Haddox, J. D. (1989). Opioid pseudoaddiction–an iatrogenic syndrome. *Pain, 36*, 363–366.

Wheeler, A. D., & Tobias, J. D. (2006). Bradycardia during methadone therapy in an infant. *Pediatric Critical Care Medicine, 7*, 83–85.

Zhang, Y., Wang, D., Johnson, A. D., Papp, A. C., & Sadee, W. (2005). Allelic expression imbalance of human mu opioid receptor (OPRM1) caused by variant A118G. *The Journal of Biological Chemistry, 280*, 32618–32624.

Zhao, Z. Q., Gao, Y. J., Sun, Y. G., Zhao, C. S., Gereau, R. W., & Chen, Z. F. (2007). Central serotonergic neurons are differentially required for opioid analgesia but not for morphine tolerance or morphine reward. *Proceedings of National Academy of Sciences of the United States of America, 104*, 14519–14524.

Arlyne Kim Thung

Keywords

Opioid withdrawal • Assessment scales • Buprenorphine management • Methadone • Ultra-rapid detoxification

Introduction

Opioid therapy has long been a mainstay in the practitioner's armamentarium to alleviate the pain and anxiety associated with the hospitalization of the pediatric patient. Whether for surgical or nonsurgical pain management, maintaining hemodynamic stability (Goldstein and Brazy 1991), reducing physiological responses to stress (Chambliss and Anand 1997), or providing sedation and analgesia for invasive procedures and mechanical ventilation in the intensive care unit, the myriad uses of opioid therapy are well known and regarded by the pediatric practitioner.

In surveys assessing current sedative and analgesic practices in pediatric intensive care in the United States and the United Kingdom (Rhoney and Murry 2002; Twite et al. 2004; Jenkins et al. 2007), opioids, specifically morphine and fentanyl, along with benzodiazepines, were the most commonly administered pharmacological agents. These findings reaffirmed the conclusions formed by Marx et al (1993) in which fentanyl and morphine along with chloral hydrate and benzodiazepines

were the most frequently administered agents for the most common cited goals of decreasing patient anxiety, preventing unplanned extubations and establishing patient ventilator synchrony in the PICU.

Despite the purported benefits of opioids as analgesic and sedative agents in the pediatric population, practitioners are still faced with the ramifications of their prolonged use, that of tolerance, dependence, withdrawal, rarely addiction (Porter and Jick 1980; Kanner and Foley 1981; McGivney and Crooks 1984), and potentially pseudo-addiction (Weissman and Haddox 1989; Lusher et al. 2006). Furthermore, practitioners are challenged by conflicting evidence that opioid therapy, specifically in ventilated preterm infants, may not be as beneficial as previously thought (Anand et al. 2004; Bhandari et al. 2005) and by the lack of evidence-based studies that may guide optimal assessment, prevention and therapy of pediatric opioid withdrawal when given (Statler and Lugo 2004; Prins et al. 2006; Ista et al. 2007). This latter sentiment has been highlighted by Playfor et al (2006) who published to date the only set of consensus guidelines related to the sedation and analgesia of critically ill children. The majority of recommendations grades were notably class C and D, likely due to the lack of randomized controlled evidence-based studies.

A.K. Thung (✉)
Department of Anesthesiology, Yale University School of Medicine, New Haven, CT, USA
e-mail: Arlyne.thung@yale.edu

B.C. McClain and S. Suresh (eds.), *Handbook of Pediatric Chronic Pain: Current Science and Integrative Practice*, DOI 10.1007/978-1-4419-0350-1_22,
© Springer Science+Business Media, LLC 2011

Notwithstanding, concern for the potentialities of opioid use has prompted practitioners to develop and enact strategies to minimize harm associated with opioid use and to allow its continued administration without reservation (Tobias 2000) in warranted situations. One such strategy is opioid tapering which has become standard practice in the adult population and currently recommended by adult sedative and analgesic clinical guidelines (Jacobi et al. 2002).

The aims of this chapter are to define terms associated with opioid use that pediatric practitioners must familiarize themselves with and review mechanisms of opioid tolerance and withdrawal, commonly used assessment scales for opioid withdrawal, published opioid tapering regimens, and current pharmacological treatments for opioid withdrawal and prevention.

Definitions

An accurate understanding of the terminology associated with opioid therapy is imperative. Practitioners should be familiar with the common and rare consequences of opioid use, such as tolerance, dependence, withdrawal, addiction, and pseudo-addiction (Table 22.1) so that appropriate treatment may be provided to patients who are at risk for and demonstrate these complications of opioid use.

Tolerance occurs when repeated exposure to opioids results in diminished therapeutic effect requiring increasing doses to maintain the same effect. Subclassifications of tolerance have been

acknowledged (Collet 1998; Chang et al. 2007), namely, innate, pharmacokinetic, pharmacodynamic, and learned tolerance. Innate tolerance refers to the genetically determined lack of sensitivity to an opioid that is observed during the initial administration. Pharmacokinetic tolerance refers to changes in drug distribution or metabolism that result in reduced opioid concentration in the blood or at sites of action with repeated administration. Pharmacodynamic tolerance refers to the adaptive mechanisms that occur within systems affected by opioids (i.e., opioid receptor desensitization or opioid-induced changes in receptor density) such that reduced response and effect is evident in spite of a constant plasma concentration of drug. Finally, learned tolerance refers to the reduction of opioid effect due to learned and compensatory mechanisms.

Opioid tolerance has been reported in both the neonatal and pediatric population (Arnold et al. 1990; Tobias and Berkenbosch 2001; Crawford et al. 2006). Findings of these studies and other reports (Hovav and Weinstock 1987; Franck et al. 1988) suggest tolerance may be related to opioid type and mode of administration as tolerance was noted to develop with the use of synthetic opioids such as fentanyl and remifentanil and continuous intravenous infusion. Furthermore, the onset of tolerance may be rapid. Studies in animal models show that a time period of 3–4 h may elapse before the onset of opioid tolerance with either intravenous or single-dose administration (Cox et al. 1968; Yano and Takemori 1977; Hovav and Weinstock 1987).

Table 22.1 Definitions

Tolerance	Diminished therapeutic effect requiring increasing doses to maintain the same effect with repeated exposure to drug
Physical dependence	Potential for withdrawal or abstinence syndrome after abrupt cessation or reduction of the drug
Physiological dependence	Craving for a substance due to its euphoric effects
Withdrawal/abstinence syndrome	Constellation of symptoms that occur with abrupt cessation or reduction of a drug
Addiction	Complex behavioral pattern of drug use characterized by overwhelming involvement and compulsive use of a drug with associated antisocial and criminal behavior with obtaining the drug
Pseudo-addiction	Iatrogenic syndrome resulting from poorly treated pain often misinterpreted as addiction

Physical or physiological dependence is defined as the potential for withdrawal or abstinence syndrome after abrupt cessation or reduction of the drug, whereas psychological dependence is defined by the craving for a substance due to its euphoric effects.

Withdrawal or abstinence syndrome is the group of symptoms that occur with abrupt cessation or reduction of a drug. In published reports, the incidence of pediatric opioid withdrawal has ranged from 13% to 57% (Arnold et al. 1990; French and Nocera 1994; Katz et al. 1994, Fonsmark et al. 1999, Bicudo et al. 1999; Jenkins et al. 2007). In a retrospective study looking at adults who received analgesic and sedative medications, the incidence of withdrawal was noted to be 32.1% (Cammarano et al. 1998). Onset of withdrawal symptoms also may be variable, with studies reporting anywhere between 1 h and 6 days after a decrease in sedative and analgesic agents (Norton 1988; French and Nocera 1994; Carnevale and Ducharme 1997; Franck et al. 2004).

Withdrawal continues to be a familiar and feared complication of opioid therapy. In their survey of sedative and analgesic practices in PICUs, Twite et al (2004) reported that 94.3% of respondents reported the occurrence of drug withdrawal in their units with a 100% of respondents weaning sedatives and analgesic drugs for withdrawal prevention. This was a significant change from the 1989 survey where Marx et al (1993) reported that only 23.5% of respondents routinely tapered drugs for withdrawal prevention.

Addiction is the complex behavioral pattern of drug use characterized by overwhelming involvement and compulsive use of drug, associated antisocial and criminal behavior with obtaining the drug, and a high tendency to relapse after drug addiction treatment. Although the occurrence of addiction is considered rare with pain management, practitioners should not avoid administering analgesic and sedative drugs in the pediatric population if appropriate.

Pseudo-addiction is a term used to describe an iatrogenic syndrome resulting from poorly treated pain. The term was introduced by Weissman and Haddox (1989) when they described a 17-year-old male with leukemia, pneumonia, and chest wall pain exhibiting behavior perceived by caregivers as signs of addiction (escalated demands for analgesics and repeated complaints of aches and pains). Further review by the medical team led to the realization that the patient's pain was real and his behavior a result of inadequately treated pain originally misinterpreted as addiction. Management of pseudo-addiction includes recognition of pseudo-addiction, establishment of trust between the patient and medical team, and administration of opioids in appropriates doses and schedules (Weissman 2005).

Clinical Signs and Symptoms of Opioid Withdrawal

The study of care given to newborns of drug-addicted mothers established the foundation for the current understanding of withdrawal in the pediatric population (Finnegan and MacNew 1974; Finnegan et al. 1975a). In the 1980s, case reports of opioid withdrawal began to surface in older children (Hasday and Weintraub 1983; Miser et al. 1986). Nevertheless, the clinical manifestations demonstrated by these earlier infants provided the framework for the systemic classification of opioid withdrawal.

Symptoms of withdrawal are typically categorized as neurological, gastrointestinal, and sympathetically mediated (Table 22.2), although other symptoms such as choreoathetoid movements (Lane et al 1991), and stridor (Tobias 1997) have also been described. Benzodiazepine withdrawal has been regarded as differing from opioid withdrawal in the relative absence of gastrointestinal symptoms (Franck et al. 2004; Anand and Ingraham 1996). In infants and in older children, the symptoms of feeding intolerance, vomiting and diarrhea may be the most frequent or only manifestations of opioid withdrawal (Katz et al. 1994; Carnevale and Ducharme 1997; Tobias 2000; Franck et al. 2004; Ista et al. 2007) The author maintains, along with Tobias (2000) and Ista et al (2007), that withdrawal is a diagnosis of exclusion, as signs and symptoms of withdrawal may mimic other treatable systemic disorders (Schecter et al. 2003).

Table 22.2 Clinical features of opioid withdrawal

CNS
Sleep disturbances
Tremors
Increased muscle tone
Irritability
Seizures
Gastrointestinal
Vomiting
Poor feeding
Abdominal pain
Diarrhea
Sympathetic
Increased sweating
Yawning
Nasal congestion
Fever
Tachycardia
Hypertension
Tachypnea
Miscellaneous
Choreoathetoid movements
Stridor

Potential Risk Factors for Withdrawal

In the 1990s, studies examining newborns and children who received fentanyl infusions provided insight into potential risk factors for withdrawal. Arnold et al. (1990) reported that withdrawal signs exhibited by newborns on fentanyl infusions for extracorporeal membrane oxygenations were associated with the total dose and duration of the fentanyl infusion. In this retrospective study examining 37 neonates, NAS (neonatal abstinence syndrome) was observed in 21 neonates (57%) based on the abstinence scoring system by Finnegan (1975b). A total fentanyl dose of 1.6 m/kg or ECMO duration of >5 days predicted a higher likelihood of abstinence. The authors also suggested that the symptoms of NAS could be attributed to the rapid tapering of opioid therapy to facilitate enteral feeding.

Katz et al. (1994) looked at the occurrence of withdrawal prospectively in 23 critically ill children (aged from 1 week to 22 months) who received fentanyl by continuous infusion.

Withdrawal was observed in 57% of the study population. A total fentanyl dose of 1.5 mg/kg and a duration of 5 days of continuous fentanyl infusion were both associated with a >50% chance of developing withdrawal. Fentanyl doses ≥2.5 mg/kg and fentanyl infusion duration ≥9 days were, however, 100% predictive of the occurrence of opioid withdrawal. The association between withdrawal and fentanyl therapy (intravenous administration, dose, duration) has also been confirmed by other studies (Franck et al. 1988; French and Nolera 1994; Bicudo et al. 1999).

Continuous vs. Intermittent Opioid Therapy

Given the use of continuous intravenous fentanyl as an associated risk factor for opioid withdrawal, results from other randomized controlled trials looking at continuous versus intermittent opioid therapy are worth noting. Lynn et al. (2000) looked at 83 infants (0–1 years) who received either continuous morphine or prn intermittent morphine boluses postoperatively. The results showed that the IV morphine group resulted in better analgesia although it was noted that the intravenous morphine group received a statistically higher total morphine dose. Follow-up studies by Bouwmeester et al. (2001) and van Djik et al. (2002) showed different results. In Bouwmeester's group, 204 children aged from 0 to 3 years were stratified in four age groups (0–4 weeks, 4–26 weeks, 26–52 weeks, and 1–3 years) and randomized to receive either continuous morphine (10 mcg/kg/h) or intermittent boluses (30 mcg/kg every 3 h) for postoperative analgesia. Plasma concentrations of epinephrine, norepinephrine, insulin, glucose, and lactate were measured before, at the end of surgery, and 6, 12, 24 h after surgery. Results indicated that there were no significant differences in catecholamine concentrations in the bolus versus intermittent morphine groups although age-related differences were noted with the neonate group with neonates showing significantly higher preoperative norepinephrine plasma concentrations and lower postoperative epinephrine concentrations indicating different age-related patterns of surgical stress responses. Similarly, in assessing the efficacy of continuous versus intermittent morphine in 181 infants aged from 0 to 3 years by COMFORT behavior and VAS scores, van Djik et al. found no statistical significance between the continuous morphine and intravenous morphine groups although differences in pain responses and actual morphine dose were between neonates and infants aged 1–6 months with neonates showing lower pain responses.

The results of these larger randomized controlled studies are noteworthy, but ultimately create more questions for the practitioner. Is morphine more efficacious than fentanyl for pain management in the pediatric patient? Is the risk of withdrawal greater, less, or the same with continuous versus bolus dosing with morphine versus fentanyl? Should practitioners move toward opioid therapy that is dose adjusted based on the age group given these recent results? Such questions highlight the need for continued adequately pow ered well-designed studies so that educated decisions may be made for pediatric patients at risk for the potential complications of opioid therapy.

Assessment of Opioid Withdrawal

The correct assessment by clinicians for opioid withdrawal is a critical component in the appropriate care of the pediatric patient. To date, multiple assessment tools have been published and utilized (Kahn et al. 1969; Finnegan et al. 1975b; Green and Suffet 1981; Zahorodny et al. 1998; Wesson and Ling 2003) for pediatric and adult patients. Kahn et al. (1969) introduced one of the earliest scoring systems for opioid withdrawal of infants of heroin-addicted mothers that differentiated withdrawal severity as mild, moderate, or severe. Finnegan et al. (1975b) followed with the NAST (Neonatal Abstinence Score Tool) in which scores were given to various signs and symptoms attributed to opioid withdrawal, with total scores >6–8 indicative of withdrawal and need for treatment. The use of NAST showed an interobserver reliability coefficient of 82%. In contrast to the widespread use of the NAST, Suresh and Anand (2001) reported the use of an adapted version of the

neonatal withdrawal index (NWI) due to its simplicity, clinical utility, greater application to iatrogenic opioid dependence and withdrawal, and greater inter-rater reliability (0.89–0.98) compared with the NAST (0.70–0.88) (54).

Although the use of NAST (Table 22.3) has been validated in the neonatal population, its use

Table 22.3 Neonatal abstinence score

Signs/symptoms	Score
Cry	
Excessive	2
Continuous	3
Sleep	
<1 h	3
<2 h	2
<3 h	1
Moro reflex	
Hyperactive	2
Marked	3
Tremors	
Mild (disturbed)	1
Moderate–severe	2
Mild (undisturbed)	3
Moderate–severe	4
Hypertonia	2
Frequent yawning	1
Excoriation	1
Seizures	5
Sweating	1
Fever	
37.2–38.4 Cel	1
>38.4	2
Mottling	1
Nasal stuffiness	1
Sneezing	1
Nasal flaring	2
Respiratory rate	
>60	1
>60 (retractions)	2
Excessive sucking	1
Poor feeding	2
Regurgitation	2
Projectile vomiting	4
Stools	
Loose	2
Watery	3

Total scores >6–8 are indicative of withdrawal and the need for treatment has not been validated in older children (Ista et al. 2007). The inclusion of the Moro reflex as a symptom of opioid withdrawal in NAST in assessing the older pediatric population is one feature that diminishes its validity in this age group, given that the reflex typically disappears after 3–4 months of age. To date, a modified version of the NAST (Tobias 1999), the use of self-designed observation lists (Fonsmark et al. 1999; Siddappa et al. 2003), OBWS (Opioid Benzodiazepine Withdrawal Scale) (Franck et al. 2004), SWS (Sedation Withdrawal Scale) (Cunliffe et al. 2004), and WAT-1 (Withdrawal Assessment Tool-1) (Franck et al. 2008) have all been utilized in the assessment of older children for opioid withdrawal.

The OBWS is a 21-item checklist that rates the frequency and severity of withdrawal symptoms. In obtaining 693 assessments of 15 children aged from 6 weeks to 28 months, the authors found the OBWS to have a sensitivity of 50%, specificity of 87%, and inter-rater reliability of 80%. As with NAST, the OBWS as a valid tool for assessing withdrawal in older children is questionable, given the incorporation of the Moro reflex in the scale.

The SWS is a scoring system incorporating 12 clinical features of withdrawal with a score given for each feature (0 = absent, 1 = mild, 2 = severe), with 24 as the maximum score. Based on the calculated score, the authors provide recommendations (i.e., continue current regimen, not to reduce a regimen, revert to a former regimen, or seek advice). Although the authors view SWS as a useful tool to assess withdrawal in children receiving opioids and/or other sedatives, reasoning for point cutoffs and validity, specificity, and sensitivity of the scoring system is not explained or provided by the authors.

The practice at the author's institution is the use of WAT-1 in assessing opioid and benzodiazepine withdrawal in patients admitted to the pediatric intensive care unit (PICU). WAT-1, an 11-item (12 point) scale is performed twice a day, has shown excellent psychometric performance when developed to measure withdrawal symptoms in PICU patients (Franck et al. 2008) and is the assessment tool being utilized in the Randomized Evaluation of Sedation Titration for Respiratory Failure (RESTORE) trial, the ongoing multi-center NIH-sponsored study evaluating the use of sedative medications in pediatric patients with acute respiratory failure.

With WAT-1, patients are assessed for (1) the absence or presence of gastrointestinal disturbances such as loose/watery stools and vomiting/wretching/gagging in a 12-h period; (2) the presence or absence of tremor, sweating, uncoordinated/repetitive movements, yawning or sneezing, and the general state of the patient noted 2 min before the patient is to be physically stimulated; (3) the presence of increased muscle tone and whether he/she startles to touch 1 min following the physical stimulus; and (4) time to gain a calm state as defined by an SBS (Sedation Behavioral Scale) ≤0, following the physical stimulus with the SBS being a scale used to assess the level of sedation/agitation in intubated infant and children on mechanical ventilation (Curley et al. 2006).

Tapering Regimens

The use of opioid tapering continues to be a common practice in the treatment of patients with opioid withdrawal. Given the close association between tolerance and withdrawal to the duration of opioid receptor occupancy (Arnold et al. 1990), opioid tapering allows the gradual removal of opioids without excessive excitation of physiologically dependent neurons which could lead to signs of withdrawal. Goals of opioid tapering, as previously outlined by Anand and Ingraham (1996), are to (1) decrease the severity of the withdrawal syndrome to a clinically tolerable degree; (2) ensure that the patient is not agitated or distressed, displaying signs or symptoms of withdrawal; and (3) ensure that the patient is able to sleep undisturbed for adequate amounts of time.

The widespread use of opioid tapering was highlighted in Twite et al.'s (2004) survey assessing sedative and analgesic practices in the United States, in which 100% of respondents reported they gradually tapered sedative and analgesic drugs to prevent withdrawal. Drugs were tapered over several days to >2 weeks or were weaned depending on the length of time that the child had been on the original drug. This was a marked contrast to an earlier survey by Marx et al. (1993) who noted that only 23.5% centers routinely tapered drugs with a duration ranging from 2 to 6 weeks to prevent withdrawal.

To date, various opioid tapering regimens have been described (Carr and Todres 1994; Anand and Arnold 1994; Yaster et al. 1996; Suresh and Anand 1998; Robertson et al. 2000). The American Pain Society (1999) stated that opioids may be tapered by giving one half of the previous daily dose in 6 h doses for the first 2 days, then reducing the dose by 25% every 2 days. The schedule is continued until a total dose of 30 mg/day of oral morphine (or the equivalent) in an adult or 0.6 mg/kg day in a child is reached. After 2 days at this minimum dose, opioid use can be discontinued

Other opioid weaning strategies directed at pediatric patients have involved distinguishing short-term opioid therapy patients (<3–7 days) from long-term therapy (>1 week) patients. Carr and Todres (1994) and Anand and Arnold (1994) recommended reducing opioid dose by 25–50% per day for short-term therapy and reducing the opioid dose 20% over the first 24 h, followed by a 10% reduction every 12 h as tolerated for long-term therapy (Table 22.4). Tobias (1994, 2000) recommended a 10–15% wean every 6–8 h in brief therapy patients and 5–10% decrease per day for long-term therapy.

Ducharme et al. (2005) looked the optimal rates at which opioids and benzodiazepines should be weaned in order to prevent withdrawal reactions in the PICU. Twenty-seven patients were enrolled aged from <1 month to 17–19 years who received opioid and/or benzodiazepine infusions ranging from 1 to >21 days. Signs of behavioral distress (tremors/twitching/jitteriness, inconsolable crying, grimacing, agitation/irritability/fussiness, gagging/vomiting, poor feeding, difficulty sleeping) were used to identify adverse reactions to weaning. The authors reported that adverse withdrawal reactions were

Table 22.4 Suggested algorithm used for prevention and treatment of opioid withdrawal (Adapted with permission from Wolters Kluwer Health. Anand and Arnold 1994)

Opioid analgesics	
A. Short-term therapy, <1 week	Reduce 25–50%; discontinue as tolerated
B. Long-term therapy, >1 week	Reduce 20% over initial 24 h
	Reduce 10% q8–12 h as tolerated
	Treat withdrawal with
	Benzodiazepines
	Clonidine
	Phenothiazines
	Barbiturates
	Convert to oral meds
	Morphine
	Methadone
	Codeine
	Tinc. opium

prevented when the daily rate of weaning did not exceed 20% for children receiving therapy for 1–3 days, 13–20% for 4–7 days, 8–13% for 8–14 days, 8% for 15–21 days, and 2–4% for more than 21 days. However, limitations of the study included the absence of a validated measurement tool for withdrawal and the uneven distribution of patients when grouped into therapy duration, with 11 patients noted to receive opioid therapy <1 day and 1 patient receiving opioid therapy 15–21 days.

Methadone

Given the potential requirement for slow weaning and long-term intravenous access in patients with extended opioid therapy, the conversion from intravenous to oral medication for opioid tapering, particularly methadone, is desirable. The advantages of methadone include its long half-life (12–24 h), oral bioavailability of 75–100%, equipotency with morphine, and ease of administration (intravenous and enteral).

Tobias et al. (1990) first described the use of methadone for iatrogenic opioid dependency in the pediatric population. Three patients with congenital heart disease aged from 10 days to 4 months who required prolonged postoperative mechanical ventilation were administered fentanyl and morphine for sedation. Signs and symptoms of withdrawal after opioid cessation were treated with methadone (0.1 mg/kg) every 12 h through the NG tube and decreased by 10–20% every week. The authors reported no recurrence of withdrawal symptoms or the need for additional narcotics.

To date, studies have looked at methadone dose, methadone weaning duration, and the efficacy of standardized opiate weaning protocol using methadone in the pediatric population. Robertson et al. (2000) reported success using a standardized methadone weaning protocol (Table 22.5) in pediatric patients with protocol patients weaned more rapidly than non-protocol patients. Siddappa et al. (2003) looked retrospectively at the care of 30 children who received an opioid infusion >7 days and who subsequently received methadone for opioid withdrawal. The patients were examined to evaluate the efficacy and the optimal dose of methadone for withdrawal prevention. Signs and symptoms of withdrawal were confirmed by the PICU physician although the authors did not specify a formal withdrawal assessment. A recommended initial methadone dose was calculated by a formula consisting of the patient's fentanyl daily dose, fentanyl potency, fentanyl duration (45 min), and the methadone duration (Table 22.6). The authors concluded that 80% of the suggested methadone dose, a dose equivalent to 2.5 times the daily fentanyl dose, was effective in minimizing withdrawal symptoms.

Meyer and Berens (2001) assessed duration of methadone weaning in preventing opioid withdrawal in pediatric patients. Efficacy of a 10 day enteral methadone weaning protocol was evaluated by the authors in a prospective observational study involving 29 children aged from 1 day to 19 years who previously received continuous fentanyl infusions. After calculating a conversion from the patient's hourly intravenous fentanyl dose to an enteral methadone dose, therapy was initiated with converted methadone dose given every 12 h for three doses and then weaned daily by 10% of the initial dose. Using the NAS to evaluate for withdrawal, 86% of the patients were successfully weaned using the 10-day enteral methadone protocol.

Berens et al. (2006) followed this earlier observational study with a randomized double-blind controlled study in which pediatric patients were treated with a 5-day versus 10-day methadone weaning protocol. To date, this was the first prospective double-blind randomized controlled study comparing two opioid weaning protocols in the pediatric population. Similar to the previous study, patients were assessed using the NAS and converted to an initial methadone dose from fentanyl (using the same conversion calculation) or morphine. No differences were noted in the number of agitation events requiring opioid rescue in either wean group with the authors concluding that pediatric patients could be weaned successfully in 5 days once conversion to oral methadone was achieved.

Buprenorphine

Buprenorphine is a synthetic partial mu-opioid receptor agonist and a mixed partial agonist/antagonist administered sublingually used for the treatment of opioid dependence and withdrawal in adults and adolescents (Marsch et al. 2005; Gowing et al. 2006; Levy et al. 2007). Advantages of buprenorphine include its safety profile, low abuse potential, particularly when combined with naloxone (Fudala et al. 2003; Mendelson and Jones 2003) and a validated assessment scale (Wesson and Ling 2003). In a Cochrane review by Gowing et al. (2006) assessing the effectiveness of buprenorphine in managing opioid withdrawal, buprenorphine was found to be more effective than clonidine for opioid withdrawal. When compared with methadone, buprenorphine showed no significant differences with respect to withdrawal severity or adverse effects.

To date, no studies have been published looking at the use of buprenorphine for the treatment

Table 22.5 Opiate Weaning Schedule (Reprinted with permission from Wolters Kluwer Health. Robertson et al. 2000)

Morphine or fentanyl continuous infusion of 7–14 days:

1. Use current 1-h dose of morphine or fentanyl to convert to an equipotent dose of methadone.

2. Day 1, give determined methadone dose intravenously every 6 h × 24 h

3. Day 2, decrease original daily dose by 20% and give orally every 8 h × 24 h

4. Day 3, decrease original daily dose by 20% and give orally every 8 h × 24 h

5. Day 4, decrease original daily dose by 20% and give orally every 12 h × 24 h

6. Day 5, decrease original daily dose by 20% and give orally every 24 h × 24 h

7. Day 6, discontinue methadone

The maximum daily dose of methadone is not to exceed 40 mg per day.

Morphine or fentanyl continuous infusion of >14 days:

1. Use 1-h dose of morphine or fentanyl to convert to an equipotent dose of methadone.

2. Day 1, give determined methadone dose intravenously every 6 h × 24 h

3. Day 2, give same dose from day 1 orally every 6 h × 24 h

4. Day 3, decrease original daily dose by 20% and give orally every 6 h × 48 h

5. Day 5, decrease original daily dose by 20% and give orally every 8 h × 48 h

6. Day 7, decrease original daily dose by 20% and give orally every 12 h × 48 h

7. Day 9, decrease original daily dose by 20% and give orally every 24 h × 48 h

8. Day 11, discontinue methadone

The maximum daily dose of methadone is not to exceed 40 mg per day.

B. Example 1: A 20 kg child receiving continuous fentanyl infusion at 2 μg/kg/h (40 μg/h) for 8 days:

1. $$\text{Conversion} = \frac{\text{fentanyl } 0.0001\text{mg} / \text{kg}}{\text{Methadone } 0.1\text{mg} / \text{kg}} = \frac{0.04\text{mg} / \text{h}}{\text{X}}$$

$$\text{X} = 4 \text{ mg}$$

2. Day 1, give methadone 4 mg iv every 6 h × 24 h (Daily dose = 16 mg)

3. Day 2, give methadone 4.3 mg orally every 8 h × 24 h (Daily dose = 12.9 mg)

4. Day 3, give methadone 3.2 mg orally every 8 h × 24 h (Daily dose = 9.6 mg)

5. Day 4, give methadone 3.2 mg orally every 12 h × 24 h (Daily dose = 6.4 mg)

6. Day 5, give methadone 3.2 mg orally every 24 h × 24 h (Daily dose = 3.2 mg)

7. Discontinue methadone on Day 6.

C. Example 2: 20 kg child on continuous morphine at 0.1 mg/kg/h (2 mg/h) for >14 days:

1. $$\text{Conversion} = \frac{\text{morphine } 0.1\text{mg} / \text{kg}}{\text{Methadone } 0.1\text{mg} / \text{kg}} = \frac{2\text{mg} / \text{h}}{\text{X}}$$

2. Day 1, give methadone 2 mg iv every 6 h × 24 h (Daily dose = 8 mg)

3. Day 2, give methadone 2 mg orally every 6 h × 24 h (Daily dose = 8 mg)

4. Day 3 & 4, give methadone 1.6 mg orally every 6 h × 48 h (Daily dose = 6.3 mg)

5. Day 5 & 6, give methadone 1.6 mg orally every 8 h × 48 h (Daily dose = 4.8 mg)

6. Day 7 & 8, give methadone 1.6 mg orally every 12 h × 48 h (Daily dose = 3.2 mg)

7. Day 9 & 10, give methadone 1.6 mg orally every 24 h × 48 h (Daily dose = 1.6 mg)

8. Discontinue methadone on Day 11

of iatrogenic opioid withdrawal in the pediatric population although its use in animal models has been studied (Stoller and Smith 2004; Bruijnzeel et al. 2007). Stoller and Smith (2004) reported that both single and repeated doses of 1 mg/kg of buprenorphine effectively blocked spontaneous morphine withdrawal in morphine-dependent infant rats and concluded its use may be suitable for treating opioid withdrawal in human infants. However, given the scarcity of literature of

Table 22.6 Fentanyl to methadone conversion

Methadone dose (mg)
= [fentanyl daily dose (mg) × fentanyl potency (100) × duration of action of fentanyl(0.75 h)]/duration of action of methadone (24 h)
= fentanyl dose × 100 × 0.75/24
= fentanyl daily dose × 3

buprenorphine in the pediatric group, the role of buprenorphine remains unclear for the treatment of opioid withdrawal in this younger patient population.

Naloxone

Although often used for the reversal of acute opioid overdose in the pediatric and adult patient, naloxone has extended into a technique to minimize the side effects of opioid therapy and for the treatment of opioid withdrawal. Suresh and Anand (2001) reported the practice of concomitant use of morphine or fentanyl infusions with ultra low-dose naloxone (0.1–0.5mcg/kg/h) for analgesia efficacy and prevention of acute tolerance via selective opioid receptor blockade of stimulatory G proteins and cAMP pathway activation associated with opioid tolerance and dependence mechanisms.

Although the use of low-dose naloxone has shown conflicting results in the adult population (Gan et al. 1997; Cepeda et al. 2002; Sartain et al 2003), the benefit of low-dose naloxone with concomitant opioid therapy has been reported by Cheung et al (2007) and Maxwell et al (2005) in the pediatric population. In a retrospective case control study comparing 14 PICU patients receiving naloxone (patients receiving <1.0 mcg/kg/h included in study with a median dose at 0.1 mcg/kg/h) and opioid infusions with 12 patients receiving opioid infusions alone for analgesia and sedation, Cheung et al. (2007) suggested that low-dose naloxone infusions may reduce opioid tolerance following opioid therapy for longer than 4 days as the naloxone group required less opioid therapy after the naloxone infusion while opioid doses were unchanged in the control group.

In a prospective double-blind randomized controlled trial, Maxwell et al. (2005) looked at 46 postoperative children (aged from 6 to 17 years) who were randomized to either saline or naloxone (0.25 mcg/kg/h) along with an IV morphine PCA. The naloxone group showed a decreased incidence of severity of pruritus and nausea with no reported differences in morphine consumption, pain scores at rest, and pain scores with coughing.

Management of opioid withdrawal has not only consisted of the use of long-acting opioids with gradual tapering, but non-opioid approaches such as rapid detoxification (RD) and ultra-rapid opioid detoxification (URD) techniques (O'Connor and Kosten 1998). Rapid detoxification shortens detoxification by causing withdrawal through the administration of naloxone or naltrexone. Purported advantages include the minimization of relapse and the early initiation of treatment consisting of naltrexone maintenance and psychosocial interventions (Cook and Lipsedge 1987). Ultra-rapid opioid detoxification, a variant of RD, consists of naloxone-induced withdrawal while under general anesthesia or heavy sedation. The use of URD in pediatric patients was reported by Greenberg (2000) who first described two children (aged at 9 and 18 months) with congenital heart disease and severe and intractable opioid dependency. Ultra-rapid detoxification was performed as the patients were unable to tolerate conventional opioid weaning. Greenberg reported that both children were successfully detoxified at the end of the URD procedure which was achieved with concomitant infusions of propofol (starting dose at 150 mcg/kg/min), naloxone (10 mcg/kg/h), and clonidine (given prior to emergence). To date, no additional cases or studies have been published describing or supporting the pediatric use of ultra-rapid detoxification.

Alpha-2 Agonists

Alpha-2 adrenergic receptor agonists have long been described and used in the treatment of opioid withdrawal, particularly in the adult population.

The ability of the alpha-2 agonists to moderate the signs and symptoms of opioid withdrawal is believed to occur through noradrenergic pathways, as increased firing of noradrenergic neurons in the locus ceruleus are demonstrated during periods of opioid withdrawal (Aghajanian 1978). Alpha-2 agonists such as clonidine have been shown to reduce this increased firing in animal models (Aghajanian 1978), an effect now thought to mediate its amelioration of opioid withdrawal in humans (Gold et al. 1981). Other mechanisms of actions involving the alpha-2 agonists include augmentation of inhibitory neurons, particularly g-aminobutyric acid (Doze et al. 1989; Correa-Sales et al. 1992; Nelson et al. 2003) accounting for its sedative and anxiolytic property and analgesic effects through modulation of substance P release and activation of alpha-2-adrenergic receptors in the dorsal horn of the spinal cord.

The widespread use of alpha-2 agonists for the treatment of opioid withdrawal has been further established by Gowing et al. (2003) in a Cochrane review, where the use of alpha-2 agonists such as clonidine and lofexinide showed no significant differences from a methadone tapering regimen over a period of around 10 days for the management of withdrawal from heroin and methadone in an adult population. Although the use of clonidine has been described for the treatment of neonatal abstinence syndrome (Hoder et al. 1981), the lack of controlled clinical studies, non-intravenous administration, and long half-life of 12–24 h have made its role in pediatric opioid withdrawal treatment suboptimal.

Dexmetomidine, a newer alpha-2 agonist, is administered intravenously, exhibits a specificity to the alpha2:alpha1 receptor eight times more than clonidine and has a shorter half-life (2–3 h vs 12–24 h) allowing for a level of titration. These characteristics along with its absence of toxic and nonactive metabolites and predictable pharmacokinetics (Diaz et al. 2007) in preliminary studies have accounted for dexmedetomidine's increased use in the pediatric population despite its potential side effects (Table 22.7) and FDA approval for short-term use (<24 h) in critically ill adult patients.

Table 22.7 Potential adverse effects of dexmedetomidine

Cardiovascular
Hypotension
Hypertension
Bradycardia
Sinus arrhythmia
Respiratory
Hypoxia
Apnea
Bronchospasm
Hypercapnia
Pulmonary edema
Central nervous system
Headache
Agitation
Pain
Fever
Dizziness
Gastrointestinal
Nausea
Abdominal pain
Diarrhea
Vomiting

The use of dexmedetomidine in the pediatric population has garnered attention for its multiple clinical uses. In a review discussing the clinical applications of dexmedetomidine, Tobias (2007) reported these applications have included intraoperative use during neurosurgical procedures (Ard et al. 2003; Everett et al. 2006) sedation during mechanical ventilation (Tobias and Berkenbosch 2004; Hammer et al. 2005; Chrysostomou et al. 2006), sole or adjuvant sedative agents for both invasive and noninvasive procedures such as cardiac catheterization, fiberoptic intubation, radiological imaging (Berkenbosch et al. 2005; Jooste et al. 2005; Mason et al. 2006, Korogulu et al. 2006; Tosun et al. 2006, Munro et al. 2007), treatment and prevention for emergence delirium following general anesthesia (Ibacache et al. 2004; Guler et al. 2005; Shukry et al. 2005; Isik et al. 2006), and treatment due to substance withdrawal (Maccioli 2003; Multz 2003; Finkel and Elrefai 2004; Finkel et al. 2005; Baddigam et al. 2005; Tobias 2006). In addition to these multiple clinical applications, Mukhtar et al. (2006) reported the intraoperative use of dexmedetomidine in pediatric cardiac surgery in a randomized controlled study with 30 children with the dexmedetomidine group showing a statistically significant attenuation in heart rate and blood pressure through skin incision and decreased circulating plasma cortisol, epinephrine, norepinephrine, blood glucose, following sternotomy and cardiopulmonary bypass.

Currently, the role of dexmedetomidine in the treatment of opioid withdrawal has been largely viewed through case reports and small case series (Maccioli 2003; Multz 2003; Finkel and Elrefai 2004; Finkel et al. 2005; Baddigam et al. 2005; Tobias 2006; Farag et al. 2006) with authors reporting success in managing opioid withdrawal with dexmedetomidine loading doses ranging from 0.5– to 1 mcg/kg and continuous infusions ranging from 0.2 to 1 mcg/kg/h. In the largest pediatric case series looking at the use of dexmedetomidine to treat opioid withdrawal in seven infants ranging in age from 3 to 24 months (Tobias 2006), dexmedetomidine was administered for withdrawal (documented by a Finnegan score ≥12) with loading doses of 0.5 mcg/kg/h followed by an infusion of 0.5 mcg/kg/h. Tobias reported success with all patients and noted no adverse hemodynamic or respiratory events.

Despite reports of safety with its long-term use (Hammer et al. 2005; Walker et al. 2006; Enomoto et al. 2006) and known desirable sedative, analgesic, and anxiolytic properties, dexmedetomidine remains a relatively nascent pharmacological agent that requires further investigation in the pediatric population, particularly with its prolonged use. Recently, Weber et al. (2008) reported an episode of acute withdrawal syndrome attributed to dexmedetomidine in a 2-year-old male with hypoplastic left ventricle following Fontan procedure after tachycardia, hypertension, and emesis were observed immediately after discontinuation of a 6-day infusion of dexmedetomidine which were refractory to lorazepam (the patient also received a midazolam infusion for sedation) but resolved with restarting dexmedetomidine. The infusion was gradually weaned every 8 h without incident with the authors suggesting that gradual tapering may even be warranted for dexmedetomidine withdrawal prevention.

Conclusions

Although significant advances have been made in the area of understanding mechanisms, risk factors and treatment of opioid tolerance, and dependence and withdrawal, much work remains ahead so that optimal care can be given to the pediatric patient at risk for opioid withdrawal. The absence of a validated measurement tool with high sensitivity and specificity for assessing opioid withdrawal particularly in older children remains an obstacle in the care of the opioid-dependent pediatric patient. Furthermore, despite the theoretical and practical benefits of opioid weaning, published weaning protocols appear variable likely due to the lack of well-powered, evidence-based studies. Future investigations focused on the search for the optimal withdrawal assessment scale, standardized weaning protocols, and continued research in the pharmacological and non-pharamcological therapy for opioid withdrawal management and prevention are needed so that continued use of opioids as analgesic and sedative agents can be administered to these vulnerable patients without hesitation.

References

Aghajanian, G. K. (1978). Tolerance of locus ceruleus neurones to morphine and suppression of withdrawal response by clonidine. *Nature, 276*(5684), 186–188.

American Pain Society. (1999). *Principles of analgesic use in the treatment of acute pain and cancer pain* (4th ed.). Glenview: American Pain Society.

Anand, K. J., & Arnold, J. H. (1994). Opioid tolerance and dependence in infants and children. *Critical Care Medicine, 22*(2), 334–342.

Anand, K. J., & Ingraham, J. (1996). Pediatric. Tolerance, dependence, and strategies for compassionate withdrawal of analgesics and anxiolytics in the pediatric ICU. *Critical Care Nurse, 16*(6), 87–93.

Anand, K. J., Hall, R. W., Desai, N., et al. (2004). Effects of morphine analgesia in ventilated preterm neonates: primary outcomes from the NEOPAIN randomized trial. *Lancet, 363*(9422), 1673–1682.

Ard, J., Doyle, W., & Bekker, A. (2003). Awake craniotomy with dexmedetomidine in pediatric patients. *Journal of Neurosurgical Anesthesiology, 15*(3), 263–266.

Arnold, J. H., Troug, R. D., Orav, E. J., et al. (1990). Tolerance and dependence in neonates sedated with fentanyl during extracorporeal membrane oxygenation. *Anesthesiology, 73*(6), 1136–1140.

Baddigam, K., Russo, P., Russo, J., et al. (2005). Dexmedetomidine in the treatment of withdrawal symptoms in cardiothoracic surgery patients. *Journal of Intensive Care Medicine, 20*(2), 118–123.

Berens, R. J., Meyer, M. T., Mikhailov, T. A., et al. (2006). A prospective evaluation of opioid weaning in opioid-dependent pediatric critical care patients. *Anesthesia and Analgesia, 102*(4), 1045–1050.

Berkenbosch, J. W., Wankum, P., & Tobias, J. D. (2005). Prospective evaluation of dexmedetomidine for noninvasive procedural sedation in children. *Pediatric Critical Care Medicine, 6*(4), 435–439.

Bhandari, V., Bergquist, L. L., Kronsberg, S. S., et al. (2005). Morphine administration and short-term pulmonary outcomes among ventilated preterm infants. *Pediatrics, 116*(2), 352–359.

Bicudo, J. N., de Souza, N., & Mangia, C. M. (1999). Withdrawal syndrome associated with cessation of fentanyl and midazolam in pediatrics. *Revista da Associação Médica Brasileira, 45*(1), 15–18.

Bouwmeester, N. J., Anand, K. J. S., van Dijk, M., et al. (2001). Hormonal and metabolic stress responses after major surgery in children aged 0–3 years: a double-blind, randomized trial comparing the effects of continuous versus intermittent morphine. *British Journal of Anaesthesia, 87*(3), 390–399.

Bruijnzeel, A. W., Marcinkiewcz, C., Isaac, C., et al. (2007). The effects of buprenorphine on fentanyl withdrawal in rats. *Psychopharmacology, 191*(4), 931–941.

Cammarano, W. B., Pittet, J. F., Weitz, S., et al. (1998). Acute withdrawal syndrome related to the administration of analgesic and sedative medications in adult intensive care unit patients. *Critical Care Medicine, 26*(4), 676–684.

Carnevale, F. A., & Ducharme, C. (1997). Adverse reactions to the withdrawal of opioids and benzodiazepines in the paediatric intensive care. *Intensive Critical Care Nurse, 13*(4), 181–188.

Carr, D. B., & Todres, I. D. (1994). Fentanyl infusion and weaning in the pediatric intensive care unit: toward science-based practice. *Critical Care Medicine, 22*(5), 725–727.

Cepeda, M. S., Africano, J. M., Manrique, A. M., et al. (2002). The combination of low dose naloxone and morphine in PCA does not decrease opioid requirements in the postoperative period. *Pain, 96*, 73–79.

Chambliss, C. R., & Anand, K. J. S. (1997). Pain management in the pediatric intensive care unit. *Current Opinion in Pediatrics, 9*(3), 246–253.

Chang, G., Chen, L., & Mao, J. (2007). Opioid tolerance and hyperalgesia. *The Medical Clinics of North America, 91*(2), 199–211.

Cheung, C. L., van Dijk, M., Green, J. W., et al. (2007). Effects of low-dose naloxone on opioid therapy in pediatric patients: a retrospective case-control study. *Intensive Care Medicine, 33*(1), 190–194.

Chrysostomou, C., Di Filippo, S., Manrique, A. M., et al. (2006). Use of demedetomidine in children after cardiac and thoracic surgery. *Pediatric Critical Care Medicine, 7*, 126–131.

Collet, B. J. (1998). Opioid tolerance: the clinical perspective. *British Journal of Anaesthesia, 81*(1), 58–68.

Cook, C. C., & Lipsedge, M. S. (1987). The pros and cons of naltrexone detoxification. *British Journal of Hospital Medicine, 38*, 79–80.

Correa-Sales, C. M., Rabin, B. C., & Maze, M. (1992). A hypnotic response to dexmetedomidine, an alpha-2 agonist, is mediated in the locus ceruleus in rats. *Anesthesiology, 76*(6), 948–952.

Cox, B. M., Ginsburg, M., & Osman, O. H. (1968). Acute tolerance to narcotic analgesic drugs in rats. *British Journal of Pharmacology and Chemotherapy, 33*(2), 245–256.

Crawford, M. W., Hickey, C., Zaarour, C., et al. (2006). Development of acute opioid tolerance during infusion of remifentanil for pediatric scoliosis surgery. *Anesthesia and Analgesia, 102*(6), 1662–1667.

Cunliffe, M., McArthur, L., & Dooley, F. (2004). Managing sedation withdrawal in children who undergo prolonged PICU admission after discharge to the ward. *Paediatric Anaesthesia, 14*(4), 293–298.

Curley, M. A., Harris, S. K., Fraser, K. A., et al. (2006). State Behavioral Scale: a sedation assessment instrument for infants and young children supported on mechanical ventilation. *Pediatric Critical Care Medicine, 7*(2), 107–114.

Diaz, S. M., Rodarte, A., Foley, J., et al. (2007). Pharmacokinetics of dexmedetomidine in postsurgical pediatric intensive care unit patients: preliminary study. *Pediatric Critical Care Medicine, 8*(5), 419–424.

Doze, V. A., Chen, B. X., & Maze, M. (1989). Dexmetedomidine produces a hypnotic-anesthetic action in rats via activation of central alpha-2 adreno-receptors. *Anesthesiology, 71*(1), 75–79.

Ducharme, C., Carnevale, F. A., Clermont, M. S., et al. (2005). A prospective study of adverse reactions to the weaning of opioids and benzodiazepines among critically ill children. *Intensive & Critical Care Nursing, 21*(3), 179–186.

Enomoto, Y., Kudo, T., Saito, T., et al. (2006). Prolonged use of dexmedetomidine in an infant with respiratory failure following living donor liver transplantation. *Paediatric Anaesthesia, 16*(12), 1285–1288.

Everett, L. L., Van Rooyen, I. F., Warner, M. H., et al. (2006). Use of dexmedetomidine in awake craniotomy in adolescents: report of two cases. *Paediatric Anaesthesia, 16*, 338–342.

Farag, E., Chahlavi, A., Argalious, M., et al. (2006). Using dexmedetomidine to manage patients with cocaine and opioid withdrawal, who are undergoing cerebral angioplasty for cerebral vasospasm. *Anesthesia and Analgesia, 103*(6), 1618–1620.

Finkel, J. C., & Elrefai, A. (2004). The use of dexmedetomidine to facilitate opioid and benzodiazepine detoxification in an infant. *Anesthesia and Analgesia, 98*(6), 1658–1659.

Finkel, J. C., Johnson, Y. J., & Quezado, Z. M. (2005). The use of dexmedetomidine to facilitate acute discontinuation of opioids after cardiac transplantation in children. *Critical Care Medicine, 33*(9), 2110–2112.

Finnegan, L. P., & MacNew, B. A. (1974). Care of the addicted infant. *The American Journal of Nursing, 74*(4), 685–693.

Finnegan, L. P., Kron, R. E., Connaughton, J. F., et al. (1975a). Assessment and treatment of abstinence in the infant of the drug-dependent mother. *International Journal of Clinical Pharmacology and Biopharmacy, 12*(1–2), 19–32.

Finnegan, L. P., Connaughton, J. F., Jr., Kron, R. E., et al. (1975b). Neonatal abstinence syndrome: assessment and management. *Addictive Diseases, 2*(1–2), 141–158.

Fonsmark, L., Rasmussen, Y. F., & Carl, P. (1999). Occurrence of withdrawal in critically ill sedated children. *Critical Care Medicine, 27*(1), 196–199.

Franck, L. S., Villardi, J., Durand, D., et al. (1988). Opioid withdrawal in neonates after continuous infusions of morphine or fentanyl during extracorporeal membrane oxygenation. *American Journal of Critical Care, 7*(5), 364–369.

Franck, L. S., Naughton, I., & Winter, L. (2004). Opioid and benzodiazepine withdrawal symptoms in the paediatric intensive care patients. *Intensive & Critical Care Nursing, 20*(6), 344–351.

Franck, L. S., Harris, S. K., Soetenga, D. J., et al. (2008). The Withdrawal Assessment Tool-1 (WAT-1): an assessment instrument monitoring opioid and benzodiazepine withdrawal symptoms in pediatric patients. *Pediatric Critical Care Medicine, 9*(6), 573–80.

French, J. P., & Nocera, M. (1994). Drug withdrawal symptoms in children after continuous infusions of fentanyl. *Journal of Pediatric Nursing, 9*(2), 107–113.

Fudala, P. J., Bridge, T. P., Herbert, S., et al. (2003). Office-based treatment of opiate addiction with a sublingual-tablet formulation of buprenorphine and naloxone. *The New England Journal of Medicine, 349*(10), 949–958.

Gan, T. J., Ginsberg, B., Glass, P. S., et al. (1997). Opioid-sparing effects of a low-dose infusion of naloxone in patient-administered morphine sulfate. *Anesthesiology, 87*, 1075–1081.

Gold, M. S., Pottash, A. C., Extein, I., et al. (1981). Neuroanatomical sites of action of clonidine in opiate withdrawal: the locus coeruleus connection. *Progress in Clinical and Biological Research, 71*, 285–298.

Goldstein, R. F., & Brazy, J. E. (1991). Narcotic sedation stabilizes arterial blood pressure fluctuations in sick premature infants. *Journal of Perinatology, 11*(4), 365–371.

Gowing, L., Farrell, M., Ali, R., & White, J. (2003). Alpha2 adrenergic agonists for the management of opioid withdrawal. *Cochrane Database Systematic Reviews (Online), 2*, CD002024.

Gowing, L., Ali, R., & White, J. (2006). Buprenorphine for the management of opioid withdrawal. *Cochrane Database Systematic Reviews (Online), 2*, CD002025.

Green, M., & Suffet, F. (1981). The Neonatal Narcotic Withdrawal Index: A device for the improvement of care in the abstinence syndrome. *The American Journal of Drug and Alcohol Abuse, 8*(2), 203–213.

Greenberg, M. (2000). Ultrarapid opioid detoxification of two children with congenital heart disease. *Journal of Addictive Diseases, 19*(4), 53–58.

Guler, G., Akin, A., Tosum, Z., et al. (2005). Single-dose dexmedetomidine reduces agitation and provides smooth extubation after pediatric adenotonsillectomy. *Paediatric Anaesthesia, 15*(9), 762–766.

Hammer, G. B., Philip, B. M., Schroeder, A. R., et al. (2005). Prolonged infusion of dexmedetomidine for sedation following tracheal resection. *Paediatric Anaesthesia, 15*, 616–620.

Hasday, J. D., & Weintraub, M. (1983). Propoxyphene in children with iatrogenic morphine dependence. *American Journal of Diseases of Children, 137*(8), 745–748.

Hoder, E. L., Leckman, J. F., Ehrenkranz, R., et al. (1981). Clonidine in neonatal narcotic-abstinence syndrome. *The New England Journal of Medicine, 305*(21), 1284.

Hovav, E., & Weinstock, M. (1987). Temporal factors influencing the development of acute tolerance to opiates. *The Journal of Pharmacology and Experimental Therapeutics, 242*(1), 251–256.

Ibacache, M. E., Munoz, H. R., Brandes, V., et al. (2004). Single dose dexmedetomidine reduces agitation after sevoflurane anesthesia in children. *Anesthesia and Analgesia, 98*(1), 60–63.

Isik, B., Arslan, M., Tunga, A. D., et al. (2006). Dexmedetomidine decreases emergence agitation in pediatric patients after sevoflurane anesthesia without surgery. *Paediatric Anaesthesia, 16*(7), 748–753.

Ista, E., van Dijk, M., Gamel, C., et al. (2007). Withdrawal symptoms in children after long-term administration of sedatives and/or analgesics: a literature review. "Assessment remains troublesome.". *Intensive Care Medicine, 33*(8), 1396–1406.

Jacobi, J., Fraser, G. L., Coursin, D. B., et al. (2002). Clinical practice guidelines for the sustained use of sedatives and analgesics in the critically ill adult. *Critical Care Medicine, 30*(1), 119–141.

Jenkins, I. A., Playfor, S. D., Bevan, C., et al. (2007). Current United Kingdom sedation practices in pediatric intensive care. *Paediatric Anaesthesia, 17*(7), 675–683.

Jooste, E. H., Ohkawa, S., & Sun, L. S. (2005). Fiberoptic intubation with dexmedetomidine in two children with spinal cord impingement. *Anesthesia and Analgesia, 101*(4), 1238–1248.

Kahn, E. J., Neumann, L. L., & Polk, G. A. (1969). The course of the heroin withdrawal syndrome in neonates treated with phenobarbital or chlorpromazine. *Jornal de Pediatria, 75*(3), 495–502.

Kanner, R. M., & Foley, K. M. (1981). Patterns of narcotic drug use in a cancer pain clinic. *Annals of the New York Academy of Sciences, 362*, 161–172.

Katz, R., Kelly, H. W., & His, A. (1994). Prospective study on the occurrence of withdrawal in critically ill children who receive fentanyl by continuous infusion. *Critical Care Medicine, 22*, 763–767.

Korogulu, A., Teksan, H., Sagir, O., et al. (2006). A comparison for the sedative, hemodynamic and respiratory effects of dexmedetomidine and propofol in children undergoing magnetic resonance imaging. *Anesthesia and Analgesia, 103*(1), 63–67.

Lane, J. C., Tennison, M. B., Lawless, S. T., et al. (1991). Movement disorder after withdrawal of fentanyl infusion. *Jornal de Pediatria, 119*(4), 649–651.

Levy, S., Vaughan, B. L., Angulo, M., et al. (2007). Buprenorphine replacement therapy for adolescents with opioid dependence: early experience from a children's hospital-based outpatient treating program. *The Journal of Adolescent Health, 40*(5), 477–482.

Lusher, J., Elander, J., Bevan, D., et al. (2006). Analgesic addiction and pseudoaddiction in painful chronic illness. *The Clinical Journal of Pain, 22*(3), 316–324.

Lynn, A. M., Nespeca, M., Bratton, S. L., et al. (2000). Intravenous morphine in postoperative infants: intermittent bolus dosing versus targeted continuous infusion. *Pain, 88*(1), 89–95.

Maccioli, G. A. (2003). Dexmedetomidine to facilitate drug withdrawal. *Anesthesiology, 98*(2), 575–577.

Marsch, L. A., Bickel, W. K., Badger, G. J., et al. (2005). Comparison of pharmacological treatments for opioid-dependent adolescents: a randomized controlled trial. *Archives of General Psychiatry, 62*(10), 1157–1164.

Marx, C. M., Rosenberg, D. I., Ambuel, B., et al. (1993). Pediatric intensive care sedation: survey of fellowship training programs. *Pediatrics, 91*(2), 369–378.

Mason, K. P., Zgleszewski, S. E., Dearden, J. L., et al. (2006). Dexmedetomidine for pediatric sedation for computed tomography imaging studies. *Anesthesia and Analgesia, 103*(1), 57–62.

Maxwell, L. G., Kaufmann, S. C., Bitzer, S., et al. (2005). The effects of a small-dose naloxone infusion on opioid-induced side effects and analgesia in children and adolescents treated with intravenous patient-controlled analgesia: a double-blind, prospective, randomized, controlled study. *Anesthesia and Analgesia, 100*(4), 953–958.

McGivney, W. T., & Crooks, G. M. (1984). The care of patients with severe chronic pain in terminal illness. *Journal of the American Medical Association, 251*, 1182–1188.

Mendelson, J., & Jones, R. T. (2003). Clinical and pharmacological evaluation of buprenorphine and naloxone combinations: why the 4:1 ratio for treatment? *Drug and Alcohol Dependence, 70*, S29–S37.

Meyer, M. M., & Berens, R. J. (2001). Efficacy of an enteral 10-day methadone wean to prevent opioid withdrawal in fentanyl-tolerant pediatric intensive care unit patients. *Pediatric Critical Care Medicine, 2*(4), 329–333.

Miser, A. W., Chayt, K. J., Sandlund, J. T., et al. (1986). Narcotic withdrawal syndrome in young adults after the therapeutic use of opiates. *American Journal of Diseases of Children, 140*(6), 603–604.

Mukhtar, A. M., Obayah, E. M., & Hassona, A. M. (2006). The use of dexmedetomidine in pediatric cardiac surgery. *Anesthesia and Analgesia, 103*(1), 52–56.

Multz, A. S. (2003). Prolonged dexmedetomidine infusion as an adjunct in treating sedation induced withdrawal. *Anesthesia and Analgesia, 96*(4), 1054–1055.

Munro, H. M., Tirotta, C. F., Felix, D. E., et al. (2007). Initial experience with dexmedetomidine for diagnostic and interventional cardiac catheterization in children. *Paediatric Anaesthesia, 17*(2), 109–112.

Nelson, L. E., Lu, J., Guo, T., et al. (2003). The alpha-2 adrenoreceptor agonist dexmedetomidine converges on an endogenous sleep-promoting pathway to exert its sedative effects. *Anesthesiology, 98*(2), 428–436.

Norton, S. J. (1988). Aftereffects of morphine and fentanyl analgesia: a retrospective study. *Neonatal Network, 7*(3), 25–28.

O'Connor, P. G., & Kosten, T. R. (1998). Rapid and ultra rapid opioid detoxification techniques. *The Journal of the American Medical Association, 279*(3), 229–234.

Playfor, S., Jenkins, I., Boyles, C., et al. (2006). Consensus guidelines on sedation and analgesia in critically ill children. *Intensive Care Medicine, 32*(8), 1125–1136.

Porter, J., & Jick, H. (1980). Addiction rate in patients treated with narcotics. *The New England Journal of Medicine, 302*(2), 123.

Prins, D., van Dijk, M., & Tibboel, D. (2006). Sedation and analgesia in the PICU: many questions remain. *Intensive Care Medicine, 32*(8), 1103–1105.

Rhoney, D. H., & Murry, K. R. (2002). National survey on the use of sedatives and neuromuscular blocking agents in the pediatric intensive care unit. *Pediatric Critical Care Medicine, 3*(2), 129–133.

Robertson, R. C., Darsey, E., Fortenberry, J. D., et al. (2000). Evaluation of an opiate-weaning protocol using methadone in pediatric intensive care unit patients. *Pediatric Critical Care Medicine, 1*(2), 119–123.

Sartain, J. B., Barry, J. J., Richardson, C. A., et al. (2003). Effect of combining naloxone and morphine for intravenous patient-controlled analgesia. *Anesthesiology, 99*, 148–151.

Schecter, N. L., Berde, C. B., & Yaster, M. (2003). *Pain in infants, children, and adolescents* (2nd ed.). Philadelphia: Lippincott Williams & Wilkins.

Shukry, M., Clyde, M. C., Kalarickal, P. L., et al. (2005). Does dexmedetomidine prevent emergence delirium in children after sevoflurane-based general anesthesia? *Paediatric Anaesthesia, 15*(12), 1098–1104.

Siddappa, R., Fletcher, J. E., Heard, A. M., et al. (2003). Methadone dosage for prevention of opioid withdrawal in children. *Paediatric Anaesthesia, 13*(9), 805–810.

Statler, K. D., & Lugo, R. A. (2004). Surveying sedation and analgesia in the pediatric intensive care unit: discomforting date raise further questions. *Pediatric Critical Care Medicine, 5*(6), 582–583.

Stoller, D. C., & Smith, F. L. (2004). Buprenorphine blocks withdrawal in morphine-dependent rat pups. *Paediatric Anaesthesia, 14*(8), 642–649.

Suresh, S., & Anand, K. J. (1998). Opioid tolerance in neonates: mechanisms, diagnosis, assessment and management. *Seminars in Perinatology, 22*(5), 425–433.

Suresh, S., & Anand, K. J. (2001). Opioid tolerance in neonates: a state-of-the-art review. *Paediatric Anaesthesia, 11*(5), 511–521.

Tobias, J. D., Schleien, C. L., & Haun, S. E. (1990). Methadone as treatment for iatrogenic narcotic dependency in pediatric intensive care unit patients. *Critical Care Medicine, 18*(11), 1292–1293.

Tobias, J. D., Deshpande, J. K., & Gregory, D. F. (1994). Outpatient therapy of iatrogenic drug dependency following prolonged sedation in the pediatric intensive care unit. *Intensive Care Medicine, 20*(7), 504–507.

Tobias, J. D. (1997). Opioid withdrawal presenting as stridor. *Journal of Intensive Care Medicine, 12*, 104–106.

Tobias, J. D. (1999). Subcutaneous administration of fentanyl and midazolam to prevent withdrawal after prolonged sedation in children. *Critical Care Medicine, 27*(10), 2262–2265.

Tobias, J. D. (2000). Tolerance, withdrawal, and physical dependency after long-term sedation and analgesia of children in the pediatric intensive care unit. *Critical Care Medicine, 28*(6), 2122–2132.

Tobias, J. D., & Berkenbosch, J. W. (2001). Tolerance during sedation in a pediatric ICU patient: effects on the BIS monitor. *Journal of Clinical Anesthesia, 13*(2), 122–124.

Tobias, J. D., Berkenbosch, J. W., Tobias, J. D., & Berkenbosch, J. W. (2004). Sedation during mechanical ventilation in infants and children: dexmedetomidine vs. midazolam. *The Southern Medical Journal, 97*, 451–455.

Tobias, J. D. (2006). Dexmedetomidine to treat opioid withdrawal in infants and children following prolonged sedation in the Pediatric ICU. *Journal of Opioid Management, 2*(4), 341–346.

Tobias, J. D. (2007). Dexmedetomidine: applications in pediatric critical care and pediatric anesthesiology. *Pediatric Critical Care Medicine, 8*(2), 115–131.

Tosun, Z., Akin, A., Esmaoglu, A., et al. (2006). Dexmedetomidine-ketamine and propofol-ketamine combinations for anesthesia in spontaneously breathing pediatric patients undergoing cardiac catheterization. *Journal of Cardiothoracic and Vascular Anesthesia, 20*(4), 515–519.

Twite, M. D., Rashid, A., Zuk, J., et al. (2004). Sedation, analgesia, and neuromuscular blockade in the pediatric intensive care unit: survey of fellowship trained programs. *Pediatric Critical Care Medicine, 5*(6), 521–532.

van Djik, M., Bouwmeester, N. J., Duivenvoorden, H. J., et al. (2002). Efficacy of continuous versus intermittent morphine administration after major surgery in 0-3 year old infants; a double-blind randomized controlled trial. *Pain, 98*(3), 305–313.

Walker, J., MacCallum, M., Fischer, C., et al. (2006). Sedation using dexmedetomidine in pediatric burn patients. *Journal of Burn Care & Research, 27*(2), 206–210.

Weber, M. D., Thammasitboon, S., & Rosen, D. A. (2008). Acute discontinuation syndrome from dexmedetomidine after protracted use in a pediatric patient. *Paediatric Anaesthesia, 18*(1), 87–88.

Weissman, D. E., & Haddox, J. D. (1989). Opioid pseudoaddiction–an iatrogenic syndrome. *Pain, 36*(3), 363–366.

Weissman, D. E. (2005). Pseudoaddiction #69. *Journal of Palliative Medicine, 8*(6), 1283–1284.

Wesson, D. R., & Ling, W. (2003). The Clinical Opiate Withdrawal Scale (COWS). *Journal of Psychoactive Drugs, 35*(2), 253–259.

Yano, I., & Takemori, A. E. (1977). Inhibition by naloxone of tolerance and dependence in mice treated acutely and chronically with morphine. *Research Communications in Chemical Pathology and Pharmacology, 16*(4), 721–734.

Yaster, M., Kost-Byerly, S., Berde, C., et al. (1996). The management of opioid and benzodiazepine dependence in infants, children, and adolescents. *Pediatrics, 98*(1), 135–140.

Zahorodny, W., Rom, C., Whitney, E., et al. (1998). The neonatal withdrawal inventory: a simplified score of newborn withdrawal. *Journal of Developmental and Behavioral Pediatrics, 19*(2), 89–93.

The Role of Nurse Practitioner in Chronic Pain Management

23

Rae Ann Kingsley and Suzanne Porfyris

Keywords
Nurse Practitioner • Roles • Certification • Licensure • Models of practice • Pediatric chronic pain NP

Introduction

As an integral member of the health-care team, the Nurse Practitioner (NP) brings a unique knowledge and set of skills to the management of specialized health problems. In the 1960s, the NP role was developed as a needful response to the precarious shortage of trained primary health-care clinicians in the workforce. With an emphasis on primary care, the NP role functioned to provide well-child care and address common childhood health problems for select underserved populations (Silver 1967). The decade that followed supported the impetus of equal access to health care for all and substantiated the need for a greater influx of primary care providers. During this period of time, NP training programs grew both in number and educational requisites. By 1980, NP practice had firmly established itself as a recognized specialization within the nursing profession. NP practice saw a shift toward clinical diversification during the 1980s, incorporating the historical primary care foundation with an expansion of clinical expertise into specialty settings. The 1990s brought further augmentation of the scope of NP practice (Dunn 1997; Kline et al. 2007; Ludder-Jackson et al. 2001; Reider-Demer et al. 2006; Sherwood et al. 1997; Silver et al. 1968). Today, nurse practitioners are found in all health-care settings: primary, tertiary, and specialty care. The current directive within the nursing profession is to strive for a paradigm shift and be a catalyst for change in the health care of individuals regardless of practice settings.

Currently, domains of practice for the Nurse Practitioner include the provision of direct, comprehensive care; the support of systems that promote innovative patient care and facilitate optimal progression of patients through the health-care system; the enhancement of patient care through the dissemination of knowledge; the generation of knowledge and the integration of research findings into clinical practice; and involvement in professional activities (Ackerman et al. 1996; Brady and Neal 2000; Kenward 2007).

Primary care NP education focuses extensively on health promotion, health maintenance,

S. Porfyris (✉)
Anesthesia Pain Service, Department of Anesthesiology, Children's Memorial Hospital, 2300 Children's Plaza, Box 19, Chicago, IL 60614, USA
e-mail: sporfyris@childrensmemorial.org

and management of both acute and chronic illness states (AANP 2007c). As the characteristics and settings of practice have expanded, so have the NP role functions. Like the original NP primary care practice model, specialty NPs hold an advanced degree in nursing, but also incorporate an accumulation of specialized clinical experiences and knowledge into their repertoire (Brundige 1997). This is evidenced by the acquisition of a distinct expertise to practice within the physical, psychosocial, environmental, and technical domains of specialty practice, including the arena of chronic pain. This blend of experience in both primary care and specialty care allows chronic pain NPs to provide unequaled, dedicated services to this particular patient population (Keane and Angstadt 1999). The fundamental clinical attributes of the pediatric chronic pain Nurse Practitioner are the ability to recognize and accept the child's pain as real, the intuitive prowess to be present and available to the child, the desire to advocate and speak on the child's behalf, the adeptness to display nonjudgmental empathy, and the proficiency to provide patient education beyond that which is customary of primary care providers.

In response to the changing needs of the consumer and health-care community, the evolution of the NP role has ensued. During times of increasing patient complexity, there has been practice expansion into specialty tracks within a variety of settings. Accepting these new clinical responsibilities and being accountable with shared decision making are all inherent components of the NP specialty role.

Advanced Practice Nurse Practice Issues

Multiple roles and responsibilities exist for Nurse Practitioners, dependent on location, resources, and scope of practice limitations. The NP functions as an autonomous provider within a collaborative network of health-care providers and is uniquely qualified to resolve unmet needs in health care. The NP serves as an individual's point of first contact with the health-care system. This contact

establishes a personalized, patient-oriented, and comprehensive continuum of care. However, the NP's degree of autonomy and scope of practice differs in accordance to the state in which the NP practices (Pearson 2009 Table 23.1).

Scope of Practice

Individual State Boards of Nursing or state-designated regulatory bodies govern the scope of NP practice. State statutes address the broad categories of prescriptive authority, title recognition, educational requisites, and licensing requirements. The underpinnings of these regulatory bodies are to determine and set the standards to regulate the practice of nursing, thereby protecting the public safety and welfare. Each state has a Nurse Practice Act, which outlines the legal State Board regulations detailing the professional scope of practice. These regulations allow advanced practice nursing to exist within the purview of the Board of Nursing or Board of Medicine, either individually or collectively. Moreover, clinical practice can be further regulated by the hospital/clinic bylaws in which the NP practices. The regulations of the Nurse Practice Act and the hospital/clinic bylaws can change in response to shifts in practice conditions and societal needs to allow the NP to provide congruent care (Sherwood et al. 1997). This scope of practice encompasses the activities NPs are educated and authorized to perform. This is the standard to which clinical care is compared.

Licensure

Licensure for the Nurse Practitioner is granted by the state within which the NP is practicing. Licensure is the legal permission to practice within a specific scope of practice once minimum requirements for that practice have been met (Kamajian et al. 1999). Although most states require a Master's degree level of educational preparation and appropriate certification by a nationally recognized agency as prerequisites for licensure, the amount of actual clinical independence that

Table 23.1 Overview of diagnosing and treating aspects of NP practice

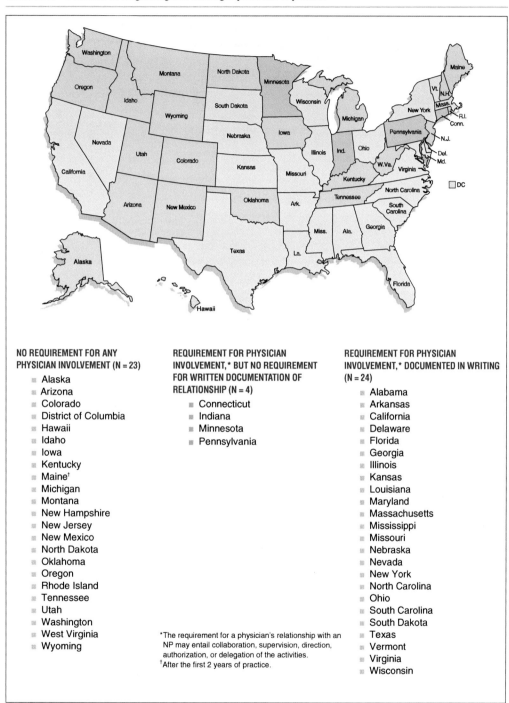

NO REQUIREMENT FOR ANY PHYSICIAN INVOLVEMENT (N = 23)

- Alaska
- Arizona
- Colorado
- District of Columbia
- Hawaii
- Idaho
- Iowa
- Kentucky
- Maine[†]
- Michigan
- Montana
- New Hampshire
- New Jersey
- New Mexico
- North Dakota
- Oklahoma
- Oregon
- Rhode Island
- Tennessee
- Utah
- Washington
- West Virginia
- Wyoming

REQUIREMENT FOR PHYSICIAN INVOLVEMENT,* BUT NO REQUIREMENT FOR WRITTEN DOCUMENTATION OF RELATIONSHIP (N = 4)

- Connecticut
- Indiana
- Minnesota
- Pennsylvania

REQUIREMENT FOR PHYSICIAN INVOLVEMENT,* DOCUMENTED IN WRITING (N = 24)

- Alabama
- Arkansas
- California
- Delaware
- Florida
- Georgia
- Illinois
- Kansas
- Louisiana
- Maryland
- Massachusetts
- Mississippi
- Missouri
- Nebraska
- Nevada
- New York
- North Carolina
- Ohio
- South Carolina
- South Dakota
- Texas
- Vermont
- Virginia
- Wisconsin

*The requirement for a physician's relationship with an NP may entail collaboration, supervision, direction, authorization, or delegation of the activities.
[†]After the first 2 years of practice.

Table 23.1 illustrates the state requirements for NP diagnosing and treating

Copyright 2009, *The American Journal for Nurse Practitioners* accompanies licensure varies greatly (Kenward 2007). Dependent upon the individual state, NP practice can be completely independent or may require proof of a collaborative MD agreement for licensure (Pearson 2009). Each individual state chooses licensure titles for NPs, that is, APRN, ARNP, ANP, RNP, CRNP, NP, etc. (Table 23.2).

The current direction in nursing education is to endorse educational preparation at the doctorate level. The AACN (American Association of Colleges of Nursing) advocates the Doctor of Nursing Practice (DNP) degree as the distinct model of practice-focused educational preparation

to bestow the acquisition of a terminal degree in the nursing discipline. This evolution to doctoral degree education is more consistent with the stringent preparation of Nurse Practitioners and more accurately reflects current clinical competencies. The DNP prepares Nurse Practitioners for the changing health-care system and places the NP more congruently aligned with other health-care providers (ACNP 2008; Clinton 2008). Currently, following matriculation from a defined course of study, NPs are awarded the academic credentials of MSN, PhD, DNP, etc. (AANP 2007c).

Table 23.2 Nurse practitioner summary of licensure titles, diagnosing, treating, and prescribing aspects of practice

State	NP title used	Physician involvement in NP diagnosing and treating[a]	Physician involvement in NP prescribing[a]	NP authorized to prescribe controlled substances	Schedules allowed
Alabama	CRNP	Yes	Yes	No	
Alaska	ANP	No	No	Yes[b]	II–V
Arizona	RNP	No	No	Yes	II–V
Arkansas	ANP, RNP	Yes	Yes	Yes	III–V
California	APRN, NP	Yes	Yes	Yes	II–V
Colorado	APN, NP	No	Yes	Yes	II–V
Connecticut	APRN, NP	Yes	Yes	Yes	II–V
Delaware	APN, NP	Yes	Yes	Yes	II–V
DC	APRN, CNP, CRNP, NP	No	No	Yes	II–V
Florida	ARNP, NP	Yes	Yes	No	
Georgia	APRN, NP	Yes	Yes	Yes	III–V
Hawaii	APRN, NP	No	Yes	Yes[b]	II–V
Idaho	APPN, NP	No	Yes	Yes	II–V[b]
Illinois	APN, CNP	Yes	Yes	Yes	II–V[b]
Indiana	APN, NP	Yes	Yes	Yes	II–V[b]
Iowa	ARNP, CNP, NP	No	No	Yes	II–V
Kansas	ARNP	Yes	Yes	Yes[b]	II–V[b]
Kentucky	ARNP, NP	No	Yes	Yes[b]	II–V[b]
Louisiana	APRN, NP	Yes	Yes	Yes[b] No for chronic pain	II–V[b]
Maine	APRN, CNP	Yes	Yes	Yes	II–V
Maryland	CRNP, NP	Yes	Yes	Yes	II–V
Massachusetts	NP	Yes	Yes	Yes	II–V
Michigan	NP	No	Yes	Yes	II–V[b]
Minnesota	APRN, CNP	Yes	Yes	Yes[b]	II–V
Mississippi	APRN, NP-BC	Yes	Yes	Yes[b]	II–V[b]
Missouri	APRN, NP	Yes	Yes	Yes	III–V[b]
Montana	APRN, NP	No	No	Yes[b]	II–V
Nebraska	APRN, NP	Yes	Yes	Yes	II–V
Nevada	APN	Yes	Yes	Yes[b]	II–V
New Hampshire	ARNP	No	Yes	Yes	II–V

(continued)

Table 23.2 (continued)

State	NP title used	Physician involvement in NP diagnosing and treating[a]	Physician involvement in NP prescribing[a]	NP authorized to prescribe controlled substances	Schedules allowed
New Jersey	APN	No	Yes	Yes[b]	II–V
New Mexico	CNP, NP	No	No	Yes	II–V
New York	NP	Yes	Yes	Yes	II–V
North Carolina	NP	Yes	Yes	Yes[b]	II–V
North Dakota	APRN, NP	No	Yes	Yes	II–V[b]
Ohio	CNP, CRNP	Yes	Yes	Yes	II–V[b]
Oklahoma	ARNP, APN	No	Yes	Yes	III–V[b]
Oregon	NP	No	No	Yes	II–V
Pennsylvania	CRNP	Yes	Yes	Yes	II–V[b]
Rhode Island	RNP	No	No	Yes	II–V
South Carolina	APRN, NP	Yes	Yes	Yes	III–V
South Dakota	CNP	Yes	Yes	Yes[b]	II–V[b]
Tennessee	APN, NP	No	Yes	Yes	II–V[b]
Texas	NP (+specialty)	Yes	Yes	Yes	III–V[b]
Utah	APRN, RNP, NP	No	Yes	Yes	II–V
Vermont	APRN	Yes	Yes	Yes	II–V
Virginia	LNP, APN, NP	Yes	Yes	Yes	II–V
Washington	ARNP	No	No	Yes	II–V
West Virginia	ANP	No	Yes	Yes	III–V[b]
Wisconsin	APNP	Yes	Yes	Yes[b]	II–V[b]
Wyoming	APRN	No	No	Yes	II–V

Table 23.2 lists the licensed Nurse Practitioner titles recognized by the state of practice, individual state requirements for physician involvement as related to diagnosing, treating, and prescribing, and the regulations surrounding prescription of controlled substances according to the individual state of practice

Information contained within the above cells are based upon 2008 data

[a] The requirements for physician involvement vary according to individual state statutes and regulations

[b] Certain provisions exist surrounding controlled substance prescribing and vary according to individual state statutes and regulations

ANP advanced nurse practitioner
APN advanced practice nurse
APNP advanced practice nurse prescriber
APPN advanced practice professional nurse
APRN advanced practice registered nurse
ARNP advanced registered nurse practitioner
CNP certified nurse practitioner
CRNP certified registered nurse practitioner
NP nurse practitioner, RNP registered nurse practitioner

Certification

Certification provides validation of a predetermined, standard level of knowledge and skills within a given specialty. Certification is a process by which an independent, nongovernmental agency recognizes an individual nurse's qualifications and mastery of knowledge for a given specialty (Kamajian et al. 1999). Certification is defined by the American Board of Nursing Specialties (2005) as the "formal recognition of the specialized knowledge, skills, and expertise demonstrated by the achievement of standards identified by a nursing specialty to promote optimal health outcomes." National Nurse Practitioner certification is offered through various nursing organizations. NPs certified as either Pediatric Nurse Practitioners (PNP) or Family Nurse Practitioners (FNP) can deliver care to pediatric patients both in general and specialty practices. Each respective certifying body grants certification after completion of specialized education, experience in specialty nursing practice and upon satisfactory completion of a rigorous and psychometrically sound qualifying examination, thereby ensuring a basic entry level of knowledge. Ultimately, the aims of certification are to assure national consistency of standards and conduct, provide the public an understanding of the professional's scope of practice, impose standard titles, and provide a venue for the public to raise practice grievances (American Association of Colleges of Nursing 1998).

The Pediatric Nursing Certification Board (PNCB) and the American Nurses Credentialing Center (ANCC) are the two pediatric Nurse Practitioner certifying agencies. The National Association of Pediatric Nurse Practitioners (NAPNAP) position statement on certification (2006) attests to the necessity of professional certification to "assure consumers, colleagues, and the public at large the highest quality pediatric nursing care." Certification validates the practitioner's minimum level of competence. Furthermore, studies have demonstrated the positive benefits of nursing certification, both professionally and personally. Certified PNPs promote optimal health outcomes and have a positive impact on the quality of health care to children and families (Cary 2001; American Association of Colleges of Nursing 1998; Hermann and Zabramski 2005).

The maintenance of certification is accomplished through a variety of relevant mechanisms including periodic reexamination, proof of continuing education, self-assessment exercises, and documentation of ongoing clinical practice. Certification maintenance seeks to assure the public that the certificant has continued to achieve an optimal level of knowledge, as well as provide evidence of ongoing participation in activities that support the maintenance of competence in the specialty (American Board of Nursing Specialties 2005). Certification identifiers for Nurse Practitioners vary. Commonly used designations are PNP, FNP, NP-C, PNP- AC, etc.

Additional certification in pain management nursing may be achieved after completion of a specialty focused examination that is offered year-round at approved testing centers. The American Society of Pain Management Nurses (ASPMN) was conceived in the spring of 1990 by a group of seven registered nurses, who specialized in pain management. These founding nurses exchanged their vision with the American Pain Society (APS), and other related groups – the American Society of Anesthesiologists and American Society of Regional Anesthesiologists. After appraising the utility of forming a special interest group within the APS, it was determined that there was an inherent need for a separate nursing organization. The first annual meeting was held the following spring in 1991 and the first pain management certification examination was offered in October 2005 through a partnership between the ASPMN and the American Nurses Credentialing Center (ANCC). The purpose of the examination is to validate the individual's knowledge of pain management specialty. The examination addresses the core content areas of pain pathophysiology, pain assessment and intervention, side effects, education and counseling of patients, families and specialty populations, and collaborative/institutional issues.

Eligibility criteria to sit for the certification exam are as follows: possess a current RN license; practiced an equivalent of 2 years as a full-time registered nurse; practiced at least 2,000 h in the prior 3 years in a nursing role which involves aspects of pain management; and completed at least 30 h of continuing education in the prior 3 years, 15 h of which are related to pain management. Maintenance of pain management certification requires renewal every 5 years via documentation of predetermined professional development activities, and either providing evidence of 1,000 h of nursing practice in pain management or choosing to retake and pass the certification examination.

The ASPMN mission is "to advance and promote optimal nursing care for people affected by pain by promoting best nursing practice through education, standards, advocacy and research."

Credentialing

Credentialing is a reference to both the academic degree and the administrative process that collects and verifies information regarding NP training and experience and parallels the medical staff model (NAPNAP 2003). Credentialing is the process of verifying and assessing the licensure and certification of a health-care practitioner to provide patient care services within a particular setting. Administrative credentialing involves the collection of relevant facts not only on educational preparation but also on practice experience, licensure and certification history, professional memberships, and professional liability history (Rustia 1997). The credentialing process requires periodic review and reappointment, as is the case with medical staff credentialing. The goal of NP credentialing by the hospital or health-care organization is to achieve an optimal degree of quality care with the appropriate utilization of resources, while also allowing for accountability and encouraging high standards of practice. Credentialing determines whether a professional is authorized to practice within a health-care organization or to participate on a managed care provider network and what specific activities the professional is authorized to perform within that setting (Kamajian et al. 1999).

Privileging

The Joint Commission (2001) mandates require that practitioners be granted clinical privileges prior to delivering patient care. Privileging is the process of authorizing a health-care professional to order or perform specific diagnostic or therapeutic services (Kamajian et al. 1999; NAPNAP 2003). Privileging outlines the clinical services and activities each NP can perform and is held accountable for. Licensure, certification, and clinical experience are essential requirements needed to obtain privileges to practice in a given medical setting. Privileging establishes credibility within the medical and health-care communities and is a professional-level quality assurance

activity. The decision to grant privileges is made by professional peer judgment based upon history of clinical competence, level of skill, and ability to perform selected therapeutic procedures (Rustia 1997). Delineation of privileges defines which medical conditions may be treated by each practitioner, which procedures may be performed, and the accountability of each practitioner. Once the delineation is completed, the NP may perform these tasks in a legally defensible manner and provide quality patient care. Privileges are granted and reviewed at predetermined periods of time. Practitioners desiring to perform new procedures and treatment modalities need to document the necessary proctoring or supervision process utilized to become skilled in those procedures and treatments. As a result of being granted practice privileges, the NP has the legal responsibility to know and abide by the regulations and bylaws governing all aspects of practice within the privileging body of the provider institution and the state statutes.

Prescriptive Authority

The ultimate determination of prescriptive authority or restriction is granted by the individual state in which the NP practices and is delineated in the Nurse Practice Act. Federal Drug Enforcement Agency (DEA) licensure can be obtained by the NP, considered a mid-level practitioner, to allow prescription of scheduled drugs within the scope of practice defined by the individual state. There is little national uniformity in the prescriptive autonomy of Nurse Practitioners (Pearson 2009, Table 23.3). State recognition of Nurse Practitioner prescriptive autonomy varies from the endorsement of independent advanced nursing practice with full prescriptive privileges of medication classes and schedules to the requirement for increasing levels of physician supervision (Brady and Neal 2000, Kenward 2007). There can be practice-associated administrative barriers against the Nurse Practitioner's prescriptive autonomy, even when the legal authority is provided by the individual state (Kaplan et al 2006, Mahoney 1995). State regulations and practice barriers regarding prescriptive authority can either

Table 23.3 Overview of prescribing aspect of NP practice

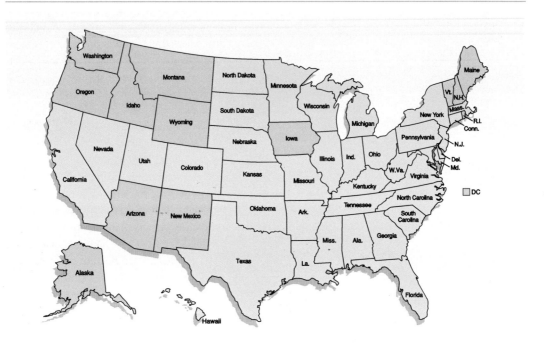

ABSOLUTELY NO REQUIREMENT FOR ANY PHYSICIAN INVOLVEMENT (N = 13)

- Alaska
- Arizona
- District of Columbia
- Idaho
- Iowa
- Maine[†]
- Montana
- New Hampshire
- New Mexico
- Oregon
- Rhode Island
- Washington
- Wyoming

REQUIREMENT FOR PHYSICIAN INVOLVEMENT,[*] DOCUMENTED IN WRITING (N = 38)

- Alabama
- Arkansas
- California
- Colorado
- Connecticut
- Delaware
- Florida
- Georgia
- Hawaii
- Illinois
- Indiana
- Kansas
- Kentucky

- Louisiana
- Maryland
- Massachusetts
- Michigan
- Minnesota
- Mississippi
- Missouri
- Nebraska
- Nevada
- New Jersey
- New York
- North Carolina
- North Dakota

- Ohio
- Oklahoma
- Pennsylvania
- South Carolina
- South Dakota
- Tennessee
- Texas
- Utah[‡]
- Vermont
- Virginia
- West Virginia
- Wisconsin

[*]The requirement for a physician's relationship with an NP may
entail collaboration, supervision, direction, authorization, or delegation of the activities.
[†]After the first 2 years of practice.
[‡] Collaboration required only for prescribing Schedules II-III drugs.

Table 23.3 identifies the states in which there is no requirement for physician involvement in contrast to those states that have some degree of required physician involvement for Nurse Practitioner prescribing

Copyright 2009, *The American Journal for Nurse Practitioners*

support or limit the inherent clinical decision-making capability of Nurse Practitioners. As a result, appropriate pharmacologic management in chronic pain clinic settings often requires coor-dination by multiple caregivers. To address pre-scriptive limitations and provide all-inclusive patient care, the use of approved practice protocols are one effective way in which the NP can assume responsibility for the pharmacologic management of these patients (Kamajian et al. 1999; Keane and Angstadt 1999).

Practice protocols are a predefined algorithm of reasonable treatment (Paul 1999). These protocols establish parameters that drive the ability to manage patients under an organized method of analysis based upon scientific evidence, acuity of patients, expert consensus, experience of the NP, and longevity of the physician/NP relationship.

Billing and Reimbursement

For many years, Nurse Practitioners have been able to directly bill for services rendered. As the focus of patient care has become more complex and the Nurse Practitioner role has expanded, the billing for various forms of care provided has also evolved. Federal legislative mandates have followed suit to better regulate billing practices. Building on federal foundations, the actual formulas for assessing reimbursement often vary by individual state, payor source, practice location, and type of services provided.

Federally funded programs have defined the minimum eligibility criteria for NP billing and dictate that Nurse Practitioners be issued a National Provider Identifier (NPI) and meet the required criteria as determined by Medicare for billing eligibility. These criteria state that the NP must be a registered professional nurse authorized to perform services in the state in which the NP practices, hold national certification as an advanced practice nurse and possess a Master's degree in Nursing. In order to qualify for state reimbursement, the NP must also meet any additional state stipulations for reimbursement above and beyond that of the federal guidelines (NAPNAP 2004).

Medicare billing may be submitted under three classifications of NP services provided; independent, incident-to, or shared visit. Billing by the NP may result in reimbursement of the full submission of charges or a percentage thereof, depending on the provider services rendered and the state within which the provider practices. The Nurse Practitioner may bill independently for coverage of services legally authorized to perform by using the assigned Medicare billing number. The next category of billing, incident-to, are for those services and supplies covered by Medicare that are furnished incident to a physician or other practitioner's services. Incident to billing describes charging for services rendered in an office setting where a collaborating physician is present within the office and is readily available if needed. The reimbursement for this form of billing is paid at 100% of the physician fee schedule. Documentation must include either a relevant addition to the medical record by the physician or the NP must indicate that the patient was seen while under the supervision of the corresponding physician. Shared visit billing is submitted under the stipulation that the NP and physician must have an employment or contractual business relationship. The claim is billed under the physician's unique billing identification number at 100% of the physician fee schedule. This provision can apply in the office setting, as well as in the inpatient setting. An important exception to note is that shared visit billing cannot be applied to consultations, procedures, or critical care evaluation and management services (Kleinpell et al. 2007, Medicare Claims Processing Manual, Chapter 12). Reimbursement for services provided by Nurse Practitioners is covered through Medicare Part B, but very few pediatric patients are covered, unless receiving dialysis or kidney transplant services (Medicare Benefit Policy Manual, Chapter 15)

In 1997, Congress mandated that all states must cover services provided by Nurse Practitioners. Medicaid, the program for eligible low-income individuals and families, is the jointly funded state/federal insurance program with coverage varying by state, and usually compensates at lower reimbursement than other insurance carriers or groups (ANA 2007; NAPNAP 2004).

Documentation for services rendered is the same as that required for physicians and requires current procedural terminology (CPT) coding. All billable procedures, services, and supplies must be appropriately coded; otherwise proper reimbursement will be compromised. Precise utilization of both CPT codes and diagnostic codes (ICD-9) for procedures billed is essential. The medical record of each service rendered must include the necessary documentation, with the greatest level of specificity, to substantiate the services and procedures billed for. Carelessness in coding and documentation can result in significant financial and legal ramifications.

Models of Practice

There are two major models of practice in which the Nurse Practitioner may function, a collaborative professional practice model or a nursing-based model. In the collaborative practice model, the Nurse Practitioner practices within a specialty physician practice plan, such as a Chronic Pain Service, with direct reporting lines to the physician partners in the practice plan and an indirect reporting line to the nursing staff and nursing organization. This comprehensive model is patient centered and allows for joint development of the plan of care. The goal for providers is to ensure optimal outcomes and patient satisfaction (Hermann and Zabramski 2005). However, obstacles to collaboration may exist in some settings. Such barriers may take place within patient/family, professional, economic, regulatory, or legal realms. Practice limitations can be encountered from patients and families who are not familiar with the role and clinical autonomy of the Nurse Practitioner. The NP may also encounter resistance from physicians outside the chronic

pain clinic practice, which may be related to a lack of understanding about the role and/or scope of practice of the NP and may lead to the perception that the NP is a competitor rather than a collaborator (Heitz and Van Dinter 2000).

In the nursing-based model, the Nurse Practitioner may have both clinical and service-based responsibilities, such as being in charge of the outpatient clinic where the NP practices (Calkin 1984). In this case, there might be dual-reporting responsibilities to both the nursing service organization for nursing care issues and to the physician who is responsible for medical management of patients. The NP practicing under this model may have conflict in prioritizing their day-to-day activities. They often have pressures from the nursing organization to accomplish tasks such as hiring, employee management and evaluation, staff education, budgets, quality assurance activities, and management of physical facilities, leaving little time for patient-centered activities.

Role Division and Core Functions

Patient care is coordinated in the clinical setting by the practicing NP through six core role functions (Table 23.4). These roles include clinician, educator, consultant, researcher, case manager,

Table 23.4 Nurse practitioner core functions

Clinician	History & physical
	Developmentally appropriate pain examination
	Assessment/diagnosis
	Order & interpret lab & diagnostic tests
	Prescribe developmentally appropriate interventions/CAM treatments
	Prescribe pharmacological agents and non-pharmacological therapies
	Perform procedures
	Re-assessment
Educator	Target audience: staff, patient, & community
	Education needs/material development
	• Learning styles
	• Pain anatomy and physiology
	• Treatments
	• Medications
	• Health promotion
	• Anticipatory guidance and counseling
Consultant	Professional resource for individuals, families, communities
	perform/request consultative intervention
	• Gather data
	• Recommendations

(continued)

Table 23.4 (continued)

Researcher	Evidenced-based practice • Literature review • Perform studies • Critical thinking • Publish data
Case manager	Coordinate/schedule services & referrals • Pre-authorization • Triage School liaison Treatment contract supervision Family support and comforting • Active listening, • Understanding • Affirmation • Guidance • Reassurance Follow-up calls/contacts with parents
Professional leader/ mentor	Continuing education/professional development Mentor/role model Organizational structuring/policy development Community/legislative intercession Professional organization participation Quality improvement Case conference presentation

Table 23.4 Ocharacterizes the comprehensive and diverse functions inherent to the nurse practitioner role

Table 23.5 Nurse practitioner role functions

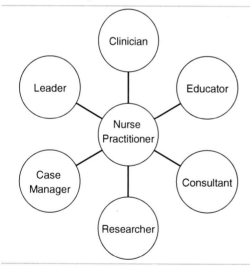

Table 23.5 depicts the integrated patient care roles of the nurse practitioner

and professional leader/mentor (AANP 2007d, St. Marie 2002). Each of these functions can intertwine and overlap without exclusion, particularly within the specialty of chronic pediatric pain management (Table 23.5). Utilizing the various role functions and a broad knowledge base of pediatric patients of all ages, the NP can engage in and be successful with the complexities of pediatric chronic pain care (Table 23.6).

Today, Nurse Practitioners are mainstream providers essential to many specialty services, in both acute and chronic care, with direct access to patients and increased decision-making scope, authority, and accountability (AANP 2007c, Keane and Angstadt 1999). Advanced theoretical and practical knowledge and a high degree of autonomy in decision making are qualities inherent in the Nurse Practitioner role. The advanced practice model of care combines the nursing model which is focused on caring, supporting, teaching, and comforting with the medical model that centers on diagnosis, treatment, and cure (Czarnecki et al. 2007). As a result, a unique model of care is created, with research-verified outcomes of high levels of patient safety, satisfaction, and improved compliance (Table 23.6).

Pediatric patients with chronic pain require a global emphasis on clinical care. Central to the role of the NP is the ability to provide excellent patient care arising from an all-encompassing

Table 23.6 Advanced practice nursing model of care

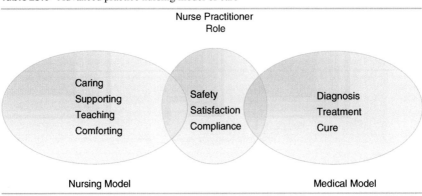

Table 23.6 portrays the nursing and medical model elements comprising the advanced practice nursing model of care

holistic framework (Wells-Federman et al. 2002). The Nurse Practitioner working in the pediatric chronic pain setting is often part of a multidisciplinary team. The chronic pain Nurse Practitioner has the ability to offer patients, families, consultants, and staff members a resource for evaluation, communication, continuity, and comprehensiveness of care that is essential for this challenging patient population (Shay et al. 1996).

The NP approaches patient care encouraging autonomous and patient-centered health promotion. Nursing has long been seen in the healthcare field as the necessary foundation for the realization of patient-centered care. Comparatively, allopathic medicine has been viewed as the cerebral underpinnings of disease treatment. The integration of these two elements is now the mantra of modern health care evidenced by the evolution of specialty NP roles.

Expert Clinician

The NP has the foundation of primary care as the basis of practice and it is this foundation of developmentally appropriate health promotion and maintenance that guides patient care. The accumulative clinical experiences of the specialty NP augment prior didactic instruction and nursing practice. The pediatric chronic pain NP has been expertly trained to gather a detailed pain history by listening closely and recording subjective descriptors. A thorough pain history includes location, intensity, quality, onset, duration, aggravating and alleviating factors, prior treatment modalities and responses, and the outlining of a chronological account of painful events. Additional intake information also encompasses any previous medical and surgical histories, current medications, naturopathic remedies, food and drug allergies, and relevant family and social histories. A thorough review of systems is obtained as determined by the presenting complaint(s). Finally, a comprehensive pain-focused examination is performed. Additional subjective data can be gathered from pain questionnaires and functional and psychosocial questionnaires (Table 23.7).

Based on both the subjective and objective data gathered from the initial history and physical examination, a working list of differential diagnoses is formed. As indicated from this list, the NP can then order and subsequently interpret laboratory and diagnostic studies and implement individualized pharmacologic and non-pharmacologic treatments and procedural interventions (Brady and Neal 2000, Kenward 2007, Wells-Federman 2002). As care continues, clinical reassessments assist in the continued management of pain and evaluation of treatment response (Royal Prince Alfred Hospital 2005).

Continuing experience augments prior knowledge and improves understanding of the proper management of the pediatric patient with chronic pain. Experience and specialized knowledge

Table 23.7 Pediatric chronic pain clinic intake form

 Children's Memorial Hospital

Department of Anesthesia
Chronic Pain Service
Chicago, IL 60614
CHILD QUESTIONNAIRE

PTRH

Medical Record Number
Patient Name
Birthdate

Background Information

	Office Use:
Name: _____ Date ___/___/___	1.
School: _____ Grade in School: _____	3.

Pain History

1. What words do you use to describe your pain or hurt?

_____
_____
_____
_____
_____

2. Please mark on the pictures below where you are having pain:

FRONT   BACK   FRONT   BACK

3. Think about the pain that bothers you most. From the list below, please circle the words that best describe the way it feels when you are hurt or in pain. You may circle as many as you like.

cutting	pounding	tingling	tiring	deep	hot
beating	squeezing	throbbing	horrible	stabbing	spreading
burning	pulling	sickening	biting	screaming	punishing
scraping	aching	uncomfortable	cold	tugging	scared
pricking	cruel	warm	miserable	stretching	lonely
pinching	unbearable	sad	itching	terrible	bad
stinging	cool	sore	flashing	pressing	
fearful	pins & needles	sharp	jumping	tight	

(continued)

Table 23.7 (continued)

Department of Anesthesia	
Children's Memorial Hospital — Chronic Pain Service, Chicago, IL 60614, **CHILD QUESTIONNAIRE**	Medical Record Number Patient Name Birthdate

	Office Use:

4. How frequently do you have pain?
 	
    1. Daily
    2. 1-2 times a week
    3. 3-7 times a week
    4. 1-2 times a month
    5. Every few months
	6.
	
	7.

5. When you have pain, how long does it usually last?

   1. Less than 15 minutes
   2. About 15-30 minutes
   3. 30 minutes to 1 hour
   4. Several Hours (How many? _____)
   5. All day
   6. 1-2 days
   7. 3-5 days
   8. 6-10 days
   9. I always have pain, it never goes away

	Office Use:
6. On a scale of 0-10 (0 = No pain; 10 = Severe pain), how severe is your pain on average? _____	8.
7. What other symptoms (if any) do you have when you are in pain? Please list: _____ _____ _____ _____	9.
8. Please list anything you have noticed that makes your pain better or worse. For example: lack of sleep, change in eating habits, exercise. **Makes pain better** **Makes pain worse**	25. 26.

_____   _____
_____   _____
_____   _____
_____   _____
_____   _____

Your Activities	Office Use:
1. Do you like school? Yes No	27.
2. On average, how do you do in school? Poor Average Good Excellent	28.
3. Has anything happened recently that has been stressful for you? Please list:	32.

(continued)

Table 23.7 (continued)

Department of Anesthesia Chronic Pain Service Chicago, IL 60614 **CHILD QUESTIONNAIRE**	Medical Record Number Patient Name Birthdate

Does your pain get in the way of you doing any of the following?

Activity	Not Applicable	Never	Hardly Ever	Some-times	Often	Very Often
Eating						
Seeing/visiting friends						
Enjoying being with the family						
Playing sports						
Sleeping						
Watching TV						
Reading						
Attending school						
Doing homework						
Extracurricular activities						
Bathing or showering						
Using the toilet						
Using the computer						
Going to the movies						
Going to a party						
Going to religious services						
Traveling in a car/bus/train						
Working at a paid job						
Doing household chores						
Doing a favorite activity (specify)						
Doing a disliked activity (specify)						

(continued)

Table 23.7 (continued)

Children's Memorial Hospital

Department of Anesthesia
Chronic Pain Service
Chicago, IL 60614
CHILD QUESTIONNAIRE

Medical Record Number
Patient Name
Birthdate

When in pain I ...	Never	Hardly Ever	Sometimes	Often	Very Often
1. Ask questions about the pain					
2. Focus on the pain to see how to make it better					
3. Talk to a friend about how they feel					
4. Tell myself "don't worry-everything will be ok"					
5. Go and play					
6. Forget the whole thing					
7. Say mean things to people					
8. Worry I will always be in pain					
9. Ask a nurse or doctor questions					
10. Think about what needs to be done to make the pain better					
11. Talk to someone about how I am feeling					
12. Say to myself "be strong"					
13. Do something fun					
14. Ignore the pain					
15. Argue or fight					
16. Keep thinking about how much it hurts					
17. Find out more information					
18. Think of different ways to deal with the pain					
19. Tell someone how I feel					
20. Tell myself, "It's not so bad"					
21. Do something I enjoy					

(continued)

Table 23.7 (continued)

Department of Anesthesia
Chronic Pain Service
Chicago, IL 60614
CHILD QUESTIONNAIRE

Children's Memorial Hospital

Medical Record Number
Patient Name
Birthdate

When in pain I ...	Never	Hardly Ever	Sometimes	Often	Very Often
22. Try to forget it (the pain)					
23. Yell to let off steam					
24. Think that nothing helps					
25. Learn more about the way my body works					
26. Figure out what I can do about the pain					
27. Talk to a family member about how I feel					
28. Say to myself, "things will be okay"					
29. Do something active					
30. Put the pain out of my mind					
31. Get mad and throw things or hit something					
32. Think that the pain will never stop					
33. Try different ways to make the pain better until finding one that works					
34. Let my feelings out to a friend					
35. Tell myself, "I can handle anything that happens"					
36. Do something to take my mind off the pain					
37. Don't think about the pain					
38. Curse or swear out loud					
39. Worry too much about the pain					

	Never	Hardly Ever	Sometimes	Often	Very Often
When you are in pain, how often do you think you can do something about it?					
How often do you think you can do something to change your mood or feelings when you are in pain?					

(continued)

Table 23.7 (continued)

 Children's Memorial Hospital

Department of Anesthesia
Chronic Pain Service
Chicago, IL 60614
**PARENT/GUARDIAN
QUESTIONNAIRE**

PTRH

Medical Record Number
Patient Name
Birthdate

Child's Background

	Office Use:
	1. 2.

Child's Name _____   Date___/____/_____

Your Name _____   Mother/Father/Guardian (circle)

Child's School: _____

Grade in School: _____   3.

Referring Doctor: _____   Phone: _____   4.

Is there any pending legal case regarding your child's pain problem?   5.
No   Yes*   * If yes, is case settled?   Yes   No

Pain History

1. Please describe what brings your child to the pain clinic

_____
_____
_____
_____
_____
_____
_____

2. How did your child's pain first start?

_____
_____
_____
_____
_____
_____

3. How frequently does your child have pain?

Office Use:

6

   1. Daily
   2. 1-2 times a week
   3. 3-7 times a week
   4. 1-2 times a month
   5. Every few months

4. When your child has pain, how long does it usually last?

7.

   1. Less than 15 minutes
   2. About 15-30 minutes
   2. 30 minutes to 1 hour
   4. Several Hours (How many? _____)
   5. All day
   6. 1-2 days
   7. 3-5 days
   8. 6-10 days
   9. Child always has pain, it never goes away

(continued)

Table 23.7 (continued)

5. On a scale of 0-10 where 0 = No pain and 10 = Severe pain, how severe is your child's pain on average? _____

6. What other symptoms (if any) does your child have when he/she is in pain? Please list:

Office Use:
8. (/10)
9.

_____
_____
_____
_____
_____

7. Please mark on the pictures below where your child is having pain.

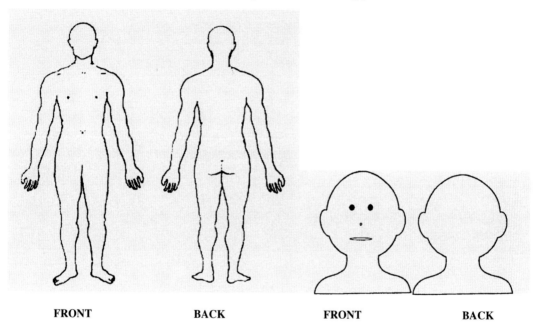

FRONT   BACK   FRONT   BACK

8. Is your child <u>currently</u> receiving any treatment for his/her pain? Please list below:

				Office Use:
a. Medications 1._____	Does it help?	Yes	No	10.
2 _____		Yes	No	
3 _____		Yes	No	
4 _____		Yes	No	
b. Physical therapy/exercise	Does it help?	Yes	No	11.
c. Surgery		Yes	No	12.
d. Nerve Blocks		Yes	No	13.
e. Behavioral Pain Management (relaxation, biofeedback, stress management)		Yes	No	14.
f. Other (Specify _____)		Yes	No	15.

(continued)

Table 23.7 (continued)

		Office Use:
9. What treatments have you tried <u>in the past</u> for his/her pain? Please list below:		
a. Medications 1. _____ Did it help? Yes No		16.
2. _____ Yes No		
b. Physical therapy/exercise Yes No		17.
c. Surgery Yes No		18.
d. Nerve Blocks Yes No		19.
e. Behavioral Pain Management Yes No		20.
(relaxation, biofeedback, stress management etc)		
10. Please list any other medical problems that your child has.		21.
11. Please list any other medications your child is currently taking.		22.
12. Please list any family history of pain or other medical disorders.		23.
13. Please list any family history of psychological disorders or problems with alcohol or drugs.		24.

Please list anything else you have noticed that makes your child's pain better or worse. For example: lack of sleep, change in eating habits, exercise.

		Office Use:
<u>Make pain better</u>	<u>Makes pain worse</u>	25. 26.

Child's Activities

			Office Use:
1. Does your child like school?	No	Yes	27.
2. On average, how does your child do in school? Poor Average Good Excellent			28.
3. Does he/she receive any special services? (resource teacher etc)	No	Yes	29.
4. Is your child in an accelerated academic program at school (e.g., AP classes)	No	Yes	30.
5. Does your child have close friends?	No	Yes	31.
6. Has the child had any recent major stressors (within past 6 months)? Please list:			32.

_____

_____

_____

_____

_____

(continued)

Table 23.7 (continued)

Does your child's pain get in the way of his/her doing any of the following?

Activity	Not Applicable	Never	Hardly Ever	Some-times	Often	Very Often
Eating						
Seeing/visiting friends						
Enjoying being with the family						
Playing sports						
Sleeping						
Watching TV						
Reading						
Attending school						
Doing homework						
Extracurricular activities						
Bathing or showering						
Using the toilet						
Using the computer						
Going to the movies						
Going to a party						
Going to religious services						
Traveling in a car/bus/train						
Working at a paid job						
Doing household chores						
Doing a favorite activity (specify)						
Doing a disliked activity (specify)						

Table 23.7 (continued)

On the next two pages are some things people might say, do or think when they are hurt or in pain. We are interested in the things that your child does when in pain.

When in pain my child....	Never	Hardly Ever	Sometimes	Often	Very Often
1. Asks questions about the pain					
2. Focuses on the pain to see how to make it better					
3. Talks to a friend about how they feel					
4. Tells his/herself "don't worry-everything will be ok"					
5. Goes and plays					
6. Forgets the whole thing					
7. Says mean things to people					
8. Worries they will always be in pain					
9. Asks a nurse or doctor questions					
10. Thinks about what needs to be done to make the pain better					
11. Talks to someone about how they are feeling					
12. Says to themselves "be strong"					
13. Does something fun					
14. Ignores the pain					
15. Argues or fights					
16. Keeps thinking about how much it hurts					
17. Finds out more information					
18. Thinks of different ways to deal with the pain					
19. Tells someone how they feel					
20. Tells themselves, "It's not so bad"					
21. Does something they enjoy					

(continued)

Table 23.7 (continued)

When in pain my child....	Never	Hardly Ever	Sometimes	Often	Very Often
22. Tries to forget it (the pain)					
23. Yells to let off steam					
24. Thinks that nothing helps					
25. Learns more about the way their body works					
26. Figures out what they can do about the pain					
27. Talks to a family member about how they feel					
28. Says to themselves, "things will be okay"					
29. Does something active					
30. Puts the pain out of their mind					
31. Gets mad and throws or hits something					
32. Thinks that the pain will never stop					
33. Tries different ways to make the pain better until finding one that works					
34. Lets their feelings out to a friend					
35. Tells themselves, "I can handle anything that happens"					
36. Does something to take their mind off the pain					
37. Doesn't think about the pain					
38. Curses or swears out loud					
39. Worries too much about the pain					

	Never	Hardly Ever	Sometimes	Often	Very Often
When your child is in pain, how often does your child think they can do something about it?					
How often does your child think they can do something to change their moods or feelings when in pain?					

Table 23.7 includes both child and parent/guardian versions of a multidimensional, chronic pain assessment tool to be completed at the time of initial consultation

equip the NP with the ability to address a greater range of problem complexity. The greatest asset of the NP is the invaluable ability to provide supportive interventions through active listening, understanding, affirmation, guidance, and reassurance. The combination of these abilities allows the NP to effectively manage, alleviate, or prevent pain. As such, the NP has the innate ability to know the patient and family and better assess the patterns of response to prescribed pain management interventions (Running et al. 2006).

In the specialty of pediatric chronic pain, developmental considerations make pain assessment more difficult than with adults. Careful consideration is given to the child's self-report and pain descriptors as well as the descriptors as stated by the family. Younger children and children with developmental delays have varying levels of difficulty communicating their degree of pain, which puts them at greater risk of unrecognized, untreated, or undertreated pain. The pediatric chronic pain NP has the ability to assess the cognitive skills of the patient and use age-appropriate language to establish an effective patient–provider relationship. The NP also has experience with maladaptive predictive responses to significant stressors, such as regression, avoidance behavior, acting out, etc. One unique aspect in the management of chronic pain in children is the interaction that occurs between the patient and the family. The NP can obtain pain histories from both the child and family, either separately or together, by asking open-ended questions that focus on the child. This process allows the NP to better understand the unique family dynamics. Families often express concerns about the child's development while debilitated with pain, the long-term effects of pain medications and treatment modalities and family support networks while caring for a child with chronic pain. Once the concerns are identified, ongoing education and guidance can be provided to families.

The NP in specialty practice approaches the patient with chronic pain from a holistic point of view. This approach encompasses the physical, biological, social, cultural, psychological, spiritual, economic, and ethical domains of the patient's pain experience. The NP is sensitive to the culture, language, and cognitive and developmental level of the chronic pain patient and explores the patient through functional and behavioral assessment/ screening, utilization of appropriate pain tools/ scales, and conversational interviewing during clinical interactions. In essence, the NP and the patient are able to make decisions together to formulate and prioritize treatment goals.

Emotional support and reassurance are essential skills employed by the Nurse Practitioner when dealing with families and children with chronic conditions. Pain is disruptive of family life and of activities of daily living such as school attendance and social encounters (Dampier and Shapiro 2003).

Educator

In the pediatric chronic pain care setting, the NP plays the role of educator in many diverse ways. Providing education in a systematic manner and addressing needs for pain patients and families are important components of the clinical skills of the NP. Education is an ongoing process. Initial assessment of the education needs of the patient includes identification of the desire to learn and the presence of motivating factors, as well as any barriers or limitations to learning. Methods of teaching include written, verbal, audio, visual, and tactile interactions. Next, clear short- and long-term goals that are specific, measurable, attainable, and realistic are set with the patient. Finally, the Nurse Practitioner implements the education plan, followed by evaluation of the intervention.

Initially, the pediatric chronic pain patient and family will need age-appropriate explanation of the anatomy and physiology of pain pathways and classifications. Once an understanding of the pathophysiology of the pain mechanisms has occurred, treatment rationale can be discussed. When prescribing medication, education is focused on the pharmacologic mechanisms of medications, classification, dosage, instructions for administration, side effects, expected responses, and the importance of adherence to the individualized treatment plan. Specific education is warranted about the hazards of chronic opioid use. The patient and family need to be counseled on the proper and safe use of opioids, as well as receive accurate information about tolerance, dependence, and addiction. Adjuvants frequently aid in the medication management of many chronic pain syndromes. Adjuvants are non-opioid supplemental treatment medications that may be prescribed to augment other pharmacological treatments. The rationale and correct use of adjuvants must also be discussed with the patient and family. In the course of educating the patient and family, the NP provides reassurance that the pain can be adequately treated even if a cause cannot be found.

The pediatric chronic pain NP provides considerable anticipatory guidance and counseling. The patient and family need to be well informed about possible painful exacerbations and receive prevention techniques, as well as direction on what to do when an exacerbation occurs and how to cope effectively. In addition, proper explanation of what pain is and the necessary reassurance that the perceived pain is not signaling an injury is part of NP guidance. Pain can be so severe and debilitating that it may lead to impairment of normal childhood, diversion of child activity, alteration of family dynamics, school absenteeism, and maladaptive behaviors. These behaviors are frequently misinterpreted by the family. The NP helps families understand that the child is not "bad" because he is not attending school and living his life as previously. The child may need to learn coping strategies that will help him engage in his life, including maintaining friendships and school attendance (Dampier and Shapiro 2003). When working with families dealing with chronic pain, the role of the NP as educator and clinician thus overlap.

The NP assists the chronic pain patient in accomplishing the goals of achieving and maintaining a level of well-being within the mental, physical, and spiritual dimensions of the individual. As educator and counselor, the chronic pain NP encourages the patient to engage in physical and cognitive self-care activities and promotes self-awareness to monitor for negative thoughts that amplify hopelessness and despair. A significant component of anticipatory guidance is to avoid fostering false expectations, but rather integrate the ability to adapt to stumbling blocks and to build the necessary coping skills to foster hope. Pediatric chronic pain is viewed within the context of the whole family. In order to focus on patient wellness and restore functional status, reassurance and education is often necessary to allay parental feelings of guilt and frustration. Finding successful treatment strategies can be challenging, but can also be an ultimately rewarding component of the NP–patient relationship. It is the fervent goal of the NP that the patient will display the necessary understanding and self-determination needed for the management of the pain syndrome.

Consultant

Being a consultant is another role function of the chronic pain Nurse Practitioner. Consultation can be any form of interaction between professionals. The NP can be the consultant or can request consultation with other professionals for their expertise. These interactions may be formal or informal and most often lead to assistance with management interventions or decision making when an identified concern arises. A collegial collaboration forms as a result of consultation that benefits both the patient and the care providers. As a consultant, the NP is expected to gather relevant data to accurately and thoroughly assess the problem, and then make reasonable, clearly articulated recommendations. The recommendations are supported as standards of care within the field of pain management as a result of evidenced-based findings or at the minimum, the consensus of expert opinion. The recommendations are then given to the appropriate medical staff for discussion and implementation. The NP is then available for further assistance as continuing patient care dictates.

The NP may be asked to discuss a chronic pain topic with faculty, staff, students, and/or the general public. Educative endeavors have the best results when specific learning needs are identified and an appropriate curriculum is formulated. Specific needs can be addressed by means of classroom didactics, in-service training, written updates, self-learning modules, grand rounds presentations, and interviews with the media for public consumption. The opportunity to address students in the classroom environment or new staff during orientation can be invaluable for all parties involved. Patient care can be greatly benefited when faculty, staff, and students are educated regarding appropriate pain assessment and management techniques. In addition, the NP can help to correct any chronic pain care misconceptions and communicate current pain management research findings.

Nurse Practitioners in the specialty of chronic pain garner a great deal of clinical experience and autonomy and are able to relate this expertise respectfully to others. The NP is able to add significant input to the multidisciplinary pain team and can lead to identification of alternative approaches to treatment and successful pediatric chronic pain management.

Researcher

Standard of care dictates that high-quality, cost-effective, evidence-based medicine should be the expected norm in pain management. The chronic pain Nurse Practitioner interprets and evaluates pertinent medical literature. Subsequently, the NP applies the appropriate findings into patient care.

The NP can be an active participant in research endeavors, within the specialty of pediatric pain management. Beginning with inspection and review of the available medical and nursing literature, the NP can bring about the planning and execution of research projects, followed by the evaluation and interpretation of data for quality, accuracy, validity, and application to practice. Being versatile, the NP can serve as both a mentor and collaborator with others in project development. The NP can be an important contributor to original research by being a part of the research process as primary investigator, coinvestigator, coordinator, or data collector. The NP can also assist in research endeavors by authoring and submitting IRB proposals, conducting or directing bedside interventions, and compiling and writing study findings for eventual publication in peer-reviewed journals and presentation to others at major conferences. Types of research in which NPs are likely participants include clinical research, either quantitative or qualitative; outcomes based research; and applied research.

By staying current with relevant medical information and by contributing to research efforts, the NP can practice at the leading edge of chronic pain management. Nurse Practitioners have developed and will continue to develop evidence-based process improvements related to patient care. These efforts serve to support existing expertise and assist in the generation of new knowledge to advance the practice of pediatric chronic pain management.

Case Manager

The Nurse Practitioner has the training background to carry out the role of case manager and provide the overall management and coordination of care utilizing a multitude of administrative services. At the initial consultation, the NP begins coordinating fundamental services necessary for patient care and continues with this undertaking through discharge. As case manager, the NP may encounter many potential barriers to the provision of seamless care and must navigate through these obstacles to achieve the greatest good and least harm for the patient. During the intake history, the NP can attempt to assess the social environment of each individual patient. Armed with the pertinent social information, attempts to organize all aspects of care can facilitate a successful and individual treatment plan. The goal of the NP as case manager is to develop a clear, focused management plan that is understandable, easy to follow, and can lead to a fruitful outcome.

The chronic pain NP, acting as case manager, creates patient contracts, which are verbal and written treatment agreements. The patient becomes an active participant in the discourse of treatment and agrees to comply with contract expectations. In return, the NP agrees to listen and reevaluate as dictated by patient response. In chronic pain management, written contracts are crucial, especially concerning opioids. When the treatment plan includes prescribing opioids, guidelines for long-term therapy should be stipulated in an opioid contract and followed by the patient (Table 23.8). These provisions should state that the patient will use the medication only as directed, obtain the medication

Table 23.8 Sample opioid contract

Yale University School of Medicine
YNHH- CHILDREN'S HOSPITAL
PEDIATRIC CHRONIC PAIN CLINIC

SECOND FLOOR WEST PAVILLION - SPECIALTY CLINICS

333 CEDAR STREET, P.O. BOX 208051
NEW HAVEN, CONNECTICUT 06520-8051
(203) 785-3892   Fax: (203) 785-6664

Brenda C. McClain, M.D., DABPM
Director of Pediatric Pain Management Services
Pediatric Chronic Pain Clinic
Section of Pediatric Anesthesiology

Pain Management Agreement

The purpose of this Agreement is to prevent misunderstandings about certain medicines you will be taking for pain management. This is to help both you and your doctor to comply with the law regarding controlled pharmaceuticals.

I understand that this Agreement is essential to the trust and confidence necessary in a doctor/patient relationship and that my doctor undertakes to treat me based on this Agreement.

I understand that if I break this Agreement, my doctor will stop prescribing these pain-control medicines.

In this case, my doctor will taper off the medicine over a period of several days, as necessary to avoid withdrawal symptoms. Also, a drug-dependence treatment program may be recommended.

I will communicate fully with my doctor about the character and intensity of my pain, the effect of the pain on my daily life, and how well the medicine is helping to relieve the pain.

I will not use any illegal controlled substances, including marijuana, cocaine, etc.

I will not share, sell or trade my medication with anyone.

I will not attempt to obtain any controlled medicines, including opioid pain medicines, controlled stimulants, or anti-anxiety medicines from any other doctor.

I will safeguard my pain medication from loss or theft. Lost or stolen medicines will not be replaced.

I agree that refills of my prescriptions for pain medicine will be made only at the time of an office visit or during regular office hours. No refills will be available during evenings or on weekends.

I agree to use _____ Pharmacy, located at _____,
telephone number _____, for filling prescriptions for all of my pain medicine.

I authorize the doctor and my pharmacy to cooperate fully with any city, state or federal law enforcement agency, including this state's Board of Pharmacy, in the investigation of any possible misuse, sale or other diversion of my pain medicine. I authorize my doctor to provide a copy of this Agreement to my pharmacy. I agree to waive any applicable privilege or right of privacy or confidentiality with respect to these authorizations.

I agree that I will submit to a blood or urine test if requested by my doctor to determine my compliance with my program of pain control medicine.

I agree that I will use my medicine at a rate of no greater than the prescribed rate and that use of my medicine at a greater rate will result in my being without medication for a period of time.

I will bring all unused pain medicine to every office visit.

I agree to follow these guidelines that have been fully explained to me. All of my questions and concerns regarding treatment have been adequately answered. A copy of this document has been given to me.

This Agreement is entered into on this _____ day of _____, _____.

_____
Patient signature

_____
Physician signature

_____
Witnessed by:

Table 23.8 is a pain management agreement that defines the mutual expectations of both the prescriber and the patient from only one prescriber, have the medication filled and dispensed from only one pharmacy, and agree to random toxicology screening.

Another important case manager function is to provide coordination of services. Chronic pain management clinic visits often result in patient referrals to various ancillary services such as rehabilitation services, mental health providers, complimentary and alternative therapy providers, nutritionists, child life specialists, home health-care agencies, social workers, hospice, and other pain consultants. It can be an all-encompassing

responsibility to coordinate these referrals; how-ever, the NP is unequivocally qualified to accom-plish this difficult task. An additional vital component of care coordination occurs via tele-phone triage that may take place between the chronic pain Nurse Practitioner and the patient and family, or any number of involved ancillary services (Table 23.9).

A unique concern associated with pediatric chronic pain is patient school attendance or absenteeism. Chronic pain places great pressure on family dynamics and additional stressors, such

Table 23.9 Chronic pain service intake screening guidelines

CHRONIC PAIN SERVICE INTAKE SCREENING GUIDELINES

APPOINTMENT #:

PROVIDERS:

SUMMARY OF SERVICES:

Any patient with chronic pain, for example, chronic headache, RSD (CRPS), sickle cell pain, neuropathic pain, fibro-myalgia, back pain, recurrent abdominal pain, or cancer pain. Modalities of treatment offered include medications, behavioral pain management, nerve block, and physical therapy referrals. The following services are not available at this time: biofeedback, spinal cord stimulators, chiropractic, magnet therapy, herbal medications, or complimentary/alternative medicine treatment. Outside referral may be available for some of these services.

SPECIAL INSTRUCTIONS:

Patients must be under 18 years of age by the time they have initial NEW patient appointment in Pain Clinic. Patients must have a physician referral with a presumptive diagnosis. Referring physicians must fill out and return the patient referral sheet (see attached). Parents/patients must fill out and return the screening questionnaire (see attached). This can be returned by e-mail, fax, or mail. E-mail should be sent to ( ) Fax number is ( ). Address is ( ) Patients/parents must bring in all current medications and reports of diagnostic studies (MRI, X-rays, CT, laboratory/blood tests). Please prepare families for a 2–3-h initial visit. Prepare families to expect to see multiple team members including an anesthe-siologist, an advanced practice nurse, a medical psychologist, a fellow and/or resident physician in training. Services received from the medical psychologist are billed separately. Patients/parents should consult their insurance carrier for their behavioral health benefits for psychological consultation. Patients/parents should understand that the first available appointment may not be for several weeks. Patients/parents should also understand that they cannot select the attending anesthesiologist whom they will see. All patients/parents should understand that an initial evaluation will precede the scheduling of any interventional procedures.

SCHEDULING TRIAGE:

The following diagnoses should be considered urgent and should be seen at the next clinic appointment:
• RSD (CRPS), cancer pain.

Other diagnoses that should be referred elsewhere are:
• Headaches associated with nausea and vomiting or sensory changes, weakness, or vision changes should be referred to Neurology.
• Sickle cell patients with symptoms of an acute crisis should be sent to an emergency room.
• Patients with joint pain should be seen by Rheumatology/Immunology before referral to our clinic.
• Headache patients with a ventriculoperitoneal shunt must be referred by Neurosurgery.
• Headache patients who have never had a medical workup for headache should see Neurosurgery.

Table 23.9 provides a listing of clinic services as well as an algorithm for triage of new clinic referrals as repeated school absences, and only makes the situation more difficult. As case manager, the NP can attempt to minimize truancy and the familial disruptions it causes by communicating to the patient a clear set of realistic expectations and providing positive reinforcement for favorable behaviors. Of note, school attendance should be encouraged because it not only provides the child with an education but also allows for peer socialization and redirected coping mechanisms.

The NP as case manager provides much needed continuity essential for care of children, adolescents, and young adults with chronic pain and can be the metaphorical glue that holds the clinic together.

Professional Leader, Manager, Mentor

Leadership can be described as the ability to influence a group of individuals toward the successful achievement of common goals. Management, on the other hand, is the control of resources and their distribution to accomplish organizational goals (McArthur 2006). Nurse Practitioners can be both leaders and managers. The leader persona attempts to do what is right, focuses on purpose or mission, and has a long-term outlook on future endeavors. The manager persona of the NP strives to accomplish tasks while focusing on organizational structures and procedures, with a short-range view of immediate projects. In other words, the chronic pain NP is able to achieve goals while caring for the patient. The NP, as both leader and manager, can be a role model and mentor while performing the many duties of clinician, educator, case manager, etc.

As a leader in the nursing profession, the NP can initiate and facilitate service projects at the community level that may progress further to the state, national, and international arenas. At the clinical or professional level, the NP can assist in the development of policy/procedures and protocols that are congruent with established standards of care (Paul 1999). The NP can also be an agent of change in response to a perceived or communicated need and can initiate policy and procedural changes that are supported by research in response to the perceived need. Strong clinical skills,

knowledge of research, and awareness of the organizational environment and systems are the attributes of the NP as a mentor. Taking note of barriers and limitations, as well as observing the existing support systems, help in planning change and mobilizing resources (Kowal 1998).

Maintaining clinical competency and nurturing collaborative collegial relationships are the responsibilities of all health-care professionals. Authoring peer-reviewed journal articles, presenting case studies, and speaking at conferences are important means to accomplish these duties. The chronic pain NP has a professional responsibility to increase awareness and knowledge of pain management, validate the accuracy of information, and facilitate better access to care. Serving as an instigator of projects that are focused on pain management education, the NP shares and disseminates knowledge that influences clinical decision making.

Mentoring students interested in learning more about chronic pain management is another important professional role of the NP. The Nurse Practitioner has the advantageous position to supervise the clinical training of students and less-experienced professionals. Insuring the spread of effective pain management strategies and techniques to the next generation of health-care providers is definitely a worthwhile goal.

As a professional, there is also a need for accountability. The NP is accountable to participate in quality assessment and self-monitoring measures to ensure high standards of care both for the NP individually and the multidisciplinary pain team as a whole. Quality improvement and process improvement activities are required to maintain and renew credentialing and privileges.

The Clinic Setting

The Pediatric Chronic Pain Nurse Practitioner performs a variety of activities for optimal patient care, including ordering diagnostic studies, initiating and changing therapies, performing invasive procedures, and prescribing medications.

The Nurse Practitioner is uniquely qualified to manage the complex, comprehensive needs of patients with chronic pain. Providing excellent patient care arising from a holistic framework is central to the role of the NP and it is paramount that the pediatric chronic pain Nurse Practitioner translates treatment into a family-centered care approach (DiAnna-Kinder 2006). Models of family-centered care strive to organize health-care services in a respectful and supportive approach that involves family members. The assessment, care, and treatment of children must be provided in a way that accommodates the inseparability of the child and family.

Management of pain is influenced by the conceptualization of the providing individual's own pain consciousness. Pain consciousness is considered the Nurse Practitioner's ability to be aware and sensitive to a patient's pain as a problem (Droes 2004). The chronic pain NP with a high pain consciousness has a diverse understanding of pain and will treat the patient's pain regardless of whether an etiology can be determined. Education of patients and families includes understanding the causes of pain, modes of self-care, preemptive use of analgesics, and facts versus myths about addiction to pain medications.

In managing pediatric chronic pain, the NP can be seen as an expert in the eyes of parents to whom they entrust the care of their children. Parents often seek the advice of the Nurse Practitioner and listen carefully to the knowledge imparted (Wells-Federman et al. 2002). Sometimes, a parent only needs to hear a calming voice that offers reassurance.

Licensed Independent Practitioner Clinics

Outcome studies have validated effectiveness of NP run clinics (Czarnecki, et al. 2007). Nurse-managed clinics have been shown to decrease the rate of hospital admissions and ER visits (Brooten et al. 2004; Sherwood, et al. 1997). Because of the frequency and the consistent care NPs provide, they become a dependable resource for patients and develop close patient–provider relationships.

Most chronic pain management programs would, at minimum, have these desired outcomes for NP care: prompt treatment and intervention

so that pain and other symptoms are minimized, prevention and management of adverse sequelae, and prompt and appropriate referral to physician or other providers as needed. Additionally, in an effort to identify the "gold standard" of nursing excellence, an expert panel devised 18 indicators of health-care quality and outcome guidelines, of which the pediatric or family Nurse Practitioner, can adopt as a tool to measure and guide practice (Betz et al. 2007) (Table 23.10).

Table 23.10 Health-care quality and outcome guidelines

1. Children and youth have an identified health-care home.
2. The families of children and youth are partners in decisions, planning, and delivery of care.
3. Family values, beliefs, and preferences are part of care.
4. Family strengths and main concerns are obvious in the care of children and youth.
5. Children, youth, and families will have accessible health care.
6. Pregnant women will have accessible health care.
7. Family needs are identified and services are offered.
8. Children, youth, and families are directed to community services when needed.
9. Children, youth, and families receive care that promotes and maintains health and prevents disease.
10. Pregnant women, children, youth, and families have access to genetic testing and advice.
11. Children and youth receive care that is physically and emotionally safe.
12. Children, youth, and families' privacy and rights are protected.
13. Children and youth who are very ill receive the full range of needed services.
14. Children and youth with disabilities and/or special health-care needs receive the full range of services.
15. Children, youth, and families receive comfort care.
16. Children's, youth's and families' health and risky behaviors and problems are identified and addressed.
17. Children, youth, and families receive care that supports development.
18. Children, youth, and families are fully informed of the outcomes of care.

Table 23.10 is a reproduction of the health-care quality and outcome guidelines developed by the American academy of nursing expert panel on children and families. These guidelines are a collation of nursing care standards, intended to aid child and family nursing professionals in evaluating health-care quality

Copyright 2007, Journal of pediatric health care

Furthermore, it is revealed that, NPs are believed to be more adept in patient communication and preventative care, the interpersonal skills of NPs are of better quality and more personalized than those of physicians, and the merit of NP technical services and patient outcomes are equivalent to physicians. Likewise, studies have shown a high level of patient satisfaction with NP care. In a meta-analytical review done for the American Nurses Association (2007), patients of NPs demonstrated greater satisfaction with their health-care providers and greater compliance with health promotion and treatment recommendations than did patients of physicians. The NPs spent more time per visit with their patients than did physicians, contributing to high patient satisfaction, while the average number of visits per patient was equivalent.

Measurement of productivity is important in determining the worth and value of NP practice. Productivity measures are used to monitor individual performance, create incentive plans, compare departmental contributions within institutions, and monitor resources needed for patient care. In pediatric chronic pain management, productivity is measured by how well the NP meets the needs of the community of patients served. All successful NP practices build on the three A's: availability, affability, and ability. The availability of the NP to patients is crucial for productivity. Affability, the health-care experience from the patient's point of view, requires NPs to examine how pleasant, open, responsive, and approachable they are. Ability, for both the NP and the office staff, directly impacts productivity of the pain clinic practice (Rhoads et al. 2006). Because NP productivity is a measure of an NP's work or output, it is closely related to efficiency, quality of care, and service provided (AANP 2007b). The Pain Clinic Assessment Tool in (Table 23.11) aids the NP to maintain a high quality of care through accurate data gathering, assessment, and patient satisfaction.

Summary

The Nurse Practitioner performs a multitude of essential roles within the auspices of a pediatric chronic pain clinic. The NP provides an expert level of specialty care utilizing the accumulated knowledge and experiences gained from both the nursing and medical fields. The combination of critical thinking, specialty expertise, and effective patient-oriented interaction makes the NP an essential and invaluable member of the pediatric pain management team. In addition to the ability to address areas of disease prevention and health maintenance, within the realm of primary care, the NP can address the unique medical needs of the chronic pain patient, and provide developmentally appropriate care for pediatric patients. The NP begins this specialized care at the time of initial triage and continues to do so well after patient discharge. As an expert clinician and a case manager, the NP has the aptitude to conduct a thorough intake history and physical examination, make an assessment of patient presentation, order and interpret any necessary laboratory and diagnostic studies, prescribe or perform treatment interventions, provide effective patient education, make necessary referrals to other disciplines, evaluate patient progress, and, finally, conduct close follow-up with patients and families, as needed.

Outside of direct patient care, the chronic pain NP provides consultative and educative services to primary care providers, associated specialty care providers, nursing agencies, school systems, communities, and industries (D'Arcy and McCarberg 2005). The integrated philosophy of patient care is displayed through the coordination and collaborative efforts of the pediatric chronic pain NP. Interdisciplinary team conclusions are summarized by the NP and communicated to the referral source. These coordinative efforts can lead to the NP being an important source of patient care continuity. The Nurse Practitioner has the benefit of becoming a familiar and trusted provider of specialized services for the patient and family.

As researcher and leader/mentor, the NP can identify deficits in the literature and subsequently be involved in original research endeavors to help advance the specialty of pediatric pain management and strengthen reliability. Serving as a mentor, the NP role models the importance of pediatric chronic pain management as a specialty.

Table 23.11 Pain clinic assessment tool

Patient Name: Date: _____

WT: _____   HT: _____   T _____   P _____   R _____   BP _____/_____

Pain Location: _____

Pain Intensity:
Pain right now: _____ Worst pain gets: _____ Best pain gets: _____

Descriptors: _____

Alleviating Measures: _____
Aggravating Factors: _____
Associative Factors: _____

Effects of Pain:
Sleep:
Appetite:
Physical Activity:
School:
Emotions:
Other:

Physical Exam Findings:
_____
_____
_____

Current Medications/Therapies:
_____
_____
_____

Questions/Concerns:
_____
_____
_____

Assessment/Plan:
_____
_____
_____

Table 23.11 is a pain-focused assessment tool for utilization at follow-up visits

The roles of the pediatric chronic pain Nurse Practitioner have continued to evolve and expand depending upon location, resources, scope of practice, and laws/limitations. By navigating through the many potential barriers and restrictions, the NP role has now joined the forefront of providing cutting-edge specialty care. By overseeing all aspects of patient management, the NP has the ability to be a recognized expert in the field of chronic pain and an essential resource for the patient and family. The NP provides a comprehensive approach of employing clinical skills, management versatility, and quality of care that results in increased productivity, cost-effectiveness, and, even more importantly, patient satisfaction (AANP 2007a).

References

Ackerman, M. H., Norsen, L., Martin, B., Wiedrich, J., & Kitzman, H. J. (1996). Development of a model of advanced practice. *American Journal of Critical Care, 5*(1), 68–73.

American Academy of Nurse Practitioners. (2007a). Nurse practitioner cost-effectiveness.

American Academy of Nurse Practitioners. (2007b). Quality of nurse practitioner practice.

American Academy of Nurse Practitioners. (2007c). Scope of practice for nurse practitioners.

American Academy of Nurse Practitioners. (2007d). Standards of practice for nurse practitioners.

American Association of Colleges of Nursing. (1998). AACN position statement: certification and regulation of advanced practice nurse.

American Board of Nursing Specialties. (2005). A position statement on the value of specialty nursing certification.

American College of Nurse Practitioners (2008). Nurse practitioner DNP education, certification and titling. A unified statement.

American Nurses Association (2007). ANA position statement-barriers to the practice of advanced practice registered nurses.

Betz, C., Cowell, J., Craft-Rosenberg, M., Krajicek, M., & Lobo, M. (2007). Health care quality and outcome guidelines for nursing of children and families: implications for pediatric nurse practitioner practice, research and policy. *Journal of Pediatric Health Care, 21*(1), 64–66.

Brady, M. A., & Neal, J. (2000). Role delineation study of pediatric nurse practitioners: a national study of practice responsibilities and trends in role functions. *Journal of Pediatric Health Care, 14*(4), 149–159.

Brooten, D., Youngblut, J., Kutcher, J., & Bobo, C. (2004). Quality and the nursing workforce: APNs, patient outcomes and health care costs. *Nursing Outlook, 52*(1), 45–52.

Brundige, K. (1997). Preparing pediatric nurse practitioners for roles in specialty practice. *Journal of Pediatric Health Care, 11*(4), 198–200.

Calkin, J. D. (1984). A model for advanced nursing practice. *The Journal of Nursing Administration, 14*(1), 24–30.

Cary, A. (2001). Certified registered nurses: results of the study of the certified workforce. *The American Journal of Nursing, 101*(1), 44–52.

Clinton, P. (2008). Latest developments in advanced nursing practice. *Journal for Specialists in Pediatric Nursing, 13*(2), 123–125.

Czarnecki, M., Murphy-Garwood, M., & Weisman, S. (2007). Advanced practice nurse-directed telephone management of acute pain following pediatric spinal fusion surgery. *Journal for Specialists in Pediatric Nursing, 12*(3), 159–169.

D'Arcy, Y., & McCarberg, B. (2005). Field guide to pain: care after a pain management referral. *The Nurse Practitioner, 30*(11), 62–64.

Dampier, C., & Shapiro, B. (2003). Management of pain in sickle cell disease. In Berde, Schecter, & Yaster (Eds.), *Pain in infants, children, and adolescents* (pp. 489–516). Philadelphia: Lippincott Williams & Wilkins.

DiAnna-Kinder, F. (2006). Pediatric nursing: nurse practitioner provides holistic care for the entire family. *The Pennsylvania Nurse, 61*(1), 23.

Droes, N. (2004). Role of the nurse practitioner in managing patients with pain. *The Internet Journal of Advanced Nursing Practice, 6*(2).

Dunn, L. (1997). A literature review of advanced clinical nursing practice in the United States of America. *Journal of Advanced Nursing, 25*(4), 814–819.

Heitz, R., & Van Dinter, M. (2000). Developing collaborative practice agreements. *Journal of Pediatric Health Care, 14*(4), 200–203.

Hermann, L., & Zabramski, J. M. (2005). Tandem practice model: a model for physician-nurse practitioner collaboration in a specialty practice, neurosurgery. *Journal of the American Academy of Nurse Practitioners, 17*(6), 213–218.

Joint Commission on Accreditation of Healthcare Organizations (JCAHO). (2001). *Accreditation manual for hospitals*. Oak Brook: Author.

Kaplan, L., Brown, M. A., Andrilla, H., & Hart, L. G. (2006). Barriers to autonomous practice. *The Nurse Practitioner, 31*(1), 57–63.

Kamajian, M., Mitchell, S., & Fruth, R. (1999). Credentialing and privileging of advanced practice nurse. *AACN Clinical Issues, 10*(3), 316–336.

Keane, A., & Angstadt, J. (1999). The role of the acute care nurse practitioner: the emergence, maturation, and future of the acute care nurse practitioner role. In P. Logan (Ed.), *Principles and practice for the acute care nurse practitioner* (pp. 3–10). Stamford: Appleton & Lange.

Kenward, K. (2007). Report findings from the role delineation study of nurse practitioners and clinical nurse specialists. National Council of State Boards of Nursing, 30.

Kleinpell, R. M., French, K. D., & Diamond, E. J. (2007). Billing for NP provider services: updates on coding regulations. *The Nurse Practitioner, 32*(6), 16–17.

Kline, A. M., Reider, M., Rodriguez, K., & Van Roeyen, L. S. (2007). Acute care pediatric nurse practitioners: providing quality care for acute and critically ill children. *Journal of Pediatric Health Care, 21*(4), 268–271.

Kowal, N. (1998). Specialty practice entrepreneur: the advanced practice nurse. *Nursing Economics, 277*(2).

Ludder-Jackson, P., Kennedy, C., Sadler, L. S., Kenney, K. M., Lindeke, L. L., Sperhac, A. M., & Hawkins-Walsh, E. (2001). Professional practice of pediatric nurse practitioners: implications for education and training of PNPs. *Journal of Pediatric Health Care, 15*(6), 291–298.

Mahoney, D. (1995). Employer resistance to state authorized prescriptive authority for NPs. Results from a pilot study. *The Nurse Practitioner, 20*(1), 58–61.

McArthur, D. B. (2006). The nurse practitioner as leader. *Journal of the American Academy of Nurse Practitioners, 18*, 8–10.

Medicare benefit policy manual (Chapter 15). Covered medical and other health services. [Text file]. URL www.cms.hhs.gov/manuals/downloads/bp102c15. pdf.

Medicare Claims Processing Manual (Chapter 12). Physicians/nonphysician practitioners. [Text file]. URL www.cms.hhs.gov/manuals/downloads/clm104c12. pdf.

National Association of Pediatric Nurse Practitioners. (2006). *Certification*. Cherry Hill: Author.

National Association of Pediatric Nurse Practitioners. (2003a). *Credentialing and privileging for pediatric nurse practitioners*. Cherry Hill: Author.

National Association of Pediatric Nurse Practitioners. (2003b). *Prescriptive privilege*. Cherry Hill: Author.

National Association of Pediatric Nurse Practitioners. (2004). *Reimbursement for nurse practitioner services*. Cherry Hill: Author.

Pearson, L. (2009). The Pearson report. A national overview of nurse practitioner legislation and healthcare issues. *The American Journal for Nurse Practitioners, 13*(2), 8–82.

Paul, S. (1999). Developing practice protocols for advanced practice nursing. *AACN Clinical Issues, 10*(3), 343–355.

Reider-Demer, M., Widecan, M., Jones, D., & Goodhue, C. (2006). The evolving responsibilities of the pediatric nurse practitioner. *Journal of Pediatric Health Care, 20*(4), 280–283.

Rhoads, J., Ferguson, L. A., & Langford, C. A. (2006). Measuring nurse practitioner productivity. *Dermatology Nursing, 18*(1), 32–38.

Royal Prince Alfred Hospital. (2005). Nurse practitioner guidelines – role and scope of practice – pain management [Text file]. URL http://www.health.nsw.gov.au/nursing/pdf/ah_pain_mment_rpa_np_v4.pdf.

Running, A., Kipp, C., & Mercer, V. (2006). Prescriptive patterns of nurse practitioners and physicians. *Journal of the American Academy of Nurse Practitioners, 18*, 228–233.

Rustia, J., & Krajicek-Bartek, J. (1997). Managed care credentialing of advanced practice nurses. *The Nurse Practitioner, 22*(9), 90–103.

Shay, L. E., Goldstein, J. T., Matthews, D., Trail, L. L., & Edmunds, M. W. (1996). Guidelines for developing a nurse practitioner practice. *The Nurse Practitioner, 21*(1), 72–81.

Sherwood, G. D., Brown, M., Fay, V., & Wardell, D. (1997). Defining nurse practitioner scope of practice: expanding primary care services. *The Internet Journal of Advanced Nursing Practice, 1*(2), 1–13.

Silver, H. K., Ford, L. C., & Steady, S. G. (1967). A program to increase health care for children: the pediatric nurse practitioner program. *Pediatrics, 39*(5), 756–760.

Silver, H. K., Ford, L. C., & Day, L. R. (1968). The pediatric nurse-practitioner program: expanding the role of the nurse to provide increased health care for children. *Journal of the American Medical Association, 204*(4), 298–302.

St. Marie, B. (Ed.). (2002). *American society of pain management nurses: Core curriculum for pain management nursing*. Philadelphia: W.B Saunders.

Wells-Federman, C., Arnstein, P., & Caudill, M. (2002). Nurse-led pain management program: effect on self-efficacy, pain intensity, pain-related disability, and depressive symptoms in chronic pain patients. *Pain Management Nursing, 3*(4), 131–140.

Index

B.C. McClain and S. Suresh (eds.), *Handbook of Pediatric Chronic Pain:*
Current Science and Integrative Practice, DOI 10.1007/978-1-4419-0350-1,
© Springer Science+Business Media, LLC 2011

Made in the USA
Las Vegas, NV
15 November 2023